EDUCATION IN HEART
Volume 3

Series Editor

PETER MILLS

Consultant Cardiologist, London Chest Hospital

First published in 2003
by BMJ Books, BMA House, Tavistock Square,
London WC1H 9JR

www.bmjbooks.com

British Library Cataloguing in Publication Data
A catalogue record for this book is available from the British Library

ISBN 0 7279 1764 1

Typeset by BMJ Electronic Production
Printed in Malaysia by Times Offset

CONTENTS

CONTRIBUTORS

Robert H Anderson
Cardiac Unit, Institute of Child Health, London, UK

Paul J R Barton
National Heart and Lung Institute, Faculty of Medicine, Imperial College London, Heart Science Centre, Harefield, Middlesex, UK

Elijah R Behr
Department of Cardiological Sciences, St George's Hospital Medical School, London, UK

F Bellocci
Department of Cardiovascular Medicine, Institute of Cardiology, Catholic University of Rome, Rome, Italy

Martin R Bennett
Unit of Cardiovascular Medicine, Addenbrooke's Centre for Clinical Investigation, Addenbrooke's Hospital, Cambridge, UK

Y Blaauw
Cardiovascular Research Institute Maastricht (CARIM), Maastricht, The Netherlands

Peter Bloomfield
Department of Cardiology, Royal Infirmary of Edinburgh, Edinburgh, UK

N A Boon
Department of Cardiology, Royal Infirmary of Edinburgh, Edinburgh, UK

Nigel J Brand
National Heart and Lung Institute, Faculty of Medicine, Imperial College London, Heart Science Centre, Harefield, Middlesex, UK

Nigel A Brown
Department of Anatomy and Developmental Biology, St George's Hospital Medical School, London, UK

Micheal Burch
Great Ormond Street Hospital for Children NHS Trust, London, UK

John Byrne
Cardiff Vascular Unit, University Hospital of Wales, Cardiff, UK

Jamie B Conti
University of Florida, Division of Cardiovascular Medicine, UF Health Science Center, Gainesville, Florida, USA

Joyce A Cramer
Yale University School of Medicine, West Haven, Connecticut, USA

H J G M Crijns
Cardiovascular Research Institute Maastricht (CARIM), Maastricht, The Netherlands

John C S Dean
Department of Medical Genetics, Medical School, Foresterhill, Aberdeen, UK

A Dello Russo
Department of Cardiovascular Medicine, Institute of Cardiology, Catholic University of Rome, Rome, Italy

Mario C Deng
The Heart Failure Center and Division of Circulatory Physiology, Columbia University College of Physicians and Surgeons, New York Presbytarian Hospital, New York, USA

Kim A Eagle
University of Michigan Cardiovascular Center, Division of Cardiology, University of Michigan Medical Center, Ann Arbor, Michigan, USA

Maurice Enriquez-Sarano
Mayo Clinic, Rochester, Minnesota, USA

Paul A Friedman
Division of Internal Medicine and Cardiovascular Diseases, Mayo Clinic, Rochester, Minnesota, USA

James B Froehlich
UMass Memorial Medical Center, Divisions of Cardiology and Vascular Surgery, University of Massachusetts Medical School, Worcester, Massachusetts, USA

Curt D Furberg
Department of Public Health Sciences, Wake Forest University School of Medicine, Winston-Salem, North Carolina, USA

Sally C Greaves
Cardiology Department, Green Lane Hospital, Auckland, New Zealand

Christlieb Haller
Hegau-Klinikum, Medizinische Klinik I, Singen, Germany

Sheila G Haworth
Institute of Child Health, London, UK

Judith S Hochman
Division of Cardiology, St Luke's-Roosevelt Hospital Center, Columbia College of Physicians and Surgeons, New York, USA

Peter R Jackson
Section of Clinical Pharmacology and Therapeutics, Royal Hallamshire Hospital, Sheffield, UK

Peter P Th de Jaegere
Department of Cardiology, University Medical Center Utrecht, Utrecht, The Netherlands

Robert A Kloner
The Heart Institute, Good Samaritan Hospital, University of Southern California, Los Angeles, USA

John G Lainchbury
Department of Medicine, Christchurch School of Medicine and Health Sciences, University of Otago, Christchurch, New Zealand

Ian Lane
Cardiff Vascular Unit, University Hospital of Wales, Cardiff, UK

G de Martino
Department of Cardiovascular Medicine, Institute of Cardiology, Catholic University of Rome, Rome, Italy

William J McKenna
Department of Cardiological Sciences, St George's Hospital Medical School, London, UK

Venu Menon
Division of Cardiology, University of North Carolina, Chapel Hill, North Carolina, USA

John M Morgan
Wessex Cardiothoracic Centre, Southampton, UK

Steven Nissen
Department of Cardiology, The Cleveland Clinic Foundation, Cleveland, Ohio, USA

G Pelargonio
Department of Cardiovascular Medicine, Institute of Cardiology, Catholic University of Rome, Rome, Italy

M C Petch
Papworth Hospital, Cambridge, UK

Lawrence E Ramsay
Section of Clinical Pharmacology and Therapeutics, Royal Hallamshire Hospital, Sheffield, UK

Thorsten Reffelmann
The Heart Institute, Good Samaritan Hospital, University of Southern California, Los Angeles, USA

Flavio Ribichini
Universita del Piemonte Orientale, Division of Cardiology, Novara, Italy

A Mark Richards
Department of Medicine, Christchurch School of Medicine and Health Sciences, University of Otago, Christchurch, New Zealand

T Sanna
Department of Cardiovascular Medicine, Institute of Cardiology, Catholic University of Rome, Rome, Italy

Richard J Schilling
Cardiology Department, St Barts Hospital, London, UK

Paul Schoenhagen
Department of Cardiology, The Cleveland Clinic Foundation, Cleveland, Ohio, USA

Samuel F Sears
University of Florida, Department of Clinical and Health Psychology, UF Health Science Center, Gainesville, Florida, USA

Willem J L Suyker
Department of Cardiothoracic Surgery, Isala Clinics, Weezenlanden Hospital, Zwolle, The Netherlands

James D Thomas
Department of Cardiology, The Cleveland Clinic Foundation, Cleveland, Ohio, USA

Gilbert R Thompson
Metabolic Medicine, Imperial College School of Medicine, Hammersmith Hospital, London, UK

John K Triedman
Department of Cardiology, Children's Hospital, Boston, Massachusetts, USA

I C Van Gelder
Thoraxcenter, Department of Cardiology, University Hospital Groningen, Groningen, The Netherlands

Erica J Wallis
Section of Clinical Pharmacology and Therapeutics, Royal Hallamshire Hospital, Sheffield, UK

Christopher Ward
Heart Failure Clinic, South Manchester University Hospital NHS Trust, Manchester, UK

Sandra Webb
Department of Anatomy and Developmental Biology, St George's Hospital Medical School, London, UK

William Wijns
Cardiovascular Centre, OLV Hospital, Moorselbaan, Belgium

Christopher Wren
Department of Paediatric Cardiology, Freeman Hospital, Newcastle upon Tyne, UK

INTRODUCTION

Education remains close to the top of the professional agenda both locally and internationally. In the *Education in Heart* series we have worked hard to obtain a portfolio of articles that will address the relevant issues in cardiovascular medicine. Their scope is driven by the structure and content of curricula and we have commissioned work from authors who are experts in their chosen field. The result of our third year is contained in this volume; we hope it will provide a topical and relevant educational resource for those involved in continuing professional development, as well as in the arena of training in cardiology. Volume 4 is well underway!

My thanks are due to the Section Editors for their sound, and often inspired, contributions to the planning and commissioning of the manuscripts. We are all indebted to John Weller for his invaluable and reliable support of the project, and to both the British Cardiac Society and BMJ Publishing Group for their parenting skills.

PETER MILLS
SERIES EDITOR

Section Editors: Martin Cowie (heart failure), Christopher Davidson (general cardiology/hypertension), Mark de Belder (coronary disease), John Gibbs (congenital heart disease), Roger Hall (valve disease), David Lefroy (electrophysiology), Richard Schilling (electrophysiology), Iain Simpson (imaging techniques), Adam Timmis (coronary disease)

SECTION I: CORONARY DISEASE

1 CAROTID ARTERY SURGERY FOR PEOPLE WITH EXISTING CORONARY ARTERY DISEASE

Ian Lane, John Byrne

Carotid artery surgery for neurological symptoms was first reported by Eastcott and colleagues in 1954 following earlier recognition that extracranial atheroma was associated with ischaemic stroke.[1] Carotid endarterectomy rapidly established itself as one of the most frequently performed procedures in the USA, largely based on surgery for asymptomatic atherosclerosis or a carotid bruit. Practice in the UK was more cautious, awaiting the results of European and US trials to clarify management of symptomatic disease with carotid stenosis of over 70%.

▶ DIAGNOSIS OF CAROTID ARTERY DISEASE

Atherosclerosis is a generalised disease, and while symptoms may be site specific, inevitably disease elsewhere will influence the overall management of a patient. The risk of stroke is increased during coronary artery surgery for angina in the presence of asymptomatic carotid disease; conversely the risks of carotid endarterectomy are higher in patients with silent myocardial ischaemia. Early carotid artery wall disease is a predictor for coronary atherosclerosis and subsequent coronary vascular events.[2]

The primary symptoms of carotid atherosclerosis are neurological events and amaurosis fugax caused by embolisation from a plaque. Neurological events include transient ischaemic attacks and stroke and must be related to the contralateral side of the body from that of the stenosis. Events may be sensory, motor, or combined and on occasion are confined to intermittent dysarthria. Classically transient ischaemic attacks last less than 24 hours with full recovery. The 24 hour watershed is an epidemiological tool and does not necessarily imply the absence of permanent brain damage. Imaging by computed tomographic scan has demonstrated multiple cerebral infarcts in patients showing full recovery after transient ischaemic attacks. The frequency of attacks is variable and weeks or months may elapse between events. Multiple events within a timescale of hours (crescendo transient ischaemic attacks) carry a high risk of stroke as they may precede carotid artery thrombosis. Loss of consciousness, vertigo, diplopia and bilateral symptoms should not be attributed to carotid stenosis which is more likely to be a coincidental finding.

Within the population there is a high prevalence of asymptomatic carotid stenosis, often coincidental to other causes of neurological events. Disorders producing neurological events, transient or permanent, include:

▶ intracerebral arteriovenous malformations
▶ demyelinating disease
▶ lacunar infarcts
▶ intracranial tumours
▶ arrhythmias
▶ systemic hypotension.

Arterial embolisation cannot be assumed to originate from atherosclerosis of the carotid bifurcation. Alternative sources of emboli include:

▶ cardiac mural thrombosis and valve disease
▶ atrial fibrillation
▶ left atrial myxoma
▶ aortic and great vessel atherosclerosis
▶ paradoxical embolus from the lower limb
▶ intracranial atherosclerosis, particularly in the carotid siphon.

Symptoms of amaurosis fugax consist of intermittent loss of vision in one eye or part of an eye. They have the appearance of a mist or curtain obscuring vision.

The presence of a carotid bruit is not an accurate determinant of either carotid stenosis or prognosis. It merely implies the presence of turbulence of flow together with the probability of atherosclerosis. Tight arterial stenoses may allow insufficient flow to produce a bruit. Imaging of the carotid bifurcation in patients with suspected carotid artery disease is performed using colour duplex scan which is accurate and sensitive, providing information on the degree of stenosis and plaque morphology (fig 1.1). Ulcerated plaque and intraplaque haemorrhage carry a poorer prognosis than endothelialised stenosis. Duplex scanning measures stenosis according to peak velocity

4

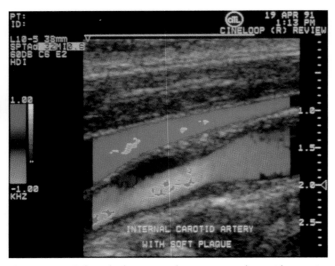

Figure 1.1 Colour duplex image showing internal carotid artery in red with a moderate stenosis characterised as soft plaque. Characterisation of plaque may be of prognostic value.

of blood flow, but the technique can also measure arterial diameter from an image. Although it does not give the same detailed information on proximal or intracranial disease as angiography, in patients with appropriate symptoms further imaging is not required before surgery. Duplex scanning may not differentiate between a tight stenosis (95%) with "trickle flow" and an occluded carotid artery. In these cases magnetic resonance angiography provides an accurate alternative to arteriography (fig 1.2). There is no indication for surgery on an occluded carotid artery as the risk of embolisation has disappeared and re-establishment of flow may propel distal thrombus into the brain. There is little need in modern practice for formal intra-arterial angiography. As well as local complications at the site of arterial puncture, there is a small but significant risk of stroke even without selective carotid catheterisation. Intravenous digital angiography has proved disappointing in providing sufficient resolution of the carotid bifurcation. Carotid imaging at the time of coronary angiography should be reserved for cases where proximal arterial or intracranial disease is suspected as a cause for symptoms.

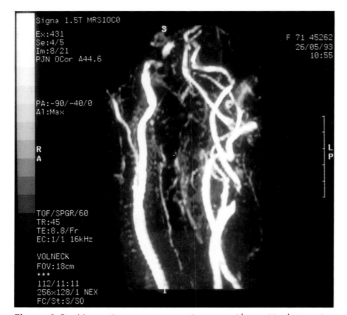

Figure 1.2 Magnetic resonance angiogram with a critical stenosis of the origin of the internal carotid artery on the right.

Duplex scan

▶ No complications
▶ Outpatient investigation
▶ No information on intracerebral circulation
▶ Requires operator expertise
▶ Provides information on plaque morphology
▶ May be inaccurate with 'trickle flow'
▶ Consider magnetic resonance angiography for tight stenoses

MANAGEMENT OF THE DISEASE PROCESS

Atherosclerosis should be treated by correction of risk factors such as hyperlipidaemia, smoking, hypertension, diabetes, and polycythaemia. In the presence of classic symptoms and appropriate carotid stenosis a decision to intervene can be based on duplex scan alone. Unless there is a contraindication, aspirin 300 mg/day will significantly reduce the incidence of further neurological events. The role of new antiplatelet agents such as clopidogrel and ticlopidine have not been subjected to trial. Anticoagulants are unproven and carry significant side effects, but may be useful when other treatment modalities have failed.

CAROTID INTERVENTION

Carotid endarterectomy under general anaesthetic carries a low mortality in fit patients. Cardiac disease was responsible for 49% of deaths in one large series of patients undergoing carotid endarterectomy with mortality due to myocardial infarction.[3] Those with severe cardiac or respiratory dysfunction can be treated under cervical block or local anaesthetic, which has the advantage that neurological events are immediately identified and corrected by shunting. There is a requirement for the patient to remain immobile for the procedure which may not be tolerated, although in one series 97% of 449 patients were successfully treated under local anaesthesia.[4] In one randomised controlled trial the rate of myocardial ischaemia in those treated under local anaesthetic was half that of general anaesthetic, although the results did not reach significance. The dilemma should be resolved by the multicentre general or local anaesthesia for carotid endarterectomy (GALA) trial. Carotid angioplasty is technically possible and subject to clinical multicentre trial. While the cranial nerve injuries associated with surgery are avoided, distal embolisation following carotid mobilisation can produce stroke, although this may be prevented by synchronous distal balloon occlusion of the artery. In a multicentre study of 504 patients randomised to surgery or angioplasty the combined stroke and mortality rate at 30 days was 10% for both surgery and angioplasty.[5] There has been criticism of the high stroke rate in the surgical arm of this trial. Modern interventional techniques, including the use of stents together with cerebral protection devices, require further long term evaluation.

SURGERY FOR SYMPTOMATIC CAROTID STENOSIS

Symptomatic carotid stenosis carries a stroke risk of approximately 15% in the year following a motor or sensory neurological event, with the sequelae of amaurosis fugax having a more benign prognosis. While antiplatelet treatment will reduce the risk of further events to 8% per year, before 1992 the evidence for efficacy of carotid endarterectomy was not scientifically sound. Publications were based on personal series with poor classification of degree of stenosis, presence

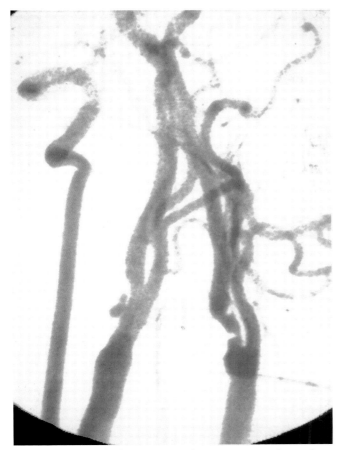

Figure 1.3 Digital subtraction carotid angiogram revealing a deep ulcerated plaque in the left carotid bulb and a severe irregular stenosis of the internal carotid artery on the right. Biplanar views are required to confirm the degree of stenosis on the right. The vertebral artery is filled on the left.

Transient ischaemic attack

▸ Correct risk factors for atherosclerosis
▸ Duplex scan
▸ Add antiplatelet treatment
▸ Consider surgery for carotid stenosis over 70%
▸ Angioplasty acceptable in high risk patients
▸ Intervention should be performed urgently
▸ Carotid restenosis is rarely symptomatic

high risk for stroke although this has recently been challenged.

The role of surgery in patients with moderate stenosis of between 50–69% is unclear, but should be considered if symptoms are uncontrolled by conventional treatment and maximum perioperative death and disabling stroke rate of 2% can be achieved.[8] Occasionally embolisation can originate from a deep ulcerated plaque in the absence of stenosis (fig 1.3). While endothelial remodelling may occur, surgery should be considered if antiplatelet medication fails to control symptoms.

Complications of surgery
The success of carotid endarterectomy to prevent stroke depends on the perioperative stroke and death rate, which should be less than 3%. Factors that increase the risk of perioperative stroke include transient ischaemic attacks rather than amaurosis fugax, contralateral carotid occlusion, and irregular or ulcerated plaque at the side of surgery. There is no significant effect of age above or below 65 years on stroke rate.[9] Patients must be provided with balanced information on the perioperative stroke rate and risk of damage to cranial nerves compared to non-operative management, in order to enable informed participation in their own management. An analysis of the North American symptomatic carotid endarterectomy trial revealed an overall perioperative stroke and death rate of 6.5%, with permanently disabling stroke combined with death of 2.0%. The risk of cranial nerve injuries was 8.6%, affecting the facial, hypoglossal, and vagus nerves, although the majority were described as mild in severity.[9]

MANAGEMENT OF ASYMPTOMATIC CAROTID STENOSIS
Asymptomatic carotid stenosis carries a stroke risk of approximately 2% per year. This stroke risk appears related to the severity of stenosis and remains constant with time, unlike the risk following a neurological event in a symptomatic carotid stenosis.[2] A trial comparing surgery to aspirin for asymptomatic carotid stenosis showed no benefit from surgery although randomisation was incomplete.[10] In a multicentre trial of 1662 patients (asymptomatic carotid atherosclerosis study, ACAS) with over 60% asymptomatic carotid stenoses randomised to surgery or medical treatment, at five years the combined stroke and mortality rate for surgery was 5.1% compared to 11% for medical treatment.[3] Although all centres were validated for low surgical morbidity, the stroke rate associated with arteriography was considered to be high at 1.2%. There should be caution when applying the results of this trial to a wide body of surgeons, especially as the absolute risk reduction for stroke was 1% per year. While surgery carries an advantage over antiplatelet medication, 20 patients have to undergo carotid endarterectomy to prevent one stroke in every five years.[3] This compares with four endarterectomies to prevent one stroke a year in symptomatic patients.[6] Surgery for asymptomatic disease may not be appropriate

or absence of symptoms, use of antiplatelet medication, and duration of follow up.

Indications for surgery
Two multicentre randomised controlled trials have demonstrated an advantage of carotid endarterectomy combined with aspirin, compared to aspirin alone, in the prevention of stroke following a neurological event in patients with over 70% carotid stenosis. In a North American trial, patients with stroke or transient ischaemic attack within three months of entry, combined with symptomatic carotid stenosis of over 70%, were randomised to carotid endarterectomy or aspirin 1300 mg/day. The cumulative stroke risk for the surgical arm of the trial was 9% compared to 22% for medical treatment.[6] A multicentre European trial, in 80 centres, randomised patients with symptomatic carotid stenosis of over 70% to surgery or best medical treatment. The qualifying neurological event for entry into the trial had to have occurred within six months previously. The cumulative risk of stroke was 12.3% for surgery compared to 21.9% for medical treatment, although the 30 day combined stroke and mortality rate for surgery was considered high at 7.5%. This may be due to some centres performing only low numbers of carotid endarterectomies.[7] Despite minor differences between these two trials in terms of assessment of the carotid stenosis and time interval from qualifying event, the conclusions were that surgery has an advantage over medical treatment in symptomatic carotid stenoses of 70% or over. Pre-occlusive lesions are considered

6

when many healthcare systems are critically examining cost and benefit. Application of the ACAS criteria would lead to a 10 fold increase in rates of carotid endarterectomy; to put this in perspective, it is estimated that in Scotland 40 000 people would have an appropriate stenosis. The ACAS trial did not address asymptomatic stenoses in patients over 79 years old, and although many series have shown that surgery can be performed safely in octogenarians, their low life expectancy may preclude benefit from carotid endarterectomy.

CAROTID ENDARTERECTOMY IN PATIENTS UNDERGOING CORONARY ARTERY SURGERY

Coronary artery surgery carries an overall risk of stroke of 1.6% and this is increased in reoperative surgery, presence of carotid stenosis, and in those over 75 years of age.[11 12] In certain subgroups the incidence is 9% and even higher in those undergoing valve surgery. Additionally, there is an excess of late neurological events following cardiovascular surgery in the presence of uncorrected carotid stenosis.[13] The coexistence of symptomatic coronary artery disease and significant carotid artery stenosis ranges from 3.4–22% of the population.[14] Screening for carotid artery disease in patients undergoing coronary artery surgery indicated a prevalence of 8.7% stenoses of over 75%, leading to a perioperative stroke rate of 14.3% in these patients.[15] Stenoses of less than 75% were associated with a postoperative neurological deficit in 2%. Causes of stroke in the perioperative period include embolisation from the heart and great vessels, global brain ischaemia caused by hypoperfusion, air embolus, and intracranial bleeding precipitated by intraoperative anticoagulation, in addition to emboli originating from the carotid bifurcation. Increased use of off-pump coronary artery bypass may reduce the incidence of carotid related events. A prospective study of 582 patients attempted to differentiate between global and focal ischaemic events.[16] Of the 12 postoperative strokes, carotid stenosis of over 50% or occlusion was significantly associated with five of seven hemispheric events but none of the five global events. Unilateral stenosis of over 80%, bilateral stenosis of over 50% or unilateral occlusion with contralateral stenosis of over 50% was associated with a 5.3% risk of hemispheric stroke. No strokes occurred in patients with unilateral 50–79% stenosis.

Although unilateral occlusion is considered of poor prognostic significance, asymptomatic patients derived no benefit from ipsilateral carotid endarterectomy compared with medical treatment alone when analysed as part of the ACAS trial. The advantage of prophylactic carotid endarterectomy in patients with over 80% carotid stenosis was shown to be significant in a retrospective non-randomised series of 68 patients undergoing synchronous or staged coronary artery surgery.[17] Synchronous bilateral carotid endarterectomy was performed with 6.1% mortality, unrelated to primary cardiac or cerebrovascular events, in an unselected series of urgent and elective patients undergoing coronary artery surgery, but the number of cases was small and further studies are required.[13]

In patients with a primary indication for coronary revascularisation, carotid endarterectomy can be carried out safely at the time of coronary artery surgery. A retrospective analysis of 206 cases revealed a stroke or neurological deficit incidence of 3.5%.[18] In 1998 Darling and colleagues demonstrated a neurological event rate of 2.9% and operative mortality of 2.4% in a prospective series of 470 patients undergoing synchronous procedures.[19] A randomised trial of synchronous versus staged procedures revealed a higher stroke rate when carotid surgery followed coronary surgery. Conversely, the low morbidity and mortality of carotid endarterectomy alone in patients with coronary artery disease may not justify synchronous coronary revascularisation where this is not indicated primarily. Carotid endarterectomy under local anaesthesia or regional block may further reduce the cardiac risk in patients with coronary artery disease unsuitable for revascularisation, but needs confirmation by a randomised trial.

Patients requiring coronary revascularisation with symptomatic carotid disease that fulfil the indications for surgery should undergo carotid endarterectomy. In the absence of randomised trials, asymptomatic patients should be managed recognising the high stroke risk associated with carotid stenosis of over 80% and carotid occlusion. There is a need for randomised trials to clarify the need for carotid endarterectomy at the time of coronary artery surgery.

ACKNOWLEDGEMENTS

We are grateful for the advice of Dr Liam Penny (consultant cardiologist) and Professor Mark Wiles (professor of neurology) in the preparation of this article.

REFERENCES

1 **Eastcott HHG**, Pickering GW, Rob CG. Reconstruction of the internal carotid artery in a patient with intermittent attacks of hemiplegia. *Lancet* 1954;ii:994–6.
▶ **First published account of carotid artery surgery, although the stenosis was resected with end-to-end anastomosis of the carotid arteries. DeBakey had performed carotid endarterectomy one year previously although this was not reported for 19 years.**

2 **Rothwell PM**. Carotid artery disease and the risk of ischaemic stroke and coronary vascular events. *Cerebrovasc Dis* 2000;**10**:21–33.
▶ **Pathophysiological review of carotid stenosis and plaque morphology related to neurological events in an attempt to identify prognostic markers.**

3 **Executive Committee for the Asymptomatic Carotid Atherosclerosis Study**. Endarterectomy for asymptomatic carotid artery stenosis. *JAMA* 1995;**273**:1421–8.
▶ **Although surgery was beneficial, patients were selected by participants which may introduce bias. All surgeons were chosen after demonstrating low perioperative morbidity which again may skew conclusions in favour of endarterectomy.**

4 **Darling RC**, Paty PH, Shah DM, *et al*. Eversion endarterectomy of the internal carotid artery: technique and results in 449 procedures. *Surgery* 1996;**120**:635–9.

5 **CAVITAS**. Endovascular versus surgical treatment in patients with carotid stenosis in the carotid and vertebral transluminal angioplasty study (CAVATAS): a randomised trial. *Lancet* 2001;**357**:1729–37.
▶ **Although similar outcomes for the two procedures were present at 3 years, endovascular treatment avoided cranial nerve damage but appeared to be associated with more severe carotid stenosis becoming apparent.**

6 **North American Symptomatic Carotid Endarterectomy Trial Collaborators**. Beneficial effect of carotid endarterectomy in symptomatic patients with high-grade stenoses. *N Engl J Med* 1991;**325**:445–53.
▶ **Landmark study demonstrating benefit of carotid endarterectomy over medical treatment for 70–99% carotid stenosis.**

7 **European Carotid Surgery Trialists' Collaborative Group**. Randomised trial of endarterectomy for recently symptomatic carotid stenosis: final results of the MRC European carotid surgery trial (ECST). *Lancet* 1998;**351**:1379–87.
▶ **Similar outcomes to NASCET in a multicentre trial with interim results published in 1991. Criticised for a relatively high death and stroke rate at 30 days of 7.0% which may be related to low numbers of patients entered by some centres, implying need for both audit of results and critical numbers of patients.**

8 **European Carotid Surgery Trialists' Collaborative Group**. Endarterectomy for the moderate symptomatic carotid stenosis: interim results from the MRC European carotid surgery trial. *Lancet* 1996;**347**:1591–3.

9 **Ferguson GG**, Eliasziw M, Barr HW, *et al*. The North American carotid endarterectomy trial: surgical results in 1415 patients. *Stroke* 1999;**30**:1751–8.
▶ **Long term results at eight years for endarterectomy of both greater and less than 70% stenosis. Although other surgical complications are described as rarely clinically important, 8.6% of patients sustained a cranial nerve injury.**

10 **CASANOVA Study Group**. Carotid surgery versus medical therapy in asymptomatic carotid stenosis. *Stroke* 1991;**22**:1229–35.

► **Although no benefit for surgery was demonstrated, all patients with stenoses greater than 90% underwent operation.**

11 **Hogue CW**, Murphy SF, Schechtman KB, *et al*. Risk factors for delayed stroke after cardiac surgery. *Circulation* 1999;**100**:642–7.

12 **Ricotta JJ**, Faggioli GL, Castilone A, *et al*. Risk factors for stroke after cardiac surgery: Buffalo Cardiac-Cerebra study group. *J Vasc Surg* 1995;**21**:359–63.

13 **Barnes RW**, Nix ML, Sansonetti D, *et al*. Late outcome of untreated asymptomatic carotid disease following cardiovascular operations. *J Vasc Surg* 1985;**2**:843–9.

14 **Dylewski M**, Canver CC, Chandra J, *et al*. Coronary artery bypass combined with bilateral carotid endarterectomy. *Ann Thorac Surg* 2001;**71**:777–82.

15 **Fagioli GL**, Curl GR, Ricotta JJ. The role of carotid screening before coronary artery bypass. *J Vasc Surg* 1990;**12**:724–9.

► **Perioperative stroke rates in 539 patients with only 19 patients submitted to prophylactic carotid endarterectomy, thus not allowing an accurate assessment of intervention.**

16 **Schwartz LB**, Bridgman AH, Kieffer RW, *et al*. Asymptomatic carotid artery stenosis in patients undergoing cardiopulmonary bypass. *J Vasc Surg* 1995;**21**:146–53.

17 **Hines GL**, Scott WC, Schubach SL, *et al*. Prophylactic carotid endarterectomy in patients with high-grade carotid stenosis undergoing coronary bypass: does it decrease the incidence of perioperative stroke? *Ann Vasc Surg* 1998;**12**:23–7.

18 **Chang BB**, Darling RC, Shah DM, *et al*. Carotid endarterectomy can be safely performed with acceptable mortality and morbidity in patients requiring coronary artery bypass grafts. *Am J Surg* 1994;**168**:94–6.

19 **Darling RC**, Dylewski M, Chang BB, *et al*. Combined carotid endarterectomy and coronary artery bypass grafting does not increase the risk of perioperative stroke. *Cardiovasc Surg* 1998;**6**:448–52.

Additional references appear on the *Heart* website–www.heartjnl.com

2 THE "NO-REFLOW" PHENOMENON: BASIC SCIENCE AND CLINICAL CORRELATES

Thorsten Reffelmann, Robert A Kloner

To achieve early and complete reperfusion of the myocardium in acute coronary syndromes is the daily challenge for every physician in clinical cardiology. However, restoration of epicardial blood flow by thrombolysis, primary angioplasty or bypass surgery does not necessarily imply complete reperfusion, even if the target stenosis is adequately removed or bypassed. The amount of microvascular integrity may limit reperfusion to the previously ischaemic tissue despite complete restoration of epicardial vessel diameters.

A 74 year old man with acute distress is admitted to the emergency room because of acute onset of severe, substernal, crushing chest pain two hours ago. He has never suffered from similar symptoms before. The ECG shows ST segment elevation in leads I, aVL, V2–V4. After aspirin and heparin, the patient is immediately transferred to the catheterisation laboratory. Coronary angiography confirms a thrombotic occlusion of the proximal left anterior descending artery. The guide wire easily crosses the occlusion. After coronary artery balloon dilatation and stent implantation the epicardial artery appears to have gained sufficient luminal diameter. However, the contrast medium is only slowly conveyed to the distal artery and not adequately washed out. Even the final angiogram after glyceryl trinitrate in different projections shows no satisfactory flow albeit no visible flow limiting obstacles, such as coronary artery dissection or recurrent thrombus formation. The battle, undertaken to restore myocardial blood supply, seems to be lost and won, finally leading to compromised tissue perfusion despite a successful restoration of patency to the epicardial blood vessel.

A bolus of abciximab, followed by a continuous infusion, is initiated. ST segment elevations resolve only slightly during the next hours; the patient requires prolonged intensive medical care because of recurrent pulmonary oedema. Finally, the patient is stabilised on cardiovascular medication including an angiotensin converting enzyme (ACE) inhibitor, oxygen, and aspirin. The echocardiography shows a large akinetic segment of the anteroseptal wall with an apical aneurysm, and a global ejection fraction of 30%.

Angiographic no-reflow, as described above, may be one of the clinically most obvious manifestations of microvascular damage. The following discussion will set forward that the so-called "no-reflow" phenomenon is far more frequent, and has important prognostic implications. Combining results from basic science and clinical research, we try to elucidate major mechanisms of no-reflow, methods of assessing microvascular dysfunction, and its significance in the clinical setting.

WHAT IS KNOWN ABOUT NO-REFLOW FROM ANIMAL STUDIES?

Anatomical no-reflow

In experimental models of myocardial infarction, injection of various dyes to the circulation has been traditionally used to stain perfused tissue. As shown in fig 2.1, a substantial part of the myocardium, after being subjected to proximal coronary occlusion and reperfusion of the epicardial artery, may remain unstained after injection of monastral blue or thioflavin S (a fluorescent vital stain for endothelium). The resulting visual perfusion defects represent the so-called "anatomical" no-reflow. Systematic investigations in the canine model of myocardial infarction demonstrated a homogenous distribution of thioflavin S after 40 minutes of ischaemia with subsequent reperfusion. However, after 90 minutes, areas of no-reflow were identified as zones not stained by the fluorescent dye,[1] indicating that a certain duration of ischaemia is necessary for the development of no-reflow. In the canine model, these zones of no-reflow first appeared in the subendocardium.

Ultrastructural changes

Electron microscopy of these areas of no-reflow revealed swollen intraluminal endothelial protrusions and membrane bound intraluminal bodies, which appeared to be free floating and often seemed to obstruct the capillary lumen. Endothelial cells showed decreased numbers of pinocytotic vesicles and nuclear chromatin margination. After 20 minutes of reperfusion, capillaries contained tightly packed erythrocytes, endothelial gaps, sometimes plugged by platelet and fibrin thrombi, with numerous extravascular red blood cells. Occasionally, capillaries seemed to be compressed by

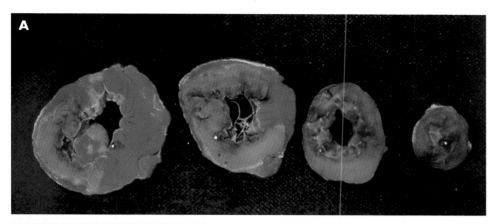

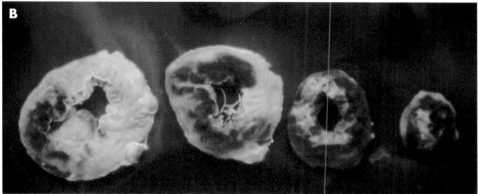

Figure 2.1 Anatomical no-reflow, visualised in a rabbit model of coronary occlusion and reperfusion. Monastral blue (A) and thioflavin S (B, photography under ultraviolet light, Minolta Y48 barrier filter) were injected into the left atrium after 120 minutes of coronary artery occlusion and 120 minutes of reperfusion. Both dyes leave a substantial part of the left ventricle unstained, indicating areas of no or low perfusion. A close look at the slices demonstrates that (although closely correlating) the area not stained by monastral blue is slightly larger than the non-fluorescent area, reflecting the ability of the two dyes to penetrate into areas of hypoperfusion.

subsarcolemmal blebs of neighbouring swollen myocytes.[1] Ultrastructural investigations after different durations (20–180 minutes) of occlusion in a dog model of coronary ligation and reperfusion demonstrated that microvascular damage (first observed after 60 minutes of occlusion) always lagged behind myocardial cell injury (first apparent after 20 minutes of ischaemia) and that microvascular alterations were always located in zones of irreversibly damaged myocytes.[2] Areas not stained by the fluorescent dye were characterised by low regional myocardial blood flow (mean (SEM) 0.13 (0.03) ml/g/min to 0.26 (0.04) ml/g/min), as assessed by radioactive microspheres.[3]

Reperfusion injury and microvascular dysfunction
The term "reperfusion injury" has been coined to describe reperfusion related worsening or expansion of various forms of ischaemic cardiac damage, including: alterations of contractile performance; the arrhythmogenic threshold; potential conversion from reversible to irreversible cardiomyocyte injury; and vascular, in particular microvascular, dysfunction. Ambrosio and colleagues demonstrated a more than twofold increase in the area of no-reflow from 2 minutes to 3.5 hours of reperfusion. This increase was accompanied by a progressive decrease of regional myocardial blood flow within the risk area after initial restoration of regional myocardial flow.[3] Thus, on the one hand no-reflow depends on the degree of the initial ischaemic damage, but on the other hand reperfusion injury at the microvascular level is a significant determinant of the final amount of no-reflow.

WHAT IS KNOWN FROM CLINICAL RESEARCH?
Angiographic no-reflow
Coronary angiography allows a semiquantitative grading of epicardial antegrade flow according to the thrombolysis in myocardial infarction (TIMI) flow grades. TIMI grade 0 refers

to no distal antegrade vessel opacification by the contrast medium, grade 1 means minimal distal flow, grade 2 partial reperfusion, and grade 3 complete reperfusion. After thrombolysis or coronary angioplasty (PTCA) for acute myocardial infarction, TIMI 0–2 grade coronary flow is associated with more complications and worse left ventricular function compared with TIMI 3 grade flow, even without evidence for obstruction of the epicardial artery. In a retrospective review of 1919 elective and emergency percutaneous interventions by Piana and colleagues, "angiographic" no-reflow, defined as TIMI grade flow less than 3 without evidence for obstruction in the proximal artery, occurred in 2% of all interventions. But the incidence varied with the technique and indication for PTCA: the highest incidence of no-reflow was found after recanalisation for acute myocardial infarction (11.5%); the incidence was significantly higher for interventions in degenerated saphenous bypass grafts (4%); and for stenting or directional atherectomy interventions (3%).[4] Recent studies demonstrated that angiographic no-reflow is a strong predictor of major cardiac complications, including congestive heart failure, malignant arrhythmias, and cardiac death after myocardial infarction.[5]

Myocardial contrast echocardiography
Myocardial contrast echocardiography (MCE) has profoundly extended our understanding of myocardial microvascular perfusion after acute myocardial infarction, and intravenous contrast application with bedside imaging is now feasible. Ito and colleagues showed that all patients with TIMI grade 2 flow after PTCA showed substantial no-reflow on MCE, defined as contrast defects after angioplasty of more than 25% of the risk zone (determined before recanalisation). But even with TIMI grade 3 flow, 16% of the patients showed no-reflow, and significant improvement of left ventricular function was only observed in the patients with reflow.[6] Comparing microvascular perfusion and regional myocardial contractile recovery,

Ragosta and associates concluded that microvascular integrity, as assessed by MCE, is closely related to myocyte viability.[7] Sakuma and colleagues demonstrated that the size of the risk area, determined before reperfusion, as well as a low peak grey scale ratio on MCE one day after primary PTCA for acute myocardial infarction, strongly predicted major cardiac events within the next 22 months.[8] Risk factors for the development of perfusion defects on MCE were not consistent in different studies, but most of them reported a higher incidence of no-reflow with longer elapsed time from onset of symptoms to reperfusion, older age, large anterior myocardial infarction, low admission blood pressure, and, interestingly, with the absence of pre-infarction angina, which might be interpreted as a clinical correlate of microvascular preconditioning.

Intracoronary Doppler flow velocity changes
Intracoronary Doppler derived flow velocity patterns showed characteristic profiles in patients with evidence for no-reflow on MCE, including early systolic retrograde flow and high diastolic deceleration rates, and a lower coronary flow reserve.[9] Iwakura and colleagues showed that patients with occurrence of these Doppler flow characteristics immediately after PTCA had longer elapsed time from onset of symptoms to reperfusion and more Q waves on the surface ECG before reperfusion. Patients with delayed (within 10 minutes) systolic retrograde flow had a higher incidence of transient ST segment re-elevation after recanalisation.[10] The delayed occurrence of these characteristics in a subgroup of patients might be a correlate of reperfusion associated progression of no-reflow.

TIMI frame count and myocardial blush grade
Other angiographic techniques, used for assessing microvascular integrity in patients with reperfused myocardial infarction, are the corrected TIMI frame count, defined as the number of angiographic frames required for the contrast medium to reach standardised distal landmarks of the coronary artery, and myocardial blush grade, as a semiquantitative description of myocardial contrast density on the final angiogram after reperfusion therapy.

Scintigraphic techniques
Visualisation of perfusion defects was also achieved by scintigraphic techniques. Intracoronary injection of macroaggregated [99m]technetium albumin after successful percutaneous recanalisation demonstrated substantial perfusion defects. In addition, evidence for a progressive impairment of tissue perfusion during reperfusion was provided by [82]rubidium positron emission in a canine model.

Magnetic resonance imaging
In magnetic resonance imaging (MRI), hypoenhancement 1–2 minutes after contrast injection is assumed to represent zones of no-reflow. A recent study validated the amount of hypoenhancement against anatomical no-reflow assessed by injection of thioflavin S and regional myocardial blood flow in a canine model of reperfused myocardial infarction.[11] Assessing hypoenhancement after contrast injection, visualised in 44 patients 10 days after acute myocardial infarction, Wu and colleagues demonstrated significant prognostic implications of microvascular obstruction for clinical outcome, even after statistical correction for the predictive value of infarct size.[12] Thus, contrast enhanced MRI might be a promising non-invasive future technique for the determination of microvascular obstruction with the opportunity of simultaneous estimation of infarct size (visible as hyperenhancement 5–10 minutes after contrast injection).

Resolution of ST segment elevation
The resolution of ST segment elevation after reperfusion therapy was shown to correlate with the amount of myocardial perfusion as visualised by MCE. The so-called ST segment elevation index refers to the sum of ST segment elevation (mV) in the different leads (excluding aVR), divided by the number of leads showing ST segment elevation. While patients without evidence of no-reflow showed a rapid reduction of the ST segment elevation index within the first 30 minutes after successful primary PTCA, ST segment elevation in patients with no-reflow resolved to a significantly lesser degree. Indeed, a (transient) re-elevation was observed in some of these patients.[13]

Biochemical markers
Serial measures of serum myoglobin, creatine kinase-MB or troponin I (or T) at baseline and 60 (or 90) minutes after reperfusion therapy have been a useful technique for the assessment of infarct related artery patency. A high ratio of

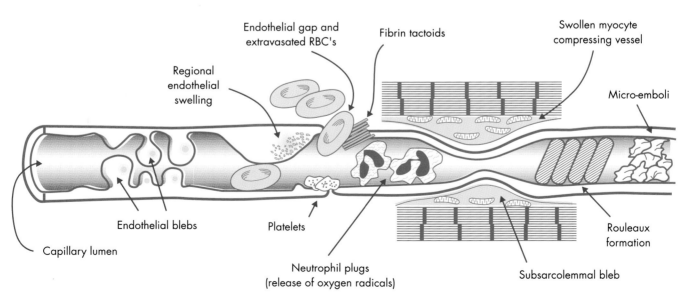

Figure 2.2 Schematic figure, summarising different mechanisms, involved in the development of no-reflow, and accompanying ultrastructural alterations of the microvascular bed (RBC, red blood cell).

the 60 minute value to the baseline value and a higher slope of increase in these markers over time are generally related to successful reopening of the epicardial occlusion, but may also reflect the completeness of microvascular tissue reperfusion. Thus, the amount of tissue reperfusion after reperfusion therapy might in part be estimated even without invasive procedures or sophisticated and expensive technical equipment.

POTENTIAL MECHANISMS OF NO-REFLOW

Although numerous potential explanations of the development of no-reflow have been put forward (fig 2.2), the significance of any single mechanism is not yet fully understood. In addition, the importance of these mechanisms might be different immediately after release of the coronary occlusion versus later during the time course of reperfusion. Mechanisms causing no-reflow in experimental mechanical coronary occlusion and reperfusion may differ from those of clinical myocardial infarction or observed during percutaneous coronary interventions (for a list of references refer to *e*Heart).

Endothelial ischaemic damage and microvascular obstruction

The pronounced ultrastructural alterations of the capillary endothelium demonstrated in the canine model suggest that morphological features of the microvascular damage related to ischaemia may directly contribute to the no-reflow phenomenon. Localised areas of endothelial swelling and endothelial protrusions (also called "blebs") were the most common findings.[1] These protrusions may act to occlude the capillary lumen, and thus play a direct role in causing regional perfusion defects, probably most important directly after reopening of the coronary artery. Following reperfusion, capillaries showed tightly packed erythrocytes suggesting that some flow must have occurred initially into these regions after release of the coronary occlusion.

Leucocytes: plugging versus interaction with endothelium, platelets, and myocytes

The pronounced increase of anatomical no-reflow during reperfusion, observed in the experiments by Ambrosio and colleagues, was accompanied by striking neutrophil accumulation within no-reflow areas.[3] Engler and associates demonstrated extensive leucocyte plugging in the microvasculature, that could not be washed out by crystalloid perfusion, after coronary occlusion and five hours of reperfusion. Leucocyte depletion or reperfusion with oxygenated perfluorochemicals led to a reduction of anatomical no-reflow in various studies. However, it should be emphasised that even in isolated saline perfused Langendorff hearts, an anatomical area of no-reflow can be visualised. Thus, leucocytes may exacerbate no-reflow, but do not appear to be a requirement for it to occur.

Even if capillary leucocyte trapping is prominent in the area of no-reflow, the effects of leucocytes are probably not solely confined to mechanical plugging, but may involve complex interactions with the endothelium, platelets, and perhaps with myocytes. Polymorphonuclear cells are able to release reactive oxygen metabolites, proteolytic enzymes, and lipooxygenase products (leukotrienes) that influence platelet and endothelial function. Endothelial cells can modulate leucocyte function by the expression of adhesion molecules—for example, intercellular adhesion molecule-1 (ICAM-1) or P-selectin—and by release of soluble factors including nitric oxide, prostacyclin, endothelin, and platelet activating factor. Platelets affect polymorphonuclear cell activation by release of

thromboxane A2, platelet derived growth factor, serotonin, lipooxygenase products, proteases, and adenosine. However, various studies addressing these questions led to partly inconsistent and contradictory results, depending upon the specific model or species investigated. Clinical trials investigating the effect of neutrophil inhibition in myocardial infarction have been in general, negative.

Reactive oxygen species

The production of oxygen-free radicals peaks during the first 2–10 minutes of reperfusion after coronary artery occlusion. Sources of oxygen free radicals include the xanthine oxidase reaction, mitochondria, and polymorphonuclear cells. The superoxide dismutase pathway, normally responsible for the clearance of superoxide anions, may be altered after an ischaemic insult. Administration of superoxide dismutase in combination with catalase led to a notable reduction of no-reflow, and ultrastructural signs of endothelial injury in animal studies[14]; also free radical scavengers were shown to prevent functional vascular dysfunction after ischaemia and reperfusion.

Functional abnormalities of the vessels

Vascular dysfunction after ischemia and reperfusion in animal models is characterised by a decreased vasodilation in response to acetylcholine or platelet derived stimuli. Functional vascular alterations were shown to persist for several weeks. Interestingly, ischaemic preconditioning can prevent functional vascular abnormalities.[15] Clinical observations confirmed a reduced coronary flow reserve after ischaemia and reperfusion. But even if impaired endothelial response to physiologic stimuli is not the primary cause of anatomical no-reflow, functional vascular abnormalities, especially long term alterations, may prevent adaptation of regional blood flow to situations with an increased oxygen or substrate demand.

Mechanical compression

Sudden myocardial cell swelling with prominent intracellular and interstitial oedema is one of the very early morphologic changes induced by reperfusion. As tissue oedema might compress the microvascular bed, the no-reflow phenomenon may in part be attributed to changes in total cross sectional vascular area. However, studies investigating the effect of increased serum osmolality to reduce tissue oedema did not show consistent results. It is likely that mechanical compression contributes in some situations, but is not the primary mechanism of no-reflow.

Coagulation, tissue factor

Ultrastructural investigations of no-reflow areas did not show direct evidence of a causal role of intravascular thrombus formation for the development of no-reflow in animal models of mechanical coronary artery occlusion and reperfusion. Some electron microscopy studies found rare microthrombi[1]; others did not find any evidence for activation of the coagulation pathway. Administration of acetylsalicylic acid, streptokinase or tissue plasminogen activator did not demonstrate any beneficial effects on microvascular integrity.

Recent observations suggest that tissue factor, a membrane bound glycoprotein that activates the extrinsic coagulation pathway (via activating factor VII) when exposed to flowing blood, contributes to the degree of no-reflow. When active site-blocked factor VII was administered during reperfusion, a pronounced reduction of no-reflow was observed,[16] which

Table 2.1 Interventions used in experimental animal models to reduce no-reflow

Intervention	Species	Methods for assessing no-reflow	Comment
Adenosine			
Adenosine, intracoronary and intravenous application during reperfusion	Dogs	Radioactive microspheres, EM	Improved regional myocardial blood flow, ultrastructural preservation of endothelial cells, less neutrophil infiltration, in one study only effective in combination with lidocaine
Calcium channel antagonists			
Nisoldipine before ischaemia	Rats	Fluorescein perfusion	Reduced area of no-reflow with nisoldipine in globally ischaemic isolated hearts
Gallopamil during ischaemia	Rabbits	Thioflavin S	Reduced no reflow with gallopamil during ischaemia, accompanied by infarct size reduction
Neutrophil depletion			
Reperfusion with neutrophil depleted blood (filter)	Dogs	Thioflavin S	Reduction of anatomical no reflow with concomitant infarct size reduction
Intraperitoneal mustin hydrochloride	Rats	Constant pressure perfusion (Langendorff)	Explanted hearts after global ischaemia for 4 hours (4°C) were transplanted into the abdomen of the recipient. After different times of in situ reperfusion, Langendorff perfusion revealed better recovery of coronary flow after leucocyte depletion
Reperfusion with intracoronary oxygenated perfluorochemical	Dogs	Thioflavin S, coloured microspheres, EM, LM	Reduced area of no-reflow, less leucocyte plugging, preservation of endothelial structure
Oxygen derived free radical scavenging			
Superoxide dismutase and catalase during reperfusion	Dogs	Radioactive microspheres, EM	Preservation of endocardial regional blood flow, less ultrastructural damage to the endothelium within myocardial necrosis, pronounced hyperaemic response in treated animals after 10 minutes of reperfusion
Active site blocked factor VIIa			
Active site blocked factor VIIa during reperfusion	Rabbits	Thioflavin S	Reduction of anatomical no-reflow and infarct size
Endothelin antagonism			
Endothelin A antagonist during reperfusion	Dogs	MCE, radioactive microspheres	Enhanced microvascular flow after 180 minutes of reperfusion by contrast echocardiography and microspheres

EM, electron microscopy; LM, light microscopy; MCE, myocardial contrast echocardiography.

might be of special interest in clinical acute coronary syndromes, associated with vascular and endothelial damage.

Microembolisation of atherosclerotic debris and thrombi

Unlike most animal models of mechanical coronary occlusion, the clinical setting probably involves microembolic events in a substantial number of cases. The transition of a stable atherosclerotic lesion to an unstable plaque, induced by inflammatory stimuli or by iatrogenic manipulation, includes the disruption of the fibrous cap with exposure of subendothelial matrix, which subsequently can lead to embolisation of lipid, matrix, endothelial cells or platelet thrombi to the distal vasculature.[17]

In unstable angina, elevation of serum troponin T is a very sensitive marker of myocardial injury, reflecting micronecrosis caused by distal coronary embolisation. The pronounced beneficial effects of glycoprotein IIb/IIIa receptor antagonists in the subgroup of patients with unstable angina and increased troponin T serum concentrations, evident in the CAPTURE (chimeric 7E3 antiplatelet therapy in unstable angina refractory to standard treatment) study, indicates a role of microembolisation followed by platelet activation in this subgroup.[18] Cyclic flow variations in stenosed coronary arteries are regarded as the consequence of the formation of platelet aggregates and subsequent dislodgement of the embolus into the microvascular bed.

Elective angioplasty procedures are associated with a certain incidence of the no-reflow phenomenon.[4] Depending on the technique, the incidence is quite variable. Patients who undergo percutaneous interventions for degenerated saphenous vein grafts have a high risk of periprocedural infarction.

Mechanical devices, designed to trap embolic debris during angioplasty, showed that embolic material could be retrieved during PTCA, especially in angioplasty interventions in degenerated venous grafts, which is "smoking-gun evidence" for the concept of PTCA associated distal embolisation. Directional and rotational atherectomy have a substantially higher risk of no-reflow compared with balloon angioplasty. Thus, microemboli significantly contribute to the no-reflow phenomenon in the clinical situation, leading to micro- and potentially macro-infarcts.

TREATMENT OF NO-REFLOW: DOES IT MAKE SENSE?

Obviously, the prevention of microembolisation or its consequences should be beneficial in the clinical setting. Glycoprotein IIb/IIIa receptor blockers, that should reduce the detrimental sequelae of coronary embolisation in the microvascular bed, have demonstrated convincing effects on clinical outcome in unstable angina and after percutaneous intervention, in addition to prevention of reocclusion of the target lesion.

However, with respect to the "classical" no-reflow phenomenon in coronary occlusion and reperfusion, the question is more difficult to answer. To date, no study could demonstrate no-reflow zones preceding myocardial necrosis. In 312 biopsies of ischaemic canine myocardium after various times of coronary occlusion (20–180 minutes), no biopsy showed microvascular damage without myocardial cell injury. In addition, ultrastructural myocyte damage greatly preceded microvascular alterations.[2] Even in the experiments of Ambrosio and colleagues, that showed a pronounced expansion of

Table 2.2 Interventions used in clinical situations to reduce no-reflow

Intervention	Clinical situation	Method for assessing no-reflow	Comment
Adenosine			
Intracoronary adenosine	Primary angioplasty for AMI	TIMI grade flow	Incidence of angiographic no-reflow could be reduced, and in one study associated with better recovery of left ventricular function and outcome
Calcium antagonists			
Intracoronary verapamil with glyceryl trinitrate	Elective and emergency PTCA for AMI	TIMI grade flow	Improvement of TIMI grade flow after verapamil in elective and emergency PTCA
Intracoronary verapamil	PTCA in AMI	MCE	Reduction of perfusion defects and increase in peak intensity, associated with better contractile recovery
Intragraft verapamil	Elective PTCA	TIMI grade flow	Improvement of flow with verapamil in PTCA in saphenous grafts, in contrast: no effect of glyceryl trinitrate
Papaverine			
Intracoronary papaverine	Elective PTCA in saphenous grafts	TIMI frame count	Papaverine reduced the number of TIMI frame counts in patients with no-reflow
Nicorandil			
Intravenous nicorandil	Anterior wall AMI	MCE	Lower incidence of perfusion defects in the nicorandil group
Nitric oxide donor			
Intracoronary nitroprusside	Elective PTCA	TIMI flow grade, modified TIMI frame count	Improvement of flow after nitroprusside in elective interventions
Glycoprotein IIb/IIIa receptor antagonism			
Intravenous abciximab	Stenting in AMI	Coronary flow velocity after 14 days	Improvement of coronary flow velocities and left ventricular function after myocardial infarction with abciximab
Intravenous eptifibatide	Elective stenting of native coronary arteries	Angiography derived flow reserve and myocardial blush	Eptifibatide improved parameters of coronary flow reserve and velocity of microvascular perfusion in elective PTCA procedures
Intravenous abciximab	Elective rotational atherectomy	Tc-99m sestamibi scintigraphy	Abciximab reduced the incidence and amount of scintigraphic perfusion defects after rotational atherectomy
Mechanical devices for prevention of microembolisation (distal temporary occlusion versus umbrella technique)			
For example, PercuSurge GuardWire temporary occlusion system, Dorros/Probing catheter, Angiogard ("umbrella" system)	Elective saphenous graft angioplasty	First experiences, feasibility	In saphenous graft interventions large amounts of atherosclerotic debris could be aspirated.

AMI, acute myocardial infarction; MCE, myocardial contrast echocardiography; PTCA, percutaneous transluminal coronary angioplasty; TIMI, thrombolysis in myocardial infarction.

no-reflow during reperfusion, the area of hypoperfusion was always confined to the area of necrosis.[3]

As there is no proof of a contribution of classical no-reflow to myocardial necrosis, one might ask whether treatment that focuses on reduction of no-reflow in necrotic tissue makes sense. In theory, improvement of tissue perfusion, even in areas of irreversibly damaged cardiomyocytes, could have beneficial effects other than myocardial salvage. Improved tissue perfusion might impede infarct expansion, ventricular remodelling or aneurysmic ventricular dilation, and promote scar healing and the delivery of pharmacological agents to the myocardium. Furthermore, blood vessels preserved in an area that might have become a no-reflow zone could serve as a source of future collateral vessels.

The MRI study by Wu and colleagues demonstrated prognostic significance of no-reflow after acute myocardial infarction independent of its relation to infarct size. The presence of microvascular obstruction in this study was significantly correlated with fibrous scar formation, left ventricular remodelling after six months, and worse clinical outcome.[12]

TREATMENT OF NO-REFLOW: WHAT TREATMENTS WORK?
Treatment strategies to reduce no-reflow have achieved increasing recognition both in basic animal research and clinical studies. However, pharmacological interventions are

not finally established except for the prevention of the detrimental effects of coronary microembolisation by special devices or therapies that reduce platelet activation. Table 2.1 summarises a selection of interventions that were shown to exhibit beneficial effects on no-reflow in animal models; table 2.2 focuses on treatment strategies used to reduce no-reflow in clinical situations. Pharmacological agents with vasodilating properties, such as adenosine, papaverine, and calcium antagonists were investigated in experimental and clinical conditions. The results from animal studies were controversial with respect to adenosine. Clinical studies mainly used angiographic no-reflow as an end point, which might not fully reflect microvascular perfusion. The beneficial effects of leucocyte depletion or oxygen radical scavenging in animal studies did not show convincing usefulness in the clinical setting. As demonstrated recently, nicorandil administered directly after the diagnosis of acute myocardial infarction was effective in both reducing the perfusion defect (MCE) and complications after infarction, accompanied by an increased recovery of left ventricular function.[19] In another study, intracoronary verapamil was also shown to reduce perfusion defects and increase peak contrast intensity in MCE after primary PTCA for acute myocardial infarction.[20]

In summary, the best treatment strategy for no-reflow has not yet been characterised, and future investigations are

13

14

No-reflow phenomenon: key points

▶ Experimental no-reflow is characterised by microvascular dysfunction, evident as distinct areas of hypoperfusion, compromised resting myocardial blood flow, and functional vascular alterations after ischaemia and reperfusion

▶ Clinical observations, using TIMI grading of coronary flow, MCE, scintigraphic, and MRI techniques show evidence for similar features of microvascular damage after acute myocardial infarction, and even after elective PTCA interventions

▶ Coronary microembolisation is an important mechanism of no-reflow in acute coronary syndromes and PTCA procedures

▶ Perfusion defects after acute myocardial infarction—for example, visualised by MCE—are closely related to lack of contractile recovery and irreversible myocyte damage

---

needed to evaluate the significance and contribution of different mechanisms responsible for no-reflow in order to provide optimal therapy.

SUMMARY AND CONCLUSIONS

Both animal models of experimental myocardial infarction and clinical studies have provided evidence of impaired microvascular perfusion after reperfusion. Characteristics of no-reflow found in basic science investigations, such as distinct perfusion defects, progressive decrease of resting myocardial flow with ongoing reperfusion and functional vascular alterations are parallelled by clinical observations demonstrating similar features. Treatment strategies of reducing no-reflow after acute myocardial infarction are under investigation. Coronary microembolisation is significantly involved in clinically observed microvascular dysfunction, and new interventional devices provide hope for capturing these emboli before they cause tissue damage. From a practical standpoint, the best way to reduce no-reflow is to reduce infarct size by early reperfusion and adequate pharmacological treatment. However, whether improvement of microvascular perfusion even in zones of irreversibly damaged myocardium—which theoretically might have beneficial effects on ventricular remodelling, infarct healing, and collateral formation—is feasible with pharmacological interventions, remains to be investigated.

REFERENCES

1 **Kloner RA**, Ganote CE, Jennings RB. The "no-reflow" phenomenon after temporary coronary occlusion in dogs. *J Clin Invest* 1974;**54**:1496–508.
▶ This is the first article describing anatomical no-reflow after experimental myocardial infarction in the canine model, using thioflavin S as a marker of anatomical no-reflow. The corresponding ultrastructural changes of the microvasculature are evaluated by electron microscopy.
2 **Kloner RA**, Rude RE, Carlson N, *et al*. Ultrastructural evidence of microvascular damage and myocardial cell injury after coronary artery occlusion: which comes first? *Circulation* 1980;**62**:945–52.
▶ The spatial and temporal distribution of ultrastructural alterations of the microvascular bed is evaluated in comparison to myocyte fine structure. Microvascular changes lagged behind myocyte changes of irreversible ischaemic damage.
3 **Ambrosio G**, Weisman HF, Mannisi JA, *et al*. Progressive impairment of regional myocardial perfusion after initial restoration of postischemic blood flow. *Circulation* 1989;**80**:1846–61.
▶ This landmark article provides evidence of reperfusion injury at the microvascular level, demonstrating a substantial increase of anatomical no-reflow with ongoing reperfusion and a progressive decrease of tissue perfusion.
4 **Piana RN**, Paik GY, Moscucci M, *et al*. Incidence and treatment of 'no-reflow' after percutaneous coronary intervention. *Circulation* 1994;**89**:2514–18.

▶ In a retrospective analysis, the incidence of angiographical no-reflow in elective PTCA procedures as well as in primary PTCA for acute myocardial infarction is evaluated.
5 **Morishima I**, Sone T, Okumura K, *et al*. Angiographic no-reflow phenomenon as a predictor of adverse long-term outcome in patients treated with percutaneous transluminal coronary angioplasty for first acute myocardial infarction. *J Am Coll Cardiol* 2000;**36**:1202–9.
6 **Ito H**, Okamura A, Iwakura K, *et al*. Myocardial perfusion patterns related to thrombolysis in myocardial infarction perfusion grades after coronary angioplasty in patients with acute anterior wall myocardial infarction. *Circulation* 1996;**93**:1993–9.
▶ Systematic analysis of the relation between TIMI grade flow and MCE and its significance for functional recovery.
7 **Ragosta M**, Camarano G, Kaul S, *et al*. Microvascular integrity indicates myocellular viability in patients with recent myocardial infarction: new insights using myocardial contrast echocardiography. *Circulation* 1994;**89**:2562–9.
8 **Sakuma T**, Hayashi Y, Sumii K, *et al*. Prediction of short- and intermediate-term prognoses of patients with acute myocardial infarction using myocardial contrast echocardiography one day after recanalization. *J Am Coll Cardiol* 1998;**32**:890–7.
9 **Iwakura K**, Ito H, Takiuchi S, *et al*. Alteration in the coronary blood flow velocity pattern in patients with no reflow and reperfused acute myocardial infarction. *Circulation* 1996;**94**:1269–75.
▶ First description of characteristic changes of intracoronary Doppler profiles in patients with no-reflow after acute myocardial infarction with a section of potential explanations of its pathophysiology (see discussion).
10 **Iwakura K**, Ito H, Nishikawa N, *et al*. Early temporal changes in coronary flow velocity patterns in patients with acute myocardial infarction demonstrating the "no-reflow" phenomenon. *Am J Cardiol* 1999;**84**:415–19.
11 **Rochitte CE**, Lima JA, Bluemke DA, *et al*. Magnitude and time course of microvascular obstruction and tissue injury after acute myocardial infarction. *Circulation* 1998;**98**:1006–14.
12 **Wu KC**, Zerhouni EA, Judd RM, *et al*. Prognostic significance of microvascular obstruction by magnetic resonance imaging in patients with acute myocardial infarction. *Circulation* 1998;**97**:765–72.
▶ Even if a substantial percentage of the included patients were not available at follow up after 16 months, this elegant study was able to relate the occurrence of microvascular obstruction, visualised as magnetic resonance hypoenhancement after contrast injection, to cardiovascular complications. This is the first study that demonstrated a prognostic significance of microvascular dysfunction independent of its relation to infarct size.
13 **Santoro GM**, Valenti R, Buonamici P, *et al*. Relation between ST-segment changes and myocardial perfusion evaluated by myocardial contrast echocardiography in patients with acute myocardial infarction treated with direct angioplasty. *Am J Cardiol* 1998;**82**:932–7.
14 **Przyklenk K**, Kloner RA. "Reperfusion injury" by oxygen-derived free radicals? Effect of superoxide dismutase plus catalase, given at the time of reperfusion, on myocardial infarct size, contractile function, coronary microvasculature, and regional myocardial blood flow. *Circ Res* 1989;**64**:86–96.
15 **Richard V**, Kaeffer N, Tron C, *et al*. Ischemic preconditioning protects against coronary endothelial dysfunction induced by ischemia and reperfusion. *Circulation* 1994;**89**:1254–61.
16 **Golino P**, Ragni M, Cirillo P, *et al*. Recombinant human, active site-blocked factor VIIa reduces infarct size and no-reflow phenomenon in rabbits. *Am J Physiol* 2000;**278**:H1507–16.
17 **Topol EJ**, Yadav JS. Recognition of the importance of embolization in atherosclerotic vascular disease. *Circulation* 2000;**101**:570–80.
▶ Excellent review on the role of coronary microembolisation in various clinical situations of unstable coronary syndromes and percutaneous interventions.
18 **Hamm CW**, Heeschen C, Goldman B, *et al*, for the CAPTURE Investigators. Benefit of abciximab in patients with refractory unstable angina in relation to serum troponin T levels. *N Engl J Med* 1999;**340**:1623–9.
▶ One of the most convincing studies on glycoprotein IIb/IIIa receptor blockade, which demonstrates the beneficial effects of glycoprotein IIb/IIIa receptor antagonism in unstable angina on clinical outcome.
19 **Ito H**, Taniyama Y, Iwakura K, *et al*. Intravenous nicorandil can preserve microvascular integrity and myocardial viability in patients with reperfused anterior wall myocardial infarction. *J Am Coll Cardiol* 1999;**33**:654–60.
▶ This study demonstrated beneficial effects of intravenous nicorandil, initiated before reperfusion therapy, on microvascular function and myocardial viability by MCE.
20 **Taniyama Y**, Ito H, Iwakura K, *et al*. Beneficial effect of intracoronary verapamil on microvascular and myocardial salvage in patients with acute myocardial infarction. *J Am Coll Cardiol* 1997;**30**:1193–9.

Additional references appear on the *Heart* website—www.heartjnl.com

3 SCREENING RELATIVES OF PATIENTS WITH PREMATURE CORONARY HEART DISEASE

Gilbert R Thompson

Used properly, screening detects metabolic time bombs before they wreak havoc; used inappropriately, screening may transform an asymptomatic individual into a modern semblance of Damocles, perpetually anxious about the future. Hence, before undertaking screening it is important to first answer the question as to whether the results are likely to influence the future management of the person screened. If the answer is no or uncertain, then it might be better to desist.

Familial occurrence of risk factors such as a raised low density lipoprotein (LDL) cholesterol is sometimes caused by a dominantly inherited disorder—for example, familial hypercholesterolaemia (FH)—but more often reflects interaction between weaker genetic traits and shared environmental influences, especially a poor diet. This review focuses mainly on metabolic risk factors causally related to the premature onset of coronary heart disease (CHD) and modifiable by alterations in diet and lifestyle or by drug treatment. Increasing evidence that certain agents, notably statins, can prevent or delay the onset of CHD makes it imperative to screen for dyslipidaemia the relatives of all patients developing or dying from CHD before the age of 55 if male or 65 if female.

▶ CATEGORIES OF RISK FACTOR

The essential criteria of a risk factor are that it shows an independent and quantitative relation with the disease in question, there is evidence of a causal mechanism and, most importantly, there is reversibility of risk. Depending on the strength of the supporting evidence risk factors can be divided into various categories, as discussed below. Factors associated with a disease which lack any of these three criteria, except age, should be regarded as risk markers rather than as true risk factors.

LDL: AN OBLIGATORY RISK FACTOR

Numerous prospective surveys have shown a positive correlation between serum cholesterol over a wide range of concentrations and the risk of developing CHD. The correlation between total cholesterol and CHD is almost entirely due to the correlation between the latter and the concentration of LDL in plasma, whether expressed as the mass of LDL particles or the concentration of LDL cholesterol. LDL has been shown to be atherogenic in experimental animals and also in man, best exemplified by FH. Furthermore, the risk of CHD can be decreased by therapeutic reduction of LDL cholesterol concentrations. Thus, LDL not only has all the criteria of a true risk factor but its presence in plasma is obligatory for other risk factors to exert their effects.

The minimum concentration of LDL cholesterol required for coronary atherogenesis in man appears to be approximately 2 mmol/l, judging from postmortem studies showing fatty streaks[1]—precursors of raised plaques[2]—in the aorta and coronary arteries of children and young adults dying suddenly from unrelated causes (fig 3.1). As with total cholesterol the relation between LDL cholesterol and CHD risk is curvilinear, relative risk ranging from < 2 at concentrations below 4.1 mmol/l to 35 in patients with FH[3] with concentrations above 6 mmol/l throughout life.

The primacy of LDL cholesterol as a risk factor and therapeutic target was stressed in the most recent US guidelines on CHD prevention,[4] which classified risk factors other than LDL as major, life habit, and emerging. Diabetes was given a higher priority than other major risk factors and was regarded as conferring a degree of risk equivalent to the presence of pre-existing CHD.

OTHER MAJOR RISK FACTORS

Major risk factors other than LDL cholesterol and diabetes are listed in table 3.1. Age, blood pressure, and high density lipoprotein (HDL) cholesterol, as well as total cholesterol, are used as continuous variables to calculate CHD risk in the current Joint British Societies' guidelines, together with cigarette smoking and diabetes as categorical variables.[5] Alternatively age, hypertension, low HDL cholesterol, and family history of premature CHD can all be used as categorical variables to calculate risk.[4] A family history of death from CHD in either parent before age 55 conferred a relative risk of 1.3 in their progeny in the Framingham study,[6] whereas in the US nurses health study

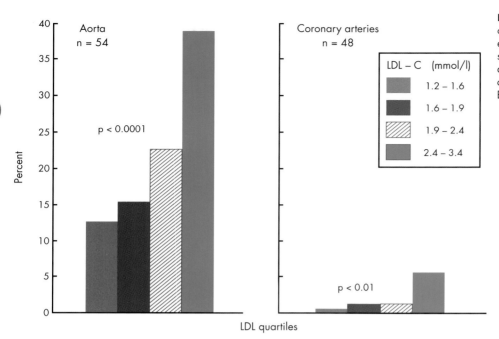

Figure 3.1 Fatty streak involvement of aorta and coronary arteries, expressed as per cent of intimal surface, in children and young adults according to quartiles of LDL cholesterol. Reproduced from Berenson et al.[1]

the relative risks of manifesting non-fatal or fatal CHD were 2.8 and 5.0, respectively, if one or other parent had developed CHD before the age of 60.[7] The effect of family history is largely independent of other major risk factors, implying the existence of a separate mechanism.

LIFESTYLE OR HABITUAL RISK FACTORS
These risk factors tend to be interdependent and are permissive in that they exert at least some of their effects via one or other of the major risk factors alluded to above.

Obesity
Obesity commonly precedes the development of hypertension, glucose intolerance, and dyslipidaemia. Several studies have shown a strong positive correlation between the degree of adiposity and fasting triglycerides, even after correcting for other variables. Plasma cholesterol is also positively correlated with body mass index, although less strongly than triglyceride, whereas HDL cholesterol is inversely correlated.

The pattern of obesity is also important in that the metabolic effects of excess fat on the abdomen differ from its effects when deposited on the thighs. Abdominal obesity and the accompanying glucose intolerance, hypertension, hypertriglyceridaemia, and low HDL cholesterol has been termed the "metabolic syndrome" [4]; additional features are hyperinsulinaemia and small, dense LDL particles.

Physical inactivity
A comparison of sedentary and highly active individuals showed that their relative risk for CHD death was 1.6. Risk was particularly increased in the lowest quintile of fitness, suggesting that even mild-to-moderate fitness may be protective. The main effect of aerobic exercise is to enhance physical fitness, but it has potentially beneficial effects also on blood pressure and serum lipids.

Atherogenic diet
An atherogenic diet exerts adverse effects on other CHD risk factors. Caloric excess promotes obesity and a sedentary state, both of which lead to hypertriglyceridaemia and a low HDL cholesterol and, eventually, to diabetes. Excessive intake of saturated fat increases LDL cholesterol whereas trans fatty acids both raise LDL and lower HDL. Excess cholesterol in the diet is hypercholesterolaemic in individuals who are efficient absorbers and blunts their response to statin treatment.[8]

EMERGING RISK FACTORS
These risk factors include Lp(a) lipoprotein, homocysteine, prothrombotic factors, impaired glucose tolerance, proinflammatory factors, and subclinical atherosclerosis.

Impaired glucose tolerance
Impaired glucose tolerance predicts cardiovascular events whether or not this is manifested as overt diabetes. Hyperinsulinaemia is a common accompaniment of impaired glucose tolerance and, as mentioned earlier, the two are frequently associated with other risk factors such as hypertension, obesity, and dyslipidaemia in the metabolic syndrome.

Table 3.1 Major risk factors for CHD, other than LDL cholesterol and diabetes.[4]

▶ Cigarette smoking
▶ Hypertension (≥140/90 mm Hg or on antihypertensive medication)
▶ Low HDL cholesterol (<1 mmol/l; HDL >1.55 mmol/l acts as a "negative" risk factor)
▶ Family history of premature CHD (CHD in male first degree relative <55 years of age, in female first degree relative <65 years of age)
▶ Age (men ≥45 years; women ≥55 years)

Abbreviations

CHD: coronary heart disease
CRP: C reactive protein
CT: computed tomography
FH: familial hypercholesterolaemia
HDL: high density lipoprotein
LDL: low density lipoprotein
NCEP: US National Cholesterol Education Program
PAI-1: plasminogen activator inhibitor

Table 3.2 Causes of increased homocysteine concentrations[3]

▶ Aging

▶ Smoking: greater effect in women
▶ High alcohol intake
▶ High coffee intake
▶ Poor nutrition: deficiency of folate, B6, B12
▶ Endocrine: diabetes, hypothyroidism, postmenopausal
▶ Renal failure
▶ Autoimmune: rheumatoid arthritis
▶ Enzyme mutations: methylenetetrahydrofolate reductase, cystathionine β synthase
▶ Iatrogenic: methotrexate, phenytoin, metformin, fibrates

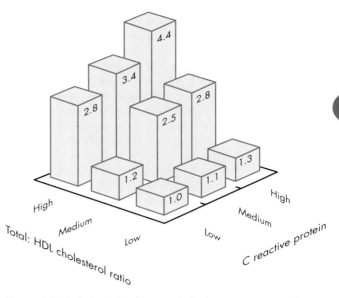

Figure 3.2 Relative risks of myocardial infarction in apparently healthy men according to tertiles of total: HDL cholesterol ratio (high, > 5.01; middle, 3.78–5.01; low, < 3.78) and C reactive protein (high, > 1.69 mg/l; middle, 0.72–1.69 mg/l; low, < 0.72 mg/l). Reproduced from Ridker *et al*,[9] with permission.

Prothrombotic factors

Several prospective studies have demonstrated an association between fibrinogen and CHD. Increased concentrations are associated with glucose intolerance, cigarette smoking, and hypercholesterolaemia. A fibrinogen concentration of > 3.1 g/l is associated with relative risks of CHD of 1.6 in men and 2.9 in women.

Case control studies have shown an association between increased concentrations of tissue plasminogen activator inhibitor (PAI-1) and CHD although prospective data are lacking. Concentrations of PAI-1, like those of factor VII, are strongly correlated with serum triglycerides, which may explain the known association between hypertriglyceridaemia and hypercoagulability. An increased frequency of factor V Leiden has been reported in patients with premature myocardial infarction but normal coronary arteries.

Lp(a) lipoprotein

Lp(a) lipoprotein consists of an LDL particle covalently linked to a molecule of apolipoprotein(a). The importance of Lp(a) as a risk factor for cardiovascular disease remains controversial. Case control studies have suggested that risk increases with Lp(a) concentrations above 30 mg/dl whereas in a large prospective study the risk of future myocardial infarction increased steeply only at concentrations above 60 mg/dl. No studies have been done which show therapeutic benefit from lowering Lp(a) per se, but reduction of concomitantly raised LDL cholesterol mitigates the risk associated with an increased concentration of Lp(a).

Hyperhomocysteinaemia

Homocysteine is a sulphur containing amino acid produced during the metabolism of methionine. Men with homocysteine concentrations in the upper 5% of the reference range (5–15 μmol/l) have a threefold increase in risk of myocardial infarction when compared with the lower 90%. Folic acid supplements have been shown to reduce raised homocysteine concentrations, whatever the cause (table 3.2). The place of homocysteine measurement in cardiovascular disease prevention should become clearer when the results of intervention trials using folate supplementation of the diet are available.

C reactive protein

C reactive protein (CRP) is a non-specific marker of inflammation and concentrations are raised in a wide variety of inflammatory disorders. High sensitivity assay methods allow accurate measurement of small increases in CRP and there is evidence that raised concentrations are an independent risk factor for myocardial infarction, peripheral vascular disease, and stroke. The reference range for CRP is 0–2.5 mg/l

and, although assay of CRP is not yet an established part of routine cardiovascular risk assessment, recent research suggests that it adds to the predictive value of the total:HDL cholesterol ratio[9] (fig 3.2).

Subclinical atherosclerosis

Non-invasive methods for detecting subclinical atherosclerosis either identify abnormalities of vascular structure or provide evidence of vascular or myocardial dysfunction. The former includes ultrasound examination of the carotid and femoral arteries, and electron beam computed tomographic (CT) scanning for coronary calcification. Electron beam CT has been claimed to detect coronary calcification in over 90% of patients with angiographically proven coronary artery disease, but the prognostic significance of this finding for clinical events is disputed. Non-invasive methods used to detect myocardial ischaemia or vascular dysfunction include electrocardiography, measurement of the ankle:arm blood pressure ratio, and flow mediated arterial dilatation. Evidence that the presence of pre-clinical disease predicts an increased risk of CHD has come from the cardiovascular health study in which asymptomatic individuals over the age of 65 years with an abnormal carotid ultrasound examination, reduced ankle:arm pressure ratio or major electrocardiographic abnormality had a relative risk of developing coronary events double that of individuals without these abnormalities.[10]

The ε4 allele

Inheritance of an ε4 allele (that is, having an apoE3/4 or 4/4 genotype or phenotype) occurs in approximately 25% of the population and is associated with a relative risk of CHD of 1.5 (table 3.3). The increased risk of CHD is caused in part by an accompanying increase in LDL cholesterol, although the severity of coronary atherosclerosis is greater than can be accounted for on this basis alone. Individuals with an ε4 allele tend to hyperabsorb cholesterol and hence respond poorly to statin treatment.[8]

Table 3.3 Prevalence of lipid risk factors, relative odds, and population attributable risk (PAR) for CHD[3]

Factor	Prevalence (%)	Relative odds for CHD	PAR for CHD (%)
Familial hypercholesterolaemia	0.2	35	6.4
ε4 allele	24	1.53	11
HDL cholesterol <0.90 mmol/l	23	2.39	24
LDL cholesterol >3.4 mmol/l	67	1.34	18
LDL cholesterol >4.1 mmol/l	30	1.41	11

PREVALENCE OF RISK FACTORS IN PATIENTS WITH PREMATURE CHD

A large study of the prevalence of modifiable risk factors in US men with angiographically documented coronary artery disease before the age of 60 showed that virtually all had one or more risk factors.[11] Compared with controls, the frequency of hypertension was 41% v 19%, of diabetes 12% v 1%, of cigarette smoking 67% v 28%, and of a low HDL cholesterol 63% v 19%. However, the frequency of a raised LDL cholesterol was similar in the two groups, 26% v 26%, reflecting the high prevalence of hypercholesterolaemia in the general population.

A subsequent study[12] revealed that more than 50% of such patients had a familial dyslipidaemia, the most common being a low HDL cholesterol accompanied by either hypertriglyceridaemia or mixed dyslipidaemia; next came a raised Lp(a), which evinced greater heritability than other familial dyslipidaemias, apart from FH.

Premature CHD is especially common in Asians in whom low HDL cholesterol, raised Lp(a), and hyperinsulinism appear to be more important risk factors than raised cholesterol or triglyceride.

PREVALENCE OF RISK FACTORS IN ASYMPTOMATIC RELATIVES OF PATIENTS WITH PREMATURE CHD

A large US study of persons developing CHD before the age of 60 showed that an LDL cholesterol concentration of ≥ 4.1 mmol/l was more than twice as common in their asymptomatic siblings below the age of 60 as in the population at large (38% v 16%).[13] Analogous but much less pronounced differences were observed in the European atherosclerosis research study (EARS) which investigated young adults with a paternal history of myocardial infarction before the age of 55.[14] In this study the best lipoprotein discriminants were plasma apoB and triglyceride concentrations, which were higher in those with a positive family history of premature CHD than in age and sex matched controls. This study also confirmed the importance of hypertension as a familial risk factor for CHD.

Studies aimed at detecting subclinical atherosclerosis have shown associations between a family history of premature CHD and coronary calcification on electron beam CT, increased frequency of carotid plaques on ultrasound, and impaired endothelium dependent dilatation of the brachial artery. The precise mechanism whereby family history exerts its effect remains to be determined.

In actual practice family screening for risk factors is undertaken in less than 20% of patients who sustain a CHD event before the age of 55.[15] Hopefully this will improve in the light of the results of a survey of over 130 000 families in the USA, where families with a history of premature CHD represented only 14% of the general population but accounted for over 70%

of reported cases of CHD in men and women before the ages of 55 and 65, respectively.[16]

PRACTICAL RECOMMENDATIONS FOR SCREENING

Screening individuals with a family history of premature CHD is encouraged by all the current guidelines on CHD prevention, namely the Joint British Societies,[5] the Joint European Societies,[17] and the US National Cholesterol Education Program (NCEP).[4] Each advocates using risk factors to calculate the 10 years absolute risk of a CHD event although they differ in the methodology used and the level of risk above which drug treatment should be commenced. The Joint European Societies guidelines are flawed by omitting HDL cholesterol from the risk calculation, whereas the NCEP's Framingham based point scoring system is more laborious than the Joint British Societies', which is also Framingham derived but computerised. Levels of risk above which lipid lowering drugs are advocated range from 15%[5] to 20% per 10 years,[4 17] the latter value being the more realistic in current circumstances.

The National Service Framework for CHD recommends screening all those under the age of 75 with a family history of hyperlipidaemia or premature CHD,[18] as illustrated in fig 3.3. However, the level of risk above which drug treatment is advocated in those whose total cholesterol is 5–7.9 mmol/l, 30% per 10 years, is too high and based on economic constraints rather than on scientific evidence. As stated previously, 20% per 10 years is currently regarded as an appropriate criterion for primary prevention with statins. Risk factors not mentioned by the National Service Framework for CHD which can contribute to the overall assessment of risk are measurement of Lp(a), CRP, and fibrinogen, the latter especially in subjects found to be hypertriglyceridaemic. This has therapeutic relevance in that most fibrates lower both triglyceride and fibrinogen concentrations. Also, in dyslipidaemic subjects whose risk is borderline, detection or exclusion of subclinical atherosclerosis may influence decisions on whether to treat.

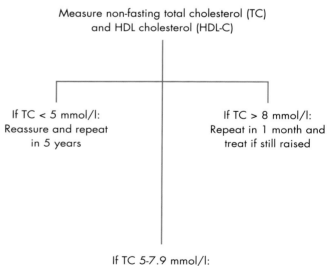

Figure 3.3 Recommendations of the National Service Framework on CHD for screening lipids in subjects with a family history of premature CHD.[18]

Screening relatives of patients with premature CHD: key points

- ► Early lesions of atherosclerosis are apparent in childhood, their extent and severity reflecting plasma lipid concentrations
- ► The premature onset of CHD in adults is usually associated with the presence of one or more underlying risk factors
- ► A family history of premature CHD is a risk factor in its own right and a marker for other risk factors, genetic and environmental
- ► Dyslipidaemia, especially raised LDL, is an important risk factor, detectable on family screening and reversible by lifestyle modification or drug treatment
- ► The National Service Framework for CHD recommends screening the lipids of relatives under the age of 75 of men who have developed CHD before 55 or women before 65

Screening in childhood

A family history of premature CHD or dyslipidaemia, or both, is generally accepted as valid grounds for paediatric screening, although there are some who consider it unjustified even then. The most common indication is FH, where there is a 50:50 chance that the child will be affected if one of the parents is a known heterozygote. A provisional diagnosis can be made at birth by demonstrating an LDL cholesterol concentration of > 1.1 mmol/l in cord blood, although this must be confirmed by further testing, preferably in a lipid clinic. Values of total and LDL cholesterol of > 6.7 mmol/l and > 4.0 mmol/l, respectively, in at least two fasting blood samples taken between the ages of 1–16 are regarded as diagnostic of FH.[19]

Other inherited disorders include familial hypertriglyceridaemia and familial combined hyperlipidaemia, both of which carry an increased risk of CHD,[20] as does type III hyperlipoproteinaemia, which is commonly caused by homozygous inheritance of the $\epsilon2$ allele. These three disorders show delayed penetrance and are best screened for after puberty. Family screening of children for inherited dyslipidaemias is more cost effective than population screening but is often neglected, despite its relevance to the prevention of premature CHD.

CONCLUSION

The potential yield from family screening in identifying high risk individuals is considerable but increased resources are needed to carry this out properly. Although the recommendations of the National Service Framework for CHD are aimed at general practitioners, the initial identification by cardiologists of risk factors in a patient with premature CHD is crucial, not least because it provides a powerful incentive to primary health care teams to screen the rest of the family.

REFERENCES

1 **Berenson GS**, Wattigney WA, Tracy RE, et al. Atherosclerosis of the aorta and coronary arteries and cardiovascular risk factors in persons aged 6 to 30 years and studied at necropsy (the Bogalusa heart study). *Am J Cardiol* 1992;**70**:851–8.
2 **Pathobiological Determinants of Atherosclerosis in Youth (PDAY) Research Group**. Natural history of aortic and coronary atherosclerotic lesions in youth. Findings from the PDAY study. *Arterioscler Thromb* 1993;**13**:1291–8.
3 **Thompson GR**, Dean J, Wilson PWF. *Dyslipidaemia in clinical practice.* Martin Dunitz: London, 2002.
▶ Newly published book on the pathogenesis, role, and management of dyslipidaemia in relation to the treatment and prevention of CHD.
4 **Expert Panel on Detection, Evaluation, and Treatment of High Blood Cholesterol in Adults.** Executive summary of the third report of the National Cholesterol Education Program (NCEP) expert panel on detection, evaluation and treatment of high blood cholesterol in adults (adult treatment panel III). *JAMA* 2001;**285**:2486–97.
▶ Most recent US guidelines on screening for, assessing severity of, and managing dyslipidaemia in primary and secondary prevention of CHD.
5 **British Cardiac Society, British Hyperlipidaemia Association, and British Hypertension Society.** Joint British recommendations on prevention of coronary heart disease in clinical practice. *Heart* 1998;**80**(suppl 2):S1–29.
▶ Joint British Societies' guidelines which provide a convenient method for calculating absolute risk of CHD.
6 **Myers RH**, Kiely DK, Cupples A, et al. Parental history is an independent risk factor for coronary artery disease: the Framingham study. *Am Heart J* 1990;**120**:963–9.
7 **Colditz GA**, Stampfer M, Willett W, et al. A prospective study of parental history of myocardial infarction and coronary heart disease in women. *Am J Epidemiol* 1986;**123**:48–58.
8 **Thompson GR**, O'Neill F, Seed M. Why some patients respond poorly to statins and how this might be remedied. *Eur Heart J* 2002;**23**:200–6.
▶ Review of the role of metabolic factors responsible for interindividual variability in LDL lowering response to statins.
9 **Ridker PM**, Glynn RJ, Hennekens CH. C-reactive protein adds to the predictive value of total and HDL cholesterol in determining risk of first myocardial infarction. *Circulation* 1998;**97**:2007–11.
▶ Analysis of the physicians health study which first demonstrated the predictive value for CHD of measuring CRP in conjunction with serum lipids.
10 **Kuller LH**, Shemanski L, Psaty BM, et al. Subclinical disease as an independent risk factor for cardiovascular disease. *Circulation* 1995;**92**:720–6.
11 **Genest JJ**, McNamara JR, Salem DN, et al. Prevalence of risk factors in men with premature coronary artery disease. *Am J Cardiol* 191;**67**:1185–9.
▶ Case control study demonstrating the high frequency of risk factors in men with premature CHD, especially a low HDL cholesterol.
12 **Genest JJ Jr**, Martin-Munley SS, McNamara JR, et al. Familial lipoprotein disorders in patients with premature coronary artery disease. *Circulation* 1992;**85**:2025–33.
13 **Allen JK**, Young DR, Blumenthal RS, et al. Prevalence of hypercholesterolemia among siblings of persons with premature coronary heart disease. Application of the second adult treatment panel guidelines. *Arch Intern Med* 1996;**156**:1654–60.
14 **Rosseneu M**, Fruchart JC, Bard JM, et al. Plasma apolipoprotein concentrations in young adults with a parental history of premature coronary heart disease and in control subjects. The EARS study. European atherosclerosis research study. *Circulation* 1994;**89**:1967–73.
15 **Swanson JR**, Pearson TA. Screening family members at high risk for coronary disease. *Am J Prev Med* 2001;**20**:50–5.
16 **Williams RR**, Hunt SC, Heiss G, et al. Usefulness of cardiovascular family history data for population-based preventive medicine and medical research (the health family tree study and the NHLBI family heart study). *Am J Cardiol* 2001;**87**:129–35.
▶ Large US study showing the potential value of family screening for preventing CHD and stroke.
17 **Wood D**, De Backer G, Faergeman O, et al, together with members of the Task Force. Prevention of coronary heart disease in clinical practice: recommendations of the second joint task force of European and other societies on coronary prevention. *Atherosclerosis* 1998;**140**:199–270.
▶ Joint European Societies' guidelines on CHD prevention. More detailed but less up to date than other current guidelines.
18 **Department of Health**. *National service framework for coronary heart disease. Modern standards and service models.* London: Department of Health, 2000.
▶ Department of Health recommendations for reducing morbidity and mortality from coronary heart disease in England and Wales by 2010.
19 **Wray R**, Neil H, Rees J. Screening for hyperlipidaemia in childhood. *J R Coll Phys London* 1996;**30**:115–18.
▶ Guidelines of the British Hyperlipidaemia Association on screening children for familial dyslipidaemias.
20 **Austin MA**, McKnight B, Edwards KL, et al. Cardiovascular disease mortality in familial forms of hypertriglyceridaemia: a 20-year prospective study. *Circulation* 2000;**101**:2777–82.

Additional references appear on the *Heart* website— www.heartjnl.com

19

4 ACUTE MYOCARDIAL INFARCTION: REPERFUSION TREATMENT

Flavio Ribichini, William Wijns

The decision over whether to treat acute myocardial infarction (AMI) with a balloon or infusion of fibrinolytics remains controversial. During the past few years profound changes in both treatment modalities[1-3] [w1] [w2] have substantially changed the arguments surrounding this long-standing debate.[w3-5] The evidence shows that the alternative use of primary angioplasty or fibrinolysis is rarely an option, either because angioplasty is simply not available or because the patient is not eligible for fibrinolysis. This evidence reflects the difference in "applicability" of each treatment—that is, the proportion of patients in whom only one of the treatments would be suitable versus patients in whom either treatment would be appropriate. As a matter of fact, primary angioplasty is applicable to almost all victims of AMI (82–90% of patients randomised to primary angioplasty actually undergo the procedure), but it is not available to the majority of patients. Conversely, fibrinolysis is a widely available treatment but "applicable" to a variable percentage of patients which does not reach 50%. The large number of patients with AMI to whom fibrinolysis is not administered represents a big challenge for the future, and perhaps the most rational and undisputed argument in favour of the use of primary angioplasty.

The best reperfusion treatment is one that achieves the highest rate of early, complete and sustained infarct related artery patency in the largest number of patients, but with the lowest rate of undesirable effects. The results obtained with both treatments, in the way they were applied before the latest breakthroughs in the field, can be represented by a geometrically opposing relation between "applicability" and "efficacy" (fig 4.1).

▶ UNCONTROVERSIAL EVIDENCE IN FAVOUR OF FIBRINOLYTIC TREATMENT

Clinical trials and experience have identified the following landmarks in the reperfusion treatment of ST segment elevation AMI.

- ▶ The daily administration of 162.5 mg of aspirin orally from the first day of AMI and continued for 30 days reduces the 30 day vascular mortality rate by 23% without risk of stroke.[w6]
- ▶ Intravenous infusion of streptokinase within six hours after AMI onset reduces 30 day total vascular mortality by 25%, but at the cost of 2–3 strokes per 100 patients treated and 3 severe bleedings requiring transfusion per 1000 patients treated. Combined treatment with aspirin has synergistic effects and will prevent 52 vascular deaths per 1000 patients treated and reduce significantly the risk of reinfarction.[w6]
- ▶ The initial benefit of streptokinase treatment on mortality is maintained at 10 year follow up.[4]
- ▶ The use of recombinant tissue plasminogen activator (rt-PA) using the "accelerated" dosing schedule plus heparin (instead of streptokinase) prevents another 10 deaths but causes two more strokes per 1000 patients treated.[5]
- ▶ Pre-hospital fibrinolysis can reduce one year mortality[w7] and should be considered when transport time exceeds 60 minutes.[w8]
- ▶ The combination of full dose of abciximab and half dose reteplase reduces non-fatal complications of AMI, but yields similar mortality rate compared with reteplase alone.[6]

EVIDENCE IN FAVOUR OF PRIMARY ANGIOPLASTY: CONSENSUS STATEMENTS

All the randomised clinical trials of primary angioplasty have shown a reduced incidence of stroke, recurrent ischaemia, and need for new target vessel revascularisation (TVR) compared to fibrinolysis, even in low risk patients.[7] In selected subsets, primary angioplasty preserves left ventricular ejection fraction[w4] [w9] and benefits patients with anterior AMI treated up to 24 hours after symptom onset.[w10] The favourable effects on mortality and reinfarction appear to be more pronounced among high risk patients, in particular those with haemodynamic evidence of failure.[8] Benefits in this setting are also apparent from non-randomised data.[9] A quantitative overview by Weaver and colleagues[10] pooling 2606 patients showed that the mortality reduction obtained with primary angioplasty compared to fibrinolysis was approximately 32% (table 4.1). If this result can be reproduced everywhere, the magnitude of such treatment effect would be similar to that observed when fibrinolysis was used instead of placebo. However, these excellent results

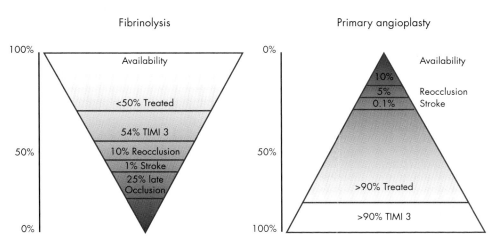

Figure 4.1 Nearly all patients with acute myocardial infarction (AMI) could potentially benefit from reperfusion treatment with fibrinolytics, but less than 50% will actually be treated; only 50–60% of those will achieve a TIMI 3 grade coronary flow, 10% will suffer from early reocclusion, 1% will have a stroke, and 20–30% will have late reocclusion. On the other hand, angioplasty can be offered to only 10% of patients with AMI, but more than 90% of these will actually be treated; 90% will achieve a TIMI 3 grade coronary flow, less than 5% will have reocclusion, and less than 0.1% will have a stroke.

derive from the experience of selected centres working under the specific requirements of randomised investigation and may not be easily achieved in the community setting, as is suggested by the results of large national registries[9] [w11] [w12]

The GUSTO II-B trial[7] addressed this particular issue by testing the effect of angioplasty when performed mainly in low volume centres on a low risk population. In fact, GUSTO II-B showed a less favourable outcome of angioplasty than expected from other trials, which was caused by a higher event rate in the angioplasty arm rather than by a lower event rate in the fibrinolysis arm. Furthermore, 36% of patients allocated to fibrinolysis received an angioplasty before discharge, which may blunt the differences between the two strategies at six months. Crossover to angioplasty in patients initially randomised to pharmacological treatment is a common and important confounding factor when analysing differences in long term outcome.[w11] Long term benefit of angioplasty has been observed in the one year analysis of the SHOCK trial.[8]

The mortality reduction obtained with the emergency revascularisation strategy compared to the approach involving initial medical stabilisation was not significant at 30 days (46.7% v 56%, p = 0.11), but became so at six months (50.3% v 63.1%, p = 0.027) and increased further at one year (55% v 70%, p = 0.008). Albeit a negative study statistically, the number of lives saved per 1000 patients treated with the strategy of emergency revascularisation is the highest ever reported in a reperfusion trial (tables 4.1 and 4.2). The recent availability of long term results of primary angioplasty trials confirms the long lasting efficacy of the invasive approach also in patients without haemodynamic failure, despite some initial concern that early benefit may not be sustained[w13] (table 4.2).

NEW PERSPECTIVES IN REPERFUSION THERAPY
It is recognised that the success rate and durability of mechanical revascularisation procedures and the efficacy and safety of fibrinolytics have both improved. Primary angioplasty has been

Table 4.1 Event rate at short term follow up, number needed to treat, and events avoided per 1000 patients treated in randomised clinical trials comparing primary angioplasty and fibrinolysis.

30-day events	PTCA (%, n)	Lysis (%, n)	p Value	OR (95%CI)	ARR%	NNT	NEA × 1000
Mortality							
Weaver[10]	4.4%, 57/1290	6.5%, 86/1316	0.02	0.66 (0.46 to 0.94)	2.1	47	21/1000
GUSTO II-B[7]	5.7%, 32/565	7.0%, 40/573	0.37	0.80 (0.49 to 1.30)	1.3	77	13/1000
SHOCK[8]*	46.7%, 71/152	56%, 84/150	0.11	0.83 (0.67 to 1.04)	9.3	11	91/1000
C-PORT[w46]	5.3%, 12/225	6.2%, 14/226	0.7	Not available	0.9	111	9/1000
DANAMI-2†	6.6%, 52/790	7.6%, 59/782	0.35	Not available	1.0	100	10/1000
Mortality or non-fatal reinfarction							
Weaver	7.2%, 94/1290	11.9%, 156/1316	<0.001	0.58 (0.44 to 0.76)	4.7	21	48/1000
GUSTO-IIB	9.6%, 54/565	12.2%, 70/573	0.08	0.72 (0.49 to 1.05)	3.1	32	31/1000
C-PORT‡	9.8%, 22/225	16.8%, 38/226	0.03	0.52 (0.30 to 0.89)	7	14	71/1000
DANAMI-2†‡	8.0%, 63/790	13.7%, 107/782	0.0003	Not available	5.7	18	55/1000
Stroke							
Weaver	0.7%, 9/1290	2.0%, 26/1316	0.007	0.35 (0.14 to 0.77)	1.3	77	13/1000
PAMI[w27]	0	3.5%, 7/200	0.01	Not available	3.5	29	34/1000
Zijlstra[16]	0.7%, 1/152	2.0%, 3/149	0.6	0.32 (0.01 to 4.08)	1.3	77	13/1000
GUSTO II-B	1.1%, 6/565	1.9%, 11/573	0.34	0.54 (0.17 to 1.63)	0.8	125	8/1000
C-PORT	1.3%, 3/225	3.5%, 8/226	0.13	Not available	2.2	45	22/1000
DANAMI-2†	1.1%, 8/790	2.0%, 15/782	0.15	Not available	0.9	111	9/1000
Haemorrhagic stroke							
Weaver	0.1%, 1/1290	1.1%, 15/1316	<0.001	0.07 (0.0 to 0.43)	1	100	10/1000
PAMI	0	2.0%, 4/200	0.05	Not available	2	50	20/1000
Zijlstra	0.7%, 1/152	1.3%, 2/149	0.98	0.49 (0.01 to 9.47)	0.6	166	6/1000
GUSTO-IIB	0	1.4%, 8/573	0.007	Not available	1.4	71	14/1000

*The SHOCK trial did not compare PTCA with lysis, but a strategy of emergency revascularisation versus initial medical stabilisation.
†Data not published. Presented at the scientific sessions of the American College of Cardiology, March 2002.
‡Includes disabling stroke.
ARR, absolute risk reduction; NEA × 1000, number of events avoided per 1000 patients treated; NNT, number needed to treat.

Table 4.2 Event rate at long term follow up, number needed to treat, and events avoided per 1000 patients treated in randomised clinical trials comparing primary angioplasty and fibrinolysis

Long term events	PTCA (%)	Lysis (%)	p Value	Odds ratio (95% CI)	ARR	NNT	NEA × 1000
Mortality							
Weaver 6 months*	6.1	8.1	0.055	0.73 (0.52 to 0.98)	2	50	20/1000
PAMI 2 years[w29]	6.2	9.5	0.21	Not available	3.3	30	33/1000
Zijlstra 5±2 years[16]	13.4	23.9	0.01	0.54 (0.36 to 0.87)	10.5	10	100/1000
SHOCK 6 months[8]†	50.3	63.1	0.027	0.80 (0.65 to 0.95)	12.8	8	125/1000
SHOCK 1 year†	55	70	0.008	Not available	15	7	143/1000
C-PORT 6 months[w46]	6.2	7.1	0.72	Not available	0.9	111	9/1000
Reinfarction							
Weaver 6 months	4.4	9.7	0.0001	0.43 (0.3 to 0.6)	5.3	19	53/1000
PAMI 2 years	10.8	16.0	0.01	Not available	5.2	19	53/1000
Zijlstra 5±2 years	6	22	0.0001	0.27 (0.15 to 0.52)	6	6	167/1000
C-PORT 6 months	5.3	10.6	0.04	Not available	5.3	19	53/1000
Mortality or non-fatal reinfarction							
Weaver 6 months	6.8	13.4	0.0001	0.47 (0.43 to 0.7)	6.6	15	67/1000
PAMI 2 years	14.9	23	0.034	Not available	8.1	12	83/1000
Zijlstra 5±2 years	22	46	0.0001	0.13 (0.43 to 0.91)	24	4	250/1000
C-PORT 6 months‡	12.4	19.9	0.03	0.57 (0.34 to 0.95)	7.5	13	77/1000
New revascularisation							
PAMI 2 years	32.8	54	0.001	Not available	21.2	5	200/1000
Zijlstra 5±2 years	46.4	71.1	<0.001	Not available	24.7	4	300/1000
Recurrence of ischaemia							
PAMI 2 years	36.4	48	0.026	Not available	11.6	9	111/1000
Zijlstra 5±2 years	52	89.5	<0.001	Not available	37.5	3	333/1000

*Data on 2635 patients. Presented at the American Heart Association meeting in Atlanta, October 1999.
†The SHOCK trial did not compare PTCA with lysis, but a strategy of emergency revascularisation versus initial medical stabilisation.
‡Includes disabling stroke.
For explanation of abbreviations see table 1.

enhanced by the use of coronary stents[w14] and the availability of glycoprotein IIb/IIIa inhibitors,[2] or the combined use of both,[11 12 w15] while new fibrinolytic regimens offer better results than those obtained with streptokinase or even with front loaded rt-PA.[1 w1 w16]

New infusive schemes
New fibrinolytic drugs are being developed and evaluated with the aim of improving pharmacological reperfusion.[1 13 w1 w16] Initial studies suggested that lytic therapy may be as effective as primary angioplasty.[w17]

Efficacy
The combined use of fibrinolytics with glycoprotein IIb/IIIa inhibitors appears encouraging at first glance. In the TIMI 14 trial[1] a high rate of TIMI 3 flow grade was observed at 90 minutes after the infusion of 50 mg of alteplase and a full dose of abciximab plus low dose heparin. This promising finding relates to only 87 patients included in the dose finding and dose confirmation phases of the study, which included angiography at 90 minutes. Out of the 34 patients studied in the dose finding phase, a TIMI 3 flow was observed in 22 patients (76%), 3% of patients died, 3% suffered major bleeding, and 27% needed an urgent revascularisation procedure. Moreover, 59% of these patients underwent angioplasty before discharge, 18% as an emergency rescue procedure.

The IMPACT-AMI trial[w18] failed to detect a dose–response relation using a combination of eptifibatide (Integrilin) and 100 mg of alteplase. On the contrary, the group treated with eptifibatide had a tendency towards increased incidence of in-hospital adverse events (51% v 39%) and mortality (11% v 0%), despite a significantly higher rate of TIMI 3 flow grade at 90 minutes (66% v 39%). Despite the discrepancy between the excellent angiographic results and the less impressive clinical outcome in these small sized studies, these preliminary results primed a new large scale trial which was recently published.[6]

GUSTO V was powered to detect a 15% reduction in mortality and randomised 16 588 patients to either standard lytic treatment with reteplase or a combination of half dose reteplase with full dose abciximab. The results obtained with the combination therapy did not lower the mortality rate (5.6%) compared to standard fibrinolysis (5.9%). Non-fatal complications of AMI were significantly reduced, at the cost of higher rates of non-intracranial bleeding. Thus, the relation between patency and survival is not as straightforward as initially anticipated; furthermore, the failure to reduce mortality in the megatrials performed in this new era of reperfusion has diverted attention to the reduction in non-fatal clinical events.

Drug delivery
Ease and speed of delivery of fibrinolytic drugs have been improved with the use of a single bolus of mutant forms of rt-PA. Recently, the results of two megatrials (ASSENT-2 and InTime-II) have been presented.[w19] Both studies confirmed that the bolus injection of TNK-tPA and lanoteplase was as effective as the long lasting infusion of rt-PA. However, lanoteplase caused a significantly higher rate of intracranial bleeding compared to rt-PA in InTime-II (1.13% v 0.62%, p = 0.003); that was not the case for TNK-tPA (0.93%) when compared to rt-PA (0.94%) in ASSENT-2.

Safety
Clinical studies aimed at assessing the efficacy and safety of combinations of potent thrombolytic treatments have caused thousands of intracranial bleeds.[w20] Furthermore, the inappropriate administration of a fibrinolytic agent may not be without complications.[w21] Indeed, nearly 4.1% of patients who receive fibrinolysis have non-coronary syndromes and the 30 day mortality of these patients was 9.5% versus 1.2% of those allocated to placebo in the ASSET trial (p < 0.01).[w22] The underutilisation of fibrinolytics in the real world as shown in NRMI-2[w2] may reflect a certain "fear to treat", particularly in

high risk patients. This concern will lead physicians to accept the natural history of the disease rather than to prescribe the reperfusion treatment that is available to most cardiologists, which can be lifesaving, but will potentially induce a severe complication. From a safety standpoint, lytic treatment may therefore be perceived as being more hazardous than the invasive approach.

Primary stented angioplasty and new antiplatelet agents

The systematic use of coronary stents during primary angioplasty was shown to reduce the incidence of reocclusion and the need for new TVR compared to balloon dilatation. The rate of TIMI 3 flow grade did not improve nor did systematic stent implantation reduce the incidence of reinfarction and mortality in the large STENT-PAMI and CADILLAC trials.[w14 w15] Similarly, initial experience with the use of IIb/IIIa receptor inhibitors in association with primary angioplasty has yielded contradictory results between some small studies[11 12] and the larger RAPPORT[2] and CADILLAC trials.[w15] In RAPPORT, the use of abciximab or placebo with primary angioplasty did not affect the incidence of death, reinfarction or TVR at six months; similarly, the CADILLAC trial yielded identical incidence of the primary end point (mortality, reinfarction, ischaemic TVR, and stroke) at six months in patients undergoing stented angioplasty with or without administration of abciximab (11.5% and 10.2%, respectively). In both studies, stent implantation offered better results than balloon dilatation independently of the use of abciximab.

The concept of facilitated angioplasty or combined "pharmaco-mechanical reperfusion" was evaluated by the PACT investigators[3]; a bolus of 50 mg rt-PA or placebo was given on admission, followed by immediate angiography and angioplasty unless TIMI 3 flow was observed. This use of fibrinolytic agents differs from the concept of "rescue angioplasty" for failed lysis and, unlike rescue procedures, offers better preservation of the left ventricular function without complications secondary to the lytic bolus. Although some benefit can be expected from the combined form of reperfusion on "soft" end points, such as preservation of left ventricular ejection fraction and a reduced need for urgent TVR, there is no evidence so far that this form of combined pharmaco-mechanical strategy will reduce mortality or widen the window of opportunity for reperfusion.

CONTEMPORARY ANGIOPLASTY AND FIBRINOLYSIS: ARE THEY TRULY EQUIVALENT?

Whenever primary angioplasty and fibrinolysis are to be evaluated as potentially equivalent,[w18] the following issues should be considered.

Time delay

Setting up for and performing primary angioplasty requires more time than starting an intravenous infusion. In randomised clinical trials, the in-hospital delay in starting fibrinolysis was on average 45–50 minutes shorter than the time needed to start angioplasty.[10] The in-hospital procedure related delay for primary angioplasty must be no longer than 90 minutes according to the American Heart Association/American College of Cardiology recommendations.[w8] In nearly 90% of cases, the invasive strategy results in immediate TIMI 3 flow grade of the infarct related artery, while with lytic agents there is an additional delay before their effect starts. In the TIMI-14 study[1] the administration of a bolus of alteplase alone or a bolus followed by a 30 minute infusion of rt-PA and abciximab was far less effective (TIMI 3 flow grade at 90 minutes: 48% and 62%, respectively) than the same bolus followed by a 60 minute infusion (TIMI 3 flow grade 74%, p < 0.02). Even with the addition of abciximab, this indicates that the concentration of the lytic agent must be maintained for at least 60 minutes. Therefore, the time delay needed for the optimal lytic regimen to be effective may be not much shorter than that for primary angioplasty.

Following primary angioplasty, a longer time delay could result in a larger infarct size and a lower left ventricular ejection fraction,[w23 w24] but apparently this does not adversely affect the patency rate of the infarct related artery or the six month clinical outcome.[w23] Hospital mortality rates remain low and predictable in patients treated within 12 hours of symptom onset unless they present with cardiogenic shock.[14 w25 w26] On the contrary, with lytic treatment, reperfusion rates decrease and the mortality rates increase with increasing time, in particular beyond the third to fourth hour after symptom onset.[5 14 w27] Short term mortality strongly depends on the quality and time frame of reperfusion.[15] Angioplasty yields a higher degree of TIMI 3 flow grade than fibrinolysis and this translates in a better short term outcome. Long term survival largely depends on left ventricular function[5 16]; this in turn depends on the extent of myocardial damage, which increases as reperfusion is delayed. Thus angioplasty may be better for patients admitted late—that is, more than four hours after onset of symptoms[14]—in whom 30 day mortality with angioplasty remains under 5% but rises to over 12% with lysis.[w26 w28] The transportation of high risk patients to hospitals offering invasive facilities should be considered since the additional treatment delay does not seem to jeopardise the result of mechanical reperfusion.[w23 w25 w26]

Patients subgroups

Primary angioplasty applied to selected candidates may prove more beneficial than its indiscriminate use, particularly in patients with small low risk AMI. Available data support the use of primary angioplasty over fibrinolysis in high risk patients and in patients with haemodynamic impairment (class I indication[w8]). Indirect data suggest that the mechanical approach is a better alternative than fibrinolysis in clinical subsets such as the elderly, patients with right ventricular involvement, patients with AMI caused by the occlusion of vein grafts, late presenters, or subjects who are ineligible for fibrinolysis. However, subgroup analysis should be considered with caution since data fragmentation reduces the statistical power and may cause type II errors. Proper randomised trials are needed if these indications are to be fully legitimised.

Number needed to treat and number needed to harm

The demonstration of a significant reduction in mortality of about 25% with fibrinolytic agents has required the randomisation of more than 10 000 patients in each of the initial studies. Later on, the GUSTO-I study[5] enrolled 41 021 patients to obtain a further 14.6% risk reduction in mortality with rt-PA versus streptokinase (95% confidence interval (CI) 5.9% to 21.3%, p = 0.001). Equivalence trials have randomised more than 31 000 patients to show that new fibrinolytic agents "do not cause a clinically significant excess in events".[w19] Assuming a 30 day mortality rate of 7% in patients treated with fibrinolysis, about 12 000 patients would need to be randomised to show a worthwhile 20% relative risk reduction with any alternative treatment. Primary angioplasty has been shown to have favourable effects on end points such as mortality and reinfarction, even in smaller sized studies. These considerations would support the contention that megatrials on direct angioplasty are no longer necessary, but this position has not gained universal acceptance.

Most potentially effective lytic drugs have been tested in large clinical trials which were funded by companies with a vested interest in orienting medical care at large. Regrettably, there has not been enough interest to support prospective randomised clinical trials comparing angioplasty and fibrinolysis that are large enough to provide unequivocal results. The largest randomised study of this kind, GUSTO II-b, included only 1138 patients and showed a non-significant mortality reduction of 18.6%, resulting in 13 lives saved per 1000 patients.[7]

A useful tool for the interpretation and comparison of outcomes is the "number needed to treat" (NNT). NNT is calculated as the reciprocal of the absolute outcome difference between two treatment groups and offers an ingenious measurement of the "therapeutic effort to clinical yield" ratio. The NNT to prevent one death, reinfarction, stroke or a combined end point in the short term, according to the most relevant trials comparing angioplasty and fibrinolysis, is shown in table 4.1. Similar calculations in regard to long term results are given in table 4.2.

When using angioplasty instead of fibrinolysis in 1000 patients, 21 more lives would be saved and 13 stokes avoided within the first month after AMI.[10] Even though the debated 32% mortality reduction obtained in the combined analysis of these trials may not be representative of current practice, the magnitude of the benefit obtained with angioplasty in the real world seems at least as important as the benefit obtained with front loaded rt-PA compared to streptokinase.[5 7] In GUSTO V the absolute risk reduction in mortality was 0.3, resulting in 3 lives saved per 1000 patients treated with combined therapy instead of reteplase only (NNT = 333). Long term analysis shows that angioplasty would save 20 more lives than fibrinolysis per 1000 patients at six months, 33 at two years,[w29] and 100 at five years.[16] Furthermore, 200 new TVRs would be prevented at two years and 300 at five years after the index AMI.

A similar analysis can be applied to determine the adverse effects of medical interventions ("number needed to harm"). Out of 1000 patients treated with fibrinolysis, 8 would have suffered from stroke in GUSTO II-B and 34 in PAMI (table 4.1). Such an event is fatal in 40% of patients and causes severe morbidity in the remainder,[5] reducing the net clinical benefit of fibrinolysis.

Applicability: the true frontier of reperfusion treatment in the "real world"

Because the limitations to the applicability of each form of reperfusion treatment are different, we believe that they rarely present as an equivalent alternative.

The major limitation of primary angioplasty is the difficulty in setting up the programme, performing the procedures in a timely fashion, and reproducing the results of clinical trials. However, a similar frontier exists for fibrinolytic treatment. In the NRMI-2[w2] only 31% of the 272 651 patients analysed were eligible for reperfusion, 3% had formal contraindications, 41% presented after six hours, and 25% had non-diagnostic ECG; furthermore, 24% of eligible patients were not given reperfusion treatment. Not surprisingly, unadjusted mortality in patients not receiving reperfusion treatment was nearly three times higher than in treated patients. Had angioplasty been available, these patients could have benefited from reperfusion treatment.

Results from the NRMI-2 study can be considered to be representative of cardiology practice in the USA. Despite differences between countries in eligibility criteria, time delay, lytic agents, and treatment strategies, the major findings in NRMI-2 are largely reproduced in Western Europe and Canada, confirming the under utilisation of reperfusion treatment. Overall fibrinolysis is given to only 66% of eligible patients, and the use of invasive procedures ranges from 2.5–11% of AMI patients between community and academic institutions.[17] Among European countries, the UK has reported the largest use of fibrinolytic agents: 71.6% of patients with suspected AMI, ranging from 49–85% in different hospitals,[w30] in the context of limited availability of invasive facilities.[w31] Other countries use lytic agents less often, perhaps in part because angioplasty is more readily available. In Germany fibrinolysis is given in 36–42% of patients while angioplasty is used in 10–25% of cases.[w32 w33] In France 37% of AMI patients receive reperfusion treatment,[w34] either by means of systemic lysis (32–45%) or angioplasty (13–43%).[w35 w36] Other reports from Israel, Italy, Scandinavia or Spain indicate that fibrinolysis is given to 35–45% of patients.[17 w37–41] Data from Australia and New Zealand state an eligibility rate of 53%, lytics being actually given in 43%, with a predominant use of streptokinase (78%) over rt-PA (15.7%), and a growth in surgery or angioplasty from 8.7% in 1986 to 17.4% in 1994.[w42 w43] Despite these differences in management of AMI among western countries, there are no significant differences in short term outcome,[w44] perhaps because the proportion of reperfused patients is similar. Thus in daily practice, half of the patients with AMI do not receive reperfusion treatment. Reperfusion is rarely denied because of formal contraindications but usually because of late arrival, non-diagnostic ECG changes, advanced age or other various reasons that raise a "fear to treat" in about 25–35% of potentially eligible cases.[17 w2 w44] Under all these circumstances, angioplasty, when available, is not an "alternative" to lysis but the sole opportunity for reperfusion. Paradoxically, the results of angioplasty in this large patient subgroup, which represent an ideal and undisputed setting for its use, are mostly unknown.[w45]

Therefore, increasing the availability of primary angioplasty, or shaping the triangle of fig 4.1 into a rectangle, would be a worthwhile effort. As mentioned earlier, patient transportation to high workload tertiary centres is a safe and valuable therapeutic approach and, at least in theory, it may prove a more rational and cost effective option than the emergence of a widespread network of low volume centres in which optimal results may not be achieved. Such a strategy has been investigated in a large randomised study in Europe (DANAMI-2). The study randomly assigned AMI patients to front loaded rt-PA or angioplasty in interventional centres, or to rt-PA versus transportation for angioplasty elsewhere in non-invasive centres, and was prematurely stopped on 1 October 2001 after a planned interim analysis because of the benefit observed in the invasive strategy of the study (table 4.1). In the USA, a recent small randomised trial has shown that the better outcome of angioplasty over fibrinolysis can also be obtained in community hospitals without on-site cardiac surgery.[w46]

Which yardstick for measuring treatment effect?

If reperfusion strategies are considered as nearly equivalent, then the accuracy of the measurement of their respective effects becomes of major relevance. Randomisation is the best tool for testing two treatment strategies; however, in this particular case, the method may have some pitfalls that must be acknowledged. On the one hand, randomisation precludes enrolment of patients who are ineligible for fibrinolysis. This represents a group of patients at particularly high risk in whom angioplasty is likely (but was not proven) to be beneficial. On the other hand, double blinded analysis and outcome adjudication is problematic. In patients assigned to angioplasty, information on coronary anatomy and ventricular function is immediately available and complications may be diagnosed and managed readily, leading to a more proactive management of patients treated invasively.

ANCILLARY BENEFIT OF THE INVASIVE APPROACH

While the primary goal of any kind of reperfusion therapy is to save lives by re-establishing effective myocardial perfusion, some potential additional benefits are granted *only* with the invasive approach. Admittedly, these ancillary benefits only pertain to the few patients who have prompt access to the invasive treatment.

The invasive approach enables the use of a variety of tools such as stents, ultrasound imaging, thrombectomy or aspiration devices, and provides the possibility of intracoronary or local drug delivery, all of which may in the future prove to be useful adjunctive agents to optimise reperfusion. Invasive diagnostic tools may also help to gain additional insights into the "mysteries" of reperfusion at the tissue level[18]—that is, why one out of four patients who achieve a brisk epicardial TIMI 3 coronary flow does not have tissue reperfusion.[w47]

The immediate knowledge of the coronary anatomy and left ventricular function facilitates accurate risk stratification and allows the most appropriate individual treatment strategy to be selected and implemented. New standards of care after AMI have ensued and reduced the length of hospital stay and the need for further diagnostic testing.[w48 w49]

Primary angioplasty is cost saving compared to fibrinolysis.[19 w48 w49] This is mainly because of the lower incidence of in-hospital reinfarction, recurrent ischaemia, stroke, and shorter hospital stay.[w49]

Late reocclusion of the infarct related artery with or without reinfarction occurs in nearly 30% of patients after fibrinolysis and bears a negative prognosis and a high mortality rate.[5 w50] This likely explains the lack of survival benefit between fibrinolysed and control patients 10 years after discharge in the GISSI study.[4 w20] Conversely, with contemporary primary angioplasty and stenting, reocclusion and reinfarction rates are as low as 1–5%.[w14 w15]

Reperfusion treatment for acute myocardial infarction: key points

- ▶ Reperfusion treatment for acute myocardial infarction remains largely underused
- ▶ Applicability of thrombolytic therapy and primary angioplasty is the major limitation to the use of reperfusion treatment
- ▶ Most recent efforts have aimed at "doing more for few patients". The real challenge is to "do more for more patients"
- ▶ Pre-hospital fibrinolysis shortens the duration of ischaemia and increases myocardial salvage
- ▶ Transportation of patients with acute myocardial infarction to a catheterisation laboratory must be considered after failed thrombolysis in high risk patients
- ▶ Advantages of primary angioplasty are sustained in the long term
- ▶ Combined treatment with lytics and glycoprotein IIb/IIIa inhibitors reduces complications, but not mortality
- ▶ Combined use of pharmacological and mechanical reperfusion improves secondary clinical end points, but not survival
- ▶ Clinical trials in specific patient subsets are needed to establish the advantages of primary angioplasty
- ▶ A tailored reperfusion strategy based on the risk profile at presentation may prove more rational than their indiscriminate use in the few patients who have access to all resources

---

As has been determined from postmortem examination[w51] and has been recently confirmed in vivo,[w52] AMI may not always be the consequence of a thrombotic coronary occlusion. Acute events such as plaque rupture, spontaneous dissections or intramural plaque haemorrhage associated with spasm are the cause of AMI in nearly 30% of cases, a figure which is close to the percentage of cases in which optimal lytic therapy is ineffective.[1 w17] Under those pathophysiological circumstances, fibrinolysis and antiplatelet agents, even when given at doses that go beyond their "safety ceiling", will never work, because the substratum on which these drugs act is non-existent.[20]

CONCLUSIONS AND FUTURE DIRECTIONS

Currently available evidence does not fully support the contention that either the immediately invasive approach or combined antithrombotic or pharmaco-mechanical strategies are clearly superior to fibrinolysis in reducing mortality. We need to learn from appropriately powered randomised clinical trials whether or not primary angioplasty is beneficial when applied to subgroups of patients who otherwise do not receive reperfusion treatment. When appropriate, current guidelines should be revised to incorporate specific recommendations for these specific patient subsets.

In the meanwhile, primary angioplasty cannot be advocated as the first therapeutic approach where it is not performed on a regular basis by experienced operators. Reperfusion by lytic treatment remains the therapy of choice for AMI in most cases, although its efficacy and applicability in the real world remain far from optimal.

Rather than taking a dogmatic approach to either form of reperfusion treatment, percutaneous coronary intervention and/or drugs should be used as needed to increase the overall impact of reperfusion treatment in the community, taking advantage of the best, locally available potential of each approach.[13] The real challenge is to increase the proportion of

26

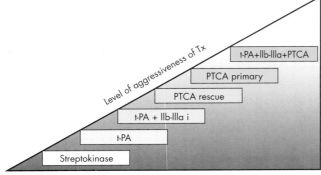

Figure 4.2 Streptokinase can still be used as a first choice treatment in low risk patients (as currently done in many patients treated in South America, UK, Australia, New Zealand, and the Netherlands), while patients presenting with higher clinical risk would benefit from the use of the more expensive recombinant tissue plasminogen activator (t-PA). The combination of recombinant t-PA and a glycoprotein IIb/IIIa inhibitor (abciximab) will reduce the clinical complications of acute myocardial infarction, but will not reduce mortality. Rescue angioplasty (PTCA) can be reserved for high risk patients who did not achieve reperfusion or have a poor clinical course. Primary angioplasty should be preferred for patients presenting with haemodynamic failure, advanced age (> 75 years) or presenting late (more than 4–5 hours after symptom onset). The previous administration of half doses of lytic treatment is desirable when it can be given out of hospital by first aid providers, or in the emergency department when access to the catheterisation laboratory is delayed. The use of stents and glycoprotein IIb/IIIa inhibitors during angioplasty does not reduce mortality. Instead of being used indiscriminately, these tools should be considered in unfavourable patient or lesion subsets, such as in the presence of a large thrombotic burden after wire crossing or suboptimal flow after angioplasty.

patients with AMI receiving reperfusion treatment and to "do more for more patients" rather than "do more for fewer patients". Pre-hospital diagnosis and treatment of AMI are important. At a time when mortality from AMI has decreased to lower levels, pre-hospital treatment will likely be the only way to reduce mortality any further. Immediate treatment with lytic and/or antiplatelet drugs and transportation for angioplasty seem to be the most rational approach. Prompt restoration of coronary flow and subsequent intervention should optimise tissue reperfusion and avoid coronary reocclusion.[3 w53] Transfer of selected patients to a centralised, high volume invasive service while reperfusion is continuing would render angioplasty applicable to a much larger patient population, shorten the duration of ischaemia, and increase the potential for myocardial salvage. Such an approach will occur when both the availability of percutaneous coronary intervention services is increased and these resources are used to treat high risk patients. To treat all AMI patients with half doses of expensive lytic agents, full doses of very expensive glycoprotein IIb/IIIa inhibitors, stents, aspiration and protection devices, followed by conventional drug treatment, would not be sensible. The available reperfusion tools should be applied selectively, tailored to the patient's risk profile and temporal presentation, as shown in fig 4.2.

There is at present little scientific evidence supporting this "common sense" line of action for the future. Widespread use of glycoprotein IIb/IIIa inhibitors in combination with lytics and an increase in the availability of invasive facilities will have a major impact on treatment costs that need to be weighed against the expected incremental reduction in mortality and postinfarction heart failure.

ACKNOWLEDGEMENT

The authors wish to thank the staff of cardiologists from their institutions for the opinions and suggestions that contributed to the preparation of this manuscript, in particular Dr Antonello Vado, from the Ospedale Santa Croce for statistical assistance. Dr F Ribichini was supported in part by a Research Fellowship of the European Society of Cardiology.

REFERENCES

1 **Antman EM**, Giugliano RP, Gibson CM, *et al* for the TIMI 14 Investigators. Abciximab facilitates the rate and extent of thrombolysis: results of the thrombolysis in myocardial infarction (TIMI) 14 trial. *Circulation* 1999;**99**:2720–32.

2 **Brener SJ**, Barr LA, Burchenal J, *et al*. Randomized, placebo-controlled trial of platelet glycoprotein IIb-IIIa blockade with primary angioplasty for acute myocardial infarction. The RAPPORT trial. *Circulation* 1998;**98**:734–41.

3 **Ross AM**, Coyne KS, Reiner JS, *et al* for the PACT Investigators. A randomized trial comparing primary angioplasty with a strategy of short-acting thrombolysis and immediate planned rescue angioplasty in acute myocardial infarction: the PACT trial. *J Am Coll Cardiol* 1999;**34**:1954–62.

4 **Franzosi MG**, Santoro E, De Vita C, *et al*, on behalf of the GISSI Investigators. Ten-year follow-up of the first megatrial testing thrombolytic therapy in patients with acute myocardial infarction. *Circulation* 1998;**98**:2659–65.

5 **GUSTO Investigators**. An international randomized trial comparing four thrombolytic strategies for acute myocardial infarction. *N Engl J Med* 1993;**329**:673–82.
► **Large reperfusion trial that showed a significant (14.6%) risk reduction in mortality with rt-PA and heparin compared to streptokinase.**

6 **GUSTO V Investigators**. Reperfusion therapy for acute myocardial infarction with fibrinolytic therapy or combination reduced fibrinolytic therapy and platelet glycoprotein IIb/IIIa inhibition: the GUSTO V randomised trial. *Lancet* 2001;**357**:1905–14.
► **The most recent megatrial of infusive reperfusion treatment in AMI that compared standard fibrinolysis with reteplase versus half dose of reteplase plus full dose of abciximab. The study showed identical mortality rates with both treatments.**

7 **GUSTO II-b Angioplasty Substudy Investigators**. A clinical trial comparing primary coronary angioplasty with tissue plasminogen activator for acute myocardial infarction. *N Engl J Med* 1997;**336**:1621–8.
► **The largest randomised trial that compared primary angioplasty with accelerated rt-PA in AMI in community hospitals. The advantages of primary angioplasty were marginal and not sustained at six months.**

8 **Hochman JS**, Sleeper LA, Webb JG, *et al* for the SHOCK Investigators. Early revascularization in acute myocardial infarction complicated by cardiogenic shock. *N Engl J Med* 1999;**341**:625–34.

9 **Tiefenbrunn AJ**, Chandra NC, French WJ, *et al*. Clinical experience with primary transluminal coronary angioplasty compared with alteplase (recombinant tissue-type plasminogen activator) in patients with acute myocardial infarction: a report from the second national registry of myocardial infarction (NRMI-2). *J Am Coll Cardiol* 1998;**31**:1240–5.
► **National registry that analyses the clinical outcome of 272 651 patients with AMI presenting at US hospitals. Very low percentage of patients eligible for reperfusion therapy (31%); similar results with lysis and angioplasty. Angioplasty is superior in patients presenting in cardiogenic shock.**

10 **Weaver DW**, Simes JR, Betriu A, *et al*. Comparison of primary coronary angioplasty and intravenous thrombolytic therapy for acute myocardial infarction. A quantitative review. *JAMA* 1997;**278**:2093–8.
► **Meta-analysis of all available randomised trials that compared fibrinolysis and primary angioplasty. The invasive strategy significantly reduces mortality by 32%.**

11 **Schömig A**, Kastrati A, Dirschinger J, *et al* for the Stent versus Thrombolysis for Occluded Arteries in Patients with Acute Myocardial Infarction Study Investigators. Coronary stenting plus platelet glycoprotein IIb/IIIa blockade compared with tissue plasminogen activator in acute myocardial infarction. *N Engl J Med* 2000;**343**:385–91.

12 **Montalescot G**, Barragan P, Wittenberg O, *et al*. Platelet glycoprotein IIb/IIIa inhibition with coronary stenting for acute myocardial infarction. *N Engl J Med* 2001;**344**:1895–903.

13 **White HD**. Future of reperfusion therapy for acute myocardial infarction. *Lancet* 1999;**354**:695–7.
► **Brief but complete summary of recent trials and thoughtful considerations about the future of reperfusion treatment.**

14 **Brodie BR**. When should patients with acute myocardial infarction be transferred for primary angioplasty? [editorial]. *Heart* 1997;**78**:327–8.
► **Comparison of differences of outcome according to time to reperfusion with primary angioplasty or fibrinolysis from the extrapolation of data from PAMI and GUSTO I trials respectively.**

15 **GUSTO Angiographic Investigators**. The effects of tissue plasminogen activator, streptokinase, or both on coronary-artery patency, ventricular function and survival after acute myocardial infarction. *N Engl J Med* 1993;**329**:1615–22.

16 **Zijlstra F**, Hoorntje JCA, de Boer MJ, *et al*. Long-term benefit of primary angioplasty as compared with thrombolytic therapy for acute myocardial infarction. *N Engl J Med* 1999;**341**:1413–19.

▶ **Impressive demonstration of the superiority of primary angioplasty over fibrinolysis on survival at long term follow up (5±2 years).**

17 **Venturini F**, Romero M, Tognoni G. Patterns of practice for acute myocardial infarction in a population from ten countries. *Eur J Clin Pharmacol* 1999;**54**:877–86.

18 **Lincoff AM**, Topol EJ. Illusion of reperfusion. Does anyone achieve optimal reperfusion during acute myocardial infarction?. *Circulation* 1993;**88**:1361–74.

▶ **Excellent editorial review that addresses the discrepancies between the complete degree of angiographic epicardial reperfusion and tissue reperfusion.**

19 **Parmley WW**. Cost-effectiveness of reperfusion strategies. *Am Heart J* 1999;**138**:S142–6.

20 **O'Neill WW**. Coronary thrombosis during acute myocardial infarction: Roberts was right! *Am J Cardiol* 1998;**82**:896–7.

▶ **Interesting observations about the non-thrombotic origin of a number of total acute coronary occlusions that may not be relieved by lytic agents.**

Additional references appear on the *Heart* website—www.heartjnl.com

27

5 OFF-PUMP CORONARY ARTERY BYPASS SURGERY

Peter P Th de Jaegere, Willem J L Suyker

Coronary revascularisation plays an important role in the management of patients with ischaemic heart disease. Its principle builds on restoring antegrade flow thereby relieving angina. As a result, the need for medication is reduced which, in turn, may improve quality of life and socioeconomic independency. Also the prognosis is beneficially affected. This is not only true for patients with severe coronary atherosclerosis such as patients with left main or three vessel disease, but also for patients with less advanced disease.[w1-3]

▶ WHY OFF-PUMP BYPASS SURGERY?

The first milestones in coronary revascularisation were surgical. It all started after the second world war with the implantation of the internal mammary artery indirectly into the cardiac muscle (the Vineberg procedure). A few years later, procedures for direct coronary artery revascularisation were designed, initially including endarterectomy, followed by the construction of an anastomosis between a donor artery or vein and the coronary artery. Interestingly, these first operations were performed on the beating heart without the use of extracorporeal circulation and cardiac arrest.[w4] The results of these early initiatives were generally unpredictable, preventing general acceptance and widespread use. It became clear that the safety and efficacy of surgical coronary revascularisation in terms of in-hospital complications and immediate and long term clinical outcome greatly depends, among other factors, on the quality of the anastomosis between the donor graft and recipient coronary artery. To predictably create these delicate and very precise hand sewn anastomoses, the surgeon needs a still and bloodless field with full exposure of the target area, enabling the required complex and coordinated manipulation of the microsurgical instruments.

In this respect, the introduction of cardiopulmonary bypass (CPB) and cardiac arrest by Favaloro in 1967 proved to be a tremendous step forward. Because basic surgical requirements could now be properly addressed, consistent high quality anastomoses could be produced by the broad majority of cardiac surgeons. Indeed, the reported excellent clinical outcome and long term results initiated a tremendous increase in the number of bypass operations reaching the clinical status of "gold standard". Earlier efforts using different techniques were completely overwhelmed and almost forgotten for nearly 30 years. Excellent long term clinical results have been reported in a wide variety of patients, especially when using the internal mammary artery.[w5 w6] The superiority of coronary artery bypass grafting (CABG) with the use of CPB and cardiac arrest—the so-called conventional CABG—with respect to angina reduction and the need for repeat revascularisation, in comparison with medical treatment and percutaneous transluminal coronary angioplasty (PTCA), is subject to little discussion.[w6-8] As a result, conventional bypass surgery has been quoted as "safe, effective, durable, reproducible, complete, versatile and teachable".[w9]

The question, however, is whether bypass surgery with CPB and cardiac arrest is indeed safe. Data from the National Cardiac Surgery Database of the Society of Thoracic Surgery encompassing 170 895 patients are summarised in table 5.1.[w10] Overall, the proportion of patients suffering no complications was only 64.3%.[1] In addition, health insurance data and data from clinical studies disclose that 10.2% do not leave the hospital within 14 days after the operation and 3.6% of the patients are discharged to a non-acute care facility.[2 w11] The scope of the problem becomes clear when one considers that bypass surgery is performed in approximately 800 000 patients/year worldwide. Conventional bypass surgery is increasingly being questioned and this has stimulated the quest for novel surgical techniques guaranteeing the good results of precise direct coronary revascularisation, but avoiding factors believed to adversely affect the outcome and, thus, leading to less perioperative morbidity, faster recovery, shorter hospital stay, and reduced costs. One of these factors may be the use of cardiopulmonary bypass.

In this paper, the clinical experience and the reasons why isolated, off-pump surgery may lead to improved outcome are addressed. Off-pump surgery is defined as CABG surgery on the beating heart without the use of CPB and cardiac arrest, irrespective of the surgical access to the heart. Isolated bypass surgery implies coronary bypass surgery without concomitant cardiac or vascular procedures at the time of bypass grafting.

Table 5.1 Perioperative complications during isolated CABG (%)

		First operation	Reoperation
Number of patients		157159	13736
Mortality		2.6	7.3
Myocardial infarction		1.1	3.4
Reoperation		4.6	7.4
	For bleeding	2.2	3.1
Stroke		2.4	3.1
	Permanent	1.7	2.2
	Transient	0.7	0.8
Pulmonary			
	Prolonged ventilation (>24 hours)	5.3	10.2
	Oedema	1.9	3.4
	Pneumonia	2.2	3.8
	Acute distress syndrome	1.4	1.8
Renal failure		2.9	5.2
	Dialysis required	0.8	1.7
Gastrointestinal complications		2.3	3.0
Multiorgan failure		0.6	1.4
Infection		4.9	6.0
	Sternal	1.3	1.5
	Leg	1.3	1.5
	Urinary tract	1.4	1.4
	Sepsis	0.9	1.6

Modified from Borst and Gründeman.[w10]
CABG, coronary artery bypass graft surgery.

DETERMINANTS OF PERIOPERATIVE MORBIDITY AND MORTALITY

Surgical risk is influenced by a number of patient related factors such as age, severity of coronary artery disease, left ventricular function, and the presence of comorbid conditions (for example, diabetes, renal insufficiency, pulmonary and peripheral vascular disease, obesity). On the basis of these demographic and clinical determinants, risk models have been developed which can be used to either calculate the surgical risk or to stratify patients into low, medium or high risk subgroups.[3] [4]

In addition to these patient related factors—which unfortunately cannot be corrected but, at best, may be modified or optimised before surgery—a number of procedure related factors play a role (table 5.2). In case of conventional bypass surgery, access to the heart must be obtained via full sternotomy, the heart and ascending aorta are cannulated for CPB, cardiac arrest is induced, and the ascending aorta is manipulated for the construction of a proximal anastomosis in case of saphenous vein or free arterial grafts. All these steps contribute to patient trauma and are likely to be associated with potential complications or may provoke biological reactions. Given their technical nature, there is ample room for improvement or innovation.

Central to the discussion is the use of CPB and the classical midsternal split. CPB requires the cannulation of the heart and the ascending aorta which may induce atherosclerotic (micro)emboli. Intraoperative transcranial Doppler monitoring has disclosed that the highest embolic load of the brain occurs during the aortic manipulation in preparation of CPB.[5] During a later stage of the operation, these emboli may not consist of particulate matter but rather of air bubbles introduced into the circuit by retrieving spilled blood from the surgical field or imperfections in the connections despite the use of arterial line filters.[5] The magnitude of the embolic load correlates with the duration of CPB and is reflected by the severity of postoperative cerebral dysfunction. Given these findings, it is conceivable that avoidance of CPB will substantially decrease the risk of perioperative neurologic complications, especially in elderly and other high risk patients. Yet, to completely avoid aortic manipulation, bypass surgery on the beating heart should also entail the exclusive use of in situ mammary grafts. For extensive coronary artery disease, more complex techniques like graft interposition between an in situ mammary artery and a coronary artery may be needed to obviate the need for aortic side clamping. Recently, automated vessel coupling systems suitable for connecting saphenous vein grafts to the aorta have started to become available. While still unproven, these systems may enable safe anastomoses on the ascending aorta in the future, simplifying the surgical procedure. Elderly patients in particular may benefit from off-pump, no-aortic touch bypass surgery since the incidence of atherosclerosis of the ascending aorta—and thus the risk of emboli—increases with age.[3] [w12]

In addition to the risk of microemboli, CPB induces a total body inflammatory response caused by the activation of the complement system due to contact of the blood with the artificial surface of the CPB circuit.[6] [w13] All organs are affected to a varying degree, potentially leading to dysfunction and/or damage of the brain, lungs, heart itself, bowel, kidneys, and coagulation system. Although the role of CPB in this response has been established and a whole body of evidence indicates that avoidance of CPB reduces oxidative stress, inflammation, and perioperative morbidity, it must be stressed that other factors such as the trauma of the surgical incision and the use of anaesthesic drugs may contribute to this inflammatory response as well.[w14–17] Thus, changes in surgical access to the heart, anaesthesiology, and pharmacology during the off-pump bypass may lead to a reduction in inflammation and postoperative morbidity.

As opposed to the heart, CPB produces a non-pulsatile flow which is thought to have an adverse effect on the microcirculation, leading to arteriolar shunting. This may contribute to postoperative organ dysfunction or failure.[w18] Non-pulsatile flow is one of the mechanisms which, in combination with the inflammatory response and the release of free radicals, is thought to be responsible for postoperative renal failure.[7]

Irrespective of the exact pathophysiology of CPB induced postoperative morbidity and mortality, these side effects have revitalised the nearly forgotten art of off-pump bypass surgery. The increasing public awareness of these complications and of less invasive alternative techniques in coronary revascularisation (PTCA) and other fields of surgery contribute to this new impetus.

Off-pump surgery on the beating heart also offers the opportunity to reduce the surgical incision and trauma to skin, soft tissue, and bone. Smaller access by means of various forms of minithoracotomy may reduce the risk of perioperative infection and enhance the speed of recovery. Sternotomy requires 6–12 weeks to heal and prevents early return to normal daily activities.[w19] Deep sternal wound infection occurs in 1–4% of the patients and is associated with a 25% mortality.[3] The determinants of deep sternal wound infections are obesity, the presence of diabetes, renal failure, redo surgery, and a number of operator related variables such as the use of more than one mammary artery and excessive use of electrocautery. Unfortunately, some of these risk factors such as obesity may not be compatible with reduced access

Table 5.2 Steps in conventional bypass surgery, consequences and potential solutions

Surgical trauma	Consequence(s)	Solution
Access to the heart Full sternotomy	Recovery time Infection (e.g. mediastinitis)	Minithoracotomy Port-access surgery Endoscopic robotic CABG
Cardiopulmonary bypass	Manipulation heart and aorta (microemboli) Inflammatory response	Off-pump CABG
Cardiac arrest Side clamping Aorta ascendens	Cell injury, necrosis Microemboli	Off-pump CABG No-touch aorta surgery (in situ arterial grafting) (graft interposition)

For details see text.

Clinical issues to be considered in CABG

- ► Effectively relieves angina (palliation)
- ► May positively affect event-free survival (prognosis)
- ► Non-negligible perioperative morbidity
- ► Cardiopulmonary bypass plays a major role in the pathophysiology of the perioperative morbidity
- ► Novel approaches such as off-pump beating bypass surgery are being proposed

---

type operations because of the prohibitive surgical difficulty of constructing a coronary anastomosis. The most benefit of a limited approach will probably be obtained in patients with diabetes, renal failure or redo heart surgery, provided that these patients do not have three vessel disease supplying viable myocardial tissue. In such a situation, full sternotomy may be more appropriate. A disadvantage of a minithoracotomy, however, is the increased amount of postoperative pain, especially when costal cartilages are traumatised as a result of substantial traction for surgical exposure or when multiple incisions are performed.[w20]

NOVEL APPROACH, NEW PROBLEMS

The potential advantages of a novel surgical approach, in this case off-pump bypass surgery, must be weighed against novel technical problems and limitations (table 5.3).

As stated before, the quality of the coronary anastomosis must be guaranteed. In the early days of off-pump bypass surgery, motion of the target area was controlled by pharmacologic reduction of global myocardial contractility and/or heart rate, with or without some primitive form of regional stabilisation by means of traction sutures. The breakthrough, however, came with the introduction of advanced regional mechanical stabilisers such as the CardioThoracic Systems Ultima device and the Utrecht Octopus in the mid 1990s.[8 w14] These devices consistently reduced the motion of the target area sufficiently to offer workable conditions for the majority of the surgical community. These stabilisers are, respectively, compressive and suction type devices that are fixed to one side of the operating table or chest wall retractor, with the other end apposed to the epicardial surface. As a result the coronary artery anastomosis can be constructed with enough surgical comfort and allow graft patency rates comparable to conventional CABG.[w10] Not surprisingly this has augmented the number of off-pump bypass operations from a negligible number in 1995 to 10% in 1999, and is expected to be 50% by 2005.[w21]

Yet, to construct a coronary anastomosis safely, the surgeon also needs a bloodless field. Therefore, the flow of the recipient coronary artery must be temporarily interrupted. For this purpose, vessel snares (suture or silicone elastomer tape) or atraumatic vascular clips are used proximally and often also distally to the coronary arteriotomy. This is invariably associated with myocardial ischaemia. Although generally well tolerated, it may occasionally provoke arrhythmia and haemodynamic instability, eventually necessitating conversion to on-pump bypass surgery and cardiac arrest. The interruption of the flow of the right coronary artery is known to provoke these complications. This can be addressed by placing an intracoronary shunt or seal when performing the anastomosis.[w22 w23] Although unproven, these mechanical solutions, as well as the coronary sutures or clips, all add to endothelial damage which may contribute to the development of late luminal narrowing.[1 w24] In addition, the clinical value of shunts is questioned since they may be cumbersome to use and, with respect to the shunt, blood flow through the shunt is only 30–50% of the native coronary flow.[1]

Ensuring a dry, bloodless field may also be hindered by back bleeding from perforating septal branches in the vicinity of the arteriotomy. This can be addressed by frequent blotting, intermittent saline infusion, or the use of high flow carbon dioxide moisturised insufflation.[9] It will be clear that, as opposed to conventional CABG, the off-pump surgeon needs an innovative and more flexible attitude to create optimal conditions consistently during surgery.

Haemodynamic instability and a drop in systemic blood pressure may occur when compressing or luxating the heart. Little displacement is required when reaching the left anterior and diagonal arteries. This is not the case when the circumflex or right coronary artery needs to be grafted. A nearly vertical displacement may be needed for the posterior wall, which is obtained by either deep pericardial traction stitches or a sling or a supporting device.[w25] Such a notable displacement is surprisingly well tolerated in most patients, but can provoke a significant drop in blood pressure and myocardial flow.[10 w26] Patients with left ventricular hypertrophy or poor ventricular function may not tolerate such a manoeuvre.[w25] Yet these patients are potentially ideal candidates for off-pump bypass surgery since a slight depression of myocardial contractility, induced by global ischaemic cardiac arrest during bypass surgery with CPB, may prohibit weaning from CPB or may lead to a low output syndrome which is the most common cause of operative mortality.[3 w27] Generally, all regions of the heart can be reached in the great majority of patients by perfect placement of the traction stitches and by improving venous

Table 5.3 Disadavantages and technical limitations of off-pump coronary artery bypass surgery

Technical issues	Proposed solutions
Motion of the heart	Pharmacologic or mechanical stabilisation
Tempory interruption of coronary flow	Luminal shunt during construction of anastomosis Arteriotomy seal Distal perfusion cannula
Blood flow in arteriotomy	Temporary luminal shunt Saline infusion Carbon dioxide gas blower
Pressure drop	Trendelenburg, inotropic support, fluid

Limited space for:
    preparation of mammary artery
    identification of coronary artery
    construction of anastomosis
	Miniaturisation of instruments
	Endoscopic video assisted surgery

Determinants of perioperative morbidity

▶ Age
▶ Extent of coronary artery disease
▶ Ventricular function
▶ Comorbid conditions
▶ Extent of the surgical trauma
▶ Use of cardiopulmonary bypass
▶ Global ischaemic cardiac arrest
▶ Manipulation and instrumentation of the ascending aorta

return by utilising the Trendelenburg position with or without additional fluid load and inotropic support.[w25]

Conventional bypass surgery via full sternotomy and CPB with a decompressed and arrested heart provides sufficient visibility and space to construct safely and adequately an anastomosis on all coronary arteries. This may be more difficult in limited access approaches and off-pump bypass surgery. Moreover, limited visibility may also interfere with identification of the target coronary artery. Therefore, training and patient selection are crucial in off-pump bypass surgery to optimise the learning curve. The left anterior descending, distal right, and proximal posterior descending arteries are relatively easy to approach with a limited anterior thoracotomy or subxyphoidal incision. Full sternotomy may be the most optimal approach for patients with three vessel disease.

Still experimental are the advanced robotic instruments capable of increasing surgical dexterity sufficiently to enable thorascopic bypass surgery, preferably with the aid of three dimensional visualisation.[w28] These systems have not yet provided the breakthrough of total endoscopic CABG (TECAB) mainly because of the still substantial technical difficulty in creating a robot-sewn anastomosis. Currently, interest seems to be shifting towards alternative, automated ways of performing the distal coronary anastomoses. While glued anastomoses certainly hold promise, most advancement has been in the area of mechanical connecting systems such as small, intraluminal stent-like structures, intraluminal magnets, and extraluminal devices with small hooks. While these connectors are already available for the larger, proximal anastomosis on the aorta, the relatively small size of the coronary arteries and their delicate, friable walls impose large obstacles for the development of reliable systems that may ultimately enable TECAB in large groups of patients.

CLINICAL EXPERIENCE

The clinical experience with off-pump bypass surgery is summarised in table 5.4. These data should be interpreted with caution since all but one originate from non-randomised observations made by pioneers in the field. Therefore selection bias, time bias, observation bias, and publication bias cannot be ruled out. Also, there is quite some variation in the definition of the outcome measures and in the consistency and methods of the acquisition of the clinical events between the studies. Taking into account these limitations, these data suggest that perioperative mortality and morbidity following off-pump bypass surgery compares favourably with those of the National Cardiac Surgery Database summarised in table 1. Only one study conducted at the University Medical Center Utrecht, using the Octopus Tissue Stabilizer, directly compared off- and on-pump bypass surgery by means of a randomised clinical trial.[11 12] This study revealed, however, no superiority in 30 day clinical outcome and only a modest superior cognitive outcome at three months which became negligible at 12 months after off-pump bypass surgery.[12]

Taking into account the expectations of off-pump bypass surgery, these findings were somewhat disappointing. The study, however, was conducted in patients of whom 50% had two vessel disease with a normal ventricular function and little comorbidity. This is also reflected by the low incidence of complications in patients who underwent on-pump bypass surgery. Two findings, however, favour off-pump CABG: there was a reduced need for blood products in the off-pump group, and there was a 41% reduction in postoperative creatine kinase MB release. The former is a consistent finding in most of the observational studies summarised in table 5.4. The latter suggests that avoiding CPB reduces the degree of myocardial necrosis which is in accordance with a significant reduction in troponin I release in off-pump patients reported previously.[13 14] Apparently local ischaemia during clamping of the coronary arteries is less harmful than global cardiac ischaemia. The clinical importance of this finding is that postoperative elevation of cardiac markers of necrosis has been identified as an independent correlate with one year clinical outcome.[w29]

Information on long term results of off-pump CABG is derived from the cases studies cited above (table 5.4) and the randomised clinical trial we directed at the University Medical Center Utrecht. Again, taking into account the limitations of

Table 5.4 In-hospital and 30 day clinical events after off-pump bypass surgery

Author (ref)	Year	Number of patients	Death	CVA	AMI	RF	Inf	Redo	AF
Subramanian[w26]	1997	182	3.8	0.5	3.8	nr	2.7	3.2	8.0
Sternik[w27]	1997	64	3.1	1.6	3.1	nr	nr	nr	nr
Diegeler[w30]	1998	209	0.5	nr	1.9	nr	nr	2.4	nr
Jansen[w31]	1998	100	0.0	2.0	4.0	nr	1.0	1.0	12.0
Magovern[w19]	1998	60	0.0	0.0	nr	nr	nr	1.7	nr
Tasdemir[w32]	1998	2052	1.9	0.8	2.9	0.2	0.5	0.9	17.0
Calafiore[w33]	1999	122	0.0	0.0	0.0	nr	nr	0.8	9.8
Arom[4]	2000	350	3.4	1.4	0.6	5.0	nr	2.8	14.0
Cartier[w34]	2000	300	1.3	1.6	4.0	nr	4.6	5.0	30.0
Koutlas[w12]	2000	53	0.0	2.2	0.0	0.0	0.0	0.0	26.0
Hart1[17]	2000	1582	1.0	0.6	1.3	0.9	0.3	1.2	15.0
Varghese[w35]	2001	35	2.9	nr	2.9	5.7	nr	nr	23.0
Yeatman[w36]	2001	75	1.3	0.0	2.7	6.7	0.0	2.7	12.0
Hernandez[18]	2001	1754	2.5	1.3	nr	nr	nr	4.5	21.0
Puskas[19]	2001	200	1.0	1.5	1.0	nr	0.0	1.5	nr
Van Dijk (39)	2002	142 off-p	0.0	0.7	4.9	0.0	5.0	4.0	20.0
		139 on-p	0.0	1.4	4.3	1.0	5.0	2.0	21.0

All events are expressed as percentage.
AF, atrial fibrillation; AMI, acute myocardial infarction; CVA, cerebrovascular accident; Inf; infection; nr, not reported; off-p, off-pump coronary artery bypass surgery; on-p, on-pump coronary artery bypass surgery; Redo, postoperative rethoracotomy for bleeding, infection or graft revision; RF, postoperative new renal failure.

Expectations and potential limitations of off-pump bypass surgery

- ► No need for cardiopulmonary bypass
- ► Reduction of surgical trauma
- ► Reduction of perioperative morbidity, recovery time, hospital stay, and costs
- ► Limited access, motion of the heart
- ► Quality of the anastomosis
- ► Haemodynamic changes, inducing organ dysfunction and reducing applicability
- ► Completeness of revascularisation

---

the observational studies, survival free from myocardial infarction after off-pump bypass surgery compares favourably with off-pump surgery. A striking feature is a higher occurrence of angina pectoris after off-pump bypass surgery and a higher frequency of percutaneous revascularisation during the follow up period.[4] This may be explained by less complete revascularisation and, thus, the learning curve of this surgically more demanding operation. This was not observed in the randomised clinical trial we conducted (Natho H, *et al*, unpublished data).

With respect to graft patency, data from observational studies in comparison with historical controls suggest similar early graft patency between off-pump (91–99 %) and on-pump (94–99%) bypass surgery.[15 16]

THE FUTURE

Doctors together with their patients now have a therapeutic spectrum of myocardial revascularisation procedures. At one end there is plain balloon PTCA which is the least invasive modality, followed by stents and other more advanced novel catheter technologies, and adjunctive pharmacologic and genetic intervention. The other end of the spectrum consists of bypass surgery. The most invasive approach, conventional CABG via full sternotomy, is now being challenged by full and limited access off-pump CABG. The slightly disappointing absence of notably better early clinical outcome after off-pump CABG draws our attention to the gap in the spectrum. This place could be filled by TECAB, the perfect intermediate between percutaneous techniques and current

surgery. While not possible for mainstream clinical use yet, this could change within a time frame of as little as five years. In the meantime, the trend towards better clinical outcome, however slight, should urge surgeons to expand carefully the use of off-pump techniques and limited size incisions whenever possible.

REFERENCES

1 **Duhaylongsod F**. Minimally invasive cardiac surgery defined. *Arch Surg* 2000;**135**:296–301.
2 **Roach G**, Kanchuger M, Mangano C, *et al*. Adverse cerebral outcomes after coronary bypass surgery. *N Engl J Med* 1996;**335**:1857–63.
 ► Observational study reporting the frequency of permanent stroke and transient neurologic dysfunction after conventional bypass surgery. The paper indirectly puts into perspective the potential role of off-pump bypass surgery.
3 **Eagle K**, Guyton R, Davidoff R, *et al*. ACC/AHA guidelines for coronary artery bypass graft surgery. *J Am Coll Cardiol* 1999;**34**:1262–347.
 ► Extensive report and summary of the American Heart Association/American College of Cardiology guidelines on bypass surgery: history, complications, outcome, and determinants.
4 **Arom K**, Flavin Th, Emery R, *et al*. Safety and efficacy of off-pump coronary artery bypass grafting. *Ann Thorac Surg* 2000;**69**:704–10.
 ► Retrospective analysis of the immediate outcome of 350 patients treated in a single centre. Patients were stratified into three risk groups. The clinical information in combination with the discussion provides insights into the potential role of off-pump bypass surgery.
5 **Mark D**, Newman M. Protecting the brain in coronary artery bypass graft surgery. *JAMA* 2002;**287**:1448–50.
6 **Edmunds L**. Why cardiopulmonary bypass makes patients sick: strategies to control the blood-synthetic surface interface. *Adv Cardiac Surg* 1995;**6**:131–67.
 ► Landmark paper on the role of cardiopulmonary bypass in the perioperative morbidity, providing insight into the pathophysiology and, thus, potential solutions.
7 **Ascione R**, Lloyd C, Underwood M, *et al*. On-pump versus off-pump coronary revascularization: evaluation of renal function. *Ann Thorac Surg* 1999;**68**:493–8.
 ► Small randomised clinical trial assessing the changes in renal function after off- and on-pump surgery. The protective effects of off-pump surgery are demonstrated.
8 **Borst C**, Jansen E, Tulleken C, *et al*. Coronary artery bypass grafting without cardiopulmonary bypass and without interruption of native coronary flow using a novel anastomosis site restraining device ("Octopus"). *J Am Coll Cardiol* 1996;**27**:1356–64.
 ► Experimental study in a pig model explaining the function of the Octopus tissue stabiliser and the histologic effects on the myocardium after application.
9 **Stanbridge R**, Hadjinikolaou L. Technical adjuncts in beating heart surgery. Comparison of MIDCAB to off-pump sternotomy: a meta-analysis. *Eur J Cardiothorac Surg* 1999;**16**(suppl 2):S24–33.
10 **Grundeman P**, Borst C, van Herwaarden J, *et al*. Hemodynamic changes during displacement of the beating heart by the Utrecht Octopus method. *Ann Thorac Surg* 1997;**63**:S898–92.
 ► Experimental study disclosing the potential adverse haemodynamic effects during the manipulation of the heart during off-pump

bypass surgery—a problem which can be adequately addressed but may still limit the use of off-pump bypass surgery.

11 **Van Dijk D**, Nierich A, Jansen E, *et al*. Early outcome after off-pump versus on-pump coronary bypass surgery. Results from a randomized study. *Circulation* 2001;**104**:1761–6.
► **First multicentre randomised clinical trial comparing off- and on-pump bypass surgery. Detailed surgical data and clinical outcome at 30 days are reported.**

12 **Van Dijk D**, Jansen E, Hijman R, *et al*. Cognitive outcome after off-pump and on-pump coronary artery bypass graft surgery. A randomized trial. *JAMA* 2002;**287**:1405–12.
► **Multicentre randomised clinical trial comparing off- and on-pump bypass surgery. Neurologic outcome and detailed information on neurocognitive dysfunction and outcome at three months are reported.**

13 **Ascione R**, Lloyd CT, Gomes WJ, *et al*. Beating versus arrested heart revascularization: evaluation of myocardial function in a prospective randomized study. *Eur J Cardiothorac Surg* 1999;**15**:685–90.
► **Small, single centre, randomised clinical trial assessing the protective effects of off-pump bypass surgery in comparison to on-pump surgery on myocardial cell damage and loss.**

14 **Kilger E**, Pichler B, Weis F, *et al*. Markers of myocardial ischemia after minimally invasive and conventional coronary operation. *Ann Thorac Surg* 2000;**70**:2023–8.
► **Non-randomised study assessing the course of the serum markers of myocardial tissue damage during off- and on-pump surgery through various routes of cardiac access. Off-pump surgery is associated with less injury in comparison with on-pump surgery.**

15 **Mack M**, Osborne J, Shennib H. Arterial graft patency in coronary artery bypass grafting: what do we really know? *Ann Thorac Surg* 1998;**66**:1055–59.

16 **Mack M**, Magovern J, Acuff T, *et al*. Results of graft patency by immediate angiography in minimally invasive coronary artery surgery. *Ann Thorac Surg* 1999;**68**:383–90.
► **A prospective, observational study reporting graft patency after LIMA insertion on the left anterior descending artery during off-pump surgery.**

17 **Hart J**, Spooner T, Pym J, *et al*. A review of 1,582 consecutive Octopus off-pump coronary bypass patients. *Ann Thorac Surg* 2000;**70**:1017–20.
► **A succinct and concise summary of the clinical outcome of a large series of patients who underwent off-pump bypass surgery with the Octopus method in seven centres in the USA and Europe.**

18 **Hernandez F**, Cohn W, Baribeau Y, *et al*. In-hospital outcomes of off-pump versus on-pump coronary artery bypass procedures: a multicenter experience. *Ann Thorac Surg* 2001;**72**:1528–34.
► **Indirect comparison of the in-hospital outcome between 1741 patients who underwent off-pump bypass surgery with 6126 patients who underwent conventional bypass surgery in four centres of the Northern New England Cardiovascular Disease Study Group.**

19 **Puskas J**, Thourani V, Marshall J, *et al*. Clinical outcomes, angiographic patency and resource utilisation in 200 consecutive off-pump coronary bypass patients. *Ann Thorac Surg* 2001;**71**:1477–84.

Additional references appear on the *Heart* website—www.heartjnl.com

6 MANAGEMENT OF CARDIOGENIC SHOCK COMPLICATING ACUTE MYOCARDIAL INFARCTION

Venu Menon, Judith S Hochman

The incidence of cardiogenic shock in community studies has not decreased significantly over time. Despite decreasing mortality rates associated with increasing utilisation of revascularisation, shock remains the leading cause of death for patients hospitalised with acute myocardial infarction (MI). Although shock often develops early after MI onset, it is typically not diagnosed on hospital presentation. Failure to recognise early haemodynamic compromise and the increased early use of hypotension inducing treatments may explain this observation.

Recently, a randomised trial has demonstrated that early revascularisation reduces six and 12 month mortality.[1 2] The current American College of Cardiology/American Heart Association (ACC/AHA) guidelines recommend the adoption of an early revascularisation strategy for patients < 75 years of age with cardiogenic shock.[3] In this article, we review the incidence, aetiology, prevention, and recognition of shock, as well as its management.

▶ INCIDENCE

The extent of myocardial salvage from reperfusion treatment decreases exponentially with time to re-establishing coronary flow. Unfortunately, there has been little progress in reducing time to hospital presentation over the past decade,[4] and this perhaps accounts for the stagnant incidence of cardiogenic shock in community studies (7.1%).[5] Cardiogenic shock also complicates non-ST elevation acute coronary syndromes. The incidence of shock in the PURSUIT trial was 2.9% (1995–97),[6] similar to the 2.5% incidence reported in the non-ST elevation arm of the GUSTO II-B trial (1994–95).[7] A number of strategies that centre on reducing the time to effective treatment may help decrease the incidence of shock. These include public education to decrease the time to hospital presentation, triage and early transfer of high risk patients to selected centres, and early primary percutaneous coronary intervention (PCI) or rescue PCI for failed thrombolysis in high risk patients.

PREDICTING AND PREVENTING SHOCK

The onset of cardiogenic shock in a patient following ST elevation MI heralds a dismal in-hospital prognosis. The 7.2% of patients developing shock in the GUSTO-I trial accounted for 58% of the overall deaths at 30 days.[8] Similarly, the 30 day death rates with non-ST elevation MI cardiogenic shock in the PURSUIT and GUSTO-II b databases were 66% and 73%, respectively. Even with early revascularisation, almost 50% die at 30 days. The prevention of shock is therefore the most effective management strategy. The opportunity for prevention is substantial, given the observation that only a minority of patients (10–15%) present to the hospital in cardiogenic shock. Whether due to pump failure or a mechanical cause, shock is predominantly an early in-hospital complication in the ST elevation MI setting. The median time post-MI for occurrence of shock in the randomised SHOCK trial was 5.0 (interquartile range 2.2–12) hours. Similarly, median time from MI onset to development of shock in the SHOCK registry was 6.0 (1.8–22.0) hours, and median time from hospital admission was 4 hours. Shock complicating unstable angina/non-Q MI occurs at a later time period. In the GUSTO-IIb trial shock was recognised at a median of 76.2 (20.6–144.5) hours for non-ST elevation MI compared to 9.6 (1.8–67.3) hours with ST elevation MI (p < 0.001), and median time to shock in the non-ST elevation PURSUIT trial was 94.0 (38–206) hours.

A primary goal in preventing shock should be an effort to reduce the large proportion of patients presenting with acute ST elevation MI who do not receive timely reperfusion treatment. Successful early reperfusion of the infarct related coronary artery while maintaining integrity of the downstream microvasculature limits ongoing necrosis, salvages myocardium, and may prevent the development of shock in many vulnerable patients. In-hospital development of shock often follows failed thrombolysis or successful thrombolysis followed by evidence of recurrent MI (ST re-elevation), infarct extension (ST elevation in new leads), and recurrent ischaemia (new ST depression). These complications may be significantly reduced by a primary PCI strategy. Currently, a minority of hospitals in the USA and an even smaller proportion worldwide possess the infrastructure and personnel to perform primary PCI effectively.

Trial acronyms

DIGAMI: Diabetes mellitus Insulin Glucose infusion in Acute Myocardial Infarction
FTT: Fibrinolytic Therapy Trialists
GUSTO: Global Utilization of Streptokinase and Tissue plasminogen activator for Occluded coronary arteries
PURSUIT: Platelet glycoprotein IIb/IIIa in Unstable angina: Receptor Suppression Using Integrilin Therapy
SHOCK: SHould we emergently revascularize Occluded Coronaries for cardiogenic shocK ?
SMASH: Swiss Multicenter trial of Angioplasty for SHock

Recognising patients at highest risk for development of shock may facilitate the early transfer of high risk patients before onset of haemodynamic instability. Early referral of high risk patients for rescue angioplasty in the setting of thrombolytic failure may also prove beneficial.

A number of scoring systems using predictive models for the development of shock have been reported to aid with this decision strategy. In the GUSTO-I study, age, systolic blood pressure, heart rate, and presenting Killip class accounted for > 85% of the predictive information. The same four variables were significant in the GUSTO III population and accounted for > 95% of the predictive information, with a validated concordance index of 0.796.[9] Major predictors of shock in the PURSUIT population included age, systolic blood pressure, ST depression on presenting ECG, heart rate, height, enrolling MI, and rales on physical examination. Although these scoring systems can be useful, the limitations of these databases need to be stressed. Patients enrolled in randomised clinical trials are themselves selected. Furthermore, positive predictive value for a patient with maximum attainable scores in the GUSTO-I and PURSUIT model are only 50% and 35%, respectively.[10]

CLINICAL RECOGNITION

Treatment cannot be initiated unless the clinical entity is recognised. Cardiogenic shock is characterised by inadequate tissue perfusion in the setting of adequate intravascular volume. Specifically, shock in the peri-infarction setting is defined as sustained hypotension (systolic blood pressure $\leqslant$ 90 mm Hg for $\geqslant$ 30 minutes), accompanied by signs of peripheral hypoperfusion (altered mental status, cool peripheries, oliguria). This clinical entity is unresponsive to fluid resuscitation alone, with a cardiac index < 2.2 l/min/m^2. Subjects requiring pharmacologic or mechanical circulatory support to maintain blood pressure are also included in this category. However, there is a wide spectrum of clinical symptoms, signs, and haemodynamic findings and variability in the severity of shock. It should be diagnosed in all patients exhibiting signs of inadequate tissue perfusion irrespective of blood pressure. Some patients, particularly those with anterior MI, develop signs of end organ hypoperfusion in the setting of unsupported blood pressure measurements > 90 mm Hg. The urine output is typically low and the heart rate > 90 beats per minute. This "pre-shock" presentation is associated with a high risk of in-hospital morbidity and mortality (43%).[11] When the physician fails to recognise that the tachycardia is caused by a pronounced reduction in stroke volume and therefore administers β blockers, frank shock may be precipitated.

In the SHOCK trial registry, 64% of patients presented typically with hypotension, evidence of ineffective cardiac output (resting tachycardia, altered mental status, oliguria, cool peripheries), and pulmonary congestion.[12] A substantial minority (28%) presented with evidence of hypoperfusion in the absence of pulmonary congestion—the "silent lung" syndrome. These latter patients have an equal distribution of anterior (50%) and non-anterior index infarctions (50%) with pulmonary capillary wedge pressure in the range of 21.5±6.7 mm Hg. Inexperienced clinicians may inappropriately treat such patients with large fluid boluses akin to the management of hypotension with right ventricular infarction.[13 14] Unadjusted in-hospital mortality for this group in the SHOCK registry exceeded that for the classical presentation (70% v 60%, p = 0.036), a difference that was non-significant after adjustment. These data highlight the clinical importance of the subjective signs of hypoperfusion obtained on physical examination in this population. In the GUSTO-I mortality model, altered sensorium (odds of dying 1.68, 95% confidence intervals (CI) 1.19 to 2.39), cold clammy skin (odds of dying 1.68, 95% CI 1.15 to 2.46), and oliguria (odds of dying 2.25, 95% CI 1.61 to 3.15) were associated with an increased 30 day mortality independent of haemodynamic variables.[15]

AETIOLOGY

There are several possible causes of cardiogenic shock in the setting of MI–left ventricular dysfunction, right ventricular dysfunction, and mechanical complications (fig 6.1). Recognition of shock should immediately lead to a quest for its cause. A combination of the history, physical findings, ECG, and a screening echocardiogram (table 6.1) will enable the clinician to arrive quickly at an accurate diagnosis. A right heart catheterisation is often not necessary for diagnosis and need only be performed when there is continued doubt or to guide management when shock does not rapidly resolve. Predominant left ventricular pump failure in the setting of a large MI is the most common aetiology. Ventricular septal rupture, severe mitral regurgitation, cardiac rupture, and tamponade should be excluded and haemorrhagic shock considered, especially in the elderly. Although the typical findings of significant right ventricular infarction are hypotension, clear lung fields, and jugular venous distension, severe right ventricular dysfunction (with or without excess fluid administration) may result in left ventricular compromise caused by right ventricular distension and septal shift, resulting in clinical evidence of pulmonary congestion. Systolic anterior motion of the anterior mitral leaflet causing left ventricular outflow tract obstruction in the MI setting has also been reported. Other masqueraders in this situation include aortic dissection and massive pulmonary embolism, which should be considered in the appropriate clinical context. The latter includes discordance between extent of ECG and haemodynamic abnormalities—that is, mild to moderate ECG abnormalities in the setting of severe haemodynamic derangement.

MANAGEMENT OF CARDIOGENIC SHOCK CAUSED BY PREDOMINANT LEFT VENTRICULAR FAILURE

Reports of dramatic declines in mortality with early revascularisation for cardiogenic shock began to emerge in the late 1980s.[16–18] Dedicated investigators in selected centres reported these single centre observations which were, however, prone to selection and publication bias. Randomised clinical trials testing the superiority and generalisability of an early

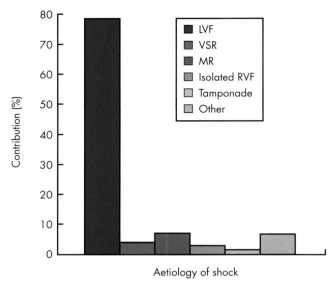

Figure 6.1 Aetiology of suspected cardiogenic shock in the combined SHOCK trial registry and trial (total n = 1422, only first 232 trial patients are included). "Other" includes shock caused by prior severe valvar disease, dilated cardiomyopathy, excess β blockade/calcium channel blockade, haemorrhage, and procedural complications. Aortic dissection, pulmonary embolism, and dynamic subaortic outflow obstruction should also be considered. LVF, left ventricular function; MR, mitral regurgitation; RVF, right ventricular failure; VSR, ventricular septal rupture.

Table 6.1 Usefulness of echocardiography in cardiogenic shock

► Evaluate left ventricular function and myocardium at risk
► Evaluate remote myocardial segments
► Screen for ventricular septal rupture
► Screen for severe mitral regurgitation and proceed to transoesophageal echocardiography as needed
► Look for tamponade/rupture
► Assess right ventricular function
► Look for aortic dissection

revascularisation strategy were clearly warranted and the National Heart, Lung, and Blood Institute funded the SHOCK trial in the USA, while the SMASH trial in Switzerland evaluated the same issue.[19][20] While SMASH failed to recruit an adequate number of patients, SHOCK reported an increase in 30 day survival from 46.7% to 56.0% by the adoption of an early revascularisation strategy, but this absolute 9% difference did not reach significance (p = 0.11). On follow up, the survival difference in favour of the early revascularisation strategy became larger and significant at six months (36.9% v 49.7%, p = 0.027) and one year (33.6% v 46.7%) for an absolute reduction of 13.2% (95% CI 2.2% to 24.1%, p < 0.03). The Kaplan-Meier survival curves for the early revascularisation and initial medical stabilisation arms are illustrated in fig 6.2. There were 10 prespecified subgroup variables examined, including sex, age, prior MI, hypertension, diabetes, anterior MI, early or late shock, and transfer or direct admission status. A benefit of early revascularisation was demonstrated for all subgroups except for the elderly. Age ⩾ 75 versus < 75 years interacted significantly with treatment effect at 30 days, six months, and one year. The benefit of early revascularisation was large for those < 75 years at 30 days (41.4% v 56.8%, 95% CI −27.8% to −3.0%), and six months (44.9% v 65.0%, 95% CI

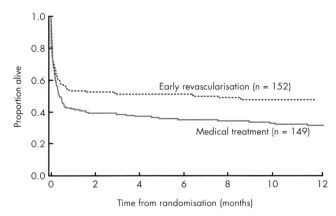

Figure 6.2 Kaplan-Meier curve showing 12 month survival in the early revascularisation and initial medical stabilisation arms of the SHOCK trial. Reproduced from Hochman et al,[2] with permission of the American Medical Association.

−31.6% to −7.1%) and was not apparent for the elderly (see below). An increased utilisation of revascularisation was also associated with improved outcome in the GUSTO-I thrombolytic trial and favourable outcomes in recent registries.[21][22] An algorithm for the management of cardiogenic shock is outlined in fig 6.3.

Step 1: immediate resuscitation measures
The goal is to prevent devastating end organ injury while the patient is being transported for definitive treatment. Maintenance of adequate mean arterial pressure to prevent adverse neurologic and renal sequelae is vital. Dopamine or noradrenaline (norepinephrine), depending on the degree of hypotension, should be initiated promptly to raise mean arterial pressure and be maintained at the minimum dose required. Dobutamine may be combined with dopamine at moderate doses or used alone for a low output state without frank hypotension. Intra-aortic balloon counterpulsation should be initiated before transportation when facilities are available. Arterial blood gas and oxygen saturation should be monitored with early institution of continuous positive airway pressure or mechanical ventilation as needed. The ECG should be monitored continuously, and defibrillating equipment, intravenous amiodarone, and lidocaine should be readily available. (Thirty three per cent of patients in the early revascularisation arm of the SHOCK trial had cardiopulmonary resuscitation, sustained ventricular tachycardia or ventricular fibrillation before randomisation.) Transcutaneous pacing electrodes as well as provisions for temporary transvenous pacing should be placed at the patient's bedside. Aspirin and full dose heparin should be administered. For ST elevation MI requiring transfer for angiography, we recommend intra-aortic balloon pump (IABP) placement at the local hospital when possible. A fibrinolytic agent should be initiated in patients with ST elevation MI if the anticipated delay to angiography is more than two hours. Thirty five day mortality for patients with systolic blood pressure < 100 mm Hg receiving thrombolysis in the FTT meta-analysis was 28.9% compared to 35.1% with placebo. This translates into 62 lives saved (95% CI 26 to 98, p < 0.001) per 1000 patients treated.[23] Augmentation of blood pressure with an IABP in this situation may facilitate thrombolysis by increasing coronary perfusion pressure. Similarly, raising blood pressure (to 130 mm Hg systole) by using vasopressor support has also shown synergism in experimental models, but this increase is difficult to achieve in patients in shock. For

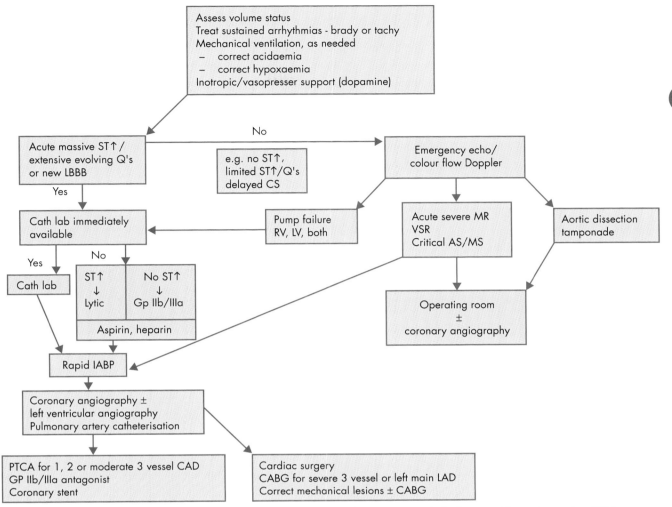

Figure 6.3 Algorithm on management of cardiogenic shock following ST elevation myocardial infarction. AS, atrial stenosis; CABG, coronary artery bypass graft; CAD, coronary artery disease; IABP, intra-aortic balloon pump; LAD, left anterior descending; LBBB, left bundle branch block; LV, left ventricle; MR mitral regurgitation; MS, mitral stenosis; PTCA, percutaneous transluminol coronary angioplasty; RV, right ventricle; VSR, ventricular septal rupture. Reproduced from Topol EJ (ed) *Textbook of cardiovascular medicine*, 2nd ed, with permission.

non-ST elevation MI cardiogenic shock awaiting catheterisation, a glycoprotein IIb/IIIa inhibitor should be initiated.

Step 2: early definition of coronary anatomy
This is the pivotal step in the management of cardiogenic shock resulting from predominant ischaemic pump failure. Patients in a community hospital setting should be emergently transferred/airlifted to an experienced designated regional tertiary care facility. The referring and accepting physician as well as the critical care transport team should be in constant communication to avoid delays in cardiac catheterisation. Prophylactic IABP placement is recommended before transfer and otherwise before angiography; radiocontrast use should be minimised. Early reversal of hypotension with IABP support serves as an excellent prognostic marker for survival, but those who do or do not respond well to IABP both derive benefit from early revascularisation. If a high quality echocardiogram has already been performed, a ventriculogram need not be repeated. Shock is characterised by a high incidence of triple vessel disease, left main disease, and impaired left ventricular function.[24] The mean (SD) left ventricular ejection fraction for patients in the SHOCK trial and registry was 29 (11)% and 34 (14)%, respectively. The extent of ventricular dysfunction and haemodynamic instability should be correlated with coronary anatomy. An isolated circumflex lesion or

a right coronary lesion should rarely manifest as shock in the absence of right ventricular infarction, left ventricular underfilling, bradyarrhythmia or prior MI or cardiomyopathy. In situations like this it is important for the clinician to immediately consider and exclude mechanical and other aetiologies of cardiogenic shock.

Step 3: perform early revascularisation
Definition of anatomy should be followed rapidly by selection of the modality of revascularisation. PCI will most often be the treatment of choice. Glycoprotein IIb/IIIa antagonists and stenting of the infarct related artery are indicated, although trial data are lacking. Recent reports suggest an additive benefit of stenting and glycoprotein IIb/IIIa antagonists in cardiogenic shock similar to the remainder of the clinical spectrum of PCI.[25] However, if there is sluggish flow despite absence of post-coronary angioplasty stenosis, we recommend waiting until flow normalises before stenting. Stenting may exacerbate distal embolisation. Glycoprotein IIb/IIIa antagonists may improve reflow. Intracoronary adenosine or nitroprusside may be tried. There is no randomised clinical evidence to support multivessel angioplasty in this setting, and the decision to perform angioplasty in the non-infarct related artery should be individualised. In selected cases, with remote ischaemia,

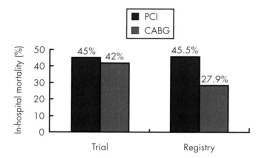

Figure 6.4 In-hospital mortality with percutaneous coronary intervention (PCI) and coronary artery bypass graft surgery (CABG) in the early revascularisation arm of the randomised SHOCK trial compared to the non-randomised larger SHOCK registry.

non-infarct related artery critical stenosis, and lack of haemodynamic improvement after infarct related artery PCI (with IABP support), revascularisation of the non-infarct territory may play a role. In patients with moderate three vessel disease, emergent PCI of the infarct related artery with consideration for later coronary artery bypass graft surgery (CABG) is preferred based on the concern that distal embolisation in non-infarct related artery segments is not tolerated in shock.

There are no trials randomising patients to PCI versus CABG in the setting of cardiogenic shock. The safety and feasibility of CABG in this situation is well documented. Severe triple vessel and left main coronary artery disease with severely impaired left ventricular function predominate in the shock setting. Emergent CABG allows the opportunity to achieve complete revascularisation and rectify severe mitral regurgitation while cardiopulmonary bypass maintains systemic perfusion. The SHOCK trial protocol recommended emergency CABG for patients with left main or severe three vessel disease. The in-hospital mortality rates with CABG in the SHOCK trial and registry were the same as the outcomes with PCI despite more severe coronary artery disease and twice the rate of diabetes in patients who underwent CABG (fig 6.4). We believe that CABG is underused in the shock setting. When dictated by anatomy, we recommend emergent CABG with pre-induction IABP support. The potential for benefit with metabolic support in this situation is large but remains formally untested in the shock setting.

Intra-aortic balloon counterpulsation support
Consistent with the current ACC/AHA guidelines, we recommend early consideration of IABP placement for patients with cardiogenic shock who are candidates for an aggressive strategy. Although randomised controlled trial data are lacking, benefit is seen across a number of observational databases.[26–29] It provides excellent temporary haemodynamic support in many patients.[30] It must also be noted that in the randomised SHOCK trial use of IABP was strongly recommended in both the early revascularisation and conservative arm. IABP utilisation was 87% in this trial and may have contributed to the improved outcomes observed in both groups compared to historical controls. The observed rates of IABP utilisation in US sites increased from 35% in GUSTO-I to 47% in GUSTO-III (p = 0.001).[31] In contrast, utilisation at non-US sites in both trials were low (7% and 10%, respectively). We believe that IABP is currently underutilised in the setting of shock and strongly recommend that community hospitals attempt to develop an IABP programme so that treatment may be initiated before transfer whenever possible.

ISSUES IN SHOCK MANAGEMENT
How should the elderly be treated?
Although there was no apparent benefit from an early revascularisation strategy in patients aged ≥ 75 years in the SHOCK trial, the total number of patients in this subgroup was small (n = 56). The 17% of 277 patients aged > 75 years in the concomitant SHOCK registry who were selected for early revascularisation appeared to derive benefit that was similar to their younger counterparts, even after covariate adjustment.[32] We do not feel there is adequate evidence to categorically deny early revascularisation to the elderly. We use an individualised approach to the elderly. A select group based on prior functional status, "physiologic" age, comorbidity, proximity of MI, duration of shock, and coronary anatomy may be offered an early revascularisation strategy. In the absence of contraindications, the remainder are treated with thrombolysis with or without IABP, or comfort care alone for those unlikely to benefit (see below). The very elderly often request comfort care alone.

Is there a therapeutic window for emergency revascularisation?
Early revascularisation should be considered as soon as possible following diagnosis of cardiogenic shock. The median time from randomisation to revascularisation was 1.4 (0.6–2.8) hours and the median time from MI to randomisation was 11 hours in the randomised SHOCK trial. However, it should be noted that patients were eligible for the trial if shock was diagnosed within 36 hours of index MI and randomisation performed within 12 hours of shock onset. There was no significant interaction between time from MI to randomisation and treatment effect. Ongoing ischaemia and stuttering necrosis are typical in the vicious cycle of ischaemia–hypoperfusion that characterise shock. Unlike primary reperfusion treatment, the window of opportunity in this setting is large. We recommend an early revascularisation strategy for shock patients up to 48 hours post-index MI and up to 18 hours post-shock. Patients who are not revascularised within 18 hours of shock onset but survive the early phase with resolution of shock should undergo coronary angiography. Revascularisation should be performed based on standard post-MI criteria—that is, triple vessel or left main disease or spontaneous or inducible ischaemia.

What is the quality of life?
Although the SHOCK trial showed that 13 lives were saved at one year per 100 patients treated with an early revascularisation strategy, it was important to document that survivors had an acceptable quality of life. It is reassuring that 83% of one year survivors (n = 90) were in New York Heart Association heart failure functional class I or II at 12 months.

Is care ever futile?
It is difficult to assess futility in the acute critical setting that characterises cardiogenic shock. It is vital to establish communication with the family as soon as the clinical entity is recognised. The patient or surrogate should play a role in the decision making process. Patients who require prolonged cardiopulmonary resuscitation and sustain presumed anoxic brain damage and those with other life shortening illnesses are not candidates for aggressive care. Although cardiac index, blood pressure, signs of hypoperfusion, and ejection fraction are independently associated with outcome, the beneficial effect of early revascularisation was noted across the spectrum of subgroups, except the very elderly. Further research is

required to develop a risk score to identify other patients with very poor outcomes despite early revascularisation. This may enable effective resource utilisation in the future and prevent heroic manoeuvres for patients unlikely to benefit.

MANAGEMENT OF MECHANICAL COMPLICATIONS

The utilisation of early reperfusion strategies has decreased the incidence of mechanical complications post ST-elevation MI.[33 34] Overall incidence of ventricular septal rupture in the GUSTO-I trial was 0.2% (84/41021) with a 30 day mortality of 73.8%.[35] Although IABP may help achieve temporary haemodynamic stability, prognosis following onset of haemodynamic collapse is grim.[36] The overall in-hospital mortality for ventricular septal rupture complicated by cardiogenic shock in the SHOCK registry was 87% (47/55) with an 81% (25/31) surgical mortality. A significant number of patients will have ventricular septal rupture without early evidence of circulatory collapse. Onset of circulatory collapse in this situation is unpredictable, and a superior surgical outcome is realised when emergent surgery is performed before the onset of cardiogenic shock. In keeping with the ACC/AHA guidelines, we recommend urgent surgery for our patients with newly diagnosed ventricular septal rupture. Similarly, all patients with mechanical mitral regurgitation and subacute rupture should be emergently considered for surgical intervention.

FUTURE DIRECTIONS

The role of L-NMMA, a selective nitric oxide inhibitor, is promising in this setting.[37] The utility of GIK (glucose, insulin, and potassium) metabolic support for cardiogenic shock patients is an intriguing but unanswered question. However, we recommend intensive insulin treatment to normalise blood glucose in those with elevated values. The DIGAMI study suggested that this strategy was beneficial for acute MI patients. In a study of intensive care unit patients, those with hyperglycaemia who were randomised to intensive insulin had reduced mortality rates.[38]

The role of selection of patients for wearable left ventricular assist devices and their clinical utility in the setting of shock following MI needs to be explored. Patients who are candidates for cardiac transplantation should receive bridging left ventricular assist devices.

CONCLUSION

Early recognition and transfer of high risk patients and adoption of a primary PCI strategy may decrease the incidence of cardiogenic shock. Establishing the aetiology of shock and early definition of coronary anatomy in the setting of pump failure are crucial. We recommend urgent revascularisation supported by IABP for patients aged < 75 years in cardiogenic shock caused by pump failure. A selective approach is advocated for the elderly. Regional care centres that are experienced in the management of shock should be designated and protocols developed for rapid transport of critically ill patients. Further research is needed in the areas of pharmacologic and mechanical haemodynamic support, refinement of revascularisation strategies, and outcome modelling.

REFERENCES

1 **Hochman JS**, Sleeper LA, Webb JG, *et al*. Early revascularization in acute myocardial infarction complicated by cardiogenic shock. *N Engl J Med* 1999;**341**:625–34.
▶ **Randomised controlled trial comparing an early revascularisation strategy to an initial medical stabilisation strategy in the setting of cardiogenic shock.**
2 **Hochman JS**, Sleeper LA, White HD, *et al*. One-year survival following early revascularization for cardiogenic shock. *JAMA* 2001;**285**:190–2.
▶ **One year follow up of the SHOCK trial.**
3 **Ryan TJ**, Anderson JL, Antman EM, *et al*. 1999 update: ACC/AHA guidelines for the management of patients with acute myocardial infarction. A report of the American College of Cardiology/American Heart Association task force on practice guidelines. (Committee on management of acute myocardial infarction). *Circulation* 1999;**100**:1016–30.
4 **Rogers WJ**, Canto JG, Lambrew CT, *et al*. Temporal trends in the treatment of 1.5 million patients with myocardial infarction in the US from 1990 through 1999. *J Am Coll Cardiol* 2000;**36**:2056–63.
5 **Goldberg RJ**, Samad NA, Yarzebski J, *et al*. Temporal trends in cardiogenic shock complicating acute myocardial infarction. *N Engl J Med* 1999;**340**:1162–68.
▶ **Large community study showing a decline in mortality but no change in incidence of shock over time.**
6 **Hasdai D**, Harrington RA, Hochman JS, *et al*. Platelet glycoprotein IIb/IIIa blockade and outcome of cardiogenic shock complicating acute coronary syndromes without persistent ST- segment elevation. *J Am Coll Cardiol* 2000;**36**:685–92.
7 **Holmes DR Jr**, Berger PB, Hochman JS, *et al*. Cardiogenic shock in patients with acute ischemic syndromes with and without ST-segment elevation. *Circulation* 1999;**100**:2067–73.
8 **Holmes DR Jr**, Bates ER, Kleiman NS, *et al*. Contemporary reperfusion therapy for cardiogenic shock: the GUSTO-I trial experience. *J Am Coll Cardiol* 1995;**26**:668–74.
9 **Hasdai D**, Califf RM, Thompson TD, *et al*. Predictors of cardiogenic shock after thrombolytic therapy for acute myocardial infarction. *J Am Coll Cardiol* 2000;**35**:136–43.
10 **Hasdai D**, Topol EJ, Califf RM, *et al*. Cardiogenic shock complicating acute coronary syndromes. *Lancet* 2000;**356**:749–56.
▶ **Recent review with emphasis on predictive modelling.**
11 **Menon V**, Slater JN, White HD, *et al*. Acute myocardial infarction complicated by systemic hypoperfusion without hypotension: report from the SHOCK trial registry. *Am J Med* 2000;**108**:374–80.
▶ **Clinical description and outcome of "pre-shock".**
12 **Menon V**, White H, Lejemtel T, *et al*. The clinical profile of patients with suspected cardiogenic shock due to predominant left ventricular failure. A report from the SHOCK trial registry. *J Am Coll Cardiol* 2000;**36**:1071–6.
13 **Swan HJ**, Forrester JS, Diamond G, *et al*. Hemodynamic spectrum of myocardial infarction and cardiogenic shock; a conceptual model. *Circulation* 1972;**45**:1097–110.
14 **Forrester JS**, Diamond GA, Swan HJC. Correlative classification of clinical and hemodynamic function after acute myocardial infarction. *Am J Cardiol* 1977;**39**:137–45.
15 **Hasdai D**, Holmes DR Jr, Califf RM, *et al*. Cardiogenic shock complicating acute myocardial infarction: predictors of death. *Am Heart J* 1999;**138**:21–31.
16 **Lee L**, Bates ER, Pitt B, *et al*. Percutaneous transluminal coronary angioplasty improves survival in acute myocardial infarction complicated by cardiogenic shock. *Circulation* 1988;**78**:1345–51.
17 **Verna E**, Repetto S, Boscarini M, *et al*. Emergency coronary angioplasty in patients with severe left ventricular dysfunction or cardiogenic shock after acute myocardial infarction. *Eur Heart J* 1989;**10**:958–66.
18 **Moosvi AR**, Khaja F, Villanueva L, *et al*. Early revascularization improves survival in cardiogenic shock complicating myocardial infarction. *J Am Coll Cardiol* 1992;**19**:907–14.
19 **Hochman JS**, Sleeper LA, Godfrey E, *et al*. Should we emergently revascularize occluded coronaries for cardiogenic shock: an international randomized trial of emergency PTCA/CABG-trial design. *Am Heart J* 1999;**137**:313–21.
20 **Urban P**, Stauffer JC, Bleed D, *et al*. A randomized evaluation of early revascularization to treat shock complicating acute myocardial infarction: the (Swiss) multicenter trial of angioplasty for shock-(S)MASH. *Eur Heart J* 1999;**20**:1030–8.
21 **Berger PB**, Holmes DR Jr, Stebbins L, *et al*. Impact of an aggressive invasive catheterization and revascularization strategy on mortality in patients with cardiogenic shock in the global utilization of streptokinase and tissue plasminogen activator for occluded coronary arteries (GUSTO-I) trial: an observational study. *Circulation* 1997;**96**:122–7.
22 **Carnendran L**, Abboud R, Sleeper LA, *et al*. Trends in cardiogenic shock: report from the SHOCK study. *Eur Heart J* 2001;**22**:472–8.
23 **Fibrinolytic Therapy Trialists (FTT) Collaborative Group**. Indications for fibrinolytic therapy in suspected acute myocardial infarction: collaborative overview of early mortality and major morbidity results from all randomized trials of more than 1000 patients. *Lancet* 1994;**343**:311–22.
24 **Wong SC**, Sanborn T, Sleeper LA, *et al*. Angiographic findings and clinical correlates in patients with cardiogenic shock complicating acute myocardial infarction: a report from the SHOCK trial registry. *J Am Coll Cardiol* 2000;**36**:1077–83.
25 **Ajani AE**, Maruff P, Warren R, *et al*. Impact of early percutaneous coronary intervention on short- and long-term outcomes in patients with cardiogenic shock after acute myocardial infarction. *Am J Cardiol* 2001;**87**:633–5.
26 **Waksman R**, Weiss AT, Gotsman MS, *et al*. Intra-aortic balloon counterpulsation improves survival in cardiogenic shock complicating acute myocardial infarction. *Eur Heart J* 1993;**14**:71–4.
27 **Kovack PJ**, Rasak MA, Bates ER, *et al*. Thrombolysis plus aortic counterpulsation: improved survival in patients who present to community hospitals with cardiogenic shock. *J Am Coll Cardiol* 1997;**29**:1454–8.
28 **Hudson MP**, Granger CB, Stebbins A, *et al*. Cardiogenic shock survival and use of intraortic balloon counterpulsation: results from GUSTO-I and III trials. *Circulation* 1999;**100**:I-370.

29 **Barron HV**, Every N, Parsons LS, *et al*. The use of intra-aortic balloon counterpulsation in patients with cardiogenic shock complicating acute myocardial infarction; data from the National Registry of Myocardial Infarction 2. *Am Heart J* 2001;**141**:933–9.

30 **Scheidt S**, Wilner G, Mueller H, et al. Intra-aortic balloon counterpulsation in cardiogenic shock: report of a cooperative clinical trial. *N Engl J Med* 1973;**288**:979–84.
▶ **Classic early paper on the utility of IABP to stabilise patients in the setting of shock.**

31 **Menon V**, Hochman JS, Stebbins A, *et al*. Lack of progress in cardiogenic shock: lessons from the GUSTO trials. *Eur Heart J* 2000;**21**:1928–36.

32 **Dzavik V**, Sleeper LA, Saucedo J, *et al*. Early revascularization is associated with improved survival in patients aged ≥75 years with acute myocardial infarction complicated by cardiogenic shock: a report from the SHOCK registry. *J Am Coll Cardiol* 2002;**39**:330A.

33 **Gertz SD**, Kragel AH, Kalan JM, *et al*. Comparison of coronary and myocardial morphologic findings in patients with and without thrombolytic during fatal first myocardial infarction. *Am J Cardiol* 1990;**66**:904–9.

34 **Honan MB**, Harrell FE Jr, Reimer KA, *et al*. Cardiac rupture, mortality and timing of thrombolytic therapy: a meta-analysis. *J Am Coll Cardiol* 1990;**16**:359–67.

35 **Crenshaw BS**, Granger CB, Birnbaum Y, *et al*. Risk factors, angiographic patterns, and outcomes in patients with ventricular septal defect complicating acute myocardial infarction. *Circulation* 2000;**101**:27–32.

36 **Menon V**, Webb JG, Hillis LD, *et al*. Outcome and profile of ventricular septal rupture with cardiogenic shock after myocardial infarction: a report from the SHOCK trial registry. *J Am Coll Cardiol* 2000;**36**:1110–6.
▶ **Largest clinical experience with ventricular septal rupture in the setting of cardiogenic shock.**

37 **Cotter G**, Kaluski E, Blatt A, *et al*. L-NMMA (a nitric oxide synthase inhibitor) is effective in the treatment of cardiogenic shock. *Circulation* 2000;**101**:1358–61.

38 **Van den Berghe G**, Wouters P, Weekers F, *et al*. Intensive insulin therapy in critically ill patients. *N Engl J Med* 2001;**345**:1359–67.

SECTION II: HEART FAILURE

7 CARDIAC TRANSPLANTATION

Mario C Deng

As a consequence of improved management in acute coronary syndromes and improved longevity of the population, the number of patients with heart failure is growing. The prevalence and incidence in industrialised countries are estimated to be around 1% and 0.15% of the population, respectively.[w1] Up to 10% of people with heart failure are at an advanced stage, amounting to 300 000 patients in the USA and 60 000 in the UK. In parallel, research [w2–5] has led to the concept of cardiac replacement by transplantation. Following the first successful heart transplantation in 1967 in the Groote-Schuur-Hospital, Kapstadt, South Africa,[w6] the first successful US heart transplant was performed in 1968 at Stanford University. In the same year, an ad hoc committee at Harvard University established the criteria of brain death.[w7] More than 55 000 cardiac transplants have now been performed in more than 200 hospitals worldwide (www.ishlt.org). The combination of good surgical success rates and the presence of a growing number of well equipped cardiac transplant programmes has created an enormous flux of heart failure patients towards these centres. Since the annual cardiac transplantation rate will likely remain below 4500 worldwide, with < 3000 in the USA and < 300 in the UK, it is evident that cardiac transplantation will continue to play only a very limited quantitative role in the treatment of the advanced heart failure syndrome.[1] Yet, its importance will continue to reside with its role as the option of last resort for patients with advanced heart failure, offered within centres with a complete spectrum of medical and surgical treatment options. The aim of this review is to outline a contemporary perspective on cardiac transplantation with respect to recipient and donor management, as well as an appropriate organisational policy. For further background reading, excellent material is available.[w8–15]

▶ EMERGING TREATMENTS IN ADVANCED HEART FAILURE

There has been progress in medical treatment including angiotensin converting enzyme (ACE) inhibitors [w16] and β blockers.[2] Surgical therapies including coronary artery bypass grafting with or without surgical anterior ventricular endocardial restoration,[w17] mitral reconstruction in cardiomyopathy patients with severe mitral regurgitation,[w18] combined with partial left ventriculectomy in idiopathic dilated cardiomyopathy,[3] [w20–24] and left ventricular assist device therapy[3] [w20–24] are evolving. The current status of surgical therapies for advanced heart failure has recently been reviewed in this series.[w25] Antiarrhythmic heart failure therapy with implantable defibrillators has also improved survival.[w26]

CURRENT SURVIVAL BENEFIT WITH CARDIAC TRANSPLANTATION

The appropriate identification of heart transplant candidates is based on the expected gain in survival and quality of life compared to all organ conserving medical and surgical treatment options in advanced heart failure. Selection criteria have been addressed in expert consensus guidelines.[4] They are a matter of increasing controversy. The assumption of a survival benefit across the entire spectrum of advanced heart failure may not be valid any longer because of two opposing trends. One trend is the increasing survival with emerging organ saving treatments. The other trend is that outcomes after cardiac transplantation have not consistently improved, due to listing of more critically ill patients, use of so-called marginal donor hearts from an extended donor pool,[1] and the initiation of new heart transplantation centres with an inevitable learning phase.[w27]

The death rates of advanced heart failure patients on the waiting list of the United Network for Organ Sharing (UNOS), the US organisation in charge of organ transplantation (www.unos.org), have decreased dramatically over time, from 432.2 per 1000 patient years in 1990 to 172.4 per 1000 patient years in 1999. For patients with advanced medical urgency status (status 1A, defined as haemodynamic instability requiring ventricular assist device implantation or high dose intravenous inotropes) in 1999, it was 581.9 per 1000 patient years, as compared with 204.7 per 1000 patient years for medical urgency status (status 1B, defined as requirement of low dose intravenous inotropes) and 130.7 per 1000 patient years for regular urgency status (status 2, defined as stable outpatient condition) registrants. In comparison to waiting list outcomes, for the 1997-98 UNOS heart transplant cohort the one year post-transplantation survival rate was 86%. Recipients

Abbreviations

COCPIT, Comparative Outcomes and Clinical Profiles In Transplantation
CMV, cytomegalovirus
HFSS, Heart Failure Survival Score
ISHLT, International Society for Heart and Lung Transplantation
LVAD, left ventricular assist device
PRA, panel reactive antibody
REMATCH, Randomized Evaluation of Mechanical Assistance for the Treatment of Congestive Heart failure
UNOS, United Network for Organ Sharing

Table 7.1 Cardiac transplantation indication criteria

1. Accepted	Heart Failure Survival Score (HFSS, Aaronson 1997[6]) high risk
	Peak VO_2 <10 ml/kg/min after reaching anaerobic threshold
	NYHA class III/IV heart failure refractory to maximal medical treatment
	Severely limiting ischaemia not amenable to interventional or surgical revascularisation
	Recurrent symptomatic ventricular arrhythmias refractory to medical, ICD, and surgical treatment
2. Probable	HFSS medium risk
	Peak VO_2 <14 ml/kg/min and severe functional limitations
	Instability of fluid status and renal function despite good compliance, daily weights, salt and fluid restriction and flexible diuretics
	Recurrent unstable ischaemia not amenable to revascularisation
3. Inadequate	HFSS low risk alone
	Peak VO_2 >15–18 ml/kg/min without other indications
	Left ventricular ejection fraction <20 % alone
	History of NYHA class III/IV symptoms alone
	History of ventricular arrhythmias alone

ICD, implantable cardioverter-defibrillator; NYHA, New York Heart Association; VO_2, oxygen consumption.

in medical urgency status 1 at the time of transplant had slightly lower one year post-transplantation survival rates (mean (SD) 84.8 (0.7)% v 87.5 (1.0)%) than those in status 2 at the time of transplant.

The International Society for Heart and Lung Transplantation (ISHLT) Registry (www.ishlt.org) indicates an improvement of one year survival after cardiac transplantation from 74.4% between 1980-86 to 85.6% between 1996-99. It does not provide data on waiting list mortality. Thus, the survival benefit with cardiac transplantation cannot be estimated from the ISHLT registry data.

The COCPIT (comparative outcomes and clinical profiles in transplantation) study by the German Transplantation Society and Eurotransplant International Foundation (www.eurotransplant.org)[5] found in a complete national cohort of all 889 adult patients listed for a first heart transplant in Germany in the year 1997 that patients with a predicted high risk of dying from heart failure according to the Heart Failure Survival Score (HFSS), using heart rate, mean blood pressure, aetiology, QRS duration, serum sodium, left ventricular ejection fraction, and peak oxygen uptake,[6] experienced not only the highest risk of dying on the waiting list (32%, 20%, 20% for high, medium, and low risk patients, respectively; p = 0.0003), but were the only group that had a survival benefit from transplantation. Limitations of this cohort study included a short observation period, and incomplete data in the HFSS which was in part a result of the fact that the COCPIT data collection was started before the HFSS was published.

All data currently available suggest that the survival benefit from cardiac transplantation is greatest in those patients who are at highest risk of dying from advanced heart failure without transplantation.

IMPROVEMENT OF MANAGEMENT COUNTERBALANCES SICKER PATIENT COHORT

Consistent with this trend, a shift toward more severely ill patients undergoing cardiac transplantation has been observed during the last 10 years.[w28] With an increasing fraction of patients undergoing orthotopic heart transplantation after previous cardiac surgery, intraoperative management has become more challenging.[w29 w30] The surgical challenges have specifically increased with an increasing fraction of patients undergoing ventricular assist implantation as bridge to transplantation.[w31 w32] Furthermore, traditional contraindications for transplant listing are being questioned—for example, with respect to a history of Hodgkin or non-Hodgkin lymphoma,[w33] elevated pulmonary vascular resistance requiring sophisticated medical bridging,[w34] increased pretransplantation panel reactive antibody (PRA) concentrations,[w35] and left ventricular

assist device (LVAD) use[w36 w37]—implying that advances in transplantation management have offset the increasing severity of transplant recipients.

CURRENT INDICATIONS/CONTRAINDICATIONS AND EVALUATION PROCEDURE

Current indication criteria are a modification of the 1993 American College of Cardiology Bethesda guidelines,[4] mainly based on the availability of the HFSS[6] (table 7.1). Conditions considered contraindications for cardiac transplantation, based on evidence of reduced short term and long term survival benefit after transplantation, are listed in table 7.2.

Patients are evaluated for transplantation after referral by a cooperating cardiologist. At the initial evaluation, a mutual long term working relationship between patient, relatives, and the team is established. The evaluation includes the tests summarised in table 7.3. The listing decision involves a recommendation by the team and decision by the patient. The complexity of the evaluation process mandates a team approach. For the patient with permanent contraindications the team offers continued care with the same intensity as for a transplant candidate, in conjunction with the primary care physician and cardiologist. At the time of listing, the patient and family are informed about the peculiarities of the waiting time, the perioperative period, the long term maintenance medication, and the rules of living with the new heart. A flexible schedule of outpatient appointments constitutes the cornerstone of waiting time surveillance. Deteriorating heart failure may precipitate organ failure. The bridging of organ function is part of the management of heart transplant candidates. If irreversible organ dysfunction ensues, the termination of life support must be considered, incorporating the patient's preferences. The patient must know that in case of a donor organ offer, acceptance of the organ depends on the judgment of donor organ quality by the donor surgical team.

EXPANSION OF DONOR CRITERIA

Donor heart acceptance criteria need to be continuously revised in order to responsibly increase the donor pool. These

Table 7.2 Cardiac transplantation contraindication criteria

Cardiac disease	Irreversible pulmonary hypertension (PVR >6 WU despite standardised reversibility testing protocol)
Other diseases	Active infection
	Pulmonary infarction within the last 6–8 weeks
	Significant chronic renal impairment with persistent creatine >2.5 or clearance <25 ml/min
	Significant chronic hepatic impairment with persistent bilirubin >2.5 or ALT/AST >×2
	Active or recent malignancy
	Systemic diseases such as amyloidosis
	Significant chronic lung disease
	Significant symptomatic carotid or peripheral vascular disease
	Significant coagulopathies
	Recent peptic ulcer disease
	Major chronic disabling disease
	Diabetes with end organ damage and/or brittle diabetes
	Excessive obesity (e.g. >30% over normal)
Psychosocial	Active mental illness
	Evidence of drug, tobacco, of alcohol abuse within the last six months refractory to expert intervention
	Psychosocial instability refractory to expert intervention
Age	> 65 years

ALT/AST, ratio of serum alanine aminotransferase to aspartate aminotransferase; PVR, pulmonary vascular resistance; WU woods units.

Table 7.3 Cardiac transplant evaluation tests

Laboratory	Creatinine, blood urea nitrogen, electrolytes, liver panel, lipid panel, calcium, phosphorus, total protein, albumin, uric acid, complete blood count with differential and platelet count, thyroid panel, antinuclear antibodies, erythrocyte sedimentation rate, rapid plasma reagin, iron binding, partial thromboplastin time, prothrombin time
	Blood type
	IgG and IgM antibodies against cytomegalovirus, herpes simplex virus, HIV, varicella-zoster virus, hepatitis B surface antigen, hepatitis C antigen, toxoplasmosis, other titres when indicated
	Prostate specific antigen (male >50 years), mammogram and pap smear (female >40 years)
	Screening against a panel of donor antigens (panel reactive antibodies) and human leucocyte antigen phenotype
	24 hour urine for creatinine clearance and total protein, urinalysis, urine culture
	Baseline bacterial and fungal cultures if indicated
Cardiac	12 lead ECG, 24 hour Holter monitor
	Echocardiogram
	Thallium scan if indicated
	Exercise stress test with oxygen uptake measurements
	Right and left heart catheterisation
	Myocardial biopsy on selected cases where aetiology of heart failure is in question
Vascular	Transcranial Doppler
	Peripheral vascular studies
	Carotid Doppler >55 years
Renal	Intravenous pyelogram if indicated
Pulmonary	Chest x ray
	Pulmonary function tests
	Chest computer tomogram >65 years (thoracic aorta)
Gastrointestinal	Abdominal ultrasound >55 years
	Upper gastrointestinal series if indicated
	Barium enema if indicated
	Liver biopsy if indicated
Metabolic	Bone densitometry
Neurologic	Screening evaluation
Psychiatric	Screening evaluation
Dental	Complete dental evaluation
Cardiothoracic surgery	Evaluation
Physical therapy	Evaluation
Social work	Patient attitude and family support, medical insurance, and general financial resources
Transplant coordinator	Education

Table 7.4 Donor contraindications

Finding	Rationale
Age >55–60 years	Reduced allograft function
Diffuse coronary artery disease	
Documented myocardial infarction	
Documented other heart disease	
Refractory ventricular arrhythmias	
Malignancies (except CNS)	Tumour spread in recipient
Refractory generalised infection	Infection spread in recipient

CNS, central nervous system.

extended criteria include advanced donor–recipient size match, donor age, donor heart dysfunction, donor heart structural changes, donor malignancies, and donor infection. A normal sized adult male (> 70 kg) donor is suitable for most recipients, despite an increased risk associated with small donor size relative to the recipient. Safe expansion of donor age criteria to >60 years has been reported.[w38] Donors older than 55 years may be used selectively in certain higher risk recipients. Other donor factors such as left ventricular hypertrophy and ischaemic time may synergistically increase the mortality risk.[w39] Donor hearts with myocardial dysfunction can recover after transplantation.[w40] Donors with mild coronary artery disease may be considered for selected higher risk recipients. A small series of donor hearts treated with bypass grafting for obstructive coronary lesions at the time of transplantation with a good long term survival has been reported.[w41] The transplantation of 37 and 363 hepatitis B surface antigen+ donor hearts and anti-hepatitis B core antibody positive donor organs, respectively, based on 13 309 heart transplants in the time period between 1994 and 1999 in the UNOS registry—on the assumption that patients were at similar risk of dying from heart failure—was associated with a similar five year post-transplantation survival.[w42] Current donor contraindications are listed in table 7.4.

DONOR MANAGEMENT PRINCIPLES

Optimal management of the haemodynamic, metabolic, and respiratory status of the donor is essential in order to maximise the yield of suitable thoracic donor organs.[7] Specifically, this has been advocated by the group at Papworth Hospital in Cambridge, UK.[w43] Brain death is associated with an "autonomic and cytokine storm". The release of noradrenaline (norepinephrine) leads to subendocardial ischaemia. Subsequent cytokine release results in further myocardial depression. This is accompanied by pronounced vasodilation and loss of temperature control. Vasodilation and myocardial depression are compounded by changes in volume status, specifically by relative hypovolaemia which is usually a consequence of aggressive diuretic treatment used to minimise donor cerebral oedema. Optimal donor haemodynamic management includes a pulmonary artery catheter to achieve the goals of euvolaemia and normal cardiac output, minimising the use of α agonists.[8] Metabolic management aims at correcting

Table 7.5 Effect of denervation on cardiac pharmacology

Substance	Effect on recipient	Mechanism
Digitalis	Normal increase of contractility; minimal effect on AV node	Direct myocardial effect; denervation
Atropine	None	Denervation
Adrenaline	Increased contractility; increased chronotropy	Denervation hypersensitivity
Noradrenaline	Increased contractility; increased chronotropy	Denervation hypersensitivity
Isoproterenol	Normal increase in contractility; normal increase in chronotropy	No neuronal uptake
Quinidine	No vagolytic effect	Denervation
Verapamil	AV block	Direct effect
Nifedipine	No reflex tachycardia	Denervation
Hydralazine	No reflex tachycardia	Denervation
β Blocker	Increased antagonist effect	Denervation

AV, atrioventricular.

acid-base imbalances and hormonal perturbations. Substitution of insulin, corticosteroids,[w44] triiodothyronine,[w45] and arginine vasopressin [w46] has been shown to be of benefit. A committed transplantation coordination network such as developed in Australia contributes to optimal donor management and recruitment.[w47]

GENERAL PRINCIPLES OF POST-TRANSPLANTATION MANAGEMENT

The post-transplantation management serves a fourfold purpose: control of allograft rejection, minimisation of side effects of immunosuppressants, coping with the transplantation process, and reintegration of the patient into society. The main challenges in the early postoperative period are the management of rejection and infection. In the long term course after transplantation, the main challenges are management of vasculopathy and malignancies. The denervation physiology characteristic of orthotopic cardiac transplantation requires a distinct modification of pharmacotherapy (table 7.5).

Allograft rejection

The alloimmune response of the recipient leads to destruction of the allograft (fig 7.1). The differentiation of this alloimmune response is orchestrated by a subtle regulation of soluble immune mediators, called cytokines.[w48] An understanding of acute allograft rejection requires an appreciation of complex, adaptive networks like the interdigitated inflammatory, immune, and physiologic processes that are at work in transplanted allografts.[w49]

Rejection management by immunosuppression

The three drug regimen of cyclosporine, azathioprine, and usually corticosteroids has been the mainstay of immunosuppression for patients undergoing cardiac transplantation since the early 1980s. However, this regimen has some inherent toxicities and does not prevent graft coronary artery disease. Thus there has been a widely perceived need for the introduction of improved immunosuppressive agents. The most commonly used drugs, their targets, selectivity, and main side effects are summarised in table 7.6.

Recently several new immune pharmacological agents have become available. For induction therapy beyond the polyclonal antithymocyte globulin or monoclonal OKT3, antibody preparations which specifically bind to the interleukin 2 (IL2) receptor, basiliximab and daclizumab, are being evaluated. The new maintenance immunosuppressive drugs are either inhibitors of de novo synthesis of purine or pyrimidine nucleotides, or are immunophilin binding drugs that inhibit signal transduction in lymphocytes. The newer inhibitors of de novo nucleotide synthesis include mycophenolate mofetil, mizoribine, brequinar, and leflunomide. The immunophilin binding drugs are cyclosporine, tacrolimus, and rapamycin. Out of these, four agents have been introduced recently into clinical cardiac transplantation. Mycophenolate mofetil is used as a substitute for azathioprine and has been shown to result in lower mortality and rejection rates in heart transplant recipients.[9] Tacrolimus can be used as a substitute for cyclosporine.[w50] Specific blockade of the high affinity IL2 receptor (CD25) with the human IgG1 monoclonal antibody daclizumab reduces the frequency and severity of cardiac allograft rejection during the induction period.[10] Rapamycin/sirolimus has been shown to reverse refractory cardiac allograft rejection.[w51]

Rejection monitoring

Several methods of rejection monitoring have evolved over the last decades (table 7.7). The endomyocardial biopsy has long

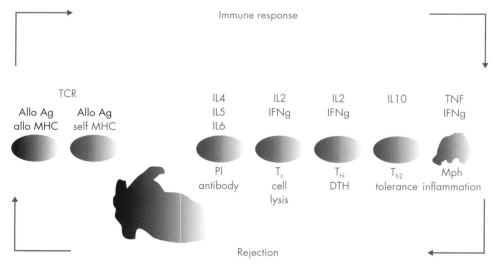

Immune response

TCR

Allo Ag allo MHC | Allo Ag self MHC

IL4 IL5 IL6 | IL2 IFNg | IL2 IFNg | IL10 | TNF IFNg

Pl antibody | T$_c$ cell lysis | T$_{h1}$ DTH | T$_{h2}$ tolerance | Mph inflammation

Rejection

Figure 7.1 The alloimmune response consists of antigen (Allo Ag) presentation in the context of major histocompatibility (MHC) molecules either by donor cells or by recipient cells to the recipient's T cells via T cell receptor (TCR). This leads to T lymphocyte differentiation to CD4 T cells of T helper1 (Th1) or T helper2 (Th2) phenotype, CD8 cytotoxic T cells (Tc), and B lymphocyte development into plasma cells producing specific clones of antibodies. These immunocompetent cells destroy the allogeneic graft cells. In addition, an inflammatory response by the innate immune system involving macrophages (Mph) participates in this networked alloimmune response. Cytokines (IL2-10, TNF, IFng) play an important role in this orchestrated response. The Th2 subset may favour graft acceptance.

Table 7.6 Commonly used immunosuppressive drugs: targets, main side effects, and selectivity

Method	Target	Major side effects	Selectivity
Steroids	Lymphocytes/RES	Osteoporosis, diabetes, psychosis, infection, obesity	+
Azathioprine	Lymphocytes	Marrow suppression, hepatopathy	++
Polyclonal antithymocyte globulin	T lymphocytes	Infection, malignancies	++
Monoclonal CD3 antibodies	CD3+ T lymphocytes	Infection, malignancies	+++
Mycophenolate	De novo purine synthesis in lymphocytes	Gastrointestinal	++++
Cyclosporine	IL2 inhibition in T lymphocytes	Nephropathy	++++
Tacrolimus	IL2 inhibition in T lymphocytes	Nephropathy	++++
Daclizumab	IL2 receptor antibodies	None	++++

RES, reticuloendothelial system.

been the preferred technique for monitoring the rejection status of the cardiac allograft,[w52] based on the ISHLT cardiac allograft rejection grading system.[11] [w53] Different non-invasive algorithms for cardiac allograft rejection monitoring have been proposed. Early after cardiac transplantation, raised concentrations of inflammatory cells and soluble inflammatory molecules and lower concentrations of immunocompetence markers are associated with impaired allograft function in the absence of cellular rejection. Based on this, an algorithm incorporating clinical status, graft function, mononuclear cell subset analysis, and endomyocardial biopsy has been proposed.[12] Use of an algorithm combining endomyocardial biopsy, lymphocyte growth assays, and anti-HLA antibody measurements enables prospective stratification of cardiac transplant recipients into risk categories for progression to high grade rejection. Low risk individuals require fewer biopsies, moderate risk individuals require an ongoing schedule of surveillance biopsies, and high risk individuals require rational organisation of interventional strategies aimed at preventing rejection.[13]

Prophylaxis and treatment of infection

Opportunistic infections after transplantation continue to constitute a challenge for management (table 7.8). Cytomegalovirus (CMV) remains the most important infection affecting heart transplant recipients. In the prevention of CMV disease, those at risk of primary disease (donor seropositive, recipient seronegative) should receive prophylaxis.[w54] In many units, oral ganciclovir is now the preferred route of prophylactic treatment. To monitor activity of CMV infection, assessment of viral load has become a valuable tool. *Legionella pneumophila* may cause pneumonia of variable severity after cardiac transplantation. Chlorination and heating of water is an important

preventive measure. Specific cultures in outbreak situations should be considered to identify less frequent *L pneumophila* serotypes and the non-pneumophila *Legionella* species.[w55] *Pneumocystis carinii* pneumonia,[w56] tuberculosis,[w57] toxoplasmosis,[w58] pulmonary aspergillosis,[w59] and other fungal infections [w60] [w61] continue to constitute challenges for the immunocompromised heart transplant recipient. Sulfamethoxazole/trimethoprine is used in most units for *P carinii* pneumonia prophylaxis.

Transplant vasculopathy

Cardiac allograft vasculopathy (CAV), an unusually accelerated and diffuse form of obliterative coronary arteriosclerosis, determines long term function of the transplanted heart and is the major cause of death in the long term after cardiac transplantation. CAV is a complicated interplay between immunologic and non-immunologic factors resulting in repetitive vascular injury and a localised sustained inflammatory response.[w62] Dyslipidemia, oxidant stress, immunosuppressive drugs, and viral infection [w63] appear to be important contributors to disease development. Endothelial dysfunction is an early feature of CAV and progresses over time after transplantation. Early identification of CAV is essential if long term prognosis is to be improved. Annual coronary angiography is performed for diagnostic and surveillance purposes. Intravascular ultrasound is a more sensitive diagnostic tool for early disease stages and has revealed that progressive luminal narrowing in CAV is in part caused by negative vascular remodelling. Because of the diffuse nature of CAV, percutaneous and surgical revascularisation procedures have a limited role. If annual coronarograms demonstrate rapid progression, retransplantation may be considered. Prevention of CAV progression is a primary therapeutic goal.[w64] Unfortunately,

Table 7.7 Methods of cardiac allograft rejection monitoring

Method	Delay	Serial assessment	Costs	Indication of rejection	Sensitivity	Specificity
History	None	Yes	+	Dyspnoea, weight gain, discomfort	+	+
Physical exam	None	Yes	+	Arrhythmia, S3, crackles, JVD, oedema	+	+
ECG	None	Yes	+	Atrial arrhythmias, low voltage	+	+
Pacemaker	Telemetry	Every night	+++	Voltage ↓ 7%	+++	+++
Echo	30 mins	Yes	+++	Isovolumic relaxation time ↓, fractional shortening ↓	+++	+++
Biopsy	24 hours	Max 1/week	+++	Cell infiltrates, haemorrhage	+++	+++
Myosin scan	24 hours	Max 1/3 month	+++	Heart/lung ratio >1.6	+++	+++
MRI	1 hour	Max 1/week	+++	Signal ↑ due to oedema	+++	+++
Immune monitoring	4 hours	Yes	+++	CD4/CD8↑, HLA-DR+/CD14 ↑, IL2↑	+++	+++

JVD, jugular venous distension.

Table 7.8 Management of opportunistic infections after cardiac transplantation

Organism	Test	Treatment
Cytomegalovirus	IE-Gene, PCR, IgM	Gancyclovir, if severe additional CMV antibodies
Herpes simplex virus	IgM	Aciclovir
Varicella-zoster virus	IgM	Aciclovir
Hepatitis B virus	IgM	Lamivudine
Legionella species	Urine antigen, x ray	Erythromycin
Mycobacterium tuberculosis	Ziehl-Neelson	Rifampicin, isoniazid, myambutol
Nocardia asteroides	Brain CT	Sulfamethoxazole/trimethoprim
Pneumocystis carinii	x ray	Sulfamethoxazole/trimethoprim
Toxoplasma gondii	X ray, IFT, CFT, IgA, IgM	Pyrimethamine + sulfadiazine, folic acid
Candida albicans	Direct	Fluconazole, itraconazole
Aspergillus fumigatus	X ray	Itraconazole, amphotericin B, flucytosine
Cryptococcus neoformans	Brain CT	Itraconazole, amphotericin B, flucytosine, or fluconazole
Listeria monocytogenes		CNS: ampicillin + gentamycin

CMV, cytomegalovirus; CT computed tomography; IFT immunofluoresence test; CFT, complement fixation test.

conventional preventative measures have limited effects. Several pharmacological agents, including the calcium channel blocker diltiazem [w65] and statins such as pravastatin[14] or simvastatin,[w66] have been shown to be effective.

Malignancies

Malignancies play a major role as cause of death after cardiac transplantation. In the long term course after cardiac transplantation, the risk of malignancies occurring is 1–2% per year. This risk is 10–100 fold higher than the risk in an age matched control population. Malignant tumours of the skin and lymphomas are the most frequent types, but any solid organ tumour may occur. The incidence of post-transplant lymphoproliferative disorder with a cyclosporine based immunosuppressive regimen is estimated to be around 2–4%[w67] (www.ctstransplant.org) and is a frequent and often fatal complication of organ transplantation. It most often results from an Epstein-Barr virus transformed B cell clone, which expresses B cell surface markers such as CD20. While these lymphomas may respond to reduction of immunosuppression, they may be successfully treated with the CD20 antibody rituximab.[w68]

TRANSPLANT CENTRE PRACTICE AND INFRASTRUCTURE

Improvements in perioperative and post-transplantation care have permitted a safe expansion of both the donor pool and recipient criteria for transplantation in experienced individual centres,[w69] and in multicentre registries such as the Cardiac Transplant Research Database.[w70] At large centres including Columbia University where more than 1200 cardiac transplants have been performed since 1977, with a one year survival rate of approximately 90% and a five year survival rate of approximately 75%, an extensive experience with recipients bridged to transplantation by mechanical assist devices has evolved.[w71] The increasing challenge of providing advanced heart failure care founded on evidence based practice patterns requires reliable outcome data including identification of between centre variability and its causes.[w72] There are only a few reports on this subject. Early data suggested an effect of centre volume,[15] potentially as a surrogate for centre experience.[w27] Recently, a total of 662 patients listed between 1992 and 1995 as UNOS status 1 for heart transplantation by four adult US cardiac transplant centres in an organ procurement organisation were analysed. These cardiac transplant centres demonstrated significant variability in the likelihood of transplantation and survival for patients listed as UNOS

status 1.[w73] In Europe, prompted by results from the German COCPIT study,[5] a Eurotransplant wide analysis of centre specific heart transplant outcomes is currently being undertaken, applying empirical Bayes methods.[w74]

ALLOCATION BASED ON MEDICAL URGENCY VERSUS WAITING TIME

The discussion on the respective roles of medical urgency and waiting time in the listing and allocation cascade was started a decade ago following the finding that the survival benefit of transplantation decreases as the waiting time lengthens.[16] Improvements in medical treatment and identification of risk factors for early mortality may make it possible to defer or avoid transplantation in many patients with advanced heart failure [w75] while selecting those patients for transplantation who are at high risk of dying from heart failure without it. To test the hypothesis that cardiac transplantation confers a higher survival benefit in patients with a high risk of dying from heart failure, randomised clinical trial designs have been discussed.[17] [w76–79] If evidence in support of this hypothesis can be established, an allocation policy may either restrict the waiting list to high risk patients from the beginning or accept all potential candidates on the waiting list and subsequently prioritise according to medical urgency, thereby decreasing the impact of waiting time in the allocation algorithm for cardiac transplantation. The latter change has been suggested by the German Transplantation Society [w80] and the US Department of Health and has been reinforced by the Institute of Medicine of the US National Institutes of Health.[18] As an example for a national allocation system incorporating medical urgency, the UK is divided into donor zones with the size of the zone allocated to each transplant centre based on their activity. Each centre then has local autonomy for allocation of donors within their zone to patients on their waiting list. In addition, approximately 15% of the donor hearts in the UK are allocated through a national high urgency system into which each centre can place a fixed number of patients depending on their transplant activity. The quota mechanism helps prevent abuse of the urgency waiting system (http://www.exeter.nhsia.nhs.uk/products/core/donor/donor.asp).

FUTURE DIRECTIONS
Cell transplantation and regrowth of heart muscle

The concept of regenerating the failing heart is in the experimental stage. Several approaches including transplantation of embryonic cardiomyocytes,[w81] cryopreserved [w82] or bioengineered fetal cardiomyocytes,[w83] neonatal cardiac myocytes, skeletal myoblasts,[w84] autologous smooth muscle cells,[w85] and dermal fibroblasts [w86] have been proposed. Current problems include chronic rejection in allogeneic cells, lack of intercellular gap junction communication, and differential patterns in excitation–contraction coupling in skeletal and cardiac myocytes. Alternatively, lineage negative bone marrow cells[19] or bone marrow derived endothelial precursor cells with phenotypic and functional characteristics of embryonic haemangioblasts have been proposed. The latter can be used to directly induce new blood vessel formation after experimental myocardial infarction, associated with decreased apoptosis of hypertrophied myocytes in the peri-infarct region, long term salvage and survival of viable myocardium, reduction in collagen deposition, and sustained improvement in cardiac function.[20]

Xenotransplantation

Xenotransplantation theoretically provides an unlimited supply of cells, tissues, and organs. The immunological challenge is that the favourite source animal of choice, the pig, and the human recipient were separated in their evolution 90 million years ago, during which time biological characteristics such as anatomy, physiology, and immunology have drifted far apart. The potential individual benefit of a xenograft has to be counterbalanced against the collective risk of xenozoonoses. Ethically, all three monotheistic religions and Hinduism support the idea of saving and improving human life with the help of an animal organ.[w87] According to a committee of the ISHLT, the current experimental results do not presently justify initiating a clinical trial, but because of the immense potential, research in xenotransplantation should be encouraged.[21]

Mechanical circulatory support

Mechanical circulatory support systems are used nowadays frequently to support patients with severe heart failure to transplantation, to recovery, or as destination therapy. While the early totally artificial hearts and ventricular assist devices were mainly driven from an external pneumatic drive unit, the current generation of assist devices are electrically powered, ultracompact, totally implantable, and have small wearable drive/control consoles, allowing patients to return to their daily activities.[w88] Successful bridging to recovery with ventricular support systems has been reported in postcardiotomy cardiogenic shock, acute myocarditis, and in the peri-infarction period. Benefit is related to reduction of left ventricular myocardial wall stress.[w89] Since the REMATCH (randomized evaluation of mechanical assistance for the treatment of congestive heart failure) trial demonstrated a survival benefit from mechanical circulatory support therapy compared to all other options in non-transplant candidates,[3] this will undoubtedly lead to a redefinition of its role in potential cardiac transplantation candidates in the near future.

Smaller rotational[w24] and completely implantable systems[w90] are under evaluation. In order to facilitate evidence based decision making in advanced heart failure therapy with mechanical circulatory support devices, the ISHLT recently inaugurated an International Mechanical Circulatory Support Device Database. This database provides the opportunity for online data entry via the internet and, as a service and motivation for every centre wordwide to participate, continuous centre specific outcome analyses enabling every participating centre to access its own data and view them in relation to the aggregate database (http://www.ishlt.org/regist_mcsd_main.htm).[22]

CONCLUSION

A little more than three decades after the successful implementation of cardiac transplantation, this revolutionary

> ### Cardiac transplantation: key points
>
> ► Advanced heart failure is an increasing epidemiological problem wordwide
> ► Cardiac transplantation has become the gold standard treatment in selected patients during the last 20 years
> ► The numerical disparity between donors and recipients requires equitable solutions
> ► Cardiac transplantation is increasingly restricted to patients at greatest risk of dying
> ► Alternative treatments include neurohormonal blockers and mechanical support devices

concept of advanced heart failure treatment has gained tremendous momentum and is considered the gold standard treatment in selected patients. More specific modalities of immunosuppression continue to decrease the impact of acute and chronic rejection and immunosuppression related side effects. The success of cardiac transplantation has led to a widespread initiation of transplant programmes and an enlargement of cardiac transplantation waiting lists. The increasing numerical disparity between waiting list size and number of donor organ supply has stimulated research to identify those patients who benefit most from cardiac transplantation, as well to develop alternative treatments for advanced heart failure. The success of these new options, specifically the comprehensive blockers of the renin–angiotensin system and adrenergic system, defibrillators, and mechanical circulatory support devices creates the new challenge for cardiac transplantation to define its contemporary role. Against this background of established advanced heart failure management, organ saving surgical approaches (revascularisation, valve repair, ventricular restoration) and new paradigms such as cell transplantation and xenotransplantation must be tested using appropriately designed studies.

REFERENCES

1 **Hosenpud JD**, Bennett LE, Keck BM, et al. The registry of the International Society for Heart and Lung Transplantation: Eighteenth official report – 2000. J Heart Lung Transplant 2001;**20**:805–15.
2 **Packer M**, Coats AJ, Fowler MB, et al for the Carvedilol Prospective Randomized Cumulative Survival Study Group. Effect of carvedilol on survival in severe chronic heart failure. N Engl J Med 2001;**344**:1651–8.
► First demonstration of survival benefit by β blockers in an advanced heart failure population considered elective cardiac transplantation candidates.
3 **Rose EA**, Gelijns AC, Moskowitz AJ, et al. for the REMATCH Study Group. Long-term use of a left ventricular assist device for end-stage heart failure. N Engl J Med 2001;**345**:1435–43.
► First study to test in a randomised design the survival benefit of mechanical circulatory support in advanced heart failure patients.
4 **Hunt SA**. 24th Bethesda conference: cardiac transplantation. J Am Coll Cardiol 1993;**22** (suppl 1):1–64.
5 **Deng MC**, De Meester JMJ, Smits JMA, et al, on behalf of COCPIT Study Group. The effect of receiving a heart transplant: analysis of a national cohort entered onto a waiting list, stratified by heart failure severity. BMJ 2000;**321**:540–5.
► First national cohort study to suggest that survival benefit of cardiac transplantation is restricted to patients at highest risk of dying from heart failure.
6 **Aaronson KD**, Schwartz JS, Chen TMC, et al. Development and prospective validation of a clinical index to predict survival in ambulatory patients referred for cardiac transplant evaluation. Circulation 1997;**95**:2660–7.
7 **Hunt SA**, Baldwin J, Baumgartner W, et al. Cardiovascular management of a potential heart donor: a statement from the Transplantation Committee of the American College of Cardiology. Crit Care Med 1996;**24**:1599–601.
8 **Wheeldon DR**, Potter CD, Oduro A, et al. Transforming the "unacceptable" donor: outcomes from the adoption of a standardized donor management technique. J Heart Lung Transplant 1995;**14**:734–42.
9 **Kobashigawa J**, Miller L, Renlund D, et al. A randomized active-controlled trial of mycophenolate mofetil in heart transplant recipients. Mycophenolate mofetil investigators. Transplantation 1998;**66**:507–15.

10 **Beniaminovitz A**, Itescu S, Lietz K, *et al.* Prevention of rejection in cardiac transplantation by blockade of the interleukin-2 receptor with a monoclonal antibody. *N Engl J Med* 2000;**342**:613-9.

11 **Billingham ME**, Cary NRB, Hammond ME, *et al.* A working formulation for the standardisation of nomenclature in the diagnosis of heart and lung rejection: heart rejection study group. *J Heart Lung Transplant* 1990;**9**:587–93.

12 **Deng MC**, Erren M, Roeder N, *et al.* T-Cell and monocyte subsets, inflammatory molecules, rejection and hemodynamics early after cardiac transplantation. *Transplantation* 1998;**65**:1255–6.

13 **Itescu S**, Tung TC, Burke EM, *et al.* An immunological algorithm to predict risk of high-grade rejection in cardiac transplant recipients. *Lancet* 1998;**352**:263–70.

14 **Kobashigawa JA**, Katznelson S, Laks H, *et al.* Effect of pravastatin on outcomes after cardiac transplantation. *N Engl J Med* 1995;**333**:621–7.

15 **Hosenpud JD**, Breen TJ, Edwards EB, *et al.* The effect of transplant center volume on cardiac transplant outcome. A report of the United Network for Organ Sharing Scientific Registry. *JAMA* 1994;**271**:1844–9.

16 **Stevenson LW**, Hamilton MA, Tillisch IH, *et al.* Decreasing survival benefit from cardiac transplantation for outpatients as the waiting list lengthens. *J Am Coll Cardiol* 1991;**18**:919–25.

17 **Finkelstein MO**, Levin B, Robbins H. Clinical and prophylactic trials with assured new treatment for those at greater risk: I. A design proposal. *Am J Public Health* 1996;**86**:691–5.

18 **Gibbons RD**, Meltzer D, Duan N, and other members of the Institute of Medicine Committee on Organ Procurement and Transplantation. Waiting for organ transplantation. *Science* 2000;**287**:237–8.

19 **Orlic D**, Kajstura J, Chimenti S, *et al.* Bone marrow cells regenerate infarcted myocardium. *Nature* 2001;**410**:701–5.

► **First demonstration of regeneration of infarcted myocardium by intracardiac injection of bone marrow derived stem cells.**

20 **Kocher AA**, Schuster MD, Szabolcs MJ, *et al.* Neovascularization of ischemic myocardium by human bone-marrow-derived angioblasts prevents cardiomyocyte apoptosis, reduces remodeling and improves cardiac function. *Nat Med* 2001;**7**:430–6.

► **First demonstration of neovascularisation and sustained functional improvement of ischaemic myocardium by peripheral venous injection of autologous bone-marrow derived angioblasts.**

21 **Cooper DK**, Keogh AM. The potential role of xenotransplantation in treating endstage cardiac disease: a summary of the report of the Xenotransplantation Advisory Committee of the International Society for Heart and Lung Transplantation. *Curr Opin Cardiol* 2001;**16**:105–9.

22 **Stevenson LW**, Kormos RL, Bourge RC, *et al.* Mechanical cardiac support 2000: current applications and future trial design. June 15-16, 2000 Bethesda, Maryland. *J Am Coll Cardiol* 2001;**37**:340–70.

Additional references appear on the *Heart* website–www.heartjnl.com

8 THE NEED FOR PALLIATIVE CARE IN THE MANAGEMENT OF HEART FAILURE

Christopher Ward

Patients with heart failure and those with advanced malignant disease, who are the main focus of palliative care specialists, share many physical, psychological, and social problems. However, it might be inferred from the respective standard textbooks that cardiology and palliative care are mutually exclusive disciplines; neither refers to the other, the former failing to mention palliative care even when detailing the management of end stage cardiac failure,[1] while the *Oxford textbook of palliative care*[2] does not envisage the extension of palliative care programmes beyond their present scope. There have, however, been a few articles from palliative care teams and cardiologists,[3] epidemiologists,[4] and psychiatrists[5] which have begun to redress this situation by highlighting the problems faced by heart failure patients during the final months and days of life. The identified deficiencies in their care are compelling and need to be addressed. Conventional cardiological treatments are demonstrably inadequate or inappropriate for solving these problems, but some of the skills and experience acquired in palliative care could be adopted, or adapted to do so.

A common misconception is that palliative care is specifically for the management of patients in the terminal stages of malignant disease. This is, in effect, a paraphrase of the *Oxford textbook of palliative care* definition[2] and reflects the origins of palliative care in the hospice movement for the care of cancer patients. The World Health Organization, while also focusing exclusively on cancer patients, elaborates on the scope of the care which should be provided: "the active total care of patients . . .control of pain, of other symptoms and of psychological, social and spiritual problems is paramount".[6] It notes that "Many aspects of palliative care are also applicable earlier in the course of the illness" and that it "offers a support system to help the family cope during the patient's illness".

Medical and lay dictionary definitions are, on the other hand, mutually identical, succinct, and unconditional—"reducing the severity: denoting the alleviation of symptoms without curing the underlying disease"[7] and "palliate and alleviate without curing".[8] Thus, collating these different definitions, palliative care is a patient management strategy which also recognises the needs of their carers, rather than simply providing disease specific treatments, and should be limited neither to cancer patients nor to those near to death. Terminal care, which is included in, but is not synonymous with, palliative care has been defined as "Turning away from active treatment . . .Concentrating on relief of symptoms and support for both patient and family".[9] All doctors caring for patients with progressive debilitating diseases will recognise the merits of the palliative approach, although they may not be familiar with the underlying concepts nor with the language used to describe them.

The cancer patients for whom treatments and communication skills have been developed in palliative care have diseases which are characterised by progressive limitations, a reduced life expectancy, intrusive symptoms and, terminally, by physical and mental distress. The objectives of this article are: (1) to present evidence which shows that these characteristics are shared by heart failure patients; (2) to identify the major needs of and the specific areas of palliative care most relevant to heart failure patients; and (3) to suggest strategies for their implementation.

▶ HEART FAILURE: PROGRESSIVE DESPITE OPTIMUM TREATMENT

The pathophysiological responses to myocardial damage dictate that recovery from congestive cardiac failure is rare. Irrespective of aetiology it is the end result of the same initially adaptive process, ventricular remodelling[10]: global or localised left ventricular hypertrophy followed by dilatation combine to maintain the cardiac output (Starling's law) in the face of an increasing afterload (for example, in hypertension) or of myocardial loss (for example, following myocardial infarction). But progressive dilatation leads to increasing wall stress (Laplace's law) with resultant further dilatation and a currently irreversible downhill cycle. Timely surgery—for example, valve replacement—sometimes permits recovery, but although angiotensin converting enzyme (ACE) inhibitors and β blockers may delay the process in other cases, they are of only temporary benefit. This is reflected in the fragmented information we have on prognosis, recently reviewed.[11] The commonly quoted figures for the mortality of heart failure, 50% after one year in severe cases and 50% after five years in milder cases, reflect the finding of studies based on different populations with varied inclusion and diagnostic criteria and which were completed before the widespread use of ACE inhibitors. Subsequently the CONSENSUS (cooperative North Scandinavian enalapril study)[12] and SOLVD (studies of left ventricular dysfunction)[13] trials showed unequivocally that ACE inhibitors improve quality of life and prognosis for patients with severe left ventricular systolic dysfunction (New York Heart Association (NYHA) functional class IV). In the CONSENSUS study the one year mortality for the enalapril treated group was 36% compared with 52% of the placebo group. This equates to a mortality reduction of 40% at six months and of 31% at one year.

Impressive though these figures are, they can be misleading as they do not indicate life expectancy—that is, months/years of remaining life. This is the most relevant figure for individual patients, but can only be derived from the mean or the median survival times.[14] The formula for calculating mean survival incorporates the time for all patients to die, and that for median survival for 50% to die, but most trials are completed before this time has lapsed; average follow up in the CONSENSUS trial was only 188 days—less than six months—at which time approximately 75% of patients were still alive. However, a 10 year review of the original cohort has been published.[15] No placebo group patients survived and only 4% of those on treatment did so. The mean increase in life span was only 260 days. Even this figure overestimates the prognosis of "real" patients. Excluded from the trial were patients with pulmonary disease, a creatinine concentration of > 300 mmol/l, an atypical presentation, and the 17% who were withdrawn "for various reasons"—and presumably also those who failed or were unable to attend hospital.

Furthermore, in practice, the majority of patients are still either prescribed an ACE inhibitor in what is regarded as a suboptimal dose or not at all. The use of ACE inhibitors was, however, credited with the observed increase in life expectancy of heart failure patients hospitalised in Scotland between 1986 and 1995 (from 1.23 years to 1.64 years—20 weeks).[16] This is probably a more realistic figure than that from the CONSENSUS trial, although it also is likely to be inaccurate—in this case because of the vagaries of the *International Classification of Diseases* (ICD) diagnostic coding used and the exclusion of patients who were not hospitalised.

The results of β blocker trials are, like those with ACE inhibitors, both impressive and deceptive.[17] The one year mortality in NYHA class II–IV patients was reduced by 30–65% by the addition of a β blocker to an ACE inhibitor, but many patients were excluded, follow up was for just 0.5 to 1.3 years, and only approximately 10% of eligible patients are currently treated. In reality the outlook for most patients with heart failure has probably changed little since these drugs were introduced and as the disease progresses, symptoms become more intrusive and the quality of life deteriorates.[18]

REPORTED SYMPTOMS AND ADEQUACY OF CONTROL

Cardiologists are used to documenting and quantifying the progressive breathlessness and fatigue in heart failure patients, but these objective clinical statements do not accurately portray quality of life (defined as "the difference between patient's perceived expectation and achievement").[19] In the UK approximately 60 000 deaths per year are attributed to cardiac failure and for many patients their final months of life are characterised by distressing and poorly controlled

Table 8.1 Common inadequately treated symptoms in heart failure patients (%)

Symptom	Terminally ill patients[4] Symptoms in final week in parentheses	Ambulant patients attending a heart failure clinic[3]
Pain	78 (63)	41
Breathlessness	61 (51)	83
Mental disturbance		
Low mood	59	41
Insomnia	45	
Anxiety	30	
Anorexia	43	21
Constipation	37	12
Nausea/vomiting	32	17
Tiredness	ND	82
Walking difficulty	ND	65
Oedema	ND	33

ND, not documented.

symptoms. This is shown by a study in which a relative or other carer of 600 patients who died from heart disease, but not necessarily cardiac failure (ICD codes 391–429) were subsequently questioned.[4] The most frequently reported symptoms are shown in table 8.1. It can be deduced from the report that:

▶ psychological or other non-cardiac symptoms were often the most distressing
▶ hospitalisation provided suboptimal or negligible symptom relief in 60–75% of patients
▶ in approximately a third of cases management plans ignored the patients wishes.

Inadequate symptom control is not confined to patients with severe heart failure. We compared the needs of patients attending South Manchester University Hospital NHS Trust heart failure clinic, two thirds of whom were in NYHA class I or II, with those of cancer patients (table 8.1).[3] Many problems were common to both groups. In the heart failure patients non-cardiac symptoms were attributable to: (1) the frequently documented co-morbidities including chronic obstructive pulmonary disease, arthropathies, and diabetes; (2) side effects of medications; and (3) the psychological and social consequences of a chronic progressive illness. We observed that even in a well established multidisciplinary clinic, approximately 60% of patients felt that one or more of their problems (cardiac, non-cardiac or psychological) were inadequately addressed. Although in some instance this occurred because of non-disclosure of a problem, it was usually because of non-documentation or from a failure to treat documented symptoms. However, appropriate action was taken in 71% of cases as a result of the study. The simple expedient of asking "What are your three most troublesome problems?" often exposed previously unrevealed symptoms.

A report from the USA, but confined to the terminally ill, provides complementary data.[20] Close relatives or other carers of 236 patients who died in hospital from cardiac failure were interviewed about symptoms during the last 48–72 hours of life. Severe symptoms had been experienced by the majority of patients (breathlessness 66%, pain 45%, and severe confusion 15%) and during the same period of time, almost 40% had had at least one major therapeutic intervention; tube feeding, ventilation or cardiopulmonary resuscitation. Many patients would have preferred comfort to aggressive treatment, but communication with patients about this was uncommon. Poor communication about patients wishes is a common theme of reports into the care of the terminally ill as was noted above.

STRATEGIES FOR IMPROVING SYMPTOM CONTROL

Conventional cardiological drugs demonstrably fail to control the predominant cardiac symptoms of heart failure patients (fatigue and dyspnoea), are not relevant for the control of the non-cardiac symptoms, and are inappropriate for terminal care. However, palliative care specialists are adept at treating many of the identified (non-cardiac) gastrointestinal problems and genitourinary and psychological symptoms for which well tried management protocols have been summarised.[21] But for many patients the distressing breathlessness of chronic pulmonary oedema remains dominant. The physiological actions of the opioids morphine and, in the UK and Canada, heroin are still poorly understood but several actions, beneficial for the treatment of left ventricular failure, have been identified[22]:

- depression of sympathetic vascular reflexes and histamine release cause arteriolar and venodilatation with resultant reduction in pre- and afterload
- reduced responsiveness of the dominant respiratory control centre, which is the carbon dioxide sensitive medullary reflex; as a result, the increase in respiratory rate in response to afferent stimuli from the lungs is decreased
- a central narcotic action reduces the usually associated mental distress.

The value of opioids in the treatment of acute left ventricular failure is unchallenged. They are also extensively employed in the palliative management of dyspnoea caused by lung tumours and by chronic obstructive pulmonary disease, but their use is not mentioned in detailed discussions of management options for intractable cardiac failure found in cardiology textbooks.[1] The reasons for this omission are unclear, but are probably related to concerns about one or more of three properties of the drugs: psychological dependence, tolerance, and physical dependence. Extensive experience in palliative care shows that such concerns are, in practice, misplaced.[23] Psychological dependence ("addiction") rarely if ever occurs in the palliative care setting. Tolerance— that is, the need for increasing the dosage of opioid to control symptoms—if it does occur, usually results from worsening of pain rather than tolerance in the pharmacological sense. It is not cited as a problem when prescribed for relief of chronic dyspnoea. Physical dependence is inevitable but irrelevant if the patient remains on treatment and is easily managed using standard detoxification protocols if continuation is not required.[24]

A dosage regimen similar to that used for long term pain control is effective[25]:

- initially 2.5 mg morphine every four hours ("by the clock") and as required at the same dose if necessary
- recalculate the four hourly dose after 1–2 days based on previous 24 hour total (four hourly dosage plus as required)
- recalculate as necessary.

The total daily dose is usually less than that used for pain control. It is essential to use concurrently a standard protocol for the management of constipation which inevitably occurs.[26]

IDENTIFICATION OF THE TERMINAL STAGE OF HEART FAILURE AND ITS MANAGEMENT

Patient management should be tailored to reflect prognosis. This is especially so when life expectation is very limited and a change from active (including palliative) treatment to terminal care is or should be considered appropriate. Palliative care specialists acknowledge that it is often difficult to judge when to do this,[27] a difficulty made worse in heart failure because of the numerous pathological scenarios, an unpredictable response to treatment, and a high incidence of sudden death. This is compounded by a valid concern that a reversible precipitant may be overlooked or that various combinations of inotropes, vasodilators, and diuretics may initiate a remission.

There has been no concerted attempt using objective criteria to identify when the end of life is imminent in individual heart failure patients, but encouraged by the need to prioritise patients for heart transplant waiting lists, efforts have been made to evaluate potential markers of long term and short term survival groups. The predictive accuracy of more than 80 variables has been assessed and comprehensively reviewed.[28] Several sources of error were identified, each common to a number of studies: small sample size, selected populations, interrelated variables (that is, different tests measuring the same phenomenon), short period of follow up, and data handling problems. The reviewers concluded that "few variables predicted consistently". Some markers, such as circulating concentrations of cytokines, endothelin-1, and hormone assays (renin noradrenaline (norepinephrine), atrial natriuretic peptide (ANP)), although useful, either have limited availability or their assay is difficult and time consuming. Some simple routine tests have, however, provided useful information.

A low serum sodium, which is inversely proportional to serum renin, has consistently predicted outcome. In a study of NYHA class IV patients[29] the median survival of those with a serum sodium less than 137 mEq/l (pre-ACE inhibitor treatment) was 164 days compared with 373 days for those with higher values. If the serum sodium was less than 130 mEq/l survival was only 99 days.

Prognosis is related to functional capacity irrespective of how it is measured: NYHA class,[30] six minute walk test,[31] or peak po_2.[32]

Assessed by echocardiography, left ventricular dilatation is predictive of outcome, but ejection fraction is not, probably because of inaccuracies inherent in the calculation used to measure it. However, its measurement by radionuclide ventriculography is useful. In one study,[33] the mortality for patients with mild (81% in NYHA II) cardiac failure was 27% after 16 months if ejection fraction was less than 20%, but only 7% with higher values.

Unfortunately, the use of these tests is often limited in clinical practice. The prognosis of hyponatraemic patients may be improved by ACE inhibitors,[29] although to a lesser extent than in the normonatraemic. Facilities for radionuclide screening are limited, and the assessment of functional capacity is often precluded by non-cardiac impairment of mobility—for example, because of chronic obstructive pulmonary disease or arthritis. Study of prognostic markers is important because it increases our understanding of the pathophysiology of heart failure and may aid treatment; however, those which have been assessed to date, while they may identify high and low risk groups, lack the predictive accuracy to indicate the imminent end of life of individual patients.

An alternative approach to the problem is therefore required. Published protocols for the management of resistant cardiac failure consist, in practice, of "check lists" to ensure that a reversible aetiology or precipitant has not been overlooked, and that all reasonable treatment options have been considered.[1 34] Cardiologists will recognise that the typical patient for whom this process is used has a very poor quality of life, with increasingly frequent hospitalisations or outpatient attendances characterised by worsening oedema and progressive renal failure in the absence of an iatrogenic cause. By this stage, the views of patient and carer on the merits of continuing active treatment should have been sought. Empirical observations (as there is no relevant objective data) suggest that assimilating these three sources of information (simple prognostic indicators, a "check list", and the patient's wishes) and their implications would be an improvement on the present situation. The findings of the SUPPORT (study to understand prognoses and preferences for outcomes and risks of treatment) group,[20] suggest that either such a strategy is not used or that if it is, its inference is ignored. The latter may be the result of a reluctance to acknowledge that a patient is terminally ill because of the implicit finality and failure. This, however, is to misunderstand the dying process which, when well managed, is a gradual and overlapping progression from active through palliative to terminal care; it does not require a sudden treatment change as active measures are often continued to aid patient comfort. This is a positive approach of doing everything possible, not a negative "there is nothing more to be done".

The protocols for patient management during these last days of life are better established than is the timing of their initiation.

Palliative care teams have devised comprehensive integrated care pathways which simply ensure that the physical and psychological problems of the dying and of their carers are conscientiously addressed. Concerns that inflexibility in these programmes may not cater for the patient who has an unanticipated remission of symptoms are unfounded since they deliver optimum care, not euthanasia. Provided cardiologists can broadly agree a process which will identify those heart failure patients who appear to be close to the end of life, there is no reason why they should not then benefit from the care and attention offered by the above protocols.

REQUIREMENTS FOR IMPROVED CARE

The quality of life of patients with all grades of heart failure could be significantly improved by applying the management principles advocated in palliative care, fundamental to which is good communication. As noted above, communication with heart failure patients is often inadequate, whereas in palliative care good communication with patients is regarded as a pre-requisite for optimum patient care. Clearly this concept of communication is not synonymous with simply asking the correct questions and taking an adequate history. In brief, there are considered to be three main components to good communication[34]: (1) active listening (not a universal attribute of doctors), the specific task of (2) breaking bad news, and (3) therapeutic dialogue. The objective of this process is to ensure that the patient understands the implications of his illness and that his concerns and aspirations are addressed. The skills required to achieve these outcomes sensitively will have to be learned. The fact that so much time is devoted to writing about and studying this topic reflects its perceived importance: "No-one who hasn't time for chat knows anything about terminal care".[35] The other relevant aspects of established palliative care, treatment schedules for the control of non-cardiac symptoms, and the management of the final days of life will need to be integrated into cardiological practice through collaboration between cardiologists and palliative care specialists.

In addition there is a need for research into the use and actions of opioids in chronic left ventricular failure. This should include the evaluation of different treatment regimens, the use of alternative opioid delivery systems (for example, nasal sprays which have been shown to relieve anxiety rapidly), and the role of newer opioids such as

Palliative care in heart failure: key points

- ▶ Heart failure and the conditions managed by palliative care specialists share many features: inexorably progressive debilitation, a deteriorating quality of life and, unless conscientiously addressed, distressing symptoms, especially at the end of life
- ▶ In end stage heart failure a strategy is urgently needed to ensure a timely progressive move away from invasive treatment towards supportive terminal care
- ▶ The views of heart failure patients on how they would prefer to be treated are often either not sought or are unheeded
- ▶ Palliative care specialists have developed treatment strategies which effectively control many of the distressing symptoms reported by heart failure patients and for which conventional cardiological treatments are ineffective or inappropriate
- ▶ There is no practical reason why the regular use of morphine should not be considered as routine for the treatment of the dyspnoea of chronic heart failure
- ▶ The basic principles of palliative care—good communication and close attention to symptom control—should be adopted to improve the quality of life of heart failure patients
- ▶ The teaching of these techniques and skills should be included in training programmes for prospective cardiologists

fentanyl. These changes are not only necessary to improve patient care, but are also important for an often ignored group—the relatives and the carers. It is a tenet of palliative care that the way in which people die remains in the memories of their survivors.[36]

It is unrealistic to expect every cardiologist to become proficient in the various aspects of palliative care. It is, however, important to acknowledge the benefits which palliative care has to offer and to encourage their adoption, either by interested cardiological colleagues, by professionals with a palliative care training, or by a combination of the two. To ensure adequate expertise among cardiologists an educational module in palliative care should be developed and incorporated into cardiology training courses. Currently many cardiologists with a major interest in heart failure devote considerable time to research. The demonstrated increasing burden of treating heart failure will dictate the need to develop heart failure as a clinical subspecialty whose practitioners would logically take on the role of developing and providing a palliative care service.

Cardiology is a speciality in which interventional treatments continue to make dramatic improvements to patient's prognosis and quality of life. At the same time, however, we should remember that: "The terminally ill fear the unknown more than the known, professional disinterest more than professional ineptitude, the process of dying rather than death itself".[37]

REFERENCES

1 **Chatterjee K**, Demarco T. Management of refractory heart failure. In: Poole-Wilson PA, *et al*, eds. *Heart failure*. Churchill Livingstone, 1997:853–74.
2 **Doyle D**, Hanks G, McDonald N. What is palliative medicine? In Doyle D, Hanks G, McDonald N, eds. *Oxford textbook of palliative medicine*. Oxford: Oxford Medical Publications, 1994:3.
3 **Anderson H**, Ward C, Eardley A, *et al*. The concerns of patients under palliative care and a heart failure clinic are not being met. *Palliative Medicine* 2001;**15**:279–86.
4 **McCarthy M**, Lay M, Addington-Hall J. Dying from heart disease. *J R Coll Phys London* 1996;**30**:325–8.
▶ Recent interest in palliative care for heart failure patients can be dated from the publication of this article.

5 **Hinton JM**. The physical and mental distress of the dying. *QJM* 1963;**32**:1–20.

6 **World Health Organization**. *Cancer pain relief and palliative care.* Technical report series 804. Geneva: WHO, 1990.

7 **Dirckx JH ed**. *Stedman's concise medical and allied health dictionary.* Baltimore: Williams & Wilkins, 1997:644.

8 **Sykes JB**, ed. *Concise Oxford dictionary*, 7th ed. Oxford: Oxford University Press, 1984:737.

9 **Saunders C**. Terminal care. In: Weatherall DJ, Ledingham JGG, Warrell DA, eds. *Oxford textbook of medicine*, 2nd ed. Oxford: Oxford Medical Publications 1987:28.1–28.13.

10 **Bozkurt B**. Medical and surgical therapy for cardiac remodelling *Curr Opin Cardiol* 1999;**14**:196–205.

11 **McMurray JJ**, Stewart S. Epidemiology, aetiology and prognosis of heart failure. *Heart* 2000;**83**:596–602.

▶ **A useful review of the major studies with valuable comments on their significance and shortcomings.**

12 **The CONSENSUS Trial Study Group**. Effects of enalapril on mortality in severe congestive heart failure. Results of the co-operative North Scandinavian enalapril study group (CONSENSUS). *N Engl J Med* 1987;**316**:1429–35.

13 **The SOLVD Investigators**. Effect of enalapril on survival in patients with reduced left ventricular ejection fractions and congestive heart failure. *N Engl J Med* 1991;**325**:293–302.

14 **Torp-Pedersen C**, Kober L. Prolongation of life with angiotensin converting inhibitor therapy. *Eur Heart J* 2000;**21**:597–8.

15 **Swedberg K**, Kjekshus J, Snapinn S, for the CONSENSUS Investigators. Longterm survival in severe heart failure patients treated with enalapril. *Eur Heart J* 1999;**20**:136–9.

16 **MacIntyre K**, Capewell S, Stewart S et al. Evidence of improving prognosis in heart failure *Circulation* 2000;**102**:1126–31.

17 **McMurray JJV**. Major β blocker mortality trials in chronic heart failure: a critical review. *Heart* 1999;**82**(suppl IV):IV14–22.

▶ **A detailed review and comparative analysis of the US carvedilol programme and of the CIBIS II and MERIT-HF trial including summaries of the findings of each study and an assessment of their significance.**

18 **Dracup K**, Walden JA, Stevenson LW, et al. Quality of life in patients with advanced heart failure. *J Heart Lung Transplant* 1992;**11**:273–9

19 **Calman KC**. Quality of life in cancer patients: an hypothesis. *J Med Ethics* 1984;**10**:124–7.

20 **The SUPPORT Investigators**. A controlled trial to improve care for seriously ill hospitalised patients. *JAMA* 1995;**274**:1591–8.

21 **Saunders C**. Terminal care. In: Weatherall DJ, Ledingham JGG, Warrell DA, eds. *Oxford textbook of medicine*, 2nd ed. Oxford: Oxford Medical Publications, 1987:28.7–28.8

22 **Ahmedzai S**. Palliation of respiratory symptoms. In: Doyle D, Hanks G, Mcdonald N. *Oxford textbook of palliative medicine*. Oxford: Oxford Medical Publications, 1994:362–4.

23 **Doyle D**, Benton TF. *Pain and symptom control in terminal care.* Edinburgh: St Colomba's Hospice, 1986:7.

24 **Inturissi CE**, Hanks G. Opioid and analgesic therapy. In: Doyle D, Hanks G, McDonald N, eds. *Oxford textbook of palliative care*. Oxford: Oxford Medical Publications, 1994:179.

25 **Grady K**, Severn A. *Key topics in chronic pain: cancer – opioid drugs.* Bios Scientific Publishers, 1997;48–52.

26 **Regnard CFB**, Tempest S. *A guide to symptom relief in advanced cancer*, 3rd ed. Manchester: Haigh & Hochland, 1992:23.

27 **Working Party on Clinical Guidelines in Palliative Care**. *Changing gear – guidelines for managing the last days of life in adults: the research evidence.* London: National Council for Hospital and Specialist Palliative Care Services, 1997.

28 **Cowburn PJ**, Cleland JGF, Coats AJS, et al. Risk stratification in chronic heart failure. *Eur Heart J* 1998;**19**:696–710.

▶ **A comprehensive review which collates the findings of approximately 200 studies. The larger studies are tabulated and ranked in order of significance based on multivariate analysis.**

29 **Lee WH**, Packer M. Prognostic importance of serum sodium concentration and its modification by converting enzyme inhibition in patients with severe chronic heart failure. *Circulation* 1986;**73**:257–67.

30 **Adams KF**, Dunlap SH, Sueta CA, et al. Natural history and patterns of current practice in heart failure. *J Am Coll Cardiol* 1993;**12**:14A–19A.

31 **Bittner V**, Weiner DH, Yusuf S, et al. Prediction of mortality and morbidity with a 6 minute walk test in patients with left ventricular dysfunction. *JAMA* 1993;**270**:1702–7.

32 **Szlachcic J**, Massie BM, Kramer BL, et al. Correlates and prognostic implication of exercise capacity in chronic congestive heart failure. *Am J Cardiol* 1985;**55**:1037–42.

33 **Gradman A**, Deedwania P, Cody R, et al. Predictors of total mortality and sudden death in mild to moderate heart failure. *J Am Coll Cardiol* 1989;**14**:564-70.

34 **Buckman R**. Communication in palliative care: a practical guide. In: Doyle D, Hanks G, McDonald N, eds. *Oxford textbook of palliative care*. Oxford: Oxford Medical Publications, 1994:47–61.

35 **Twycross R**, Lack S. *Oral morphine in advanced cancer*, 2nd ed. Beaconsfield Publishing, 1989:30.

36 **Saunders C**. Terminal care. In: Weatherall DJ, Ledingham JGG, Warrell DA, eds. *Oxford textbook of medicine*, 2nd ed. Oxford: Oxford Medical Publications, 1987:28:12.

37 **Doyle D**, Benton TF. *Pain and symptom control in terminal care.* Edinburgh: St Columba's Hospice, 1986:1.

9 EXERCISE TESTING IN THE ASSESSMENT OF CHRONIC CONGESTIVE HEART FAILURE

John G Lainchbury, A Mark Richards

Despite advances in treatment which have resulted in reductions in morbidity and mortality, heart failure remains a common condition often associated with a poor outcome. In most patients with chronic congestive heart failure, symptoms are not present at rest but become limiting with exertion. Despite this, the majority of measures used to characterise the severity of heart failure and prognosis are obtained at rest.

The New York Heart Association (NYHA) classification attempts to stratify patients according to their exercise limitation, but has a limited relation to objective measures of exercise tolerance and is a very subjective measure of disability. Self administered questionnaires which attempt to assess activity and exercise limitation are unable to measure functional capacity accurately and have only modest correlation with objective parameters such as peak oxygen uptake ($p\dot{V}_{O_2}$).

Making the diagnosis of heart failure can be difficult. Signs and symptoms lack both sensitivity and specificity. Although objective resting measures, such as left ventricular ejection fraction, can define structural cardiac abnormality, they are by no means synonymous with the diagnosis of heart failure. A further issue is the increased recognition of heart failure in subjects with normal left ventricular ejection fraction, and the difficulty of diagnosis in this patient group.

Exercise testing of patients, in combination with assessment of gas exchange parameters, is an attractive and practical method of obtaining accurate information which can aid in the diagnosis of heart failure as well as the assessment of functional limitation and prognosis.

Directly measured maximum oxygen uptake (more correctly $p\dot{V}_{O_2}$ in heart failure patients) has been shown to be a reproducible marker of exercise tolerance in heart failure and provide objective and additional information regarding patients clinical status and prognosis. Facilities for exercise testing with continuous measurement of gas exchange parameters are increasingly available.

► PRACTICAL ISSUES IN EXERCISE TESTING

Exercise testing with concurrent measurement of gas exchange parameters can be undertaken using either treadmill or bicycle exercise protocols (table 9.1). Peak $\dot{V}_{O_2}$ has been found to be 10–20% higher on treadmill exercise compared to bicycle exercise. Patient familiarity is important and subjects who are unaccustomed to riding bicycles may be unable to sustain bicycle exercise for as long because of leg fatigue. It is important that patients are given time to become accustomed to the requirements of the exercise test in order to obtain peak exercise capacity. This involves practising getting on and off the treadmill or adjusting bicycle pedals to an appropriate height, as well as becoming familiar with the mask or mouthpiece and nose clip.

In order to obtain valid data with regard to peak exercise parameters in patients with cardiac disease, it is important that subjects exceed the anaerobic threshold or that the respiratory exchange ratio (the ratio of carbon dioxide production to oxygen consumption) is greater than 1 to indicate adequate effort. With regard to this, peak exercise parameters are affected by patient motivation and perceived symptoms as well as patient familiarity, and experienced medical and technical personnel are required when performing these tests to obtain adequate data.

Ideally the exercise protocol should be individualised for each patient. Small increments in exercise load and total duration of around 8–12 minutes are ideal. Ramp protocols, where workload increases continuously, are available for both bicycle and treadmill exercise.

There may be concerns about the safety of exercise testing of patients with significant heart failure. Available data suggest a very low incidence of serious adverse events such as arrhythmias or significant hypotension. In a study of 607 patients with a history of heart failure and average left ventricular ejection fraction of 30% who underwent symptom limited exercise testing, only 10 patients' exercise tests were stopped because of arrhythmia, and only one of these subjects had ventricular tachycardia.[1] Only one exercise test was stopped because of hypotension. Commonsense precautions, such as avoiding exercising patients with unstable symptoms, active arrhythmia or critical valvar stenosis, should be taken.

Table 9.1 Suggestions for obtaining an adequate exercise test

▶ Avoid unstable patients
▶ Ensure patient familiarity with equipment and requirements of the test
▶ Individualise the protocol (ramp protocol preferred)
▶ Optimal duration 8–12 minutes
▶ Consider using submaximal data in those unable to perform maximal test—for example, early slope of ventilation versus CO_2 production, six minute walk

---

EXERCISE TESTING IN THE DIAGNOSIS OF HEART FAILURE

A normal exercise test with gas exchange monitoring virtually excludes congestive heart failure as a cause for patient symptoms.[2]

Easily obtained variables help to distinguish between cardiac and pulmonary causes of breathlessness and exercise limitation. For example, subjects with pulmonary disease often experience a decrease in oxygen saturation with exercise, while in subjects with cardiac disease oxygen saturation remains unchanged or increases (table 9.2, fig 9.1).

This ability to differentiate the cause of shortness of breath may be useful in subjects with heart failure caused by diastolic dysfunction where differentiation from other causes of shortness of breath may be very difficult.

EXERCISE TESTING IN DEFINING PROGNOSIS IN HEART FAILURE

Most investigators have found that $p\dot{V}O_2$ is the best indicator of prognosis in patients with heart failure. This well established variable can be thought of as integrating a number of factors which determine the severity of heart failure and the degree of functional limitation including cardiac reserve, skeletal muscle function, pulmonary abnormalities, and endothelial dysfunction.[3]

Peak $\dot{V}O_2$ correlates poorly with haemodynamic factors measured at rest which is consistent with the fact that these resting parameters do not reflect functional reserve. There is, however, a good correlation between maximum cardiac output and $p\dot{V}O_2$.[4]

The factors that appear to be important in determining $p\dot{V}O_2$ are outlined in table 9.3.

The measurement of $p\dot{V}O_2$ was first described by Webber and colleagues as a method for characterising cardiac reserve and functional status in heart failure.[5] Subsequently $p\dot{V}O_2$ has been shown by a number of investigators to be of prognostic significance, with lower $p\dot{V}O_2$ predicting mortality and the need for cardiac transplantation. For example, Szlachcic and colleagues studied 27 patients with heart failure and reported a 77% one year mortality rate in those with $p\dot{V}O_2 < 10$ ml/kg/min and 21% mortality rate in those with $p\dot{V}O_2$ between 10–18 ml/kg/min.[6] A further study of 201 heart failure patients found that $p\dot{V}O_2$ was an independent predictor of mortality.[7] Many other studies have confirmed these findings.

Cardiac transplantation is an important and successful treatment for end stage heart failure but its major limitation continues to be a shortage of appropriate donors. Therefore, accurate selection of those patients who will benefit most from transplantation is important. In this regard exercise parameters, in particular $p\dot{V}O_2$, have been found to be very important. Measurement of $p\dot{V}O_2$ in the assessment of subjects for cardiac transplantation is now endorsed within guidelines.[8]

In a widely quoted study Mancini and colleagues reported on 116 patients who were referred for assessment for cardiac transplantation (fig 9.2).[9] Thirty five of the patients had a $p\dot{V}O_2$ of < 14 ml/kg/min; these patients were accepted for cardiac transplantation. A further 52 patients had a $p\dot{V}O_2 > 14$ ml/kg/min and in these subjects transplantation was deferred. In addition to these two groups, a further 27 patients had $p\dot{V}O_2 < 14$ ml/kg/min but had other comorbidities which meant that they were not suitable for cardiac transplantation. One year survival in those with $p\dot{V}O_2 > 14$ ml/kg/min was 94%, while in those with $p\dot{V}O_2$ below this cut-off in whom transplantation was not carried out because of comorbidities, survival at one year was only 47%. In the subjects with $p\dot{V}O_2 < 14$ml/kg/min accepted for transplantation, one year survival while waiting for transplantation was 70%, and if urgent transplantation was counted as death one year survival was reduced to 48%. One year survival of 24 patients with a $p\dot{V}O_2 < 14$ ml/kg/min after transplantation was 83%. These results clearly demonstrate that low $p\dot{V}O_2$ identified a group of heart failure patients at high risk of death or need for urgent transplantation and that those subjects with higher $p\dot{V}O_2$ could have transplantation deferred.

Attempts have been made to use percentage of predicted $p\dot{V}O_2$ to improve the prognostic power of this measure. Percentage of predicted $p\dot{V}O_2$ may account for factors such as age, sex, and muscle mass which may have a significant impact on $p\dot{V}O_2$. In a study of 272 patients referred for transplantation, subjects were divided by strata of $p\dot{V}O_2$ uptake and percentage of predicted $p\dot{V}O_2$.[10] These strata were designed to be of similar size. In this study survival curves were found to be similar whether the strata were classified by $p\dot{V}O_2$ or percentage of predicted $p\dot{V}O_2$. Others have found that percentage of $p\dot{V}O_2$ is a better prognostic marker than $p\dot{V}O_2$, with 50% of predicted $p\dot{V}O_2$ the most significant predictor of death.[11] It is likely that in some patients, percentage of $p\dot{V}O_2$ would be more useful—for example, at the extremes of age and possibly in women.

Table 9.2 Response to exercise in cardiac versus pulmonary disease

Variable	Cardiac disease	Pulmonary disease
Peak $\dot{V}O_2$	Reduced	Reduced
Heart rate reserve	Usually none	Increased
Anaerobic threshold	Reduced (<40% predicted)	Normal or not achieved
Oxygen pulse	Reduced	Normal
$\dot{V}O_2$ workload ratio	Reduced	Normal
Peak PaO_2 or O_2 saturation	Normal	Decreased

Peak $\dot{V}O_2$, peak oxygen uptake; Heart rate reserve, difference between predicted maximum heart rate and attained heart rate with maximum exercise; Oxygen pulse, O_2 uptake divided by heart rate, represents O_2 extracted by the tissues from O_2 carried in each stroke volume; $\dot{V}O_2$ workload ratio, represents the efficiency of muscular work; PaO_2, arterial oxygen tension.

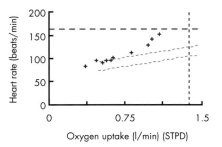

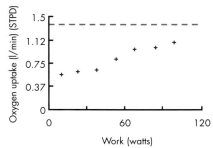

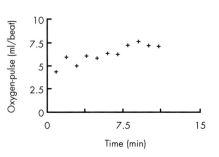

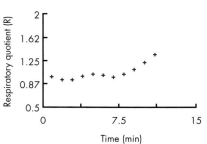

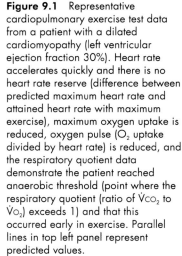

Figure 9.1 Representative cardiopulmonary exercise test data from a patient with a dilated cardiomyopathy (left ventricular ejection fraction 30%). Heart rate accelerates quickly and there is no heart rate reserve (difference between predicted maximum heart rate and attained heart rate with maximum exercise), maximum oxygen uptake is reduced, oxygen pulse (O_2 uptake divided by heart rate) is reduced, and the respiratory quotient data demonstrate the patient reached anaerobic threshold (point where the respiratory quotient (ratio of $\dot{V}CO_2$ to $\dot{V}O_2$) exceeds 1) and that this occurred early in exercise. Parallel lines in top left panel represent predicted values.

Table 9.3 Factors determining exercise capacity

▶ Central factors: resting ventricular function, chronotropic response, stroke volume response
▶ Peripheral factors: skeletal muscle mass, skeletal muscle vascular function, endothelial function, autocrine/paracrine factors
▶ Pulmonary function and pulmonary response to exercise
▶ Neurohormonal systems including sympathetic nervous system, other vasodilator and vasoconstrictor systems

---

Although a $p\dot{V}O_2$ < 14 ml/kg/min is well known as a measure for deciding on eligibility for cardiac transplantation, it has been clearly shown that there is no absolute threshold for adverse prognosis and that $p\dot{V}O_2$ uptake should be considered as a continuous variable. In terms of discriminating survivors from non-survivors, it appears that a $p\dot{V}O_2$ < 10 ml/kg/min definitely defines high risk, while a value > 18 ml/kg/min defines low risk; those values in between may represent a grey zone. Attempts have been made to stratify further the group with a $p\dot{V}O_2$ uptake of < 14 ml/kg/min. In a study of 500 patients, 154 had $p\dot{V}O_2$ < 14 ml/kg/min.[12] Using all the non-invasive parameters measured during exercise testing in a multivariate analysis including peak heart rate, systolic blood pressure, respiratory quotient, minute ventilation, $p\dot{V}O_2$, percentage of predicted $p\dot{V}O_2$, and anaerobic threshold it was found that a peak systolic blood pressure < 120 mm Hg and percentage of predicted $p\dot{V}O_2$ were significant prognostic indicators. Three year survival in those with a $p\dot{V}O_2$ < 14 ml/kg/min but > 50% of the predicted maximal value was similar to those with a $p\dot{V}O_2$ > 14 ml/kg/min. Survival was 55% if peak exercise blood pressure was < 120 mm Hg, while it was 83% with a peak systolic blood pressure of > 120 mm Hg.

A number of investigators have attempted to combine $p\dot{V}O_2$ and haemodynamic variables in an effort to improve prognostic power. Chomsky and colleagues, in a study of 185 ambulatory heart failure patients with an average $p\dot{V}O_2$ uptake of 12.9 ml/kg/min, calculated cardiac output from the $\dot{V}O_2$ data.[13] In multivariate analysis a $p\dot{V}O_2$ < 10 ml/kg/min and a reduced cardiac output response to exercise were predictive of one year survival. Directly measured haemodynamics can be added but

may considerably increase the risk and difficulty of exercise testing, and may be of limited additional benefit. End systolic stroke work index has been shown to add to the prognostic power of $p\dot{V}O_2$.[14] However, in addition to requiring invasive measurements this variable is not accurate in the presence of significant mitral regurgitation.

There has been recent interest in using the slope of the relation between minute ventilation ($\dot{V}E$) and carbon dioxide production ($\dot{V}CO_2$) in assessing the prognosis of subjects with heart failure. There is a linear correlation between minute ventilation and carbon dioxide production until anaerobic threshold is reached. Subjects with a steeper response have decreased cardiac output, increased pulmonary pressures, and increased dead space to tidal volume ratio as well as possibly augmented chemoreceptor sensitivity. The slope of the relation between $\dot{V}E$ and $\dot{V}CO_2$ has been shown to be predictive of survival in addition to $p\dot{V}O_2$.[15] Others have looked at the slope of the relation between $\dot{V}E$ and $\dot{V}CO_2$ within the first six minutes of exercise, and while this was predictive of survival it was not as strong a prognostic indicator as $p\dot{V}O_2$.[16] However, this measure may be useful if maximum exercise is not obtained. $\dot{V}O_2$ at anaerobic threshold has been considered as a prognostic marker, but it does not outperform $p\dot{V}O_2$ and problems exist with defining and determining this variable.

There are a large number of other well recognised prognostic markers in heart failure which are not exercise related. An attempt to combine these variables along with exercise data in pretransplant risk stratification has been reported.[17] A heart failure survival score was developed using 268 ambulatory patients from the University of Pennsylvania Hospital from July 1986 to January 1993. The model was subsequently validated in a group of 199 patients at Colombia Presbyterian Hospital who were followed from July 1993 to October 1995. The model contained 80 clinical variables from each patient that were derived from history, laboratory data, exercise data, catheterisation data, and physical examination. Significant univariate predictors were subsequently analysed using multivariate techniques where the variables were grouped and prognostic factors thought to represent different aspects of heart failure were incorporated into the model. One statistical model incorporated seven non-invasive parameters which

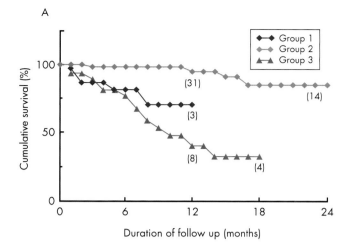

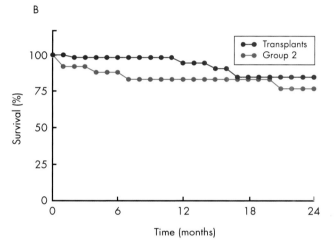

Figure 9.2 (A) Survival curves for patients with heart failure. Group 1 (n = 35) represents survival while waiting for transplantation in patients accepted for transplantation with pVo_2 < 14 ml/kg/min. Group 2 (n = 52) comprises patients with pVo_2 > 14 ml/kg/min in whom transplantation was deferred. Group 3 (n = 27) comprises patients with pVo_2 < 14 ml/kg/min rejected for transplantation because of non-cardiac problems. Survival of groups 1 and 3 are similar but significantly reduced compared to group 2. Numbers in parentheses represent number of subjects at risk. (B) Survival curves for group 1 patients after transplantation (n = 24) and for medically treated patients (group 2). Difference in survival is not significant. Reproduced from Mancini et al[9] with permission.

included the presence of ischaemic heart disease, resting heart rate, left ventricular ejection fraction, mean arterial pressure, presence of intraventricular conduction defect on ECG, serum sodium, and pVo_2. This model (the heart failure survival score, HFSS) provided excellent ability to predict survival, and in the validation group the model performed better than pVo_2 alone. Interestingly, in the sample used to derive the model pVo_2 alone performed as well as the model.

Limited data are available on serial exercise testing and prognosis. It has been suggested that increases in pVo_2 on serial tests are predictive of better survival, although this has not been supported in other studies.[18 19]

As mentioned above, measuring the slope of the relation between $\dot{V}E$ and $\dot{V}co_2$ in the initial stages of exercise may provide useful prognostic information in those unable to obtain maximum exercise, or if maximum exercise is contra-indicated. Others have attempted to predict pVo_2 from the initial stages of exercise testing. In general these measures are less predictive of prognosis than pVo_2 but may be useful when maximum exercise is not possible.

The six minute walk test has been used as a submaximal exercise test in heart failure subjects. There are some conflicting data about the value of the six minute walk test. It may be useful in discriminating high risk from low risk. In a recent study of 315 patients with moderate to severe heart failure, six minute walk distance was not related to central haemodynamics and only moderately related to exercise capacity.[20] In that study six minute walk distance was not an independent predictor of prognosis in models that contained either NYHA class or pVo_2

COMBINING EXERCISE PARAMETERS WITH OTHER NOVEL PREDICTORS OF PROGNOSIS IN HEART FAILURE

Functional reserve as defined by an increase in left ventricular ejection fraction during dobutamine infusion has been shown to be a multivariate predictor of survival in heart failure. This may be helpful in those with intermediate values of pVo_2. The ability of dobutamine assessed cardiac reserve to stratify prognosis in subjects with non-ischaemic dilated cardiomyopathy has been assessed in a study of 27 patients with pVo_2 between 10–14 ml/kg/min.[21] Dobutamine was infused at 10 µg/kg/min and the increase in ejection fraction measured. This particular range of pVo_2 was chosen as it was felt to represent a grey zone in which further risk stratification in terms of selection for transplantation may be useful. After a mean follow up of 18 months, changes in left ventricular end systolic dimension and end systolic wall stress were found to be significantly different between those who died of cardiac causes (n = 9) and those who survived (n = 18). This finding suggests that dobutamine echocardiography may be a useful prognostic indicator in addition to pVo_2 in those being considered for cardiac transplantation who have a low pVo_2 uptake.

It is known that the restrictive left ventricular filling pattern defined by transmitral Doppler echocardiography is a predictor of mortality in heart failure in those with impaired left ventricular function. This parameter has been compared to pVo_2 uptake.[22] While a restrictive filling pattern was shown to be a better predictor than ejection fraction, it did not perform as well as pVo_2 in the assessment of prognosis.

It has been known for some time that neurohormonal factors are predictive of survival in heart failure when measured at rest. Measurement of plasma natriuretic peptides in particular has often been shown to perform better as a prognostic marker than other established rest parameters such as left ventricular ejection fraction. There has been some interest in the use of these factors in combination with exercise testing in prediction of prognosis in heart failure. In a study of 264 patients with moderate heart failure, atrial natriuretic peptide (ANP), noradrenaline (norepinephrine), and endothelin-1 were measured at rest and a maximum exercise test was undertaken.[23] It was found that ANP, left ventricular ejection fraction, and noradrenaline predicted death or transplantation. In this study pVo_2 was not predictive. In a further study in which maximum exercise workload was measured, endothelin-1 and ANP measured at rest were again shown to convey independent prognostic power.[24] One study has reported both rest and peak exercise neurohormonal data.[25] Fifty five consecutive ambulatory patients with stable, moderate congestive heart failure (NYHA functional class II–III) underwent maximum symptom limited cardiopulmonary exercise testing with determination of peak oxygen

Exercise testing in assessing CHF: key points

- ► Exercise testing with monitoring of gas exchange parameters provides useful information on exercise capacity and prognosis in heart failure; in addition it is helpful in establishing the cause of exercise limitation
- ► Both treadmill and bicycle protocols are acceptable, but attention to technical aspects of exercise testing are important in order to obtain maximum exercise data
- ► Peak $\dot{V}O_2$ is probably the strongest predictor of prognosis in heart failure but other exercise, clinical, and hormonal data must be taken into account in arriving at an assessment of prognosis.
- ► In subjects unable to perform a maximal exercise test submaximal data such as the slope of the relation between $\dot{V}E$ and $\dot{V}CO_2$ may be useful
- ► Further studies of the response of neurohormones to exercise may add to the utility of exercise tests in assessing prognosis

consumption, and measurement of plasma ANP, aldosterone, and plasma renin activity at rest and peak exercise. There was no correlation between exercise parameters and hormone values either at rest or at peak exercise. At a median follow up of 724 days the most significant independent prognostic marker was the plasma concentration of ANP at peak exercise.

We have undertaken a study in 68 patients with NYHA class III–IV heart failure and average $p\dot{V}O_2$ of 13.6 ml/kg/min. Natriuretic peptide plasma concentrations were measured at rest and with peak exercise. In multivariate analysis which included $p\dot{V}O_2$, only change in brain natriuretic peptide (BNP) with exercise or a fall versus an increase in BNP with exercise added prognostic power for survival in addition to left ventricular ejection fraction at rest. Fifteen subjects had a decrease in plasma BNP with exercise and over an average follow up of two years seven (45%) of these patients died, compared with only eight out of 53 (15%) in those with a rise in BNP during exercise (p < 0.01).[26]

From the limited information available, the addition of neurohormonal data, in particular measurement of natriuretic peptide plasma concentrations and their response to exercise, offer promise in the assessment of subjects with heart failure.

CONCLUSIONS

Congestive heart failure is characterised by symptoms with activity. Exercise testing is useful in the diagnosis of heart failure, assessing functional capacity objectively, and in determining prognosis. It appears that if maximum exercise is possible, measurement of $p\dot{V}O_2$ or percentage predicted $\dot{V}O_2$ is the most useful exercise parameter. It may be that other measures are useful if maximal exercise cannot be undertaken. Prognosis should not be assessed from exercise data in isolation but other clinical factors should be also taken into account. Peak $\dot{V}O_2$ is known to be a continuous variable in terms of its ability to predict prognosis and, although much remains to be learned, it is likely that further assessment of subjects with intermediate level $p\dot{V}O_2$ will prove useful. Finally, preliminary data suggest combining maximum exercise testing with assessment of neurohormones (particularly the natriuretic peptides both at rest and at peak exercise) may be valuable.

REFERENCES

1 **Tristani FE**, Hughes CV, Archibald DG, *et al*. Safety of graded symptom-limited exercise testing in patients with congestive heart failure. *Circulation* 1987;**76**(suppl VI):VI54–8.
2 **Remme**, WJ, Swedberg K, on behalf of the Task Force for the Diagnosis and Treatment of Heart Failure. Guidelines for the diagnosis and treatment of chronic heart failure. *Eur Heart J* 2001;**22**:1527–60.
3 **HarrinGton D**, Coats A. Mechanisms of exercise intolerance in congestive heart failure. *Current Opinion in Cardiology* 1997;**12**:224–32.
4 **Clark AL**, Poole-Wilson PA, Coats A. Exercise limitation in chronic heart failure: central role of the periphery. *J Am Coll Cardiol* 1996;**28**:1092-102.
5 **Weber K**, Kinasewitz G, Janicki J, *et al*. Oxygen utilization and ventilation during exercise in patients with chronic congestive heart failure. *Circulation* 1982;**65**:1213–23.
6 **Szlachcic J**, Massie B, Kramer B, *et al*. Correlates and prognostic implication of exercise capacity in chronic congestive heart failure. *Am J Cardiol* 1985;**55**:1037–42.
► **Early description of prognostic value of $p\dot{V}O_2$ in heart failure.**
7 **Likoff MJ**, Chandler SL, Kay HR. Clinical determinants of mortality in chronic congestive heart failure secondary to idiopathic or dilated cardiomyopathy. *Am J Cardiol* 1987;**59**:634–8.
8 **Costsnzo MR**, Augustine S, Bourge R, *et al*. Selection and treatment of candidates for heart transplantation: a statement for health professionals from the committee on heart failure and cardiac transplantation of the council on clinical cardiology, American Heart Association. *Circulation* 1995;**92**:3592–612.
9 **Mancini DM**, Eisen H, Kussmaul W, *et al*. Value of peak exercise consumption for optimal timing of cardiac transplantation in ambulatory patients with heart failure. *Circulation* 1991;**83**:778–86.
► **Study designed to determine if $p\dot{V}O_2$ measurement can identify heart failure patients in whom cardiac transplantation can be deferred.**
10 **Aaronson KD**, Mancini DM. Is percentage of predicted maximal exercise oxygen consumption a better predictor of survival than peak exercise oxygen consumption for patients with severe heart failure? *J Heart Lung Transplant* 1995;**14**:981–9.
► **Comparison of $p\dot{V}O_2$ with percentage of predicted $\dot{V}O_2$ in severe heart failure.**
11 **Stelken AM**, Younis LT, Jenison SH, *et al*. Prognostic value of cardiopulmonary exercise testing using percent achieved of predicted peak oxygen uptake for patients with ischemic and dilated cardiomyopathy. *J Am Coll Cardiol* 1996;**27**:345–52.
12 **Osada N**, Chaitman BR, Miller LW, *et al*. Cardiopulmonary exercise testing identifies low risk patients with heart failure and severely impaired exercise capacity considered for heart transplantation. *J Am Coll Cardiol* 1998;**31**:577–82.
► **Peak systolic blood pressure during exercise may help stratify prognosis in those with $p\dot{V}O_2$ < 14 ml/kg/min.**
13 **Chomsky DB**, Lange CC, Rayos GH, *et al*. Hemodynamic exercise testing: a valuable tool in the selection of cardiac transplantation candidates. *Circulation* 1996;**94**:3176–83.
► **Cardiac output response to exercise and $p\dot{V}O_2$ < 10 ml/kg/min were independently predictive of survival in this group of patients with a low average $p\dot{V}O_2$.**
14 **Griffin B**, Shah P, Ferguson J, *et al*. Incremental prognostic value of exercise hemodynamic variables in chronic congestive heart failure secondary to coronary artery disease or to dilated cardiomyopathy. *Am J Cardiol* 1991;**67**:848–53.
15 **Chua T**, Ponikowski P, Harrington D, *et al*. Clinical correlates and prognostic significance of the ventilatory response to exercise in chronic heart failure. *J Am Coll Cardiol* 1997;**29**:1585–90.
► **In this study, ventilatory response to exercise added prognostic power over $p\dot{V}O_2$.**
16 **Pardaens K**, Van Cleemput J, Vanhaeke J, *et al*. Peak oxygen consumption better predicts outcome than submaximal respiratory data in heart transplant candidates. *Circulation* 2000;**101**:1152–7.
► **The submaximal ventilatory response to exercise was not as reliable as $p\dot{V}O_2$ in predicting prognosis in heart transplant candidates.**
17 **Aaronson K**, Schwartz JS, Chen T, *et al*. Development and prospective validation of a clinical index to predict survival in ambulatory patients referred for cardiac transplant evaluation. *Circulation* 1997;**95**:2660–7.
18 **Stevenson LW**, Steimie AE, Fonarow G, *et al*. Improvement in exercise capacity of candidates awaiting heart transplantation. *J Am Coll Cardiol* 1995;**25**:163–70.
19 **Gullestad L**, Myers J, Ross H, *et al*. Serial exercise testing and prognosis in selected patients considered for cardiac transplantation. *Am Heart J* 1998;**135**:221–9.
20 **Opasich C**, Pinna GD, Mazza A, *et al*. Six-minute walking performance in patients with moderate-to-severe heart failure: is it a useful indicator in clinical practice? *Eur Heart J* 2001;**22**:488–96.
► **Six minute walk test was not predictive of survival in models including NYHA class and $p\dot{V}O_2$.**
21 **Paraskevaidis IA**, Adamopoulos S, Kremastinos DT. Dobutamine echocardiographic study in patients with nonischemic dilated cardiomyopathy and prognostically borderline values of peak exercise oxygen consumption: 18-month follow-up study. *J Am Coll Cardiol* 2001;**37**:1685–91.

22 **Tabet JY**, Logeart D, Geyer C, *et al.* Comparison of the prognostic value of left ventricular filling and peak oxygen uptake in patients with systolic heart failure. *Eur Heart J* 2000;**21**:1864–87.

23 **Isnard R**, Pousset F, Trochu J, *et al.* Prognostic value of neurohormonal activation and cardiopulmonary exercise testing in patients with chronic heart failure. *Am J Cardiol* 2000;**86**:417–21.

24 **Hulsmann M**, Stanek B, Frey B, *et al.* Value of cardiopulmonary exercise testing and big endothelin plasma levels to predict short-term prognosis of patients with chronic heart failure. *J Am Coll Cardiol* 1998;**32**:1695–700.

25 **de Groote P**, Millaire A, Pigny P, *et al.* Plasma levels of atrial natriuretic peptide at peak exercise: a prognostic marker of cardiovascular-related death and heart transplantation in patients with moderate congestive heart failure. *J Heart Lung Transplant* 1997;**16**:956–63.

26 **Lainchbury JG**, Swanney MP, Beckert L, *et al.* Change in plasma brain natriuretic peptide during exercise is an important predictor of survival in systolic heart failure. *Eur Heart J* 2001;**22**(suppl):377.

▶ **Assessment of natriuretic peptides at peak exercise may add to the assessment of prognosis in heart failure.**

SECTION III: CARDIOMYOPATHY

10 HYPERTROPHIC CARDIOMYOPATHY: MANAGEMENT, RISK STRATIFICATION, AND PREVENTION OF SUDDEN DEATH

William J McKenna, Elijah R Behr

Hypertrophic cardiomyopathy (HCM) is an inherited cardiac muscle disorder disease that affects sarcomeric proteins, resulting in small vessel disease, myocyte and myofibrillar disorganisation, and fibrosis with or without myocardial hypertrophy. These features may result in significant cardiac symptoms and are a potential substrate for arrhythmias. Before the identification of disease causing genes the World Health Organization defined HCM as the presence of left or biventricular hypertrophy in the absence of any cardiac or systemic cause.[w1] When these criteria are applied to a western population the estimated prevalence of HCM is approximately 1 in 500.[1] [w2] Morphological evidence of left ventricular hypertrophy, however, may be absent in up to 20% of gene carriers.[w3] Adults are often asymptomatic but their estimated mortality rate may nonetheless be as high as 1–2% per annum.[2] [w4] This article will present the natural history of HCM and relate it to the need for medical intervention to alleviate symptoms and prevent sudden death.

▶ NATURAL HISTORY AND PROGNOSIS

The expression of disease is age related, occurring during or soon after periods of rapid somatic growth. Detectable cardiovascular abnormalities usually develop during adolescence.[w5] For this reason the regular evaluation of the offspring of carriers during puberty and early adulthood is necessary for diagnosis and risk stratification. HCM has been described in infants and young children but data are limited. Children diagnosed before 14 years of age have a worse prognosis once they reach adolescence and early adulthood with a 2–4% annual incidence of sudden death.[3] The development of clinical features of HCM in the elderly is associated with myosin binding protein C (MyBPC) mutations.[w6] Although MyBPC disease appears benign in that presentation is in the later decades, once disease develops patients are at risk of all the recognised complications of HCM including arrhythmia, stroke, and sudden death.[w7] A subanalysis of data from patients who had received an implantable cardioverter-defibrillator (ICD) indicated a higher proportion of individuals (40–50%) undergoing defibrillation in the age groups 11–20 years and > 55 years compared to the 21–55 years range.[4] Aggressive management in these higher risk age groups may therefore be required.

In adults, left ventricular hypertrophy caused by mutations in genes other than MyBPC is not progressive and in the majority is usually benign in its clinical course. Most affected individuals go unrecognised and are asymptomatic or experience only paroxysmal manifestations.[w8] Chronic exertional symptoms such as chest pain and dyspnoea can be secondary to myocardial ischaemia (table 10.1), diastolic dysfunction and/or congestive cardiac failure, and tend to deteriorate slowly with age. The classical pattern of asymmetric septal hypertrophy (ASH) may be accompanied by systolic anterior motion of the mitral valve (SAM) and dynamic left ventricular outflow tract (LVOT) obstruction that can also cause exertional symptoms of impaired consciousness, dyspnoea, and chest pain. A subset of patients, however, who represent < 5% of the total, exhibit progressive symptomatic deterioration in left ventricular systolic function with myocardial thinning and dilatation.[5] This is usually accompanied by the development of systolic cardiac failure. The severity of symptoms and exercise limitation caused by obstruction and/or cardiac dysfunction will dictate symptomatic management while the presence of arrhythmias and abnormal vascular responses will influence the need for prevention of sudden death. The risk of stroke secondary to atrial fibrillation (AF) must also be considered.

MECHANISMS OF CARDIAC ARREST

Fortuitous observations have recorded several mechanisms for the generation of ventricular fibrillation (VF). These include paroxysmal AF, sinus tachycardia with abnormal vascular responses and/or myocardial ischaemia, sustained monomorphic ventricular tachycardia (VT), rapid atrioventricular (AV) conduction via an accessory pathway, and AV block. Recent data have reported that appropriate discharges by ICDs (that is, probable aborted sudden death) were related to the occurrence of monomorphic VT, VF preceded by VT, and VF alone.[4] ICD Holter data, however,

Table 10.1 Possible mechanisms for myocardial ischaemia in HCM

Increased myocardial oxygen demand	Reduced myocardial perfusion
Myocardial hypertrophy	Small vessel disease
Diastolic dysfunction	Abnormal vascular responses
Myocyte disarray	Myocardial bridges
Left ventricular outflow obstruction	Increased coronary vascular resistance
Arrhythmia	

Abbreviations

AF, atrial fibrillation
ASH, asymmetric septal hypertrophy
AV, atrioventricular
HCM, hypertrophic cardiomyopathy
ICD, implantable cardioverter-defibrillator
LVOT, left ventricular outflow tract
MyBPC, myosin binding protein C
NSVT, non-sustained ventricular tachycardia
SAM, systolic anterior motion of the mitral valve
SVT, supraventricular tachycardia
VF, ventricular fibrillation
VT, ventricular tachycardia
WPW, Wolff-Parkinson-White

may not establish the importance of a trigger—for example, an abnormal vascular response or preceding ischaemia, in precipitating cardiac arrest. In the young this may be related to the haemodynamic changes of paradoxical vasodilatation in the presence of sinus tachycardia or primary atrial and ventricular arrhythmias. The development of a sustained ventricular arrhythmia would then represent a terminal event.[6 w9]

SYMPTOMATIC TREATMENT

The diagnosis of HCM relies on the demonstration of otherwise unexplained electrocardiographic (ECG) and two dimensional echocardiographic (echo) abnormalities (see accompanying article in this series, by Wigle *Heart* 2001;**86**:709–14). Echo is also of use in the assessment of diastolic and systolic dysfunction. The measurement of peak oxygen consumption during maximal upright exercise with continuous ECG and blood pressure monitoring facilitates symptomatic assessment of the HCM patient and provides an objective measure of functional limitation, vascular responses, and ischaemia. This helps to identify those patients with subclinical involvement and provides a useful objective correlate for subjective symptoms that may be particularly difficult to evaluate in young patients. The detection of a significant LVOT gradient either at rest or during exercise will guide symptomatic treament (fig 10.1). Angiography is usually necessary to exclude coronary artery disease in older patients with chest pain or ECG abnormalities.

Obstructive HCM: medical treatment

β Blockers are the first line treatment in patients with LVOT obstruction. The majority of patients show improvement upon treatment although high doses are often required. Side effects, however, can limit utility as well as induce pharmacological chronotropic incompetence, blunting the heart rate response to exercise and causing symptomatic deterioration. Verapamil is best avoided in individuals with obstruction because of possible peripheral vasodilatation and haemodynamic collapse. Unfortunately much of the data on verapamil or β blockers is observational and uncontrolled.[w10]

Disopyramide has been evaluated more systematically and is also effective in gradient and symptom reduction, probably because of negative inotropism.[w11] It may have a superior effect on exercise tolerance compared to β blockers.[7] They are, however, best used in combination as disopyramide alone tends to accelerate AV node conduction and increase the potential risk from supraventricular arrhythmias. Disopyramide should be administered in the maximum tolerated dose; the limiting factor is usually the anticholinergic side effects.

Obstructive HCM: non-medical treatment

Surgical septal myectomy remains the gold standard for those individuals with drug refractory symptoms and a resting gradient of ≥ 50 mm Hg. The aim is to widen the outflow tract, eliminating systolic mitral leaflet septal contact. There is a success rate of > 80% that can be achieved with a perioperative mortality rate of 2% or less. Long term symptom relief is maintained in up to 70% of patients.[8 w12] The operation should be tailored to the patient's anatomy including the severity of hypertrophy, the location and size of papillary muscles, and mitral valve anatomy. Mitral regurgitation can develop secondary to SAM and obstruction, and cause significant dyspnoea because of pulmonary oedema. The requirement for mitral valve surgery and/or myectomy needs to be individualised and can be guided by careful preoperative as well as intraoperative echocardiography.

Two other modalities have been developed for the treatment of LVOT obstruction: dual chamber pacing and alcohol septal ablation. The efficacy of pacing is controversial. Adult HCM patients were evaluated in randomised double blind trials of DDD or AAI pacing.[9 w13] Gradient reduction during active DDD pacing was approximately 50%. No other differences in objective measures were detected between the two pacing modalities. While 60% felt better with DDD pacing, 40% experienced symptomatic improvement with the pacemaker effectively turned off.[9] This suggested a substantial placebo effect.[9 w14 w15]

Alcohol ablation in experienced hands is effective and safe.[10] The technique involves injection of alcohol into the perforators of the left anterior descending coronary artery to cause a limited septal myocardial infarction.[w16] This reduces septal hypertrophy and the associated obstruction.[w16] Experienced centres are vital for good results as these are dependent on appropriate patient selection as well as good technique in order to ensure the delivery of alcohol is to the correct areas.[w16] The extent of myocardial perfusion by septal vessels is variable and may include papillary muscles and wide areas of both ventricles. Accurate definition by contrast echo of the area perfused is vital to avoid diffuse myocardial damage, particularly to papillary muscles.

Non-obstructive HCM: medical treatment

Agents such as β blockers, verapamil, and diltiazem are used to treat chest pain and dyspnoea and improve exercise tolerance. The mechanism probably involves improvement of left ventricular diastolic function and myocardial ischaemia. The response can be suboptimal although those patients with severe chest pain often benefit from high doses of verapamil or diltiazem. Pulmonary congestion has been treated with diuretics but there is a risk of decompensation in individuals with severe diastolic dysfunction. Diuretics should only be used judiciously and if possible only in the short term, as

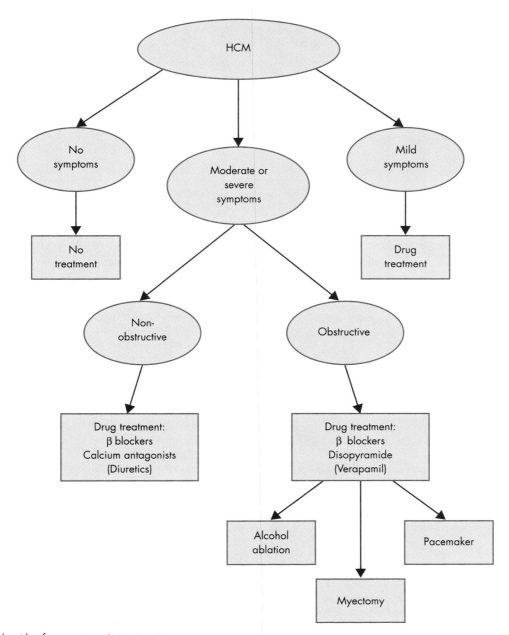

Figure 10.1 Algorithm for symptomatic treatment

chronic prescription tends to result in a reduction in stroke volume and cardiac output that ultimately lowers exercise capacity.[w8]

The subset that develops systolic impairment should receive treatment for conventional cardiac failure, including angiotensin converting enzyme (ACE) inhibitors, β blockers, digoxin, spironolactone, and if necessary cardiac transplantation.

SUPRAVENTRICULAR ARRHYTHMIAS

Supraventricular arrhythmias are common in HCM. They are related to left atrial enlargement and fibrosis developing in the context of chronically elevated filling pressures as a consequence of obstruction, diastolic dysfunction, and/or mitral valve dysfunction.[w8] Paroxysms of supraventricular tachycardia (SVT) and AF can be detected on Holter monitoring in up to 30% of adults, although the incidence in the young is closer to 5–10%. Sustained or symptomatic episodes are much less common and warrant treatment with amiodarone, which is

usually effective in reducing recurrences and attenuating the development of permanent AF.[11] The threshold for starting anticoagulation should be low to minimise embolic complications.[w17]

Established AF is uncommon in the young, while in adults the prevalence can be up to 30%.[11] It is more common in elderly HCM patients and has been associated with a poorer overall prognosis, an enlarged atrial size, and increased risk of thromboembolism including stroke.[6 11 w17 w18] Its onset is associated with an acute deterioration in symptoms that usually reverses with control of the ventricular response.[11] The long term outlook, with appropriate treatment to control heart rate and prevent emboli, is usually good.[12 w17 w19] Repeated cardioversions to restore sinus rhythm are not warranted. In most HCM patients the contribution of atrial systoles to stroke volume is negligible by the time AF develops—that is, patients have a palpable atrial beat but no fourth heart sound.

A slurred upstroke to a broad QRS complex is a common surface ECG finding in HCM patients. In less than 5% of these

Table 10.2   The recognised markers of risk in HCM and their sensitivity, specificity, positive and negative predictive accuracy (PPA and NPA)

Risk factor	Sensitivity (%)	Specificity (%)	PPA (%)	NPA (%)
Abnormal blood pressure response: <40 years old[19]	75	66	15	97
NSVT: adult <45 years old[18]	69	80	22	97
NSVT: ≤21 years old[23]	<10	89	<10	85
Inducible VT/VF: High risk population[w30]	82	68	17	98
*Syncope: <45 years old[3]	35	82	25	86
*Family history: at least one unexplained sudden death ± HCM[3]	42	79	28	88
†LVH ≥3 cm[17]	26	88	13	95
†‡Two or more risk factors[2]	45	90	23	96

*Figures provided are for the risk of death from all causes rather than sudden death only.
†Figures provided are for risk of sudden death and/or appropriate ICD discharge.
‡In this data set from Elliott and colleagues, family history and syncope were combined in order to achieve statistical significance of relative risk.
LVH, left ventricular hypertrophy; NSVT, non-sustained ventricular tachycardia; VF, ventricular fibrillation; VT, ventricular tachycardia.

Table 10.3   Five year survival rates free of death, cardiac arrest or appropriate ICD discharge in studies of HCM patients treated for secondary prevention of cardiac arrest or haemodynamically compromising ventricular arrhythmias

Study	5 year survival rates (95% CI)
Cecchi 1989[14]	65% (18%)
Elliott 1999[15]	59% (25%)
Maron 2000[4]	45% (CI unavailable)

CI, confidence interval.

patients, however, is an accessory pathway found at electrophysiological testing.[13] This may then be amenable to radiofrequency ablation. Enhanced AV nodal conduction may be more frequent in HCM and may facilitate the rapid conduction of pre-excited arrhythmias and so precipitate VF.[w20]

SUDDEN DEATH: RISK ASSESSMENT

All patients should undergo non-invasive risk factor stratification with a clinical history, Holter monitoring, and maximal exercise testing regardless of symptomatic status or the apparent severity of morphological disease.

History
Syncope and symptoms
Unexplained, exertion related syncope is a predictor of risk in all age groups, but especially in children and adolescents with severe symptoms.[3] This is an insensitive measure, however, as most patients who die suddenly have no prior history of syncope. In adults the severity of symptoms of chest pain and dyspnoea does not add to the predictive value (table 10.2).[3]

Prior cardiac arrest
Early evidence suggested that the short and medium term prognosis after a cardiac arrest was not as ominous as expected. The data indicated that roughly one third of survivors died within seven years while receiving non-systematic medical or surgical treatment.[14] The most recent ICD data, however, suggests a poorer prognosis with appropriate discharge rates of approximately 10% in survivors of cardiac arrest (table 10.3).[4 15]

Family history
Unpublished tertiary referral centre data indicates that 25% of HCM patients have a family history of premature sudden

death (< 45 years old) while less than 5% had two or more HCM related sudden deaths in the family. Family history of premature sudden death is also an insensitive but relatively specific marker of risk (table 10.2). The combination of a history of syncope with a family history of sudden death, however, does increase significantly the overall positive predictive accuracy for sudden death (Cox model multivariate relative risk 5.3, 95% confidence interval (CI) 1.9 to 14.9).[2 3]

Echocardiogram
Early echocardiographic and Doppler data has not suggested any predictive value from the degree of hypertrophy or severity of outflow tract obstruction.[w21] More recent studies have, however, identified severe (≥ 3 cm) hypertrophy as a risk factor for sudden death.[16 17] Spirito and colleagues had concluded that severe hypertrophy alone justified ICD insertion, particularly in the young.[16] This has been criticised, however, for failing to consider the distribution of left ventricular hypertrophy (LVH) and the fact that the majority of patients with maximal wall thicknesses ≥ 3 cm survived without prophylactic treatment. The data from Elliott and colleagues support a significantly increased risk of sudden death or ICD discharge associated with a maximal hypertrophy ≥ 3 cm (Cox model relative risk 2.1, 95% CI 1.0 to 4.2) but argues against prophylactic treatment solely on the basis of left ventricular wall thickness.[17] All the individuals with a mean left ventricular wall thickness ≥ 3 cm who died suddenly had additional risk factors, while those without other risk factors all survived.[17] In addition, 74% of Elliott's and 82% of Spirito's subgroups who died suddenly had hypertrophy of less than 3 cm.[16 17] The severity of wall thickness in isolation has insufficient predictive accuracy to guide decisions regarding prophylactic treatment.

Holter monitor
Twenty per cent of adult HCM patients exhibit non-sustained ventricular tachycardia (NSVT) during Holter monitoring. In adults it is the most sensitive marker for increased risk of sudden death, conferring a doubled relative risk in a selected low risk population and an eightfold increase in relative risk in a consecutive referral centre population.[18 w22] The absence of NSVT in adults is particularly reassuring because of its high negative predictive accuracy (table 10.2).

NSVT, however, is seen infrequently in adolescents and rarely in children, but when detected is more ominous and specific with an up to eightfold increase in relative risk for sudden death.[18 19] The relative rarity of ventricular arrhythmias

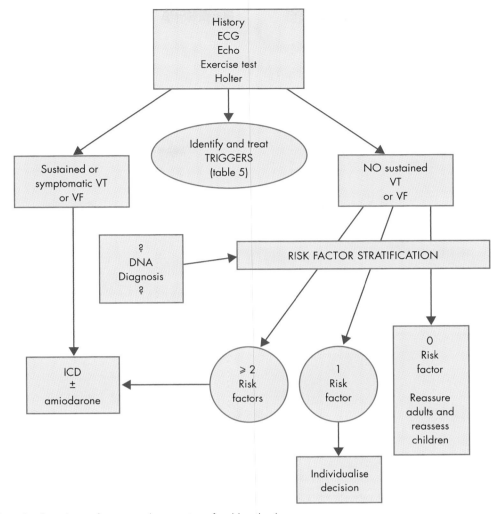

Figure 10.2 Algorithm for risk stratification and prevention of sudden death.

in children limits its utility in this population. In the young little reassurance is provided by the absence of NSVT while its presence even in isolation warrants prophylactic treatment.

SVT and AF have been observed as antecedent events in the development of VF and sudden death. Prophylaxis may therefore have an additional benefit in the reduction of the risk of sudden death.

Blood pressure response to exercise testing

During upright exercise HCM patients commonly demonstrate an abnormal blood pressure response, with either a fall or failure of blood pressure to rise.[w23] [w24] Inappropriate arterial vasodilatation in non-exercising muscles has been documented and it is postulated that this is related to activation of left ventricular baroreceptors by wall stress or ischaemia.[w23] [w25]

An abnormal blood pressure response during exercise is defined as a failure to either augment and/or sustain a systolic blood pressure of > 25 mm Hg above the resting systolic blood pressure during exercise. It can be detected in 25% of HCM patients and thus its positive predictive accuracy for sudden death is low at 15% (table 10.2).[20] [w24] It is a more sensitive indicator of risk in younger patients (< 40 years old) and is associated with sudden death, although the relative risk is low (1.8).[2] [20] Therefore a positive result should be used in conjunction with other risk factors. The absence of an abnormal blood pressure response is reassuring, however, as its negative predictive value for sudden death is 97% (table 10.2) and in

the young, in the absence of other risk factors, permits accurate reassurance.

Other investigations

Thallium cardiac perfusion scanning reveals reversible thallium defects in young HCM patients with histories of prior cardiac arrest or syncope.[w26] These findings have not been borne out in larger mixed groups of prospectively studied patients although in a small subset of patients ischaemia is important.[w27]

An angiographic study of children with HCM suggested that myocardial bridging was a significant risk factor for sudden death.[w28] These children were a highly selected group by virtue of having to undergo angiography and were examined retrospectively, making these findings difficult to extrapolate to the general paediatric HCM population. The significance of myocardial bridging and ischaemia in triggering secondary arrhythmias remains unknown but the available data do not provide sufficient justification for routine angiography.

Other non-invasive electrophysiological investigations have been assessed in risk stratification with little success.[w8] Signal averaged ECGs and heart rate variability studies are commonly abnormal in HCM patients, but there is no association with increased risk. QT interval analysis, including QT dispersion, has provided contradictory results. Beat to beat QT variability has been studied in β myosin mutations and was found to be increased in patients with Arg403Gln mutations of the β

Table 10.4 Recognised markers of increased risk of sudden death in HCM

Risk factor
1. Previous cardiac arrest
2. Non-sustained VT on Holter or exercise
3. Abnormal exertional blood pressure response
4. Unexplained syncope
5. Family history of premature sudden death
6. Severe left ventricular hypertrophy ⩾3 cm

Table 10.5 Triggers for sudden death and their associated treatment

Factor/trigger	Treatment
Paroxysmal atrial fibrillation	Amiodarone ± anticoagulation
Sustained monomorphic VT	ICD ± amiodarone
Conduction system disease	Permanent pacemaker
Accessory pathway	Radiofrequency ablation
Myocardial ischaemia	High dose verapamil

myosin heavy chain gene, but there are no data as yet on follow up and outcomes.[w29]

Invasive electrophysiological investigations have been used as research and potential clinical tools. Programmed stimulation studies using aggressive protocols have suggested that inducible VT is associated with a higher risk of future sudden death (table 10.2).[w30] These protocols, however, result in a low positive predictive accuracy similar to non-invasive methods. Therefore the hazard and inconvenience of electrophysiological studies cannot be justified.

Genetic testing

Recent studies have suggested that some mutations in HCM may carry prognostic significance. Troponin T mutations can be exceptionally lethal and appear to be more homogenous in their high level of risk than the prognostic allelic heterogeneity which characterises the other sarcomeric gene abnormalities.[21] Troponin T patients tend to exhibit subtle or absent hypertrophy but with significant myocyte disarray, and thus may be at risk without conspicuous evidence of disease.[w31] β Myosin mutations are heterogeneous in their associated levels of risk. Arg403Glu and Arg453Cys mutations appear to predispose to sudden death while the Val606Met mutation appears to carry a better prognosis.[21]

Nevertheless the genotype–phenotype relation has to be clarified further to allow proband risk prediction as the existing data have been elicited from selected groups of patients and their families. In addition there may be pronounced heterogeneity of disease within a family with the same mutation. For example, a MyBPC mutation has demonstrated a wide variation in expression in a large German family.[w7] Only a minority of the family exhibited full expression, which was partly age related, and once disease developed placed them at high risk of syncope, arrhythmias, and sudden death. In addition, DNA diagnosis is limited by the lack of clinical testing outside of research institutions.

Recently mutations in the gene PRKAG2 encoding the gamma-2 subunit of an AMP activated protein kinase have been identified in families with Wolff-Parkinson-White (WPW) syndrome with premature conduction disease and HCM.[w32 w33] Genetic testing may prove useful as this phenotype has a high incidence of pre-excitation, paroxysmal AF, and flutter and the development of premature conduction disease.

SUDDEN DEATH: PROPHYLAXIS

It is accepted practice to treat aggressively those patients who have experienced cardiac arrest and/or sustained or symptomatic ventricular arrhythmias (secondary prevention) using ICDs because of their high risk (table 10.3).[4 15] Most cardiac arrest victims with HCM do not survive the initial event, making it imperative to evaluate all HCM patients for risk and institute primary prevention accordingly (fig 10.2).

There are several recognised markers for risk of sudden death (table 10.4). Individually they all have low positive predictive accuracy (table 10.2). The proposed risk management algorithm (fig 2) advocates reassurance of individuals with no risk factors and no evidence of ischaemia. This is justifiable given the high negative predictive accuracy seen in patients without risk factors (table 10.2).[2] Individuals with two or more risk factors have annual sudden death rates of 3% (95% CI 2% to 7%) and should be offered prophylaxis with ICD and/or amiodarone.[2] Individuals with only one risk factor have annual sudden death rates of approximately 1% but with wide confidence limits (95% CI 0.3% to 1.5%); their management should therefore be tailored according to age, genotype, intensity of the risk factor, and the acceptability of risk for each individual.[2] For example, a patient's only risk factor may be a family history of premature sudden death, but if the proportion of affected individuals in a pedigree who suffer premature sudden death is high the justification for prophylaxis is greater than if the proportion was low.

Triggers

In approximately 30% of patients risk factor stratification identifies potential triggers for sudden death which are usually amenable to specific treatments (table 10.5).

Lifestyle

Over 60% of cases of sudden death in HCM die during or immediately after mild to moderate exertion.[w21] In addition, necropsy studies of sudden death in young athletes have shown that the majority had HCM and that two thirds of them died during or immediately after exertion.[22] It is therefore reasonable to advise those at risk of sudden death not to undertake strenuous exercise or competitive sports which require extreme physical exertion.[22]

Drug and device treatment

In the absence of a recognised trigger, treatment of high risk patients is limited to ICD and/or amiodarone.[4 23] There are limited data to define who should receive which treatment. In those at the highest risk an ICD is appropriate while amiodarone may be prescribed in lower risk patients. Amiodarone is also recommended if there is evidence of additional features that require prophylaxis such as paroxysmal supraventricular arrhythmia.

The use of amiodarone in children and adolescents may be complicated by anxiety about the potential dose/duration side effects. It can be used temporarily, however, as bridging therapy to delay ICD insertion in high risk young individuals in whom a device is thought to be the long term treatment of choice. In addition it can provide prophylaxis during a period of high risk until adulthood is reached and a lower risk profile is achieved.[4 w34] A recent retrospective and non-randomised paediatric study suggested a 5–10 fold reduction in risk with

Management of HCM: key points

► Symptomatic relief:
  - in non-obstructive HCM treatment relies on calcium channel antagonists and β blockers
  - in obstructive HCM pharmacological treatment relies on β blockers and disopyramide initially
  - myectomy, alcohol ablation, and dual chamber pacing are alternative interventions in obstructive HCM in the drug refractory patient
► Atrial fibrillation should be treated aggressively to minimise the risks of thromboembolism
► Sudden death prophylaxis:
  - all HCM patients should undergo risk stratification for sudden death
  - patients suffering prior cardiac arrest or sustained ventricular arrhythmia warrant prophylactic treatment
  - patients with two or more recognised risk factors warrant prophylaxis (table 10.4)
  - patients with one risk factor require individualised decision making in relation to the strength of the risk factor (table 10.4)
  - effective prophylactic treatment includes the use of ICD and/or amiodarone
► Clarification of the genotype–phenotype relation in HCM may ultimately assist decision making

It is still necessary to determine which prophylactic treatment is appropriate for which patient. Thus a continued registry of ICD and amiodarone treatment in HCM, incorporating genetic testing and risk stratification, may be the only definitive way to guide therapy in relation to genotype and phenotype.

71

CONCLUSION

The management of HCM remains an important clinical challenge necessitating regular longitudinal follow up of young individuals. Treatment of obstruction offers several effective options but symptom relief can be difficult, particularly in non-obstructive patients. Stratification of the risk of sudden death is feasible using available non-invasive techniques. Ultimately, genotyping may further refine our predictive abilities. The potential benefit of risk assessment also includes the reassurance of low risk individuals, while for high risk individuals there are prophylactic treatments available. The weight of evidence supports the judicious use of amiodarone and ICD therapy in primary prevention. Secondary prevention data support ICD therapy as mandatory. Data on treatment in the younger age groups are limited despite their relatively high risk of sudden death.

high dose β blockade.[w35] Interpretation of these data is limited by the small sample size derived from a heterogeneous population of young patients (all diagnosed < 19 years old), which included a high proportion of patients with "HCM" unrelated to sarcomeric contractile protein gene mutations (38% Noonan's syndrome). The sudden death risk of "HCM" caused by mitochondrial disease, Noonan's, Freidrich's ataxia, and Fabry's disease is likely to be different to the risk of HCM caused by mutations in contractile protein genes.

More recently retrospective registry data on ICD therapy have become available from US and Italian investigators.[4] The risk profile of the patients is incomplete but the primary prevention data suggest that individuals not at excessively high risk were treated. Extrapolation to a 10 year period suggested an annual appropriate discharge rate of 2.5%. This correlates with the experience of the European ICD registry (M Borggrefe MD, personal communication).

The complications of ICD therapy, however, appear to be greater in patients with HCM compared to high risk dilated cardiomyopathy or coronary artery disease patients. For example, 25% of the whole Italo-American group and 22% of European registry patients suffered inappropriate discharges and 15% had significant complications caused by lead failure or local effects of insertion (for example, infection, haemorrhage, and subclavian thrombosis). Amiodarone may reduce the frequency and rate of ventricular and supraventricular tachycardias and hence reduce the number of inappropriate and appropriate discharges. In the Italo-American population, however, it was used less frequently than one might have expected (25%). In addition the young are also more at risk of complications. Children are more likely to require insertion in an abdominal position with redundant intra-atrial loops of lead required to allow for further growth.[w34] Adolescents often have psychological problems adapting to the device, while young people in general will require multiple box and lead placements resulting in difficult vascular access and an increase in complications.[w34]

REFERENCES

1 **Maron BJ**, Gardin JM, Flack JM, *et al*. Prevalence of hypertrophic cardiomyopathy in a general population of young adults. Echocardiographic analysis of 4111 subjects in the CARDIA study. Coronary artery risk development in (young) adults. *Circulation* 1995;**92**:785–9.
2 **Elliott PM**, Poloniecki J, Dickie S, *et al*. Sudden death in hypertrophic cardiomyopathy: identification of high risk patients. *J Am Coll Cardiol* 2000;**36**:2212–18.
► **This study demonstrated the clinical utility and statistical validity of risk stratification using recognised risk factors to identify high risk patients.**
3 **McKenna W**, Deanfield J, Faruqui A, *et al*. Prognosis in hypertrophic cardiomyopathy: role of age and clinical, electrocardiographic and hemodynamic features. *Am J Cardiol* 1981;**47**:532–8.
4 **Maron BJ**, Shen WK, Link MS, *et al*. Efficacy of implantable cardioverter-defibrillators for the prevention of sudden death in patients with hypertrophic cardiomyopathy. *N Engl J Med* 2000;**342**:365–73.
► **The registry data presented, although retrospective, are the first to describe the utility and complications of ICD treatment in a large group of HCM patients.**
5 **Spirito P**, Maron BJ, Bonow RO, *et al*. Occurrence and significance of progressive left ventricular wall thinning and relative cavity dilatation in hypertrophic cardiomyopathy. *Am J Cardiol* 1987;**60**:123–9.
6 **Nicod P**, Polikar R, Peterson KL. Hypertrophic cardiomyopathy and sudden death. *N Engl J Med* 1988;**318**:1255–7.
7 **Pollick C**. Disopyramide in hypertrophic cardiomyopathy. II. Noninvasive assessment after oral administration. *Am J Cardiol* 1988;**62**:1252–5.
8 **McCully RB**, Nishimura RA, Tajik AJ, *et al*. Extent of clinical improvement after surgical treatment of hypertrophic obstructive cardiomyopathy. *Circulation* 1996;**94**:467–71.
► **A comprehensive retrospective assessment of the efficacy and safety of surgical myectomy according to the Mayo Clinic experience.**
9 **Nishimura RA**, Trusty JM, Hayes DL, *et al*. Dual-chamber pacing for hypertrophic cardiomyopathy: a randomized, double-blind, crossover trial. *J Am Coll Cardiol* 1997;**29**:435–41.
10 **Seggewiss H**, Faber L, Gleichmann U. Percutaneous transluminal septal ablation in hypertrophic obstructive cardiomyopathy. *Thorac Cardiovasc Surg* 1999;**47**:94–100.
► **The largest series to demonstrate clearly the safety and efficacy of alcohol ablation.**
11 **Cecchi F**, Olivotto I, Montereggi A, *et al*. Hypertrophic cardiomyopathy in Tuscany: clinical course and outcome in an unselected regional population. *J Am Coll Cardiol* 1995;**26**:1529–36.
12 **Robinson K**, Frenneaux MP, Stockins B, *et al*. Atrial fibrillation in hypertrophic cardiomyopathy: a longitudinal study. *J Am Coll Cardiol* 1990;**15**:1279–85.
13 **Fananapazir L**, Tracy CM, Leon MB, *et al*. Electrophysiologic abnormalities in patients with hypertrophic cardiomyopathy. A consecutive analysis in 155 patients. *Circulation* 1989;**80**:1259–68.
14 **Cecchi F**, Maron BJ, Epstein SE. Long-term outcome of patients with hypertrophic cardiomyopathy successfully resuscitated after cardiac arrest. *J Am Coll Cardiol* 1989;**13**:1283–8.

15 **Elliott PM**, Sharma S, Varnava A, *et al*. Survival after cardiac arrest or sustained ventricular tachycardia in patients with hypertrophic cardiomyopathy. *J Am Coll Cardiol* 1999;**33**:1596–601.

16 **Spirito P**, Bellone P, Harris KM, *et al*. Magnitude of left ventricular hypertrophy and risk of sudden death in hypertrophic cardiomyopathy. *N Engl J Med* 2000;**342**:1778–85.

17 **Elliott PM**, Gimeno BJ, Mahon NG, *et al*. Relation between severity of left-ventricular hypertrophy and prognosis in patients with hypertrophic cardiomyopathy. *Lancet* 2001;**357**:420–4.

▶ **Elliott and colleagues provide convincing evidence that hypertrophy alone should not be used as an indicator of high risk but as part of full risk stratification.**

18 **Maron BJ**, Savage DD, Wolfson JK, *et al*. Prognostic significance of 24 hour ambulatory electrocardiographic monitoring in patients with hypertrophic cardiomyopathy: a prospective study. *Am J Cardiol* 1981;**48**:252–7.

19 **McKenna WJ**, Franklin RC, Nihoyannopoulos P, *et al*. Arrhythmia and prognosis in infants, children and adolescents with hypertrophic cardiomyopathy. *J Am Coll Cardiol* 1988;**11**:147–53.

20 **Sadoul N**, Prasad K, Elliott PM, *et al*. Prospective prognostic assessment of blood pressure response during exercise in patients with hypertrophic cardiomyopathy. *Circulation* 1997;**96**:2987–91.

▶ **An abnormal blood pressure response to exercise was shown to be a useful predictor of risk of sudden death, particularly in the young.**

21 **Watkins H**, McKenna WJ, Thierfelder L, *et al*. Mutations in the genes for cardiac troponin T and alpha-tropomyosin in hypertrophic cardiomyopathy. *N Engl J Med* 1995;**332**:1058–64.

22 **Maron BJ**, Roberts WC, McAllister HA, *et al*. Sudden death in young athletes. *Circulation* 1980;**62**:218–29.

23 **McKenna WJ**, Oakley CM, Krikler DM, *et al*. Improved survival with amiodarone in patients with hypertrophic cardiomyopathy and ventricular tachycardia. *Br Heart J* 1985;**53**:412–16.

Additional references appear on the *Heart* website—www.heartjnl.com

SECTION IV: VALVE DISEASE

11 TIMING OF MITRAL VALVE SURGERY

Maurice Enriquez-Sarano

Mitral valve surgery has changed considerably in the past decades and is now indicated mostly for pure or predominant mitral regurgitation. This is the result of the regression of rheumatic disease, of the efficacy of mitral balloon valvuloplasty for mitral stenosis, and of the aging of the population with increasing degenerative or ischaemic disease causing mitral regurgitation. Mitral regurgitation can be "organic" (that is, caused by intrinsic mitral disease such as rheumatic disease, ruptured chord, perforation of leaflet) or be "functional" (that is, where a normal valve regurgitates because of ventricular dysfunction).

The timing of mitral surgery has remained one of the most vexing problems of clinical cardiology because symptoms can remain absent or minimal despite severe regurgitation caused by adaptive remodelling of left ventricle and atrium, or because of patient adaptation to the disease. However, recent advances in the understanding of the natural history of the disease and of the impact of left ventricular dysfunction on outcome, in the echocardiographic evaluation of mitral diseases and in the risk and success of mitral repair, have resulted in a widespread evolution towards earlier surgery.

► POOR OUTCOME OF SEVERE MITRAL REGURGITATION

Mitral regurgitation is a progressive disease

The new quantitative techniques have allowed the progression of mitral regurgitation to be defined. As was clinically suspected, mitral regurgitation is a progressive disease,[1] with an increase on average of 7.5 ml per year for regurgitant volume and of 5.9 mm^2 per year for the effective regurgitant orifice. The determinants of progression are anatomic changes, with more rapid progression in patients with mitral valve prolapse, in particular new flail leaflet, and in patients with an enlarging mitral annulus.[1] Importantly, progression is not uniform and if half of the patients see notable progression, 11% see also spontaneous regression of mitral regurgitation, related to improved loading conditions. The progression of mitral regurgitation also causes progression of left ventricular remodelling leading to the development of left ventricular dysfunction.[2]

The worrisome natural history of severe mitral regurgitation

Widely disparate estimates of long term survival in patients with mitral regurgitation—between 97–27% at five years—have been reported.[3][4] We analysed the natural history of mitral regurgitation caused by flail leaflets because these patients present with severe mitral regurgitation in more than 85% of cases.[5] We observed that, in comparison to the expected survival, an excess mortality was noted (6.3% yearly) (fig 11.1). A high morbidity was also present with a 10 year incidence of atrial fibrillation of 30%, and of heart failure of 63%. Furthermore, at 10 years 90% of patients were either dead or had undergone surgery, which means that the operation is almost unavoidable. Patients with New York Heart Association (NYHA) functional class III or IV symptoms, even transient, displayed a considerable mortality (34% yearly) if not operated upon, but even those in class I or II had a notable mortality (4.1% yearly). Patients with ejection fraction < 60% also displayed an excess mortality as compared to those with ejection fraction ≥ 60%, but no group at very low risk under medical treatment could be defined.

Sudden death is a catastrophic event, responsible for approximately a quarter of the deaths occurring under medical treatment.[6] The determinants of higher rates of sudden death are mostly severe symptoms and reduced ejection fraction, but most sudden deaths occur in patients with no or minimal symptoms and normal left ventricular function.[6] The rate of sudden death is 1.8% per year overall; even in patients without risk factors it is 0.8% per year. These data underscore the serious prognostic implication of severe mitral regurgitation, suggesting that surgery should be considered early in the course of the disease.

Left ventricular dysfunction: frequent and poorly predictable

How to assess left ventricular function in mitral regurgitation is the subject of an ongoing debate and research. The increased diastolic inflow volume increases preload. During systole, the regurgitant flow towards the left atrium suggests a decreased impedance to ejection, but end

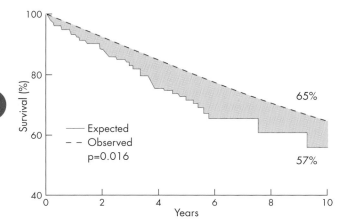

Figure 11.1 Survival in patients with medically treated mitral regurgitation caused by flail mitral leaflets. Note the excess mortality as compared to the expected survival (red screen). Reproduced from Ling et al, *N Engl J Med* 1996;**335**:1417–23, with the authorisation of the Massachusetts Medical Society.

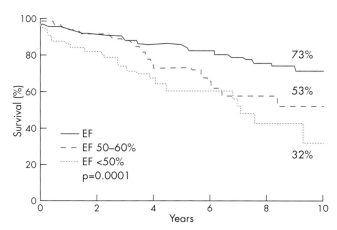

Figure 11.2 Long term postoperative survival according to the preoperative echocardiographic ejection fraction. Note the excess mortality in patients with ejection fraction < 50% but also with "low normal" ejection fraction 50–59%. Reproduced with the authorisation of the American Heart Association.

systolic wall stress is usually normal. Multiple methods of correction of the measured left ventricular function indices have been suggested, showing that there is no wide consensus on how to measure intrinsic left ventricular function in mitral regurgitation.

Clinically, left ventricular dysfunction is a major source of poor outcome under conservative management[5] or postoperatively.[7] Although it currently represents a rare cause of perioperative death due to the progress of anaesthesia and myocardial protection, it is the most frequent cause of late death after surgery.[7] The ejection fraction decreases significantly immediately after surgical correction of mitral regurgitation by approximately 10%.[2] Therefore, despite symptomatic improvement, postoperative left ventricular dysfunction (ejection fraction < 50%) is frequent, occurring in close to a third of the patients successfully operated upon for organic mitral regurgitation. Postoperative left ventricular dysfunction is associated with poor survival[2 8] and high but delayed incidence of heart failure.[9]

Preoperative ejection fraction is the best predictor of long term mortality under conservative management[5] and after surgery[7] (fig 11.2), of congestive heart failure,[9] and of postoperative residual left ventricular function.[2] The end systolic dimension is also a significant predictor of the postoperative left ventricular function.[2] Therefore, either an ejection fraction < 60% or an end systolic diameter ⩾ 45 mm are considered as demonstrating overt left ventricular dysfunction and should be immediately considered for surgery in the absence of major comorbidities.[10]

However, reduced left ventricular function, even pronounced, should not be considered as a contraindication to surgery in patients with organic mitral regurgitation, because operative mortality is not excessive is these patients[7] and because the postoperative clinical complications are often delayed after surgery. Also, the precision of the prediction of outcome is imperfect, with a relatively wide range of error for the prediction of postoperative left ventricular function.[2 8 11] As the best outcome is observed in patients with an ejection fraction ⩾ 60%, this stage of the disease appears to represent the best opportunity for surgery. Therefore, the concept of waiting for signs of early decline of left ventricular function is rigged with a notable risk of "unexpected" left ventricular dysfunction,[2] and appears defensible mostly when the mitral

Aetiology and mechanism of mitral regurgitation

Mechanism	Aetiology	
	Non-ischaemic	Ischaemic
Organic	Rheumatic, prolapse, flail leaflet, endocarditis, etc	Ruptured papillary muscle
Functional	Cardiomyopathy	Post-myocardial infarction functional mitral regurgitation

regurgitation is not severe enough to warrant immediate surgery, the operative risk is high, or the chances of a valve repair are low.

Ischaemic mitral regurgitation: a group at high risk
The high risk associated with ruptured papillary muscle is well known.[12] After a myocardial infarction, mitral regurgitation can develop without ruptured papillary muscle as a consequence of left ventricular remodelling, due to the apical and inferior displacement of the papillary muscles leading to incomplete coaptation of tenting leaflets.[13] The strong impact of this "functional" mitral regurgitation on the outcome post-myocardial infarction has been underscored in two recent studies, showing that its mere presence is associated with poor survival.[14 15] Quantitative measurements show that higher degrees of regurgitation are associated with worse outcome independently of the ejection fraction.[15] Therefore, even though the murmur may not be loud,[16] an aggressive surgical approach should be considered in these patients.

MITRAL SURGERY: RECENT PROGRESS
The operative risks, results, and improvements are essential considerations in the appraisal of the timing of surgery.

The operative mortality is of considerable importance but was too high to consider surgery in asymptomatic patients in the past. However, for patients with organic mitral regurgitation, operative mortality has considerably decreased recently,[17] and in our institution is currently around 1% in patients younger than 75 years whether repair or replacement is performed.[7] Conversely, the operative mortality in patients

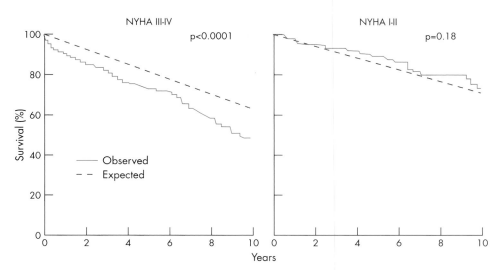

Figure 11.3 Comparison of observed and expected survival after surgical correction of mitral regurgitation separately in patients preoperatively with severe symptoms (left graph) and no or minimal symptoms (right graph). There is excess mortality in patients operated on with severe symptoms but no excess mortality in patients who had no or minimal symptoms, suggesting that in the latter group the long term consequences of mitral regurgitation have been suppressed. Reproduced with the authorisation of the American Heart Association.

≥ 75 years old, or in patients operated on for ischaemic mitral regurgitation, although improved recently, remains relatively high, between 3.5–12% depending on the preoperative presentation.[18]

The availability of valve repair is of crucial importance. Previous studies suggested a lower operative mortality and a better long term survival after valve repair than replacement,[19–21] but it was unclear whether this was due to a better preoperative condition of patients undergoing valve repair or to the procedure itself. In our experience, taking into account all differences at baseline between valve repairs and replacements, valve repair is indeed an independent predictor of a better outcome after surgery for mitral regurgitation, with a lower operative mortality and a better long term survival than valve replacement.[22] This benefit is noted whether or not an associated coronary bypass surgery is performed.[22] A major reason for the improved outcome after valve repair is a better left ventricular function than after valve replacement.[22] The conservation of the subvalvar apparatus certainly plays a role in the preserved left ventricular function after valve repair, as it does after valve replacement without transsection of chordae. The improved survival after valve repair is not accomplished at the expense of an increased risk of reoperation.[22]

Intraoperative transoesophageal echocardiography is an essential component of the success of valve repair and should be performed by experienced physicians, to monitor the repair procedure and help with intraoperative decisions.[23]

Therefore, valve repair has become extremely popular[24] and currently a successful repair can be performed in 85–90% of patients with isolated mitral regurgitation. This high percentage of repair has been achievable after the initial learning phase of this difficult procedure through the utilisation of special techniques, such as the transposition of chordae or insertion of artificial cords, in particular for the rupture chords of the anterior leaflet.[25 26] However, the repairability of rheumatic lesions is not as consistent as that of degenerative lesions.[27] Despite these high feasibility rates, the repair of the mitral valve should not be considered as a panacea and does not eliminate the risk of myocardial dysfunction. In patients with an ejection fraction < 60%, an excess mortality is noted whether repair or replacement is performed.[22] Therefore, the ability to perform repair in a high percentage of patients should be considered as an incentive to perform surgery because of its low risk and good survival, and not as an incentive to delay surgery and encounter the risk of more left ventricular dysfunction.

OUTCOME AFTER SURGICAL CORRECTION OF MITRAL REGURGITATION

To make appropriate decisions, it is important to analyse the postoperative outcome, in particular the implications of delaying surgery until overt alterations occur.

Waiting for left ventricular dysfunction (ejection fraction < 60%, end systolic diameter ≥ 45 mm) imposes an excess rate of mortality[7] and of heart failure[9] compared to patients with more normal function at surgery.

Waiting for severe symptoms to occur before surgery is also not benign. In the Mayo experience, the more severe the preoperative symptoms were, the lower the postoperative ejection fraction[2] and the higher the incidence of congestive heart failure[9] were during follow up. Adjusting for age at surgery and all other determinants of outcome, severe preoperative symptoms are associated with a worse long term survival[18 28] and excess incidence of heart failure.[9] Even in the privileged subgroup of patients with an ejection fraction ≥ 60% where the survival is not different from the expected survival, patients operated at an early stage with minimal symptoms have a better survival than patients with severe symptoms.[7] Therefore, waiting for severe symptoms is associated with a higher incidence of complications after the surgery is performed (fig 11.3)

Waiting for atrial fibrillation to occur and persist more than three months before surgery was associated with a high risk of postoperative persistence of atrial fibrillation and therefore of requiring long term anticoagulation. Conversely, recent atrial fibrillation tends to revert to sinus rhythm postoperatively.[29] Therefore, waiting for chronic atrial fibrillation preoperatively is associated with residual postoperative morbidity.

There is no randomised trial comparing the outcome after early surgery for organic mitral regurgitation to the outcome with medical management. In patients with flail mitral leaflets the long term outcome after early surgery was compared to that of patients managed conservatively and operated on whenever it was judged necessary. Although many patients initially treated conservatively eventually underwent surgery, the early surgical approach was associated with an improved long term survival through a pronounced reduction in cardiac mortality, and a decreased morbidity (less heart failure and less atrial fibrillation) during follow up.[30] These results underline the potential for eliminating most of the cardiac complications caused by mitral regurgitation through an early surgical approach as long as the operative mortality remains low (< 2%).

Timing of surgery in organic mitral regurgitation

	Prompt mitral surgery decision
Severe mitral regurgitation	
Symptoms or LV dysfunction present	Yes
No symptoms and n LV dysfunction	
AF or VT or PHTN	Yes
No AF, no VT, no PHTN	
Repairable = No	Usually no
Massive MR (regurgitant volume ≥100 ml)	Possible yes
Pronounced left atrial enlargement	
Repairable = Yes and	
Low risk	Usually yes
High risk or severe comorbidity	Usually no
Not severe mitral regurgitation	
Regurgitant volume <45 ml	No
Regurgitant volume 45–60 ml	Usually no
VT or AF or LV dysfunction and repairable = yes	Possible yes
Other cardiac operation scheduled and repairable = yes	Possible yes

AF, atrial fibrillation; LV, left ventricle; MR, mitral regurgitation; PHTN, pulmonary hypertension; VT, ventricular tachycardia.

Timing of surgery in ischaemic mitral regurgitation

	Prompt mitral surgery decision
Ruptured papillary muscle	Yes
Functional mitral regurgitation	
Bypass surgery indicated for angina	
MR severe (ERO ≥ 20 mm^2)	Yes
MR mild or moderate (ERO < 20 mm^2)	Possible yes
MR trace	No
Bypass surgery not indicated for angina but possible	
MR severe	Yes
MR mild to moderate	
History of CHF (or class III) and viable myocardium	Possible yes
No or mild symptoms or no viability	Uncertain
MR trace	No
Bypass surgery not possible	
MR severe (ERO ≥20 mm^2)	
Regurgitant volume ≥50–60 ml, EF >35% and low comorbidity	Possible yes
Regurgitant volume <50 ml or EF <30–35%	Uncertain
High comorbidity	No
MR mild to moderate	No
MR trace	No

CHF, congestive heart failure; EF, ejection fraction; ERO, effective regurgitant orifice; MR, mitral regurgitation.

WHAT INFORMATION IS NEEDED TO DEFINE THE TIMING OF MITRAL SURGERY?

Symptoms

The severity of symptoms is defined by history but as many patients limit progressively their physical activity, performing exercise testing in "asymptomatic" patients,[31] in particular with oxygen consumption measurement, may unveil unexpected exercise limitations.

Left ventricular function

Left ventricular function is usually assessed by echocardiography. An ejection fraction < 60% or left ventricular end systolic diameter ≥ 45 mm are considered as signs of overt left ventricular dysfunction.

Degree of mitral regurgitation–haemodynamics

Although the extent of the jet of mitral regurgitation by colour flow imaging or the density of dye in the left atrium by angiography are useful to observe, these methods have numerous pitfalls.[32 33] The comprehensive assessment of the degree of mitral regurgitation can be performed by quantitative Doppler echocardiography. The most widely used method of quantitation of mitral regurgitation is the PISA method, based on the analysis of flow convergence region proximal to the regurgitant orifice.[34 35] The Doppler measurement of mitral and aortic stroke volumes is also useful but more cumbersome to master.[36] Both methods allow calculation of the regurgitant volume (RVol) and effective regurgitant orifice (ERO).[37] The respective thresholds for severe mitral regurgitation are ≥ 60 ml for RVol and ≥ 40 mm^2 for ERO. Haemodynamics can also be characterised by measuring the cardiac output by Doppler and the right ventricular systolic pressure by use of the tricuspid regurgitant velocity.

Aetiology–repairability

The mitral lesions can be reliably defined by echocardiography (fig 11.4),[38] and usually transthoracic echocardiography is sufficient but when imaging is mediocre, transoesophageal

Information needed to determine timing of mitral surgery

- ▶ Symptoms or signs of heart failure, if unclear exercise test
- ▶ Left ventricle:
  - – left ventricular function (ejection fraction, end systolic diameter)
- ▶ Left atrium:
  - – atrial fibrillation?
  - – size
- ▶ Haemodynamics:
  - – pulmonary hypertension (Doppler—rarely catheterisation needed)
- ▶ Degree of mitral regurgitation:
  - – clinical examination: intensity of murmur, thrill, S3
  - – quantitative Doppler echocardiography, if inconclusive
  - – transoesophageal echocardiography or angiography
- ▶ Repairability:
  - – aetiology, mechanism
  - – calcifications, anterior leaflet involvement
  - – surgeon's skills
- ▶ Surgical risk:
  - – age
  - – heart failure
  - – comorbidity

echocardiography can be helpful (fig 11.5).[38] Rheumatic lesion or massive calcifications of the valve or annulus are often difficult to repair and in the vast majority of cases mitral prolapse is repairable. The repairability is highly dependent on the skills and experience of the surgeon and should be defined based on both patient and institution based criteria. New methods have extended the field of application of repair, particularly with anterior leaflet flail segments,[26] but if local experience is limited, it is important to refer patients to centres with more extensive experience.

Surgical risk
The operative risk is mostly determined by age ≥ 75 years,[7] by the presence of severe preoperative heart failure,[18] by the presence of coronary disease,[39] and by the severity of comorbid

conditions. A composite assessment of the risk is essential for clinical decision making, but the risk in asymptomatic patients ≤ 75 years old is usually low—between 0.1–0.2% in most advanced centres.

TIMING OF SURGICAL CORRECTION OF MITRAL REGURGITATION
The timing of mitral surgery translates into a simple categorical answer when the patient is seen—that is, should we advise the patient to have mitral surgery promptly or should we advise follow up with conservative management? This process can be stratified according to aetiology and severity of mitral regurgitation.

Organic mitral regurgitation
Severe mitral regurgitation: patient has overt symptoms or left ventricular dysfunction
These patients with severe mitral regurgitation with overt severe consequences should be offered surgery, even in relatively high risk patients and irrespective of repairability of the mitral valve. Although surgery performed with this type of presentation results in symptomatic improvement, it is associated with notable excess postoperative risk,[7][18] but the postoperative outcome is far better than the outcome under medical treatment.[5]

Severe mitral regurgitation: patient has neither overt symptoms nor left ventricular dysfunction
Irrespective of repairability, some recent events before the visit are a strong incentive to propose surgery immediately: atrial fibrillation, even paroxysmal, ventricular tachycardia at rest or during exercise, or the observation of pulmonary hypertension by echocardiography are such events.[10]

With low probability of repair, patients are usually not referred to surgery if there are no clinical risk factors. However, patients with a massive degree of mitral regurgitation (regurgitant volume ≥ 100 ml/beat) or with pronounced left atrial enlargement may be considered for surgery if at low risk for surgery.

With high probability of valve repair, our approach,[30] and the current guidelines,[10] have become much more aggressive

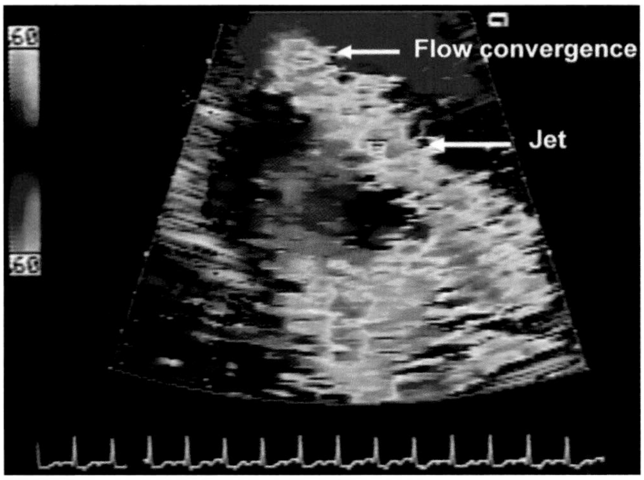

Figure 11.4 Echocardiographic long axis apical view of the left atrium with colour flow imaging of the jet of mitral regurgitation in a patient with flail posterior leaflet. Note the eccentric jet occupying only a portion of the left atrium despite the severe regurgitation with a large proximal flow convergence.

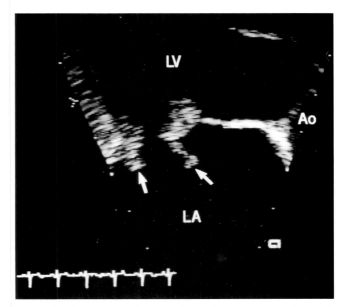

Figure 11.5 Transoesophageal echocardiographic view of the left atrium (LA), left ventricle (LV) and aorta (Ao) in a patient with bileaflet mitral valve flail segments (arrows) and ruptured chordae.

80

towards surgery, even if there are no symptoms or signs of left ventricular dysfunction, if the operative risk is low. This aggressive approach will require a randomised clinical trial in the future to define the magnitude of its benefit.

Mitral regurgitation not severe

For regurgitant volumes < 45 ml/beat there is almost never a need for surgery; furthermore, there is concern that a failed repair attempted during another cardiac operation (such as bypass surgery needed for angina) may result in worse mitral regurgitation than originally present.

For regurgitant volumes 45–60 ml/beat, there is usually no need for immediate surgery but in certain rare circumstances mitral surgery may be indicated. These involve valves that are repairable and patients who need a cardiac operation for a MAZE procedure, or bypass surgery or another valve operation. In some patients with mitral valve prolapse and ventricular tachycardia at rest or with exertion we have indicated a mitral valve repair to suppress the volume overload. The comparison of a surgical approach to medical treatment and even the determination of the benefit of medical treatment under those circumstances remains to be defined.[10]

Ischaemic mitral regurgitation

The timing of surgery in ischaemic mitral regurgitation is more complicated than in organic mitral regurgitation because the definition of what is severe mitral regurgitation (that is, mitral regurgitation with severe vital consequences) is different from organic mitral regurgitation. Indeed, patients with an ERO ≥ 20 mm^2 (and not ≥ 40 mm^2 as in organic mitral regurgitation) incur a notable excess mortality.[15] Also, despite the fact that repair is often possible, the risk of surgery is higher than in organic mitral regurgitation and still represents a limitation to early surgery.

When coronary bypass grafting surgery is deemed necessary and mitral regurgitation is present, recent data suggest that patients with ERO ≥ 20 mm^2 should be offered mitral repair. It is uncertain whether patients with trace mitral regurgitation but ERO < 20 mm^2 may benefit from repair.

When coronary bypass grafting surgery is deemed not indispensable but possible, a previous history of heart failure, the presence of viable myocardium, and mitral regurgitation ≥ 20 mm^2 all argue in favour of mitral surgery combined with revascularisation.

When coronary bypass grafting surgery is deemed not to be feasible, the indications of mitral surgery are more restrictive and frank symptoms, lack of diffuse myocardial scars, and a frank volume overload with regurgitant volume ≥ 45–50 ml appear all minimal considerations for mitral surgery. The choice of performing cardiac transplantation is to be discussed.

Therefore, the timing of mitral surgery has changed considerably from a relatively passive response to the development of severe symptoms, to an early surgery concept preceding the signs of left ventricular dysfunction. The early surgery approach requires a high repair rate and a low operative mortality; therefore currently not all patients and not all institutions are candidates to apply the early indications of surgical correction of mitral regurgitation. Nevertheless, considerable progresses have recently been accomplished for the assessment and treatment of mitral regurgitation and surgery should be considered early in the course of the disease, when severe regurgitation has been diagnosed.

REFERENCES

1 **Enriquez-Sarano M**, Basmadjian A, Rossi A, *et al.* Progression of mitral regurgitation: a prospective Doppler echocardiographic study. *J Am Coll Cardiol* 1999;**34**:1137–44.
2 **Enriquez-Sarano M**, Tajik A, Schaff H, *et al.* Echocardiographic prediction of left ventricular function after correction of mitral regurgitation: results and clinical implications. *J Am Coll Cardiol* 1994;**24**:1536–43.
3 **Delahaye J**, Gare J, Viguier E, *et al.* Natural history of severe mitral regurgitation. *Eur Heart J* 1991;**12**(suppl B):5–9.
4 **Horstkotte D**, Loogen F, Kleikamp G, *et al.* Effect of prosthetic heart valve replacement on the natural course of isolated mitral and aortic as well as multivalvular diseases. Clinical results in 783 patients up to 8 years following implantation of the Björk-Shiley tilting disc prosthesis. *Z Kardiol* 1983;**72**:494–503.
5 **Ling H**, Enriquez-Sarano M, Seward J, *et al.* Clinical outcome of mitral regurgitation due to flail leaflets. *N Engl J Med* 1996;**335**:1417–23.
▸ **A study of 229 patients with mitral regurgitation caused by flail leaflets. The study shows excess mortality under conservative management with high morbidity and 90% of patients with either death or surgery 10 years after diagnosis.**
6 **Grigioni F**, Enriquez-Sarano M, Ling L, *et al.* Sudden death in mitral regurgitation due to flail leaflet. *J Am Coll Cardiol* 1999;**34**:2078–85.
▸ **A study of sudden death in 348 patients with mitral regurgitation showing that sudden death occurs at a rate of 1.8% per year overall. The predictors of sudden death are ejection fraction, symptoms, and atrial fibrillation. In patients with no risk factors the rate of sudden death was 0.8% per year.**
7 **Enriquez-Sarano M**, Tajik A, Schaff H, *et al.* Echocardiographic prediction of survival after surgical correction of organic mitral regurgitation. *Circulation* 1994;**90**:830–7.
▸ **A large study of the outcome of mitral surgery for mitral regurgitation, analysed as a function of preoperative left ventricular function. Despite its limitation, ejection fraction was the best predictor of long term survival.**
8 **Crawford M**, Souchek J, Oprian C, *et al.* Determinants of survival and left ventricular performance after mitral valve replacement. *Circulation* 1990;**81**:1173–81.
9 **Enriquez-Sarano M**, Schaff H, Orszulak T, *et al.* Congestive heart failure after surgical correction of mitral regurgitation. A long-term study. *Circulation* 1995;**92**:2496–503.
10 **Bonow R**, Carabello B, DeLeon A, *et al.* ACC/AHA guidelines for the management of patients with valvular heart disease. *Circulation* 1998;**98**:1949–84.
▸ **A large summary of the literature on valvar heart disease and the recommendations made by the panel on that basis for surgery.**
11 **Leung D**, Griffin B, Stewart W, *et al.* Left ventricular function after valve repair for chronic mitral regurgitation: predictive value of preoperative assessment of contractile reserve by exercise echocardiography. *J Am Coll Cardiol* 1996;**28**:1198–205.
12 **Kishon Y**, Oh J, Schaff H, *et al.* Mitral valve operation in postinfarction rupture of a papillary muscle: immediate results and long term follow up of 22 patients. *Mayo Clin Proc* 1992;**67**:1023–30.
13 **Yiu S**, Enriquez-Sarano M, Tribouilloy C, *et al.* Determinants of the degree of functional mitral regurgitation in patients with systolic left ventricular dysfunction: a quantitative clinical study. *Circulation* 2000;**102**:1400–6.
14 **Lamas G**, Mitchell G, Flaker G, *et al.* Clinical significance of mitral regurgitation after acute myocardial infarction. *Circulation* 1997;**96**:827–33.
▸ **A study reporting a subset (angiographic) of the SAVE (survival and ventricular enlargement) study. Although severe mitral regurgitation was an exclusion of the SAVE trial, the presence of mitral regurgitation in these patients included early after myocardial infarction was associated with poor survival independently of all other baseline characteristics.**
15 **Grigioni F**, Enriquez-Sarano M, Zehr K, *et al.* Ischemic mitral regurgitation: long-term outcome and prognostic implications with quantitative Doppler assessment. *Circulation* 2001;**103**:1759–64.
▸ **A study of chronic ischaemic (post-myocardial infarction) heart disease with and without mitral regurgitation. The mitral regurgitation was quantified by Doppler echocardiography. The patients with mitral regurgitation had a pronounced excess mortality and the ERO was the best predictor of survival.**
16 **Desjardins V**, Enriquez-Sarano M, Tajik A, *et al.* Intensity of murmurs correlates with severity of valvular regurgitation. *Am J Med* 1996;**100**:149–56.
17 **Cohn L**, Couper G, Kinchla N, *et al.* Decreased operative risk of surgical treatment of mitral regurgitation with or without coronary artery disease. *J Am Coll Cardiol* 1990;**16**:1575–8.
18 **Tribouilloy C**, Enriquez-Sarano M, Schaff H, *et al.* Impact of preoperative symptoms on survival after surgical correction of organic mitral regurgitation: rationale for optimizing surgical indications. *Circulation* 1999;**99**:400–5.
▸ **A large recent study of patients operated on for mitral regurgitation and stratified according to their preoperative symptoms. The main result is that patients with NYHA functional class III-IV symptoms incur postoperative excess mortality whereas those operated on have a survival no different from the age and sex expected survival.**
19 **Cohn L**, Kowalker W, Bhatia S, *et al.* Comparative morbidity of mitral valve repair versus replacement for mitral regurgitation with and without coronary artery disease. *Ann Thorac Surg* 1988;**45**:284–90.

20 **Perier P**, Deloche A, Chauvaud S, *et al.* Comparative evaluation of mitral valve repair and replacement with Starr, Bjork, and porcine valve prostheses. *Circulation* 1984;**70**:I187–92.

21 **Sand M**, Naftel D, Blackstone E, *et al.* A comparison of repair and replacement for mitral valve incompetence. *J Thorac Cardiovasc Surg* 1987;**94**:208–19.

22 **Enriquez-Sarano M**, Schaff H, Orszulak T, *et al.* Valve repair improves the outcome of surgery for mitral regurgitation. *Circulation* 1995;**91**:1264–5.

▶ **A large study comparing short and long term outcome after mitral repair and replacement for mitral regurgitation. The study shows that, adjusting for all differences, repair was associated with a lower operative mortality, better long term survival, and better postoperative left ventricular function. Therefore, repair should be the preferred mode of surgical correction of mitral regurgitation.**

23 **Freeman W**, Schaff H, Khanderia B, *et al.* Intraoperative evaluation of mitral valve regurgitation and repair by transesophageal echocardiography: incidence and significance of systolic anterior motion. *J Am Coll Cardiol* 1992;**20**:599–609.

24 **Cosgrove D**, Chavez A, Lytle B, *et al.* Results of mitral valve reconstruction. *Circulation* 1986;**74**:I-82–7.

25 **Frater R**, Gabbay S, Shore D, *et al.* Reproducible replacement of elongated or ruptured mitral valve chordae. *Ann Thorac Surg* 1983;**35**:14–28.

26 **Lessana A**, Escorsin M, Romano M, *et al.* Transposition of posterior leaflet for treatment of ruptured main chordae of the anterior mitral leaflet. *J Thorac Cardiovasc Surg* 1985;**89**:804–6.

27 **Gillinov A**, Cosgrove D, Blackstone E, *et al.* Durability of mitral valve repair for degenerative disease. *J Thorac Cardiovasc Surg* 1998;**116**:734–43.

▶ **A large study of degenerative mitral regurgitation, mostly caused by prolapse, showing that the best results are obtained in pure posterior leaflet prolapse.**

28 **Sousa Uva M**, Dreyfus G, Rescigno G, *et al.* Surgical treatment of asymptomatic and mildly symptomatic mitral regurgitation. *J Thorac Cardiovasc Surg* 1996;**112**:1240–9.

29 **Chua Y**, Schaff H, Orszulak T, *et al.* Outcome of mitral valve repair in patients with preoperative atrial fibrillation. Should the maze procedure be combined with mitral valvuloplasty? *J Thorac Cardiovasc Surg* 1994;**107**:408–15.

30 **Ling L**, Enriquez-Sarano M, Seward J, *et al.* Early surgery in patients with mitral regurgitation due to partial flail leaflet: a long-term outcome study. *Circulation* 1997;**96**:1819–25.

▶ **A study comparing, exclusively in surgical candidates, conservative management (with surgery performed when needed) to immediate early surgery in patients with mitral regurgitation. Early surgery is followed by better survival and less heart failure than conservative management, even after adjustment for all baseline differences.**

31 **Leung D**, Griffin B, Snader C, *et al.* Determinants of functional capacity in chronic mitral regurgitation unassociated with coronary artery disease or left ventricular dysfunction. *Am J Cardiol* 1997;**79**:914–20.

32 **Enriquez-Sarano M**, Tajik A, Bailey K, *et al.* Color flow imaging compared with quantitative Doppler assessment of severity of mitral regurgitation: influence of eccentricity of jet and mechanism of regurgitation. *J Am Coll Cardiol* 1993;**21**:1211–9.

33 **Croft C**, Lipscomb K, Mathis K, *et al.* Limitations of qualitative angiographic grading in aortic or mitral regurgitation. *Am J Cardiol* 1984;**53**:1593–8.

34 **Enriquez-Sarano M**, Miller FJ, Hayes S, *et al.* Effective mitral regurgitant orifice area: clinical use and pitfalls of the proximal isovelocity surface area method. *J Am Coll Cardiol* 1995;**25**:703–9.

35 **Vandervoort P**, Rivera J, Mele D, *et al.* Application of color Doppler flow mapping to calculate effective regurgitant orifice area. An in vitro study and initial clinical observations. *Circulation* 1993;**88**:1150–6.

36 **Enriquez-Sarano M**, Bailey K, Seward J, *et al.* Quantitative Doppler assessment of valvular regurgitation. *Circulation* 1993;**87**:841–8.

37 **Enriquez-Sarano M**, Seward J, Bailey K, *et al.* Effective regurgitant orifice area: a noninvasive Doppler development of an old hemodynamic concept. *J Am Coll Cardiol* 1994;**23**:443–51.

38 **Enriquez-Sarano M**, Freeman W, Tribouilloy C, *et al.* Functional anatomy of mitral regurgitation: echocardiographic assessment and implications on outcome. *J Am Coll Cardiol* 1999;**34**:1129–36.

39 **Tribouilloy C**, Enriquez-Sarano M, Schaff H, *et al.* Excess mortality due to coronary artery disease after valvular surgery: secular trends in valvular regurgitation and effect of internal mammary bypass. *Circulation* 1998;**98** (suppl II):II-108–15.

12 THE MEDICAL MANAGEMENT OF VALVAR HEART DISEASE

N A Boon, P Bloomfield

Although there is very little high quality evidence to guide the medical treatment of valve disease, this is an important area of cardiology for two reasons. Firstly, there are many frail older people with symptomatic degenerative valve disease in whom the risks of surgical intervention are prohibitive and medical treatment is the only realistic option. Secondly, there is a real and exciting prospect of using medical treatment to influence the natural history of some forms of valve disease, thereby delaying or even avoiding the need for surgery.

Left ventricular systolic dysfunction caused by ischaemic heart disease was the underlying problem in the vast majority of patients who took part in the landmark trials of medical treatment (angiotensin converting enzyme (ACE) inhibitors, angiotensin receptor antagonists, vasodilators, β blockers, and spironolactone) for heart failure. However, some of these trials included patients with valve disease and the principles that have been learned may be widely applicable. Thus, it seems reasonable to assume that a small dose of spironolactone will benefit most patients with severe congestive cardiac failure including those with valvar heart disease. On the other hand it seems clear that the characteristic haemodynamic problems associated with individual valve lesions may influence the relative benefits and hazards of specific treatments. For example, vasodilator treatment may be unwise in patients with severe aortic stenosis because there is a risk that this will reduce aortic pressure and coronary perfusion without an equivalent reduction in the left ventricular afterload. In contrast, vasodilators may be particularly beneficial in patients with aortic or mitral regurgitation because they might be expected to reduce the regurgitant fraction and increase forward flow. Similarly, by prolonging diastole and left ventricular filling, β blockers may harm patients with aortic regurgitation but benefit patients with mitral stenosis.

Medical treatment might be able to alter the natural history of valve disease in two ways. Firstly, it is conceivable that outcome might be improved by treatments that suppress the disease process in the valve itself—for example, it may be possible to restrict fibrosis, scarring and calcification by using anti-inflammatory treatments in some forms of degenerative and rheumatic valve disease. Secondly, it may be possible to prevent or ameliorate the deleterious effects of secondary heart muscle disease—for example, vasodilator treatment may help to protect the myocardium in patients with left ventricular volume overload caused by chronic aortic or mitral regurgitation.

This article will review the medical treatment of the four major left heart valve lesions (aortic stenosis, mitral stenosis, aortic regurgitation, and mitral regurgitation). The optimum timing of surgery, the role of anticoagulants, and the prophylaxis of infective endocarditis have been covered in separate reviews in this series.

▶ AORTIC STENOSIS

Pathophysiology

Calcific aortic stenosis may be caused by progressive calcification of a congenitally bicuspid valve, when it typically presents in the fourth and fifth decades of life, or senile calcification of a morphologically normal tricuspid valve when it tends to present later in life (fig 12.1). The disease appears to be an active process that has much in common with atherosclerosis and is probably mediated by mechanical stress ("wear and tear"), lipid deposition, and inflammation; significant coronary artery disease is present in approximately 50% of patients with calcific aortic stenosis and the two conditions share many of the same risk factors, with a similar level of risk (table 12.1).[1 2] Rheumatic disease of the aortic valve usually causes mixed stenotic and regurgitant lesions and is commonly associated with mitral valve disease.

Acquired aortic stenosis develops slowly and the cardiac output is initially maintained at the cost of a steadily increasing gradient across the aortic valve. The left ventricle becomes increasingly hypertrophied and coronary blood flow may become inadequate; patients may therefore develop angina, even in the absence of concomitant coronary disease. The fixed outflow obstruction limits the increase in cardiac output required on exercise and effort related hypotension and syncope may occur. Eventually the left ventricle can no longer overcome the outflow tract obstruction and left ventricular failure supervenes. Patients with aortic stenosis typically remain asymptomatic for

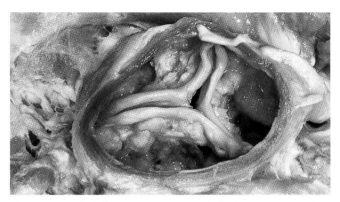

Figure 12.1 Calcific aortic stenosis: a calcified stenotic tricuspid valve.

Table 12.1   Risk factors for aortic valve calcification

Clinical
- ▶ Age
- ▶ Male sex
- ▶ Smoking
- ▶ Diabetes mellitus
- ▶ Hypertension
- ▶ Renal failure
- ▶ Hyperparathyroidism
- ▶ Paget's disease

Biochemical
- ▶ Hyperlipidaemia
  - – increased total cholesterol
  - – increased LDL cholesterol
  - – reduced HDL cholesterol
  - – increased Lp (a) lipoprotein
- ▶ Hypercalcaemia
- ▶ Increased serum creatinine

HDL, high density lipoprotein; LDL, low density lipoprotein.

many years but deteriorate rapidly when symptoms develop; thus, death usually ensues within 3–5 years of the onset of symptoms.[3]

Symptom control

Symptomatic aortic stenosis is a surgical condition and has become the most common reason for valve replacement in the developed world. However, it is also an important cause of angina and heart failure among frail elderly subjects who are unsuitable for surgery, and in these people conventional medical treatment may provide the only means of alleviating symptoms. The cautious use of β blockers and nitrates may control angina. Unfortunately, nitrates may cause symptomatic hypotension, especially if they are used shortly after exertion. Diuretics may relieve the symptoms of pulmonary congestion but it is important to appreciate that patients with severe aortic stenosis are dependent on adequate filling pressures and excessive diuretic treatment may be hazardous. Digoxin may benefit those with atrial fibrillation or depressed left ventricular systolic function. Atrial fibrillation is often poorly tolerated and in this situation attempts to restore sinus rhythm by means of early DC cardioversion, or antiarrhythmic treatment with amiodarone, should be considered.

Most doctors avoid ACE inhibitors in patients with aortic stenosis and heart failure on the grounds that these drugs are unlikely to reduce left ventricular afterload and may cause dangerous hypotension. These fears have not been substantiated by small clinical studies evaluating short term treatment with a variety of vasodilators including ACE inhibitors, prazosin, hydralazine, nitroprusside, and nitrates.[4] For example, two small clinical series describing the acute effects of captopril in severe aortic stenosis (mean aortic valve gradients 78 and 93 mm Hg) have shown not only that first dose hypotension did not occur, but that mean cardiac output increased substantially and pulmonary capillary wedge pressure decreased significantly in the majority of patients. In one of these studies mean cardiac output increased by 41% among patients with overt heart failure; moreover, symptomatic benefit from long term treatment was documented among those who had a beneficial haemodynamic response. Further studies are warranted but it seems clear that some patients with heart failure and aortic stenosis may benefit from treatment with ACE inhibitors provided that these drugs are introduced cautiously in hospital.

Secondary prevention

In established aortic stenosis, natural history studies have shown that the annual reduction in valve area is approximately 0.1 cm²/year, with an average increase in Doppler jet velocity of approximately 0.3 m/s/year (equivalent to an increase in gradient of 7 mm Hg/year)[5]; however, this varies considerably and tends to be greater in the elderly, those with heavy aortic valve calcification, and, in some studies at least, those with hyperlipidaemia. In one series of 170 consecutive patients a serum cholesterol concentration of more than 5.2 mmol/l (200 mg/dl) was associated with double the rate of reduction in aortic valve area.[6] Moreover in a recent non-randomised retrospective study the use of hydroxymethyl glutaryl coenzyme A (HMG CoA) reductase inhibitors (statins) was associated with a significantly lower rate of decrease in aortic valve area (mean (SD) 0.06 (0.16) cm²/year v 0.11 (0.11) cm²/year).[7]

These observations have obvious implications for secondary prevention in patients with calcific aortic stenosis, and several randomised controlled trials have been set up to test the hypothesis that lipid lowering treatment with HMG CoA reductase inhibitors will retard the progression, or even induce regression, of the disease. Trials of aspirin and antihypertensive treatment are also warranted.

MITRAL STENOSIS
Pathophysiology

Mitral stenosis is almost always rheumatic in origin; however, in the elderly, heavy calcification of the mitral valve apparatus can produce a similar syndrome.

The mitral valve orifice is slowly diminished by progressive fibrosis, calcification of the valve leaflets, and fusion of the cusps and subvalvar apparatus. The flow of blood from the left atrium to the left ventricle is therefore restricted and left atrial pressure rises, leading to pulmonary venous congestion and breathlessness. There is dilatation and hypertrophy of the left atrium, and left ventricular filling becomes more dependent on left atrial contraction. Any increase in heart rate shortens diastole (the time the mitral valve is open) and produces a further rise in left atrial pressure; situations that demand an increase in cardiac output will also increase left atrial pressure. Exercise and pregnancy are therefore poorly tolerated. At first, symptoms occur only on exercise; however, in severe stenosis left atrial pressure is permanently elevated and symptoms may occur at rest. Reduced lung compliance, caused by chronic pulmonary venous congestion, contributes to breathlessness, and a low cardiac output may cause fatigue.

Atrial fibrillation caused by progressive dilatation of the left atrium is very common. A minority of patients (less than 20%) remain in sinus rhythm; many of these individuals have a small fibrotic left atrium and severe pulmonary hypertension.

Symptom control

Medical treatment is a reasonable option for patients with mild symptoms but mechanical relief of the obstruction, by balloon valvuloplasty or surgery, should always be considered in patients with more severe symptoms, those with new onset atrial fibrillation, and those with evidence of moderate or severe pulmonary hypertension.[3] Diuretics will usually reduce left atrial pressure and the symptoms of pulmonary congestion (breathlessness, haemoptysis); however, they may also reduce cardiac output and worsen fatigue. β Blockers and rate limiting calcium antagonists (for example, diltiazem, verapamil) slow the heart rate, at rest and during exercise, and may improve left ventricular filling by prolonging diastole. They will often relieve effort related symptoms and are particularly effective in patients with sinus tachycardia (for example, pregnancy, anaemia), atrial fibrillation, and other tachyarrhythmias.

Atrial fibrillation

Atrial fibrillation is a common complication of mitral stenosis, particularly in older patients, and is associated with a high risk of arterial embolism, especially stroke, and an adverse prognosis (10 year survival of 25% compared to 46% for patients in sinus rhythm[3]). Although no randomised controlled trials have specifically examined the efficacy of anticoagulant treatment in mitral stenosis there is compelling evidence to support the use of anticoagulants (target international normalised ratio (INR) 2–3:1) in those with all forms of atrial fibrillation and those who have already suffered an embolic event.[8] A high proportion of emboli occur at or shortly after the onset of atrial fibrillation and it is therefore desirable to introduce anticoagulants while the patient is still in sinus rhythm. Older patients, those with severe mitral stenosis, and those with left atrial dilatation are at greatest risk and are most likely to benefit from early anticoagulation.

The onset of atrial fibrillation is often accompanied by pronounced haemodynamic deterioration precipitated by a dramatic reduction in left ventricular filling caused by the effects of tachycardia and the loss of atrial contraction. Good rate control is essential to relieve symptoms. Digoxin, β blockers, and rate limiting calcium antagonists can be used to control heart rate, at rest and during exercise, and are all effective.[8 9] However, digoxin has a narrow therapeutic index, and is inferior to β blockade in terms of preventing paroxysms of atrial fibrillation, and controlling the heart rate at the onset of atrial fibrillation and during exercise or other forms of stress. Combination drug treatment is often necessary and a few patients require atrioventricular node ablation and pacing.

Paroxysmal atrial fibrillation may respond to treatment with amiodarone or group 1c drugs such as flecainide, but usually gives way to permanent atrial fibrillation. Chemical or electrical cardioversion may have a limited role in the management of persistent atrial fibrillation but, unless the mitral stenosis is relieved by surgery or valvuloplasty, the arrhythmia invariably recurs.

Secondary prevention

There are no treatments that have been shown to retard the rheumatic process of chronic fibrosis and scarring, but eradication of streptococcal infection and prophylaxis against further attacks of rheumatic fever are thought to be beneficial. Most guidelines recommend long term treatment with 250 mg phenoxymethyl penicillin (penicillin V) orally twice daily or, if compliance is in doubt, 1.2 million units of benzathine penicillin intramuscularly every four weeks; a sulfonamide or erythromycin can be used if the patient is allergic to penicillin. The optimum duration of antibiotic prophylaxis has not been established and will depend to a large extent on practical issues such as compliance and the likelihood of coming into contact with populations that have a high prevalence of streptococcal infection. The American Heart Association/American College of Cardiology (AHA/ACC) guidelines recommend that in most patients with established rheumatic heart disease it is advisable to maintain prophylactic antibiotic treatment until the age of 40 years and for at least 10 years after the last attack of rheumatic fever.[3]

AORTIC REGURGITATION

Pathophysiology

In aortic regurgitation the main determinants of regurgitant volume are the regurgitant orifice area (which is typically fixed), the duration of diastole (a function of the heart rate), and the diastolic transvalvar pressure gradient (aortic minus left ventricular diastolic pressure).[10] Both bradycardia and hypertension are therefore undesirable and should be treated energetically.

Aortic regurgitation imposes volume overload and a high afterload on the left ventricle. In slowly progressive chronic aortic regurgitations adaptive remodelling processes, including left ventricular dilatation and hypertrophy, mean that the heart can accommodate large volumes of regurgitant flow for many years with little or no change in filling pressures or cardiac output.[11] However, eventually these adaptive processes fail and myocardial dysfunction and left ventricular failure ensue.

The potential haemodynamic benefits of vasodilator drug treatment in aortic regurgitation are obvious. Arterial vasodilators redistribute left ventricular stroke volume by increasing forward flow and reducing regurgitant flow; venodilators and diuretics diminish preload and will reduce both left ventricular end diastolic volume and pressure.[10 11] These drugs can therefore be used both to alleviate the symptoms and signs of heart failure and to preserve left ventricular function by reducing wall stress.

Symptom control

Diuretics and vasodilators remain the drugs of choice for the relief of symptoms in patients with aortic regurgitation who are considered unsuitable for aortic valve replacement because of associated comorbidity. Short term vasodilator treatment may also be given to patients with severe heart failure and severe left ventricular dysfunction to improve their haemodynamics and clinical condition before aortic valve replacement.[3]

Preservation of left ventricular function (secondary prevention)

Several studies have tested the hypothesis that vasodilators can be given chronically to asymptomatic patients with severe aortic regurgitation to reduce systolic blood pressure and afterload mismatch, and thereby preserve left ventricular function, prevent heart failure, and delay the need for aortic valve replacement.

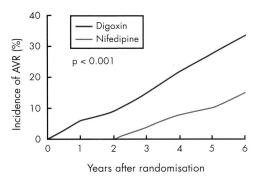

Figure 12.2 Cumulative incidence of progression to aortic valve replacement in initially asymptomatic patients with severe aortic regurgitation and normal left ventricular function randomised to treatment with digoxin 0.25 mg daily or nifedipine 20 mg twice daily. Reproduced from Scognamiglio *et al*[12] with permission of the Massachusetts Medical Society.

Scognamiglio and colleagues found that nifedipine (20 mg twice daily), compared with digoxin (0.25 mg daily), given to asymptomatic patients with severe aortic regurgitation and normal left ventricular function, reduced the number of patients developing symptoms and/or left ventricular dysfunction; at the end of a six year period only 15% had undergone aortic valve replacement compared to 34% in the digoxin group[12] (fig 12.2). Importantly, when the patients who had been receiving nifedipine came to aortic valve replacement, all survived, and left ventricular size and function improved postoperatively; therefore nifedipine did not appear to mask the development of irreversible left ventricular dysfunction. Long term treatment with nifedipine was also shown to reduce left ventricular mass in an earlier placebo controlled trial in patients with severe aortic regurgitation.[13]

Similar data have emerged from trials of hydralazine and ACE inhibitors[14–16]; in these trials hydralazine had a higher incidence of side effects than nifedipine and, in one study, was less effective than enalapril.[16] Nevertheless, the admittedly very limited trials of ACE inhibitors in asymptomatic aortic regurgitation have produced inconsistent results, possibly because plasma renin activity is not necessarily increased in this setting.[11] [14]

It is important to appreciate that the goal of protecting the left ventricle in severe aortic regurgitation depends on reducing afterload mismatch by lowering systolic blood pressure[14]; the dose of whichever drug is chosen should therefore be titrated against blood pressure. However, it is rarely possible to reduce systolic blood pressure to normal because of the high stroke volume which is characteristic of severe aortic regurgitation.

The beneficial effects of vasodilators on left ventricular remodelling in chronic aortic regurgitation are likely to be greatest in those patients with the largest and sickest hearts.[10] The clinical trials are certainly consistent with this view and there is no evidence to support the use of long term vasodilator treatment in patients with mild to moderate aortic regurgitation, or those with normal blood pressure and a normal left ventricular cavity size—all of whom have an excellent outlook anyway.

The class 1 recommendations for vasodilator treatment in chronic aortic regurgitation of the ACC/AHA task force[3] for management of patients with valvar heart disease are listed in the box below.

Choice of vasodilator

There are very few comparative trials to guide the choice of vasodilator in aortic regurgitation. However, intravenous sodium nitroprusside is usually the drug of choice in acute heart failure because its short half life and rapid onset of

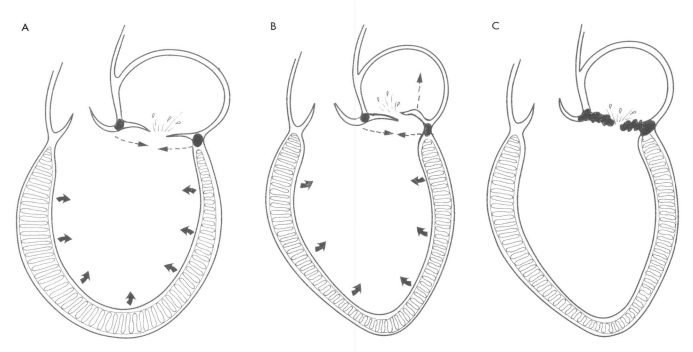

Figure 12.3 The relation between the cause of mitral regurgitation, drug induced changes in left ventricular preload, and the degree of mitral regurgitation. (A) In dilated cardiomyopathy the left ventricle is dilated and more spherical than normal. Mitral regurgitation is caused by stretching of the mitral annulus and chordal apparatus. A reduction in left ventricular preload will therefore reduce the degree of mitral regurgitation. (B) In mitral valve prolapse a reduction in left ventricular preload will reduce left ventricular volume and may increase the degree of prolapse and mitral regurgitation. (C) In rheumatic disease fibrous scarring and calcification of the mitral valve leaflets creates a fixed orifice so the degree of mitral regurgitation is not influenced by left ventricular preload.

ACC/AHA guidelines: class I* recommendations for the use of vasodilator treatment in chronic aortic regurgitation

▶ Chronic treatment in patients with severe regurgitation who have symptoms and/or left ventricular dysfunction when surgery is not recommended because of additional cardiac or non-cardiac factors

▶ Long term treatment in asymptomatic patients with severe regurgitation who have left ventricular dilatation but normal systolic function

▶ Long term treatment in asymptomatic patients with hypertension and any degree of regurgitation

▶ Long term ACE inhibitor treatment in patients with persistent left ventricular systolic dysfunction after aortic valve replacement

▶ Short term treatment to improve the haemodynamic profile of patients with severe heart failure symptoms and severe left ventricular dysfunction before proceeding with aortic valve replacement

*Conditions for which there is evidence and/or general agreement that a given procedure or treatment is useful and effective

action facilitate dose titration. In chronic aortic regurgitation ACE inhibitor treatment is particularly appealing because of the powerful evidence that these drugs reduce morbidity and mortality in patients with hypertension and/or heart failure. An ACE inhibitor is certainly the drug of choice for symptomatic patients with chronic aortic regurgitation and hypertension, poor left ventricular function or overt heart failure. Nifedipine is perhaps the best evidence based treatment that can be prescribed for patients with asymptomatic severe aortic regurgitation and well preserved left ventricular function.

MITRAL REGURGITATION
Pathophysiology
Mitral regurgitation causes chronic left ventricular volume overload, compensatory left ventricular hypertrophy and dilatation, and ultimately progressive left ventricular failure. Without surgery, the outlook for patients with severe mitral regurgitation is poor with an average annual mortality of 5%. Most deaths are caused by deteriorating left ventricular function and heart failure, but sudden, presumably arrhythmic, death is also common.[17]

The proven benefits of vasodilator treatment in aortic regurgitation do not necessarily extend to patients with mitral regurgitation for two reasons. Firstly, it is important to appreciate that, in contrast to aortic regurgitation, left ventricular afterload is typically reduced (left ventricular ejection is bi-directional in mitral regurgitation but unidirectional in aortic

regurgitation).[10] [14] Secondly, unlike aortic regurgitation, the size of the regurgitant mitral orifice is often dynamic and critically dependent on ventricular dimensions (fig 12.3).[10] Vasoactive treatment might therefore be expected to alter the regurgitant volume in some but not all settings. For example, a reduction in preload or an increase in contractility will reduce the regurgitant volume when mitral regurgitation is caused by left ventricular dilatation in ischaemic heart disease, or dilated cardiomyopathy. Conversely, a fall in preload may produce a deleterious increase in the mitral regurgitant volume in patients with hypertrophic cardiomyopathy or mitral valve prolapse. In rheumatic heart disease the mitral orifice is usually rigid or fixed and the degree of regurgitation is not therefore influenced by preload. A clear understanding of the aetiology of mitral regurgitation is therefore vital to the logical use of vasoactive treatment.

Symptom control
Mitral valve repair or replacement is strongly indicated if symptoms develop or there is evidence of impaired or deteriorating left ventricular systolic function.[17] However, medical treatment can be used to ameliorate symptoms if surgery is contraindicated by serious comorbidity or very poor left ventricular function. Venodilators, particularly nitrates, and diuretics have not been tested in formal trials but might be expected to relieve the symptoms and signs of pulmonary congestion; in our experience they are particularly valuable in patients with preload dependent mitral regurgitation (for example, ischaemic heart disease and all forms of functional mitral regurgitation).

Although there is very little high quality data on the effects of vasodilators in mitral regurgitation, ACE inhibitors are, in our experience, a valuable form of treatment in patients with heart failure and mitral regurgitation. Short term haemodynamic studies have shown a reciprocal relation between forward and regurgitant flow and demonstrated that hydralazine and ACE inhibitors will both typically reduce the degree of mitral regurgitation, and increase forward flow with little or no change in ejection fraction.[10] Long term treatment with quinalapril has been reported to improve functional class and reduce left ventricular volume and mass in a very small study of selected patients with chronic mitral regurgitation.[18] The theoretical risk that ACE inhibitors will increase the degree of mitral regurgitation in patients with mitral valve prolapse (fig 12.3) was not born out in one small study[19]; nevertheless, it seems prudent to assess the impact of vasodilator treatment in such patients by means of serial echocardiography.

Preservation of left ventricular function (secondary prevention)
There are no data to support the hypothesis that vasodilator treatment can preserve left ventricular function in asymptomatic patients with severe mitral regurgitation. There is

Table 12.2 Summary of useful medical treatments in valvar heart disease

Lesion	Symptom control	Secondary prevention and natural history
Aortic stenosis	Diuretics for heart failure. Nitrates and β blockers for angina	No proven treatment but lipid lowering therapy may slow progression of calcific aortic stenosis
Mitral stenosis	Diuretics for heart failure. Digoxin, β blockers, and rate limiting calcium antagonists for rate control in atrial fibrillation	Penicillin prophylaxis against recurrent episodes of rheumatic fever. Anticoagulants to prevent systemic thromboembolism
Aortic regurgitation	Diuretics and vasodilators (usually ACE inhibitors) for heart failure	Vasodilators (nifedipine or ACE inhibitors) to protect the left ventricular myocardium and delay the need for surgery
Mitral regurgitation	Diuretics and vasodilators (usually ACE inhibitors) for heart failure	No proven treatment

ACE, angiotensin converting enzyme.

evidence, however, that in carefully selected patients early mitral valve surgery can achieve this goal.[3] [17]

CONCLUSIONS

Medical treatment may alleviate symptoms and improve the natural history of valvar heart disease (table 12.2). An understanding of the pathophysiology of different valvar lesions and the haemodynamic changes they engender helps to guide the logical administration of drug treatment.

REFERENCES

1 **Mohler ER**. Are atherosclerotic processes involved in aortic-valve calcification? *Lancet* 2000;**356**:524–5.
▶ **A well written editorial drawing attention to the evidence that aortic stenosis and atherosclerosis have a similar pathogenesis.**
2 **Otto CM**, Kuusisto J, Reichenbach DD, *et al*. Characterization of the early lesion of "degenerative" valvular aortic stenosis: histologic and immunohistochemical studies. *Circulation* 1994;**90**:844–53.
▶ **A landmark study identifying the link between aortic sclerosis and aortic stenosis.**
3 **Bonow RO**, Carabello B, De Leon AC, *et al*. ACC/AHA guidelines for the management of patients with valvular heart disease: a report of the American College of Cardiology/American Heart Association task force on practice guidelines (committee on management of patients with valvular heart disease). *J Am Coll Cardiol* 1998;**32**:1486–588.
▶ **A superb resource that includes a comprehensive review of the literature on valve disease with 732 references and a series of authoritative and practical recommendations dealing with every aspect of the management of heart valve disease. It can be accessed in full text via www.acc.org**
4 **Cox NLT**, Abdul-Hamid AR, Mulley GP. Why deny ACE inhibitors to patients with aortic stenosis? *Lancet* 1998;**352**:111–2.
▶ **A challenging editorial that contains a review of the limited animal and human data on this subject.**
5 **Otto CM**, Burwash IG, Legget ME, *et al*. A prospective study of asymptomatic valvular aortic stenosis: clinical, echocardiographic, and exercise predictors of outcome. *Circulation* 1997;**95**:2262–70.
▶ **A careful large scale prospective study of the natural history of aortic stenosis.**
6 **Palta S**, Pai AM, Gill KS, *et al*. New insights into the progression of calcific aortic stenosis: implications for secondary progression. *Circulation* 2000;**101**:2497–502.
▶ **Probably the best of the many studies describing the risk factors for progression of aortic stenosis.**
7 **Novaro GM**, Tiong IY, Pearce GL, *et al*. Effect of hydroxymethyl glutaryl coenzyme A reductase inhibitors on the progression of calcific aortic stenosis. *Circulation* 2001;**104**:2205–9.
▶ **A non-randomised retrospective study that provides some evidence to justify prospective randomised trials of statins in aortic stenosis.**
8 **Gohlke-Barwolf C**. Anticoagulation in valvar heart disease: new aspects and management during non-cardiac surgery. *Heart* 2000;**84**:567–72.
9 **Carabello BA**, Crawford FA. Valvular heart disease. *N Engl J Med* 1997;**337**:32–41.
▶ **A succinct clinical review.**
10 **Levine HJ**, Gaasch WH. Vasoactive drugs in chronic regurgitant lesions of the mitral and aortic valves. *J Am Coll Cardiol* 1996;**28**:1083–91.
▶ **An excellent review that concentrates on the pathophysiology of left ventricular overload.**
11 **Bonow RO**. Chronic aortic regurgitation; role of medical therapy and optimal timing for surgery. *Cardiology Clinics* 1998;**16**:449–61.
▶ **Another excellent review with plenty of practical advice.**
12 **Scognamiglio R**, Rahimtoola SH, Fasoli G, *et al*. Nifedipine in asymptomatic patients with severe aortic regurgitation and normal left ventricular function. *N Engl J Med* 1994;**331**:689–94.
▶ **A landmark trial that compared the effects of nifedipine and digoxin.**
13 **Scognamiglio R**, Fasoli G, Ponchia A, *et al*. Long-term nifedipine unloading therapy in asymptomatic patients with chronic severe aortic regurgitation. *J Am Coll Cardiol* 1990;**16**:424–9.
▶ **A placebo controlled trial of nifedipine.**
14 **Grayburn PA**. Vasodilator therapy for chronic aortic and mitral regurgitation. *Am J Med Sci* 2000;**320**:202–8.
▶ **An excellent review.**
15 **Greenberg B**, Massie B, Bristow D, *et al*. Long-term vasodilator therapy of chronic aortic insufficiency: a randomised double-blinded, placebo controlled clinical trial. *Circulation* 1988;**78**:92–103.
▶ **An important placebo controlled trial of hydralazine that was ahead of its time.**
16 **Lin M**, Chiang H-T, Lin S-L, *et al*. Vasodilator therapy in chronic asymptomatic aortic regurgitation: enalapril versus hydralazine therapy. *J Am Coll Cardiol* 1994;**24**:1046–53.
▶ **A small trial among 38 patients.**
17 **Otto CM**. Evaluation and management of chronic mitral regurgitation. *N Engl J Med* 2001;**345**:740–6.
▶ **An eloquent account of the natural history, clinical evaluation, and management of mitral regurgitation.**
18 **Schon HR**, Schroter G, Barthel P, *et al*. Quinapril therapy in patients with chronic mitral regurgitation. *J Heart Valve Disease* 1994;**3**:197–204.
19 **Tischler MD**, Rowan M, LeWinter MM. Effect of enalapril therapy on left ventricular mass and volumes in asymptomatic chronic, severe mitral regurgitation secondary to mitral valve prolapse. *Am J Cardiol* 1998;**82**:242–5.
▶ **A small study of just 12 patients**

13 CHOICE OF HEART VALVE PROSTHESIS

Peter Bloomfield

It is 40 years since Starr and Edwards' description of successful prosthetic valve replacement in 1961. Some patients who underwent valve replacement with the original Starr-Edwards prosthesis in the 1960s are alive to this day. The Starr-Edwards ball and cage prosthesis, albeit in modified form, is still available commercially. Each year more than 6000 patients in the UK and 60 000 in the USA alone undergo valve replacement surgery. In the last 40 years more than 80 models of prostheses have been developed for patients requiring valve replacement.[1 2]

Mitral valvotomy for mitral stenosis predated the introduction of heart valve replacement, and valvotomy can now usually be achieved percutaneously with balloon dilatation in selected cases. Additionally techniques for repair of the diseased mitral valve, particularly mitral valve prolapse, have been developed and refined, avoiding the need for valve replacement. The morbidity, mortality, and long term results of valvotomy or valve repair in suitable patients are better than for valve replacement and should be used in preference when possible. Choice of operation and the prosthesis used for those undergoing valve replacement is important for each individual patient and ideally should be made together by the patient, cardiologist, and surgeon. This article deals with choice of prosthesis for the individual patient. Other articles in this series deal with the medical management of valvar heart disease,[3] anticoagulant control,[4] late results and late complications of valve replacement,[5] and management of endocarditis.[6]

▶ TYPES OF PROSTHESIS AVAILABLE

Mechanical prostheses
Ball valves
The original Starr-Edwards prosthesis comprised a silastic ball which seated in the sewing ring when closed and moved forward into the cage when open (fig 13.1). The original design has gone through several modifications but the basic design remains similar to the original. More than 200 000 have been implanted.

Disc valves
The Bjork-Shiley prosthesis is comprised of a single graphite disc coated with pyrolite carbon which tilts between two struts of the housing which is made of stainless steel or titanium (fig 13.1). The original design was modified in the early 1980s to increase the angle of opening and to change the disc to a convexo-concave shape (cc model). This design change in conjunction with changes in the manufacturing process led to some models of this generation of the prostheses being prone to fracture of one of the retaining struts, allowing the disc to escape with catastrophic results. Although these structural defects were corrected and modified versions of the valve were subsequently implanted for several years, the Bjork-Shiley valve is no longer manufactured. More than 360 000 Bjork-Shiley prostheses have been implanted. Other manufacturers continue to produce single disc prostheses—for example, the Medtronic-Hall and the Aortech Ultracor.

Bileaflet valves
Bileaflet valves have two semicircular leaflets which open and close creating one central and two peripheral orifices. The St Jude medical valve (fig 13.1) was introduced in 1977, and more than 600 000 have been implanted. It and similar valves produced by other manufacturers are now the most commonly implanted type of mechanical prosthesis in the world.

Biological prostheses
All mechanical prostheses have an absolute requirement for anticoagulant treatment. The potential advantage of avoiding the hazards of anticoagulation has led to the search for a valve replacement of suitable biological material which would not require long term anticoagulant treatment. A number of different approaches to the problem of finding a suitable biological valve have been made. An autologous or autogeneous valve is fashioned from the patient's own tissue such as fascia lata or pericardium. An autograft valve is one translocated from one position to another—for example, when the patient's own pulmonary valve is used to replace a diseased aortic valve. A

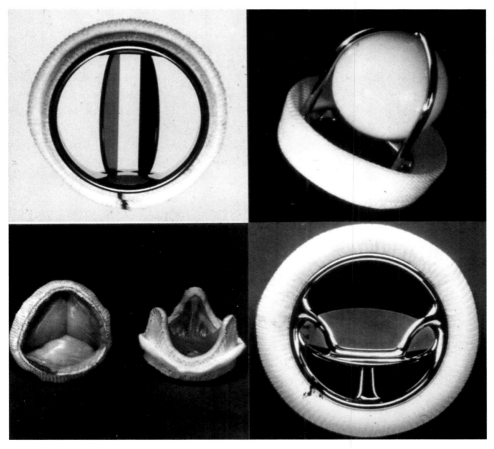

Figure 13.1 Common types of heart valve prostheses: St Jude's Medical bileaflet (top left); Starr-Edwards ball and cage (top right); Bjork-Shiley tilting disc (bottom right); stented porcine prosthesis (bottom left).

homograft (or allograft) valve is one transplanted from a human donor. A heterograft (or xenograft) valve is one transplanted from another species such as a pig, or manufactured from tissue such as bovine pericardium.

Autologous valves

In the 1970s valves were fashioned freehand from the patient's own fascia lata in the operating theatre. The procedure was technically demanding, the valves had very limited durability, and this approach has been abandoned. More recently frame mounted valves constructed from the patient's pericardium in the operating room using a commercially produced kit have been developed—for example, the Carpentier-Edwards Perimount pericardial prosthesis.

Autograft valves

Described by Donald Ross in 1967 the Ross procedure involves replacing the patient's diseased aortic valve with their own pulmonary valve which is in turn replaced by a homograft. The procedure is of particular value in children as the translocated pulmonary trunk grows with the child. Most late problems have been related to failure of the pulmonary homograft. The procedure requires a double valve replacement at operation with attendant increased surgical risk.

Homograft valves

Homografts from human cadavers (also known as allografts) have been used in some centres for aortic valve replacement for over 30 years. They are sterilised using an antibiotic solution and either stored in fixative or cryopreserved. Viable homografts are also successfully harvested from brain dead organ donors or from the explanted heart of a heart transplant patient.

Porcine heterograft (or xenograft) valves

Porcine valves are treated with glutaraldehyde which both sterilises the valve tissue and renders it biologically acceptable to the recipient—for example, the Hancock II Porcine (Medtronic) and the Biocor Porcine (St Jude Medical) prostheses. Most bioprosthesis are mounted on stents attached to a sewing ring (fig 13.1), but more recently stentless valves which are sewn in free hand have become available. Stentless valves have a greater effective orifice area compared with stented valves, but are technically more difficult to implant.

Bovine pericardial valves

These valves are fashioned from bovine pericardium mounted on a stented frame. The Ionescue-Shiley pericardial valve proved less durable than porcine valves and has been withdrawn. The Carpentier-Edwards pericardial valve is fabricated by anchoring the pericardial tissue behind the stents rather than using stitches through the tissue, as proved to be a weakness in the Ionescue-Shiley valve, but long term durability remains to be proven.

STUDIES EVALUATING DIFFERENT TYPES OF MECHANICAL PROSTHESES

Most studies of results of mechanical valve replacement have been observational studies of the results of valve replacement with one type of prosthesis. Most have shown excellent long term results for prosthesis survival, with no difference in durability between types of prosthesis. There have been few randomised controlled trials comparing outcomes after mechanical valve replacement. Thromboembolism has been reported as occurring at a higher rate following Starr-Edwards replacement than Bjork-Shiley. Bileaflet prostheses such as the St Jude valve appear to have the lowest risk of thromboembolism. Rates of thromboembolism are higher following mitral valve replacement than following aortic valve replacement.[1][2]

STUDIES EVALUATING DIFFERENT TYPES OF BIOLOGICAL PROSTHESES

As with mechanical valve prostheses, most studies have been observational, reporting results with one type of prosthesis. Several studies have identified porcine valve failure seven or more years after implantation, particularly in younger patients.[1][2][7] One study compared results with stentless porcine prostheses with stented prostheses in the aortic position in a non-randomised case–controlled study of patients undergoing aortic valve replacement, and showed apparently enhanced durability of the stentless prosthesis.[8] Advocates of the stentless prosthesis point to its superior haemodynamics with an effective valve area some 10% larger than a stented prosthesis of equivalent size. How relevant this is in clinical practice when the vast majority of patients undergoing aortic valve replacement for calcific aortic stenosis are in their 60s, 70s or 80s is doubtful. To answer properly the question of whether stentless prostheses give superior long term results, a randomised controlled trial is needed.

STUDIES COMPARING MECHANICAL WITH BIOLOGICAL PROSTHESES

There have been two large randomised trials comparing results of mechanical valve with porcine valve replacement. Both trials used the Bjork-Shiley mechanical valve before the introduction of the convexo-concave model which subsequently proved liable to strut fracture. The Department of Veterans Affairs (VA) trial randomised 575 male patients undergoing single valve replacement in 13 centres between 1977 and 1982 to receive either a Bjork-Shiley tilting disc prosthesis or a Hancock porcine prosthesis. Three hundred and ninety four patients underwent aortic valve replacement and 181 patients mitral valve replacement. All patients receiving the Bjork-Shiley prosthesis received anticoagulants, but for those patients receiving a porcine prosthesis only those requiring anticoagulants for another reason (for example, atrial fibrillation) received warfarin. After a mean duration of follow up of 15 years Hammermeister and colleagues[9] reported significantly improved survival at 15 years for those who had undergone aortic valve replacement with a Bjork-Shiley prosthesis (79% v 66%), but no significant difference for those who had undergone mitral valve replacement (fig 13.2). There was a significantly increased risk of reoperation with the Hancock prosthesis, both for patients who had undergone aortic valve and mitral valve replacement. There was no significant difference in the occurrence of thromboembolism or endocarditis, but there was a significantly greater occurrence of major bleeding with those receiving a Bjork-Shiley prosthesis as a result of the greater use of anticoagulants.

The Edinburgh heart valve trial randomised male and female patients undergoing valve replacement between 1975 and 1979 to receive a Bjork-Shiley or porcine (Hancock or Carpentier-Edwards) prosthesis.[10] After a mean follow up period of 20 years, we reported results in 533 patients; 261 patients who had undergone mitral valve replacement, 211 aortic replacement, and 61 combined aortic and mitral valve replacement.[11] We found no difference in patient survival between biological or mechanical valve recipients when all patients were considered together or when the subgroups

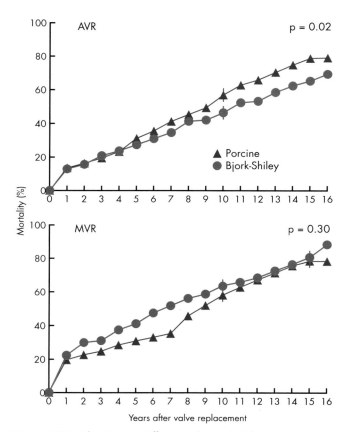

Figure 13.2 The Veterans Affairs randomised trial comparing outcome following valve replacement with a mechanical (Bjork-Shiley) versus a porcine bioprosthetic valve. Cumulative mortality curves show significantly higher mortality over 15 years of follow up with bioprostheses for those undergoing aortic valve replacement (AVR). For mitral valve replacement (MVR) cumulative mortality was initially higher with mechanical prostheses but with more prolonged follow up the mortality curves converged. Reproduced from Hammermeister K, et al. J Am Coll Cardiol 2000:36;1152–8, with permission of the publisher.

undergoing aortic valve replacement, mitral valve replacement, and combined aortic and mitral valve replacement were considered separately. As in the VA study we found an increased need for reoperation with the porcine prostheses. An actuarial analysis using death or reoperation as combined end points showed a lower event rate and therefore improved valve survival with the Bjork-Shiley prosthesis. The increased need for re-operation for valve failure occurred after 8–10 years in those who had received a porcine mitral prosthesis, and at 10–12 years in those who had received a porcine aortic prosthesis (fig 13.3). Interestingly, when a patient who had received combined aortic and mitral valve replacement with porcine prosthesis required reoperation for valve failure, it was invariably the mitral prosthesis which had failed. There was a significantly increased risk of bleeding in those with the Bjork-Shiley prosthesis. When we performed an analysis examining the combined end points of death, reoperation, endocarditis, major embolism, and major bleeding as end points, we found survival free from major events was significantly better in those who received a Bjork-Shiley prosthesis.

INFLUENCE OF PATIENT'S AGE ON DURABILITY OF PORCINE PROSTHESES

Biological valves have a higher failure rate in younger patients. Burdon and colleagues[7] found that after 15 years of follow up only a third of patients who had received a bioprosthesis for

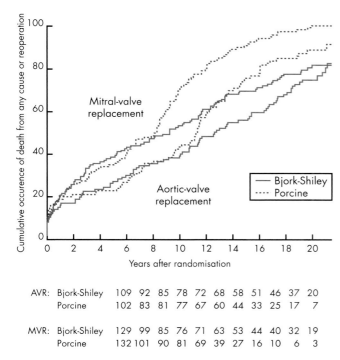

Figure 13.3 The Edinburgh heart valve trial. Cumulative occurrence of death or reoperation for patients undergoing aortic valve replacement or mitral valve replacement. Significantly more patients receiving a porcine prosthesis had one of these events compared with those receiving the mechanical Bjork-Shiley prosthesis. The curves separated at 8–10 years for mitral valve replacement and at 10–12 years for aortic valve replacement.

AVR:	Bjork-Shiley	109	92	85	78	72	68	58	51	46	37	20
	Porcine	102	83	81	77	67	60	44	33	25	17	7
MVR:	Bjork-Shiley	129	99	85	76	71	63	53	44	40	32	19
	Porcine	132	101	90	81	69	39	27	16	10	6	3

aortic valve replacement between the ages of 16–39 years remained free of structural valve deterioration, compared with more than 90% of those over 70 at the time of implantation. In the Edinburgh trial we found an increased risk of porcine valve failure in younger patients with a relative risk of approximately 1.5 for every 10 years of age. Bioprostheses for mitral valve replacement have proved less durable than for aortic valve replacement in all age groups.

Peterseim and colleagues[12] reported a large non-randomised series from a single centre of predominantly elderly patients undergoing aortic valve replacement with the patients receiving either a mechanical or porcine prosthesis. There was no difference in prosthesis survival between mechanical and porcine prostheses up to 10 years after implantation. Beyond 10 years an increased need for reoperation became apparent in the patients who had received a porcine prosthesis. The risk of bleeding was significantly increased in those who had received a mechanical prosthesis. However, at 10 years patient survival was only 50%, and in this older population with relatively limited life expectancy and low incidence of porcine prosthetic valve failure, aortic valve replacement with a porcine prosthesis appeared to confer an advantage compared with mechanical prostheses.

RISKS OF ANTICOAGULATION

The risks of anticoagulation are influenced by the intensity of treatment, the propensity for bleeding in the population studied, and the accuracy in identifying complications of anticoagulant treatment within the population studied. Before the introduction of the international normalised ratio (INR) intensity of anticoagulant treatment was not directly comparable between countries, or even within the same country. In the USA during the 1970s and 1980s higher average

doses of warfarin were prescribed compared with the UK and other European countries. This followed a switch from human brain to rabbit brain thromboplastin in commercially available kits for measuring prothrombin time. Complication rates for anticoagulant treatment from this era in the USA were often higher than those reported from the UK and Europe, and higher than present studies in the USA.[13]

In the large trials of anticoagulation for non-rheumatic atrial fibrillation, in which there was optimal surveillance of anticoagulant control, much lower complication rates for anticoagulation were reported. Of these trials, those involving a high proportion of very elderly patients and higher intensities of anticoagulation reported higher complication rates. Modern bileaflet mechanical prostheses have been shown to function safely at low levels of anticoagulation similar to those used in most of the atrial fibrillation trials. One randomised trial compared high and low intensities of anticoagulation in patients undergoing aortic valve replacement with the St Jude or Omnicarbon bileaflet mechanical prosthesis. All patients included in this trial were at low risk of thromboembolism as they were in sinus rhythm and had a small left atrium on echocardiography. The trial showed that a target INR of 2.0–3.0 was as effective as a target INR of 3.0–4.5 in preventing valve thrombosis and thromboembolism, but at a significantly lower risk of bleeding.[14] However, in unselected patients undergoing aortic valve replacement with the St Jude bileaflet mechanical prosthesis, thromboembolic events were only seen in patients with an INR of <2.5, and a target INR of 2.5–3.0 is therefore normally recommended for patients with bileaflet mechanical valves in the aortic position.[15] Patients undergoing mitral valve replacement are at a higher risk of thromboembolism than those undergoing aortic valve replacement; left atrial size is frequently increased and atrial fibrillation is common. A higher target INR of 3.0–3.5 is therefore recommended for patients with bileaflet mechanical valves in the mitral position.[15] A target of 3.0–4.5 is recommended for Starr-Edwards ball and cage and Bjork–Shiley single disc prostheses.[15]

The addition of low dose aspirin (75–100 mg daily) at these levels of anticoagulation appears to confer additional protection against thromboembolism, with only a small increased risk of bleeding. A recent meta-analysis of randomised trials comparing aspirin and warfarin with warfarin alone showed significant benefit with the combination of treatment.[16] Aspirin may be of particular advantage in patients who have undergone concomitant coronary bypass surgery at the time of valve replacement.

CHOICE OF VALVE PROSTHESIS FOR THE INDIVIDUAL PATIENT

In synthesising the results from these trials and observational studies, how should we advise individual patients on what type of prosthesis is most suitable for them? For most patients undergoing mitral valve replacement who are in atrial fibrillation and already on anticoagulant treatment the advice is easy. Bioprosthetic valves confer no advantage as the patient will continue anticoagulant treatment. Mechanical prostheses have better durability: modern bileaflet valves have good long term durability and can safely be managed with low intensity warfarin, and appear to be the optimal choice. Even for the minority of patients requiring mitral valve replacement who remain in sinus rhythm unless elderly or at risk from anticoagulant treatment, the enhanced durability of mechanical prostheses and the likelihood of atrial fibrillation developing

Table 13.1 Summary of class I and II AHA/ACC recommendations for choice of prosthetic valve

Recommendations for valve replacement with a mechanical prosthesis	Class
1. Patients with expected long life spans	I
2. Patients with a mechanical prosthetic valve already in place in a different position than the valve to be replaced	I
3. Patients in renal failure, on haemodialysis, or with hypercalcaemia	II
4. Patients requiring warfarin treatment because of risk factors* for thromboembolism	IIa
5. Patients ≤65 years for AVR and ≤70 years for MVR	IIa

Recommendations for valve replacement with a bioprosthesis	
1. Patients who cannot or will not take warfarin treatment	I
2. Patients ≥65 years needing AVR who do not have risk factors for thromboembolism*	I
3. Patients considered to have possible compliance problems with warfarin treatment	IIa
4. Patients >70 years needing MVR who do not have risk factors for thromboembolism*	IIa
5. Valve rereplacement for thrombosed mechanical valve	IIb

Class I There is evidence and/or general agreement that a given procedure or treatment is useful and effective.
Class II There is conflicting evidence and/or a disagreement of opinion about the usefulness/efficacy of a procedure or treatment.
Class IIa Weight of evidence/opinion is in favour of usefulness/efficacy.
Class IIb Usefulness/efficacy is less well established by evidence/opinion.
*Risk factors: atrial fibrillation, severe left ventricular dysfunction, previous thromboembolism, and hypercoagulable condition.
AVR, aortic valve replacement; MVR, mitral valve replacement.

with the passage of time would make a mechanical prosthesis the better choice. In replacing the valve the surgeon should try to conserve the subvalvar apparatus as this helps to preserve left ventricular function and appears to improve long term results.

For patients undergoing aortic valve replacement, choice of prosthesis is easier for the elderly patient. Bioprosthetic valves degenerate more slowly in elderly patients than in the young and the risks of anticoagulation may be higher in the very elderly. If an elderly patient would not be expected to live for more than 10 years following aortic valve replacement then a bioprosthesis would be the best choice, as the patient would avoid the risks of anticoagulant treatment. This strategy carries the risk that some patients will outlive their prosthesis and face the need for repeat surgery in their 80s with increased mortality and morbidity following reoperation at this age. It is difficult to choose an arbitrary age at which this strategy could be adopted; the American Heart Association/ American College of Cardiology (AHA/ACC) task force recommends bioprostheses for those over 65 undergoing aortic valve replacement.

For younger patients undergoing aortic valve replacement a modern bileaflet mechanical valve would seem the optimal choice. Those wishing to, or needing to, avoid anticoagulant treatment could have a bioprosthesis. Aortic homografts may be more durable than porcine bioprostheses, particularly in younger patients, and seem to produce the best results with a short harvest and implantation time when the homograft is obtained from a brain dead organ donor or a heart transplant recipient. In one large series involving 618 patients, freedom from reoperation for valve failure at 10 years was 81% and at 20 years was only 35%. Homografts from donors older than 65 years of age, or where the donor was more than 10 years older than the recipient, had poorer results. It was also found that using the homograft to replace the valve and the aortic root with reimplantation of the coronary arteries produced better long term results than using the homograft for a subcoronary valve replacement.[17] Repeat surgery for valve failure in patients with reimplanted coronaries is, however, much more demanding. Patients with renal failure, or with hypercalcaemia, have accelerated degeneration of bioprosthesis and should not receive a bioprosthesis. The AHA/ACC task force recommendations are shown in table 13.1. Additionally, some authorities advocate the use of homografts for patients with active endocarditis requiring valve replacement.

WOMEN OF CHILDBEARING AGE

For young women of childbearing age, wherever possible severe valvar lesions likely to cause problems during pregnancy should be corrected before pregnancy by treatments which avoid valve replacement—balloon valvuloplasty for mitral stenosis, mitral valve repair for mitral valve prolapse. If valve replacement is required the choice of type of prosthetic valve is difficult. Implantation of a bioprosthetic valve in the mitral position will confer the near certainty that the valve will degenerate in the patient's lifetime and require replacement, and the patient will face significant risk of mortality and morbidity at reoperation. This is likely to occur when the patient's children are still young. Pregnancy may accelerate the rate of bioprosthetic valve degeneration.

Implantation of a mechanical valve will necessitate warfarin treatment with an attendant risk of fetal loss or malformation and a maternal risk of valve thrombosis and peripartum haemorrhage. Warfarin crosses the placenta and is associated with an increased incidence of spontaneous abortion, stillbirth, prematurity, and embryopathy. The risk of warfarin embryopathy has been estimated at between 4–10% and appears to be dose dependent.[18] In a recent observational study from Italy, Vitale and colleagues reported an overall risk of fetal complications as being four times higher in women requiring an average daily dose of > 5 mg warfarin compared with those requiring 5 mg daily.[19] These authors therefore recommended for patients requiring low doses of warfarin a strategy of maintaining warfarin throughout pregnancy and an elective caesarean at 38 weeks.

Heparin does not cross the placental barrier and for this reason has been considered to be safer for the fetus. However, the risk of thromboembolic complications including fatal valve thrombosis in patients treated with subcutaneous heparin has been observed in some studies to be between 12–24%. The European Society of Cardiology guidelines for prevention of thomboembolic events in valvar heart disease therefore recommend that women at high risk because of a history of previous thromboembolism or an older generation prosthesis in the mitral position who chose not to take warfarin during the first trimester should receive continuous unfractionated heparin intravenously throughout the first trimester (table 13.2).[20] Low molecular weight heparin has been safely used for deep vein thrombosis in pregnancy, is obviously far more convenient than continuous unfractionated heparin,

Table 13.2 Recommendations[20] for anticogulation during pregnancy in patients with mechanical prosthetic valves: weeks 1–35

Indication	Class
1. The decision whether to use heparin during the first trimester or to continue oral anticoagulation throughout pregnancy should be made after full discussion with the patient and her partner; if she chooses to change to heparin for the first trimester, she should be made aware that heparin is less safe for her, with a higher risk of both thrombosis and bleeding, and that any risk to the mother also jeopardises the baby*	I
2. High risk women (a history of thromboembolism or an older generation mechanical prosthesis in the mitral position) who choose *not* to take warfarin during the first trimester should receive continuous unfractionated heparin intravenously in a dose to prolong the midinterval (6 hours after dosing) aPTT to 2–3 times control. Transition to warfarin can occur thereafter	I
3. In patients receiving warfarin, INR should be maintained between 2.0–3.0 with the lowest possible dose of warfarin, and low dose aspirin should be added	IIa
4. Women at low risk (no history of thromboembolism, newer low profile prosthesis) may be managed with adjusted dose subcutaneous heparin (17 500–20 000 U twice daily) to prolong the mid interval (6 hours after dosing) aPTT to 2–3 times control.	IIb

Class I There is evidence and/or general agreement that a given procedure or treatment is useful and effective.
Class IIa Weight of evidence/opinion is in favour of usefulness/efficacy.
Class IIb Usefulness/efficacy is less well established by evidence/opinion.
From the European Society of Cardiology guidelines for prevention of thromboembolic events in valvular heart disease.[20]
aPPT, activated partial prothrombin time; INR, international normalised ratio.

but has yet to be fully evaluated during pregnancy in patients with mechanical prosthetic valves.

The risks of anticoagulation with warfarin are increased in patients in whom compliance is poor. North and colleagues reviewed outcomes in 232 females aged 12–35 years who underwent valve replacement between 1972 and 1992 in Auckland, New Zealand.[21] The 10 year survival of patients with mechanical (n = 178), bioprosthetic (n = 73), and homograft (n = 72) valves was 70%, 84%, and 96%, respectively, with wide confidence intervals. After adjusting for other variables the relative risk of death with mechanical compared with bioprosthetic valves was approximately 2. Thromboembolism occurred significantly more commonly in patients with mechanical prostheses, with 45% having had a thrombo-embolic event by five years compared with 13% for bioprosthetic valves. The authors noted that there was a high proportion of patients in this study in whom compliance with medication was not ideal. Reoperation for valve failure occurred significantly more often in patients with bioprostheses than with mechanical or homograft prostheses. There were 132 pregnancies in 71 of the patients, and although no details of the outcome of the pregnancy were given, in this study pregnancy appeared not to increase structural deterioration or reduce survival of bioprosthetic valves.

The best management strategy for women of childbearing age requiring valve replacement remains unclear. Both they and their spouses must be fully informed of the risks of each strategy before undergoing valve replacement surgery.

ACKNOWLEDGEMENTS

I am grateful to Ole Lund for his constructive comments.

REFERENCES

1 **Vongpatanasin W**, Hillis LD, Lange RA. Prosthetic heart valves. *N Engl J Med* 1996;**335**:407–16.
▶ **A useful and up to date review of different types of prosthetic valve presently in use. This review covers the auscultatory characteristics of different types of prosthesis, and radiological and echocardiographic assessment.**
2 **Bonow RO**, Carabello B, DeLeon AC, *et al*. ACC/AHA practice guidelines. Guidelines for the management of patients with valvular heart disease. *J Am Coll Cardiol* 1998;**32**:1486–588.
▶ **A comprehensive review of all aspects of the management of patients with valvar heart disease including valve replacement surgery with more than 700 references. Available in full text from www.acc.org.**
3 **Boon NA**, Bloomfield P. Medical management of valvar heart disease. *Heart* 2002;**87**:395–400.
4 **Gohlke-Barwolf C**. Anticoagulation in valvar heart disease: new aspects and management during non-cardiac surgery. *Heart* 2000;**84**:567–72.
5 **Groves P**. Surgery of valve disease: late results and late complications. *Heart* 2001;**86**:715–21.
6 **Oakley CN**, Hall RH. Endocarditis: problems—patients being treated for endocarditis and not doing well. *Heart* 2001;**85**:47–54.
7 **Burdon TA**, Miller DC, Oyer PE, *et al*. Durability of porcine valves fifteen years in a representative North American patient population. *J Thorac Cardiovasc Surg* 1992;**103**:238–51.
▶ **A report on a large series of patients which identified an increased failure rate of porcine prostheses in younger patients.**
8 **David TE**, Puschmann R, Ivanov J, *et al*. Aortic valve replacement with stentless and stented porcine valves: a case-match study. *J Thorac Cardiovasc Surg* 1998;**116**:236–41.
▶ **A non-randomised study showing a trend to superior results with stentless prostheses.**
9 **Hammermeister K**, Sethi GK, Henderson WG, *et al*. Outcomes 15 years after valve replacement with a mechanical versus a bioprosthetic valve: final report of the Veterans Affairs randomized trial. *J Am Coll Cardiol* 2000;**36**:1152–8.
10 **Bloomfield P**, Wheatley DJ, Prescott RJ, *et al*. Twelve-year comparison of a Bjork-Shiley mechanical heart valve with porcine bioprostheses. *N Engl J Med* 1991;**324**:573–9.
11 **Oxenham H**, Bloomfield P, Wheatley DJ, *et al*. Twenty year comparison of a Bjork-Shiley mechanical heart valve with porcine bioprostheses. *Heart* (in press).
▶ **These two randomised controlled trials confirmed the increased risk of valve failure with biological valves compared with mechanical valves although with an increased risk of bleeding with mechanical valves. The VA trial demonstrated significantly better survival in those undergoing mechanical aortic valve replacement.**
12 **Peterseim D**, Can Y-Y, Cheruvu S, *et al*. Longterm outcome after biological versus mechanical aortic valve replacement in 841 patients. *J Thorac Cardiovasc Surg* 1999;**117**:890–7.
▶ **A large non-randomised series demonstrating similar long term (10 years) results with porcine prostheses compared with mechanical prostheses in the aortic position in patients over 65 years of age.**
13 **Rosendaal FR**. The scylla and charybdis of oral anticoagulant treatment. *N Engl J Med* 1996;**335**:587–9.
▶ **A succinct review of the use of warfarin treatment at different levels of intensity of anticoagulation and the relative risks of haemorrhage and thromboembolism.**
14 **Acar J**, Iung B, Boissel JP, Samama MM, *et al*. AREVA: multicenter randomized comparison of low-dose versus standard-dose anticoagulation in patients with mechanical prosthetic heart valves. *Circulation* 1996;**94**:2107–12.
▶ **This study showed that in patients at low risk of embolism (aortic valve replacement in sinus rhythm), for bileaflet mechanical valves a target INR of 2.0–3.0 was as effective as a target INR of 3.0–4.5 with a significantly lower risk of bleeding.**
15 **British Cardiac Society and Royal College of Physicians**. Valvular heart disease; investigation and management. Recommendation of a working group of the British Cardiac Society and the research unit of the Royal College of Physicians. London: Royal College of Physicians, July 1996.
▶ **A useful guideline for the management of patients with valvar heart disease.**
16 **Masssel D**, Little SH. Risks and benefits of adding anti-platelet therapy to warfarin among patients with prosthetic heart valves: a meta-analysis. *J Am Coll Cardiol* 2001;**37**:569–78.

► A useful overview and meta-analysis of the use of warfarin and aspirin in patients with prosthetic valves. It concludes that combining low dose aspirin with warfarin decreases the risk of systemic embolism or death in patients with prosthetic heart valves, with only a slightly increased risk of bleeding.

17 **Lund O**, Chandrasekaran R, Grocott-Mason H, *et al*. Primary aortic valve replacement with allografts over twenty-five years: valve-related and procedure-related determinants of outcome. *J Thorac Cardiovasc Surg* 1999;**1117**:71–91.

► One of the largest series of patients undergoing valve replacement surgery using allografts (homografts) with a very long period of follow up of the patients receiving these valves.

18 **Hanania G**. Management of anticoagulants during pregnancy. *Heart* 2001;**86**:125–6.

19 **Vitale N**, De Feo M, De Santo LS, *et al*. Dose-dependent fetal complications of warfarin in pregnant women with mechanical heart valves. *J Am Coll Cardiol* 1999;**33**:1637–41.

20 **Gohlke-Barwolf C**, Acar J, Oakley C, *et al*. Guidelines for prevention of thromboembolic events in valvular heart disease: study group of the working group on valvular heart disease of the European Society of Cardiology. *Eur Heart J* 1995;**16**:1320–30.

21 **North RA**, Sadler L, Stewart AW, *et al*. Long-term survival and valve-related complications in young women with cardiac valve replacements. *Circulation* 1999;**99**:2669–76.

► An observational study of outcome of valve replacement surgery in 255 young women, 71 of whom became pregnant and had children during the period of study.

Additional references appear on the *Heart* website–www.heartjnl.com

SECTION V: ELECTROPHYSIOLOGY

14 WHICH PATIENT SHOULD BE REFERRED TO AN ELECTROPHYSIOLOGIST: SUPRAVENTRICULAR TACHYCARDIA

Richard J Schilling

The management of supraventricular tachycardia (SVT) has changed considerably over the last 10 years, and some of the techniques that interventional electrophysiologists were using last year are now outdated. This rapid evolution means that many cardiologists who do not specialise in this field find it difficult to keep up to date with the optimum strategies for the investigation and treatment of arrhythmia. This review aims to give an update on the available treatment options and their outcomes, and provide a guide to appropriate referral to specialist interventional cardiac electrophysiologists.

▶ CLASSIFICATION AND AETIOLOGY OF SUPRAVENTRICULAR ARRHYTHMIAS

Most tachycardia has a re-entry mechanism (fig 14.1) and the classification of most arrhythmias is based on the location of this re-entry circuit. Tachycardia can be categorised as ventricular (involving the ventricle ± the His-Purkinje system only) and supraventricular (involving the supra-hisian structures with or without ventricular tissue). They can then be subdivided into regular or irregular tachycardia. Irregular SVTs—that is, atrial fibrillation (AF)—are less amenable to catheter ablation than regular SVT, but catheter ablation may be possible in selected patients. Regular SVTs can be cured by catheter ablation with high success rates (95–99%) and low complication rates (< 1%). Regular SVTs take the form of:

▶ atrioventricular re-entry tachycardias (AVRT), using the ventricle as part of the circuit; these tachycardias are dependent on the presence of an accessory atrioventricular (AV) pathway (fig 14.2)

▶ atrioventricular nodal re-entry tachycardia (AVNRT), where the re-entry circuit is within the AV node and the ventricle plays no part in maintaining the arrhythmia (fig 14.3)

▶ atrial tachycardia, where the re-entry circuit does not involve any part of the AV junction. Examples are atrial flutter (fig 14.4) or ectopic atrial tachycardia (AT) (fig 14.5).

MECHANISMS OF SVTs

Atrioventricular re-entry tachycardias
Patients with AVRT are born with an accessory pathway which usually has very different conduction characteristics from the AV node. As a result these tachycardias may present at any age, even in neonates or early childhood.

Atrioventricular nodal re-entry tachycardia
AVNRT, however, is dependent on the difference in conduction properties of the two atrial inputs into the AV node—the fast and slow pathway.[1] AVNRT, the most common regular SVT, often presents in early adulthood, probably because maturation of the AV node results in differentiation of the conduction properties of the fast and slow pathways.

Atrial flutter
As with all tachycardias with a re-entry mechanism, atrial flutter is dependent on the passage of the activation wave front around the atrium taking long enough to allow repolarisation of myocardium before the wave front completes one circuit, so that the wave front is always approaching excitable myocardium. This may happen as a result of slow conduction velocity or a long wave front path.[2-4] Stretching and scarring of the atria are likely to produce these conditions and so patients with atrial flutter present at an older age and often have concomitant disease predisposing to atrial pathology, such as atrial septal defect, previous surgery or ischaemic heart disease.

Atrial tachycardia
AT is now considered a misnomer and really refers to focal AT as opposed to atrial flutter and fibrillation.[5] It is rare and has a focal mechanism which has not been clearly defined[5]; indeed, it may be that the cause is a very small re-entry circuit, but the mapping systems used to characterise the circuit do not have adequate resolution.

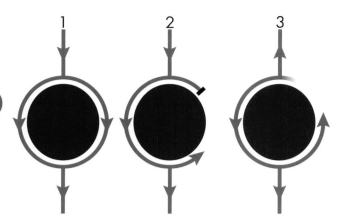

Figure 14.1 Diagrammatic representation of the mechanisms of re-entry. (1) A wavefront (arrows), initiated in a normal fashion in the sinus node, passes around an obstacle (disc) to electrical activation in a uniform fashion. This obstacle may be formed by an anatomical feature (fixed conduction block) like the tricuspid annulus, or by a physiological abnormality (functional conduction block) like an area of ischaemic myocardium, which may or may not result in block depending on a variety of conditions like vagal tone or coupling interval. (2) A premature impulse results in block of conduction on one side of the obstacle while conduction continues on the other. This is functional block because it is the result of a short electrical coupling interval which means that the myocardium in this region has not recovered its excitability in time to conduct the premature beat. (3) This wavefront takes sufficient time to circulate around the obstacle that repolarisation occurs and the area previously resulting in block recovers its excitability, so that this wavefront continually encounters excitable tissue and perpetuates as a re-entry circuit.

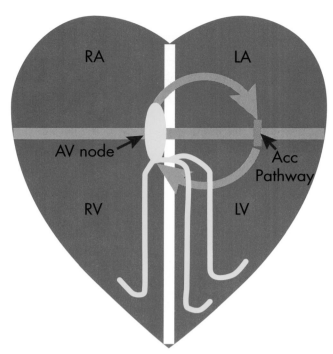

Figure 14.2 Mechanism of atrioventricular re-entry tachycardias (AVRT). The right and left atria (RA/LA) and ventricles (RV/LV) are normally electrically isolated by the fibrous rings that form the mitral and tricuspid annulus (grey line), with the only connection being the atrioventricular (AV) node. If a patient has an accessory connection (acc pathway) then the requirements for a re-entry circuit (grey arrows) are fulfilled; where the mitral/tricuspid annuli form fixed conduction block and the AV node, accessory pathway and tissue of the atria and ventricles form the re-entry circuit.

Abbreviations

AF: atrial fibrillation
AT: atrial tachycardia
AV: atrioventricular
AVNRT: atrioventricular nodal re-entry tachycardia
AVRT: atrioventricular re-entry tachycardia
EPS: electrophysiological study
RF: radiofrequency
SVT: supraventricular tachycardia

Atrial fibrillation

AF, the irregular SVT, is the most common and results from multiple re-entry circuits which can have varying degrees of randomness, so that the tachycardia may appear relatively organised or disorganised on the 12 lead ECG.[6] The re-entry is established by lines of conduction block resulting from scarring, ischaemia or stretch of the atria, and therefore AF may often be associated with hypertension, mitral valve disease, and ischaemic heart disease.[7]

INCIDENCE

The incidence of regular SVT in the population has been poorly defined. AVNRT is by far the most common regular SVT and accounts for 90% of so called "junctional tachycardias",[8] the remainder being dependent on the presence of an accessory AV connection to produce AVRT. Epidemiological studies have demonstrated an incidence of regular AVNRT or AVRT of 35/100 000 person-years and a prevalence of 2.29/1000 persons.[9] Atrial flutter has an incidence of 88/100 000 person-years and is unsurprisingly associated with increasing age, patients over 80 years having an incidence of 587/100 000.[10] AF is the most common sustained cardiac arrhythmia,[11] having a

prevalence of 6% in the population over 65 years old,[11] and is the most common cardiac cause of stroke.[12] Because of this AF represents a considerable burden on health care systems which is why enormous efforts are currently being made to develop curative treatments.

TREATMENTS FOR SVT
Palliation

Antiarrhythmic drugs act by either slowing conduction or lengthening the refractory period of cardiac tissue. Some antiarrhythmic drugs have selective actions. An example is flecainide, which has some effect on the AV node, prolonging the effective refractory period by 10% and the conduction velocity by 20%[13 14]; by contrast, it will completely block anterograde conduction in accessory pathways in approximately 40% of patients while prolonging refractory periods in 20% of the remaining cases.[15 16] For the majority of SVT pharmacological treatment results in changes to the conduction properties of all or a large proportion of cardiac conduction tissue. Therefore, when prescribing these treatments, the physician hopes that the drug will either: (a) change the conduction velocity of components of the re-entry circuit differentially, so that they no longer differ sufficiently to allow re-entry to be established; or (b) that the refractory period is lengthened so that the re-entry wave front encounters refractory tissue and is therefore extinguished. If conduction velocity is slowed in all parts of the circuit equally, or the refractory period of one part of the circuit is lengthened by a critical amount, this can be proarrhythmic, and antiarrhythmic drugs may therefore result in incessant tachycardia. A brief synopsis of drug treatment of SVT is shown in the box below.

AVRT/AVNRT

► Recurrence rate on antiarrhythmic drugs is around 20%[9]
► Useful drugs:
  – (a) AVRT: flecainide, disopyramide or β blockers
  – (b) AVNRT: verapamil, β blockers, sotalol, flecainide or disopyramide

Atrial flutter

► Recurrence rate: 55%, 6 months after DC cardioversion[17] and as high as 60% long term, even with antiarrhythmic treatment[18]
► Antiarrhythmic drugs that slow atrial conduction and lengthen refractory period (for example, flecainide, amiodarone) may have some effect on reducing atrial flutter recurrence, but drugs that reduce rate may also slow the flutter enough to allow 1:1 AV nodal conduction, resulting in a tachycardia rapid enough to cause haemodynamic compromise[19]
► Alternatively, antiarrhythmic drug strategies for atrial flutter may aim to control the ventricular response rather than maintain sinus rhythm. Because the ventricular response rate is a function of the atrial flutter rate, achieving a balance between tachycardia (2:1 AV block or 3:1 AV block causing ventricular response rates of 150 and 100 beats per minute) and bradycardia is difficult, and many opt to encourage AF and control rate response with digoxin and β blockers

Atrial fibrillation

► Recurrence rate: 20–50%[20–22]
► Useful drugs:
  – (a) Maintain sinus rhythm: flecainide (or other class Ic agents), amiodarone
  – (b) Ventricular response: digoxin, β blockers or calcium antagonists
  – (c) Stroke prevention: warfarin, aspirin (in low risk patients)

Curative therapies

Catheter ablation is a minimally invasive procedure whereby 4–8 French electrodes are passed intravascularly, most commonly to the right heart, under x ray guidance. The procedure is performed under local anaesthetic, often as a day case procedure. The general principles of catheter ablation are that an electrophysiological study (EPS) is performed first using a specifically designed pulse generator to perform programmed stimulation. The primary aim of the EPS is to induce tachycardia so that the activation sequence recorded by the diagnostic catheter electrodes can be used to determine the arrhythmia mechanism. A deflectable mapping/ablation catheter is then positioned on a portion of the re-entry circuit critical for maintenance of tachycardia that is not part of the normal cardiac conduction system. Once in a suitable location, radiofrequency (RF) energy is delivered via the ablation catheter. This results in conductive and resistive heating of the endocardium and some of the myocardium rendering a small area (2–4 mm³) electrically inactive. Most patients do not feel the energy application but some patients feel warmth or even pain in the chest during RF application. More often, patients find lying on the x ray table for the length of time required for the ablation more troublesome than the actual procedure itself; although this may result in suppression of the arrhythmia, light sedation or analgesics can help. After RF delivery, a further limited EPS is then performed to confirm successful ablation of the re-entry circuit. The targets, success rates, and complication rates for each SVT are summarised in table 14.1.

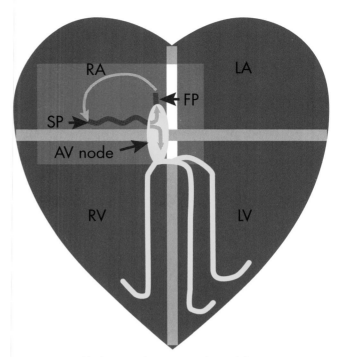

Figure 14.3 Mechanism of atrioventricular nodal re-entry tachycardia (AVNRT). Patients with AVNRT have two inputs to the AV node—a slow (SP) and fast (FP) pathway. The re-entry circuit is formed by the SP, AV node, FP and the atrial tissue intervening between the FP and SP, and most commonly activates in the direction shown by the grey arrows. Note that the ventricle activates via the AV node but is not part of the re-entry circuit (unlike in AVRT). Adenosine will block conduction through the AV node, which is part of the re-entry circuit in both AVNRT and AVRT and therefore terminates the tachycardia.

Table 14.1 Results of radiofrequency catheter ablation

Arrhythmia	Success rate (%)	Complication rate (%)	Possible additional/ maintenance therapy
AVNRT	98	0–2	None
AVRT	99	1.8	None
Atrial flutter	95	<1	None
AV node ablation for established AF	>99	<1	Permanent pacemaker
AF secondary to focal tachycardia	62	5	Antiarrhythmic drugs

This table shows the outcome of catheter ablation for arrhythmia. Some of these data are likely to be out of date; an example is focal atrial fibrillation in which the techniques are progressing rapidly enough that published data are not applicable to currently used approaches and are likely to underestimate the success rates.
AF, atrial fibrillation; AV, atrioventricular; AVNRT, atrioventricular nodal re-entry tachycardia, AVRT, atrioventricular re-entry tachycardia

Complication rates vary depending on the arrhythmia being ablated. Estimated rates for individual complications are listed in table 14.2, based on prospective data collected in the USA in 1998,[23] apart from ablation of AF secondary to focal tachycardia for which data have not yet been published (this is estimated from the data from our centre and that associated with left sided accessory pathway ablation). For newer procedures—that is, AF ablation—some of these data may already be outdated. The extra risk of developing a cancer over a lifetime from the radiation exposure associated with an hour of fluoroscopy is 480 per million patients.[24] Few ablation procedures require this degree of exposure; the doses received by patients undergoing even the most complex catheter ablation

Table 14.2 Major complications associated with ablation procedures

Arrhythmia	Heart block (%)	Vascular damage/ haematoma (%)	Other (%)	Death (%)
AVNRT	0.9	0.49	0.08 DVT 0.08 PE 0.08 Pneumothorax	0
AVRT: left sided	<0.1	3.1	1.7 Tamponade 0.2 Coronary occlusion	0
AVRT: right free wall	1 (3rd degree)	0	1 PE	0
AVRT: septal	0.5	0.5	0.5 Pneumothorax 0.5 Pericarditis	0
Atrial flutter	0.4	0.6	0.2 Tamponade 0.2 DVT 0.2 Haemothorax 0.2 TR	0
AV node ablation for established AF	N/A	0.3	0.15 TR	0.15 (pacemaker failure)
AF secondary to focal tachycardia	0	1	2 Tamponade 0.5 Embolic stroke	0

DVT, deep vein thrombosis; PE, pulmonary embolus, TR, tricuspid regurgitation. For key to rest of abbreviations see table 1.

have been reduced by modern fluoroscopy equipment or non-fluoroscopic cardiac mapping systems.

GENERAL GUIDANCE FOR REFERRAL
Regular SVT
The studies comparing catheter ablation with drug treatment are limited because it has been generally accepted for some years that catheter ablation has greater efficacy and the evolution of techniques for catheter ablation has been so rapid. Studies have shown that catheter ablation has a higher success rate than drug treatment,[25][26] patients have a higher quality of life after catheter ablation,[27] and it is more cost effective than antiarrhythmic drug treatment within 9–12 years.[25][28] Most patients warrant treatment for their arrhythmia if they find the symptoms debilitating or require recurrent attendance at hospital for termination of tachycardia. If a patient has evidence of pre-excitation and a history of tachycardia, I would offer them catheter ablation even without recurrent symptoms because of the low but definite risk of sudden death associated with AF in this group of patients.[29] Whether patients who have pre-excitation discovered incidentally should be offered ablation is more controversial, but EPS to assess the Wenckebach cycle length of the accessory pathway (to determine its potential for rapid conduction if AF occurs) may be misleading because a variety of factors affect the refractory period which may change from one day to the next. The case for catheter ablation of atrial flutter is even more compelling because the catheter ablation success rate is now considerably higher than drug treatment. In summary, all patients with regular SVT who require treatment should be referred to a cardiac electrophysiologist for consideration of catheter ablation.

Atrial fibrillation
The techniques used and the success rates of catheter ablation of AF are changing so rapidly that within one year this review will almost certainly be out of date in this regard. There are two approaches to catheter treatment of AF. The first is to

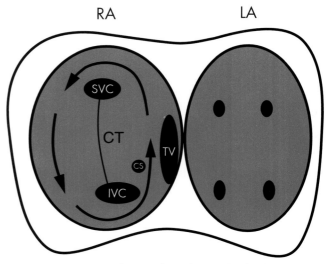

Figure 14.4 Diagram showing the pathway taken by the re-entry wavefront causing atrial flutter (arrow). The right (RA) and left atria (LA) are depicted with the anatomical landmarks in the right atria marked as follows: SVC, superior vena cava; IVC, inferior vena cava; CS, coronary sinus os; TV, tricuspid valve; CT, crista terminalis. The TV and CT form lines of conduction block which "electrically" divide the atria into two halves. The only electrical connections between these two halves are the roof and appendage of the right atrium and the isthmus between the TV and IVC. Note that the narrowest part of the re-entry circuit is this isthmus which is why this is the target for ablation of atrial flutter. The left atrium activates via conduction through the septum but is not part of the re-entry circuit.

control ventricular response rate by modifying or abolishing AV nodal conduction. AV node modification is a technique whereby the atrial inputs into the AV node with the shortest refractory periods are selectively ablated. This reduces the rate at which the AV node can conduct to the ventricle. It is a technique that has been less in vogue in recent years mainly because it is difficult to predict the outcome reliably, and

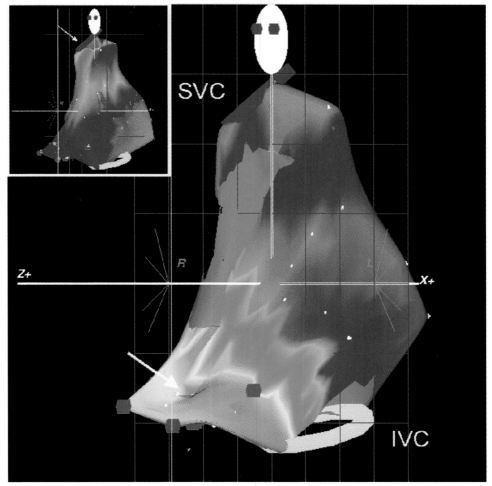

Figure 14.5 An electroanatomical map of the right atrium in a patient with focal atrial tachycardia (AT). The atrium is shown in the left anterior oblique (LAO) view with the superior (SVC) and inferior vena cava (IVC) shown as rings on the map. An isochronal map has been superimposed onto the computer generated model of the right atrium. This shows early activation in red and latest activation in purple. The earliest activation can be seen at the low lateral right atrium which is in contrast to activation during sinus rhythm (inset) which is earliest at the superior lateral right atrium, the location of the sinus node.

patients often require pacemaker implantation because of bradycardia or repeat ablation procedures because of tachycardia. Complete AV node ablation and permanent pacemaker implantation is more frequently employed when drug treatment fails to control the ventricular response rate.

The second approach to treatment of AF, used more often for paroxysmal than established AF, involves catheter ablation of the focal activity that initiates AF. This focal activation often arises from one of the pulmonary veins and electrical isolation of these veins may cure AF in up to 60% of patients long term.[30]

The complication rate of this procedure is slightly higher than for most catheter ablations because a transeptal puncture is required and the catheters are passed to the left heart. This is only a marginal risk because most interventional electrophysiologists are experienced in transeptal puncture, and transoesophageal echocardiography is performed immediately before the procedure to exclude thrombus in the left atrium that may be embolised by catheter manipulation. Patients may benefit from the opinion of an interventional electrophysiologist if they are in established AF and their ventricular rate cannot be controlled with antiarrhythmic drugs, or they have lone paroxysmal AF that cannot be abolished with class Ic antiarrhythmic treatment. Amiodarone may be a suitable alternative in this group of patients, but the side effect profile of amiodarone means that other options should at least be explored before committing the patient to lifelong treatment.

COMMON MISCONCEPTIONS

(1) Flecainide causes sudden death: Although flecainide was associated with an increased risk of sudden death in CAST (cardiac arrhythmia suppression trial)[31] in patients with impaired left ventricular function and ventricular premature beats, there is no evidence that it increases risk of sudden death when used in patients with SVT (and normal ventricles).[32]

(2) Digoxin is good at rate control: Digoxin appears to be less effective than other agents at controlling ventricular rate in AF, particularly during exercise or critical illnesses.[33][34] Moreover, in patients with paroxysmal AF, digoxin does not appear to have a significant effect on ventricular rate during paroxysms and may be associated with the occurrence of longer paroxysms.[35]

(3) Ablation of SVT is time consuming: Most catheter ablations take approximately 30 minutes to one hour. Factors that may prolong the procedure are difficulty in inducing the tachycardia, multiple accessory pathways, or large, abnormal atria requiring unusual mapping/ablation catheters.

(4) Ablation of SVT is traumatic: Most catheter ablation can be performed as a day case procedure and patients require no

Supraventricular tachycardias: key points

▶ The following groups of patients may benefit from referral to a cardiac electrophysiologist:
(1) All patients with regular SVT on antiarrhythmic drugs
(2) All patients with recurrent regular SVT
(3) Patients with established AF in whom control of the ventricular response is suboptimal
(4) Patients with lone paroxysmal AF in whom maintenance of sinus rhythm cannot be achieved with class Ic antiarrhythmics

▶ It is likely that an effective curative catheter ablation procedure for established AF will be established within the next 10 years

special follow up after the procedure. Although sedation may suppress the arrhythmia it will often alleviate the anxiety experienced by the patient before and during the procedure. (5) Ablation should be reserved for patients failing antiarrhythmic drugs: Ablation for most SVT has such a low complication rate and high success rate that it is more cost effective and may be safer than antiarrhythmic drugs.

CONCLUSION

Almost all regular SVTs can be treated simply and quickly with catheter ablation. Exceptions are those that occur as a result of structural abnormalities of the atria. The treatment of AF is evolving rapidly and at the present time the only patients that may be reliably and effectively treated are those with short frequent paroxysms of AF. Electrophysiologists may still have a role in ablating established AF if control of the ventricular response is proving difficult.

REFERENCES

1 **Jackman WM**, Beckman KJ, McClelland JH, et al. Treatment of supraventricular tachycardia due to atrioventricular nodal reentry, by radiofrequency catheter ablation of slow-pathway conduction. N Engl J Med 1992;**327**:313–8.
▶ This is the first description of the technique of slow pathway ablation for treating AVNRT, one of the more common regular SVTs. It proved to be easier to perform and have fewer complications than the previous approach of fast pathway ablation, and as such revolutionised the treatment of patients with AVNRT.
2 **Tai CT**, Chen SA, Chiang CE, et al. Characterization of low right atrial isthmus as the slow conduction zone and pharmacological target in typical atrial flutter. Circulation 1997;**96**:2601–11.
3 **Shah DC**, Jaïs P, Haïssaguerre M, et al. Three-dimensional mapping of the common atrial flutter circuit in the right atrium. Circulation 1997;**96**:3904–12.
4 **Kinder C**, Kall J, Kopp D, et al. Conduction properties of the inferior vena cava-tricuspid annular isthmus in patients with typical atrial flutter. J Cardiovasc Electrophysiol 1997;**8**:727–37.
5 **Saoudi N**, Cosio F, Waldo A, et al. Classification of atrial flutter and regular atrial tachycardia according to electrophysiologic mechanism and anatomic bases: a statement from a joint expert group from the working group of arrhythmias of the European Society of Cardiology and the North American Society of Pacing and Electrophysiology. J Cardiovasc Electrophysiol 2001;**2**:852–66.
6 **Schilling RJ**, Kadish AH, Peters NS, et al. Endocardial mapping of atrial fibrillation in the human right atrium using a non-contact catheter. Eur Heart J 2000;**21**:550–64.
7 **Kannel WB**, Abbott RD, Savage DD. Coronary heart disease and atrial fibrillation: the Frammingham study. Am Heart J 1978;**106**:389–96.
8 **Josephson M**, Buxton A, Marchlinski F. The tachyarrhythmias. In: Isselbacher K, Braunwald E, Wilson JD, et al, eds. Harrison's principles of internal medicine, 13th ed. New York: McGraw-Hill, 1994:1024–9.
9 **Orejarena LA**, Vidaillet H Jr, DeStefano F, et al. Paroxysmal supraventricular tachycardia in the general population. J Am Coll Cardiol 1998;**31**:150–7.
▶ This is one of the few studies describing the epidemiology of SVT.
10 **Granada J**, Uribe W, Chyou PH, et al. Incidence and predictors of atrial flutter in the general population. J Am Coll Cardiol 2000;**36**:2242–6.
11 **Feinberg WM**, Blackshear JL, Laupacis A, et al. Prevalence, age distribution and gender of patients with atrial fibrillation. Arch Intern Med 1995;**155**:469–73.
12 **Wellens HJ**. Atrial fibrillation - the last big hurdle in treating supraventricular tachycardia. N Engl J Med 1994;**331**:944–5.
13 **Estes NAM**, Garan H, Ruskin JN. Electrophysiologic properties of flecainide acetate. Am J Cardiol 1984;**53**(suppl B):26B–29B.
14 **Hellenstrand KJ**, Bexton RS, Nathan AW, et al. Acute electrophysiological effects of flecainide acetate on cardiac conduction and refractoriness in men. Br Heart J 1982;**48**:140–8.
15 **Hellenstrand KJ**, Nathan AW, Bexton RS, et al. Electrophysiological effects of flecainide acetate on sinus node function anomalous atrioventricular connections and pacemaker thresholds. Am J Cardiol 1984;**53**:30–8.
16 **Neuss H**, Buss J, Schlepper M, et al. Effects of flecainide on electrophysiological properties of accessory pathways in the Wolff-Parkinson-White syndrome. Eur Heart J 1983;**4**:347–53.
17 **Pozen RG**, Pastoriza J, Rozanski JJ, et al. Determinants of recurrent atrial flutter after cardioversion. Br Heart J 1983;**50**:92–6.
18 **Pozen RG**, Pastoriza J, Rozanski JJ, et al. Determinants of recurrent atrial flutter after cardioversion. Am J Cardiol 1993;**71**:710–13.
19 **Nathan AW**, Hellestrand KJ, Bexton RS, et al. Proarrhythmic effects of the new antiarrhythmic agent flecainide acetate. Am Heart J 1984;**107**:222–8.
20 **Chun SH**, Sager PT, Stevenson WG, et al. Long-term efficacy of amiodarone for the maintenance of normal sinus rhythm in patients with refractory atrial fibrillation or flutter. Am J Cardiol 1995;**76**:47–50.
21 **Horowitz LN**, Spielman SR, Greenspan AM, et al. Use of amiodarone in the treatment of persistent and paroxysmal atrial fibrillation resistant to quinidine therapy. J Am Coll Cardiol 1985;**6**:1402–7.
22 **Gold RL**, Haffajee CI, Charos G, et al. Amiodarone for refractory atrial fibrillation. Am J Cardiol 1986;**57**:124–7.
23 **Scheinman MM**, Huang S. The 1998 NASPE prospective catheter ablation registry. PACE 2000;**23**:1020-8.
▶ This is the first prospective study to describe the outcome of catheter ablation using modern techniques in large numbers of patients and centres. Using the data provided by this study may be less misleading to patients because the complications of catheter ablation are so rare it is not uncommon for individual centres to have fewer than one major complication a year.
24 **Perisinakis K**, Damilakis J, Theocharopoulos N, et al. Accurate assessment of patient effective radiation dose and associated detriment risk from radiofrequency catheter ablation procedures. Circulation 2001;**104**:58–62.
25 **Weerasooriya HR**, Murdock CJ, Harris AH, et al. The cost-effectiveness of treatment of supraventricular arrhythmias related to an accessory atrioventricular pathway: comparison of catheter ablation, surgical division and medical treatment. Aust NZ J Med 1994;**24**:161–7.
26 **Natale A**, Newby KH, Pisano E, et al. Prospective randomized comparison of antiarrhythmic therapy versus first-line radiofrequency ablation in patients with atrial flutter. J Am Coll Cardiol 2000;**35**:1898–904.
27 **Bathina MN**, Mickelsen S, Brooks C, et al. Radiofrequency catheter ablation versus medical therapy for initial treatment of supraventricular tachycardia and its impact on quality of life and healthcare costs. Am J Cardiol 1998;**82**:589–93.
28 **Ikeda T**, Sugi K, Enjoji Y, et al. Cost effectiveness of radiofrequency catheter ablation versus medical treatment for paroxysmal supraventricular tachycardia in Japan. J Cardiol 1994;**24**:461–8.
29 **Fitzsimmons PJ**, McWhirter PD, Peterson DW, et al. The natural history of Wolff-Parkinson-White syndrome in 228 military aviators: a long-term follow-up of 22 years. Am Heart J 2001;**142**:530–6.
▶ This describes the true long term outcome of unselected patients with Wolff-Parkinson-White (WPW) syndrome. These data are particularly relevant to asymptomatic patients with WPW detected at health screening, which raises the dilemma as to whether catheter ablation of this potentially life threatening condition should be performed. In fact this study shows that sudden cardiac death in patients with WPW is rare.
30 **Haïssaguerre M**, Jais P, Shah DC, et al. Electrophysiological end point for catheter ablation of atrial fibrillation initiated from multiple pulmonary venous foci. Circulation 2000;**101**:1409–17.
▶ This is one of the first descriptions of the currently employed technique for eliminating the focal triggers for paroxysmal atrial fibrillation.
31 **The Cardiac Arrhythmia Suppression Trial (CAST) Investigators.** Preliminary report: effect of encainide and flecainide on mortality in a randomized trial of arrhythmia suppression after myocardial infarction. N Engl J Med 1989;**321**:406–12 .
32 **Pritchett ELC**, Wilkinson WE. Mortality in patients treated with flecainide and encainide for supraventricular arrhythmias. Am J Cardiol 1991;**67**:976–80.
33 **Goldman S**, Probst P, Selzer A, et al. Inefficacy of "therapeutic" serum levels of digoxin in controlling the ventricular rate in atrial fibrillation. Am J Cardiol 1975;**35**:651–5.
34 **Botker HE**, Toft P, Klitgaard NA, et al. Influence of physical exercise on serum digoxin concentration and heart rate in patients with atrial fibrillation. Br Heart J 1991;**65**:337–41.
35 **Rawles JM**, Metcalfe MJ, Jennings K. Time of occurrence, duration, and ventricular rate of paroxysmal atrial fibrillation: the effect of digoxin. Br Heart J 1990;**63**:225–7.

15 ARRHYTHMIAS IN ADULTS WITH CONGENITAL HEART DISEASE

John K Triedman

103

Refinement of surgical techniques for the treatment of congenital heart disease (CHD) has created a new population of young adults with heart disease. In the USA, it is estimated that there are nearly one million CHD patients, 15–20% with disease of severity to warrant surgical intervention. As surgical mortality has fallen, the number of adults living with major congenital heart defects has increased.[1]

Arrhythmias complicate the care of many adults with CHD. Their prevalence and the difficulty of treatment have made arrhythmia a major focus of interest for physicians working in this area. The presence of longstanding CHD in an arrhythmia patient significantly alters the nature and potential severity of the arrhythmia complaint and the safety and feasibility of various treatments. In addition to analysis of the targeted arrhythmia complaint, the physician must have complete and specific knowledge of the patient's cardiovascular anatomy and the consequences of that anatomy and subsequent surgical modifications on cardiovascular function.

The arrhythmogenic substrate in adults with CHD is complex. All arrhythmias prevalent in the normal population may also occur in CHD, and some specific associations are observed—for example, Wolff-Parkinson-White syndrome and Ebstein's anomaly. However, more common are acquired arrhythmias that are rarely seen in normal young adult hearts, and that are associated with longstanding hypertrophy and fibrosis caused by cyanosis, chronic haemodynamic overload, and superimposed surgical scarring. These arrhythmias include re-entrant atrial and ventricular tachycardias, heart block, and sinus node dysfunction. This article will review the evaluation and management of these more common arrhythmia problems in adults with CHD.

► CLINICAL BACKGROUND

Although the anatomical classification of congenital heart defects is complex, three major categories constitute a large percentage of adult CHD patients with arrhythmia, because of their frequency and high incidence of arrhythmia (fig 15.1).

The spectrum of clinical consequences of arrhythmia in adults with CHD ranges from clinically occult arrhythmia to sudden death. Incessant or recurrent arrhythmia may cause gradual haemodynamic deterioration, and vice versa, often resulting in a vicious cycle of clinical decompensation. Thrombosis[2] and thromboembolic events are also associated with tachycardia. Symptoms, frequent need for hospitalisation, and the management of cardiac devices and antiarrhythmic drugs constitute a significant burden on quality of life.

In the era of effective automatic implantable cardioverter-defibrillator (AICD) therapy, assessment of risk of cardiac sudden death is an important component of clinical arrhythmia management. Patients with acquired heart disease can now be segregated into large, relatively homogeneous groups of similarly elevated risk (for example, patients in the first year after myocardial infarction, or with depressed ejection fraction). In contrast, CHD populations are small, anatomically diverse, and have relatively low rates of sudden death, with annual mortality in even "high risk" groups in the range of < 2%.[3][4] Thus, it is difficult to identify specific risk factors in CHD and to measure the effect of interventions on survival. Nonetheless, some clinical markers appear to affect outcomes adversely over a wide range of anatomical defects, including the presence of residual haemodynamic defects, performance of surgical repair later in life, and longer duration of follow up.

At the other extreme of clinical presentation, not all adults with CHD and arrhythmia are symptomatic, and some experience symptoms so subtle that the amount of the day spent in tachycardia is not easily quantified. A major area for future research will be a clarification of the natural history of arrhythmia in these patients, with attention paid to their role in the gradual deterioration of older patients with CHD.

ATRIAL TACHYCARDIAS
Intra-atrial re-entrant tachycardia
Intra-atrial re-entrant tachycardia (IART) denotes macroreentrant atrial tachycardias other than common atrial flutter occurring in the normal heart. Rare in normal hearts, IART is a common late

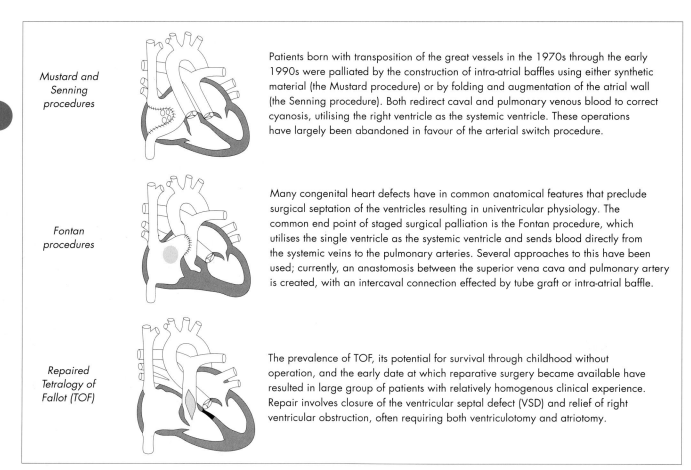

Mustard and Senning procedures	Patients born with transposition of the great vessels in the 1970s through the early 1990s were palliated by the construction of intra-atrial baffles using either synthetic material (the Mustard procedure) or by folding and augmentation of the atrial wall (the Senning procedure). Both redirect caval and pulmonary venous blood to correct cyanosis, utilising the right ventricle as the systemic ventricle. These operations have largely been abandoned in favour of the arterial switch procedure.
Fontan procedures	Many congenital heart defects have in common anatomical features that preclude surgical septation of the ventricles resulting in univentricular physiology. The common end point of staged surgical palliation is the Fontan procedure, which utilises the single ventricle as the systemic ventricle and sends blood directly from the systemic veins to the pulmonary arteries. Several approaches to this have been used; currently, an anastomosis between the superior vena cava and pulmonary artery is created, with an intercaval connection effected by tube graft or intra-atrial baffle.
Repaired Tetralogy of Fallot (TOF)	The prevalence of TOF, its potential for survival through childhood without operation, and the early date at which reparative surgery became available have resulted in large group of patients with relatively homogenous clinical experience. Repair involves closure of the ventricular septal defect (VSD) and relief of right ventricular obstruction, often requiring both ventriculotomy and atriotomy.

Figure 15.1 Congenital heart malformations commonly associated with arrhythmia.

complication in many varieties of CHD. Like atrial flutter, it tends to have a stable cycle length and P wave morphology, suggesting that it is organised by a fixed substrate. Its prevalence among patients who have undergone surgical procedures involving extensive atrial dissection and repair indicates a particular dependence on surgical injury,[5] and animal models explicitly patterned after surgeries associated with IART (for example, the Mustard and Fontan procedures) result in tachycardias similar to those observed clinically.

Frequently identified risk factors for IART include older age at operation and longer follow up. About half of those patients with "old-style" Fontans—connection of the entire right atrium to the pulmonary artery by anastomosis or conduit—will develop IART within 10 years of surgery,[6] while construction of a lateral right atrial tunnel and cavopulmonary connection are at lower risk.[7] It is anticipated that the extracardiac Fontan, performed using an intercaval tube graft, may also be low risk, but arrhythmia has been reported in early follow up of those patients.[8] Survivors of the Mustard and Senning procedures are at risk for the development of sinus node dysfunction and IART, often concurrently. IART is more prevalent in patients with repaired tetralogy of Fallot (TOF) than ventricular tachycardia, and more likely to be associated with symptoms.[9]

The first large follow up study of IART after CHD surgery revealed a mortality rate over 6.5 years of 17%, with 10% experiencing sudden death. More recently, a group of patients with atrial tachycardias and a prior surgical history of Fontan, Mustard or Senning procedures reported sudden cardiac death in 6% over an average follow up of three years. The clinical factors associated with sudden death were ongoing

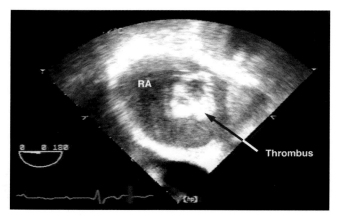

Figure 15.2 Echocardiographic image of a large thrombus identified in the giant right atrium of a patient with an "old-style" Fontan procedure using an atriopulmonary anastomosis.

and/or poorly controlled tachycardia episodes and overall poor clinical status.[5]

Reports of stroke after cardioversion of IART in CHD patients are rare. However, intravascular and intracardiac thromboses are associated with IART, and a prevalence of intracardiac thrombi in 42% of patients undergoing echocardiography before cardioversion has been reported (fig 15.2).[2] It is not clear whether atrial tachycardias actually promote such events, or are merely a concomitant problem occurring in patients with sick, prematurely aging hearts.

Drug treatment

Although some small studies have suggested otherwise, clinical experience generally has shown that antiarrhythmic drug treatment is unlikely to suppress recurrences of IART. Experimental models of atrial re-entry have given us a good understanding of the potential salutary effects of class 1C and class 3 drugs, and symptomatic arrhythmias can sometimes be suppressed in individual patients using these agents. However, proarrhythmia and adverse effects on ventricular and nodal function may limit their value. Novel antiarrhythmic drugs with pure class 3 activity have not been widely used in IART, and may prove useful.

The frequent occurrence of thrombosis in adult patients with CHD and atrial tachycardia suggests that warfarin or other potent anticoagulant treatment is indicated in most of these patients. Atrioventricular (AV) nodal blocking drugs may also be used, but are often difficult to titrate because of the relatively slow cycle length and fixed conduction ratios often seen in IART.

Pacemaker therapy

Atrial antibradycardia pacing alone sometimes results in symptomatic improvement and decreased tachycardia frequency.[10] In patients with sinus node dysfunction, this may be the result of improved haemodynamics with appropriately timed atrial activation. Automatic antitachycardia pacing has also been of value for some patients. The overall efficacy of atrial pacing is variable, and there are significant technical difficulties associated with lead placement in these patients. Few endocardial or epicardial sites are generally available and able to generate sensed electrograms of sufficient quality to ensure reliable atrial sensing. Endovascular placement of atrial leads may also increase risk of thrombosis. The potential of other innovative device therapies currently being developed for treatment of atrial fibrillation, such as dual site pacing and the atrial defibrillator, has not been explored in CHD.

Catheter ablation

A proposed curative approach to IART has been to extend or create lines of conduction block, using catheter based and/or surgical techniques. This anatomical approach to treatment involves the design of a lesion or lesions based on an understanding of the relation of macroreentrant circuits to the underlying cardiac anatomy. It has precedents in the catheter and surgical ablation procedures for ventricular tachycardia (VT) and the maze procedure for atrial fibrillation.

Acute success rates reported for radiofrequency catheter ablation for IART range from 55–90%.[11] Catheter ablation procedures usually target individual macroreentrant circuits, seeking a vulnerable site for application of a radiofrequency lesion. Review of IART ablation experience has shown that, in patients with a right AV valve, the isthmus between that valve and the inferior vena cava commonly supports IART, similar to common atrial flutter.[12] When this isthmus is present, as is the case in patients with Mustard and Senning procedures, TOF, and other biventricular repairs, techniques developed for atrial flutter may be used to perform and assess the effectiveness of the ablation. Even in these familiar anatomies, however, the

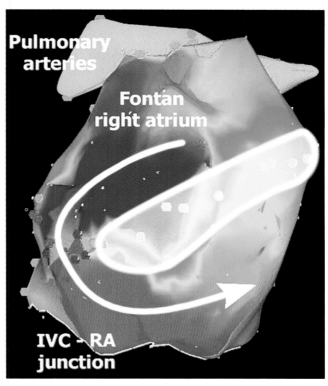

Figure 15.3 Electroanatomical map in right anterior oblique view of an intra-atrial re-entrant tachycardia circuit constructed in a patient with an older variant of the Fontan procedure. Activation times are colour coded to indicate the movement of the wavefront in this tachycardia, indicated by the white arrow. The white shaded area indicates an area of scarring and conduction block, inferred from characteristics of electrograms recorded from that region.

observation of multiple IART circuits is common, and other anatomical or surgical features relevant to ablation may be difficult to locate fluoroscopically. It may also be difficult to generate the large and confluent lesions sometimes needed to interrupt these circuits. Application of recently introduced mapping and ablation techniques, such as advanced activation mapping technologies, and application of irrigated radiofrequency lesions, is associated with improved acute success rates. Longer term follow up after ablation has revealed that arrhythmia symptoms and quality of life are improved in most patients after IART ablation, but recurrences are documented in almost half of these patients.[13] Further advances in our understanding of the arrhythmia substrate and the technology available to visualise and modify it will be necessary to improve this important clinical outcome (fig 15.3).

Surgical treatment

Attempts to revise "old style" Fontan patients to cavopulmonary type connections for haemodynamic reasons are associated with perioperative mortality in the region of 10%,[14] and in the absence of specific intervention for arrhythmia do not reliably prevent arrhythmia recurrence. More recent reports of right atrial maze procedures performed with surgical and/or cryoablative techniques and employing an empiric set of lesions have shown promising results, with no clinically significant arrhythmia recurrence in the majority of patients.[15] This suggests that maze revision of Fontan procedures can be performed at a reasonable surgical risk and may greatly reduce recurrence of postoperative IART. Additional follow up studies are needed to ascertain long term haemodynamic and arrhythmia benefit.

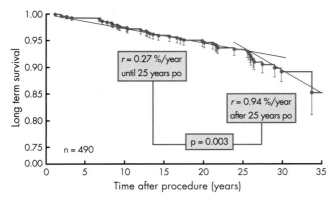

Figure 15.4 Survival curve in late follow up of adult patients with tetralogy of Fallot. Most deaths were sudden; increased mortality in late decades of follow up has also been observed in other series. Reproduced from Nollert et al[4] with permission of the publisher.

Atrial fibrillation

Atrial fibrillation occurs in as many as 25–30% of patients with CHD and atrial tachycardia. The limited information available on these patients suggests that those with residual left sided obstructive lesions or unrepaired heart disease are more prone to atrial fibrillation. Principles of management are drawn from the general adult population, including anticoagulation and rate control. Risk of thromboembolism is presumably elevated. Sinus rhythm is haemodynamically preferred in CHD, and cardioversion, prophylactic antiarrhythmic drugs, and atrial pacing are used to prevent the establishment of permanent atrial fibrillation if possible. The occurrence of atrial fibrillation in patients who also have IART reduces the likelihood that ablation will be beneficial, and may prompt consideration of a surgical maze procedure, though the efficacy of this approach to atrial fibrillation in CHD has not yet been reported. Use of internal atrial defibrillators and ablation of focal atrial fibrillation in the pulmonary veins have not been explored in CHD.

VENTRICULAR ARRHYTHMIAS

Considerable data are available on the natural history data of ventricular arrhythmias and clinical outcomes among patients with TOF, because of its prevalence in the adult CHD population and elevated incidence of ventricular arrhythmia. Mapping studies have shown that, similar to IART, VT in TOF involves a macroreentrant circuit dependant on an anatomical obstacle, in this case the right ventricular outflow tract patch and/or the conal septum.[16]

The long term prognosis for patients with repaired TOF is excellent, with nearly 90% survival at 30 years.[4] Sudden death and VT occur with a reported incidence of 1–2% over five years for young adults and an overall prevalence of sudden cardiac death of 3–6% (fig 15.4).[4 17] Although clinical presentation of adult TOF patients with sustained monomorphic VT is uncommon, such VT is inducible by programmed stimulation in 15–30% of patients,[18 19] and half have frequent and complex ventricular ectopy on ambulatory ECG.[20] Sinus node dysfunction and IART occur in 20–30% of patients with repaired TOF, and in up to 50% of symptomatic patients,[9] often mimicking VT symptoms and/or causing wide complex tachycardias. These issues make it difficult to apply standard diagnostic tools to screen individuals with clinical arrhythmia symptoms for increased risk of sudden death.

Although patients with Mustard, Senning, and Fontan procedures experience atrial tachycardias and premature mortality, they do not appear to be particularly prone to VT. Data on VT prevalence in other defects are limited. Patients with valvar aortic stenosis, pulmonary stenosis, and ventricular septal defect have been noted to have frequent ventricular ectopy. Aortic stenosis has the highest risk of sudden death among these lesions, but mortality in this defect is characterised by severity of outflow tract obstruction, rather than arrhythmia.

Risk stratification

Simple models of risk stratification for sudden death (for example, ejection fraction) do not exist for adult CHD patients. Assessment of the risk of sudden death caused by ventricular arrhythmia requires an understanding of the limited predictive values of commonly used diagnostic tests in this population. Although Holter, exercise testing, and programmed ventricular stimulation are useful for provoking and/or recording clinically documented arrhythmias, their value as screening tests is unclear. Risk assessment is further complicated by the occurrence of atrial tachycardias, which may also cause symptoms and sudden death.

Several clinical features are associated with VT and sudden death in adult CHD patients, including older age, older age at repair, and poorer haemodynamic status. Electrocardiographically, pronounced prolongation of QRS duration and prolongation dispersions of the QT and JT intervals—poorly understood indices of ventricular repolarisation—are associated with cardiomegaly, mortality, and inducible sustained VT in TOF patients.[21] These findings identify a more arrhythmogenic myocardium and suggest that both depolarisation and repolarisation are abnormal in high risk TOF patients. Because of the ubiquity of lower grades of ventricular ectopy in this population, ambulatory ECG is often abnormal, and in the absence of significant runs of VT it may be of limited value in discriminating patients at elevated risk.

The value of programmed ventricular stimulation in patients with CHD is unclear. In one large series evaluating programmed stimulation in patients with a variety of defects, inducibility of VT predicted subsequent cardiac arrest and mortality after adjustment for covariate clinical factors, but also emphasised the importance of careful selection of patients for study on the basis of those clinical features.[22] In another study of adults with TOF, no patients who subsequently died suddenly had inducible VT.[18] Both false positive studies[19] (inducible VT in patients without VT or mortality on follow up) and false negative studies (non-inducibility of patients with documented sustained VT) occur with appreciable frequency.

Management

Minimally symptomatic patients with non-sustained ventricular ectopy must be evaluated to determine whether an associated evolution of underlying abnormal haemodynamics or metabolism has occurred. If not, periodic clinical monitoring and non-invasive assessment (ECG, echo, and Holter monitoring) are probably sufficient. Event monitoring may be useful for investigation of arrhythmia symptoms. More ominous arrhythmia presentations such as syncope, near syncope with palpitation or non-sustained VT should trigger more comprehensive inquiry, including catheterisation with haemodynamic assessment and programmed atrial and ventricular stimulation. Patients with negative studies, minimal symptoms, and good haemodynamics are managed without treatment, or by using drugs with a favourable side effect profile (such as β blockers) to suppress symptomatic ectopy. Supraventricular tachycardia is treated with ablation when possible, and severe bradycardia managed with pacing. Patients with severe symptoms or inducible VT are considered for more aggressive antiarrhythmic drug treatment and AICD placement (fig 15.5).

Antiarrhythmic drugs may be useful for suppression of symptomatic ventricular arrhythmias, but have not been shown to prolong survival in CHD. AICD therapy is feasible in many patients with CHD, and its use is increasing. Catheter ablation of VT has been successful in small series of patients with CHD, and may be appropriate for patients with sustained, monomorphic VT that is haemodynamically tolerated.[23] When patients warrant surgery for haemodynamic reasons, attempts to resect potential critical zones for VT may be considered. Recently, indications have broadened for pulmonary valve replacement in patients with symptoms and/or signs of right heart failure and pulmonary regurgitation—many of whom also have prolonged QRS duration on ECG. The effect such surgical intervention may have on ventricular arrhythmia is unknown.

BRADYCARDIA
Sinus node dysfunction
Gradual loss of sinus rhythm occurs after the Mustard and Senning and all varieties of Fontan procedures.[24] Patients with heterotaxy syndromes, particularly left atrial isomerism, may also have congenital abnormalities of the sinus node independent of the effects of their surgical procedures. Paroxysmal atrial tachycardias are frequently associated with sinus node dysfunction, and loss of sinus rhythm appears to increase risk of sudden death.

Electrophysiological study of patients with the Mustard procedure have identified a variety of abnormalities of atrial electrophysiology, including prolonged sinus node recovery times, intra-atrial conduction times, and atrial refractoriness.[25] Direct surgical injury to the sinus node has been proposed as a cause of observed abnormalities of sinus node function. However, the progressive loss of sinus rhythm observed over extended follow up implies additional ongoing pathophysiological processes related to chronic haemodynamic abnormality.

AV block
Interventricular conduction abnormalities, particularly right bundle branch block, are very common after surgery for CHD. Complete postoperative heart block is caused either by direct surgical injury to the specialised conduction system or by indirect damage due to inflammatory response. It is typically associated with surgical manipulation of the ventricular septum. Patients at highest risk are those undergoing surgery for left ventricular outflow tract obstructions and patients with ventricular inversion (L-transposition of the great arteries), but it is also common after ventricular septal defect and TOF repairs. Review of clinical outcomes before cardiac pacing systems appropriate for CHD patients were available showed that postoperative heart block had a high mortality rate, even in the presence of an escape rhythm.

Complete heart block also occurs spontaneously in patients with certain structural heart defects, especially endocardial cushion defects and ventricular inversion. This may be caused by aberrant anatomy of the AV node and His bundle in these patients, rendering them vulnerable to injury. Although some of these patients present with heart block at birth, it may progress at any stage of life.

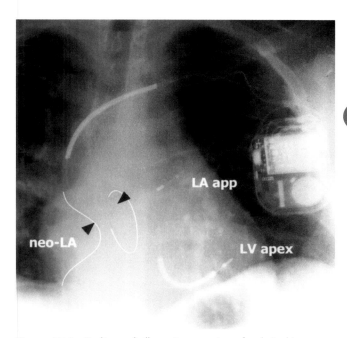

Figure 15.5 Radiograph illustrating a variety of technical issues with pacemaker placement in a patient who has undergone the Mustard procedure. The ventricular pacing lead is located in the apex of the left ventricle (LV apex), and the atrial lead in the mouth of the left atrial appendage (LA app). Both traverse the superior limb of the Mustard baffle between the superior vena cava and the left atrium, which was stenotic and required stenting (black arrows) to relieve obstruction before lead placement. The presumed locations of the lateral margin of the intra-atrial baffle, defining the pulmonary venous atrial channel (neo-LA) and the communication between left and right atria, are highlighted in white.

Pacemaker issues
While heart block is a clear indication for permanent cardiac pacing in CHD, others are less well substantiated. Many patients with CHD tolerate chronic bradycardia well, but pacing may alleviate symptoms such as fatigue, dizziness, or syncope in some patients with junctional escape rhythms, severe resting bradycardia, chronotropic incompetence, and/or prolonged pauses. Pacing may also be necessary to permit treatment with antiarrhythmic drugs.

Cardiac pacing in adults with CHD presents a variety of special challenges (fig 15.5). Congenital and acquired cardiovascular abnormalities and shunting may limit opportunities for endocardial lead placement and necessitate an epicardial or even a hybrid approach. Examples include patients with old transvenous lead systems who may have associated acquired vascular abnormalities, and Fontan patients, in whom the ventricular cavities and much or all of the atrial myocardium are surgically excluded from systemic venous pathways. Patients with the Mustard and Senning procedures may receive transvenous dual chamber pacing systems, and even AICDs, but the leads must navigate the superior limb of the intra-atrial baffle, which is prone to obstruction. Atrial lead placement in unusual sites may be difficult and must avoid inadvertent stimulation of the phrenic nerve. Because asynchronous atrial pacing may provoke IART, careful lead site selection resulting in excellent sensing of atrial electrical activity is important.

Clinical experience shows the value of AV synchrony and favours implantation of a system capable of providing a physiological heart rate response. However, the specific value of rate responsive and dual chambered pacing as compared to

Arrhythmias in adults with CHD: key points

▶ Although long term survival and clinical outcomes for adults with congenital heart disease (CHD) are generally good, arrhythmias are a significant cause of morbidity and mortality in this group of patients, especially in later decades of follow up

▶ Strategies for individual risk assessment are limited, but groups at particular risk for arrhythmia include patients with the Mustard and Senning procedure for transposition of the great vessels, patients with the Fontan procedure, and patients with repaired tetralogy of Fallot

▶ In most forms of CHD, atrial tachycardias appear to be more prevalent than ventricular tachycardias, frequently symptomatic, and associated with an increased risk of thrombosis and death

▶ Interventional strategies are currently in development for treatment of atrial and ventricular tachycardia in patients with CHD, and include innovative applications of catheter based and surgical ablative procedures, and antitachycardia and defibrillator device therapies

simpler pacing modalities is not well established in CHD. Practical limitations often require that the choice of system be adapted to patient specific problems faced with lead placement and maintenance. Exploration of the potential utility of new device technologies in CHD, such as dual site pacing for ventricular resynchronisation and atrial defibrillators, will further challenge the inventiveness of physicians caring for these patients.

CONCLUSION

Our understanding of arrhythmia in adults with CHD has progressed rapidly, through increased appreciation of the extended natural history of these patients and innovative application of treatments designed for and tested in patients without CHD. Patients with these tachycardias have poor outcomes, but the small size and anatomical diversity of this group make it difficult to determine which patients are most at risk and whether arrhythmia control will lead to measurable gains in longevity and health. Animal models and the application of evolving therapeutic technologies have provided us with valuable insights into the anatomical substrates of arrhythmia in this group, and helped to understand some of the problems with preventing their recurrence. Development of a more complete picture of the underlying pathophysiological changes in the myocardium that lead to these arrhythmias will help to focus further efforts to improve our current therapeutic outcomes.

Disclosure of potential conflict of interest: Dr Triedman is a consultant for Biosense-Webster, Inc.

REFERENCES

1 **Boneva RS**, Botto LD, Moore CA, et al. Mortality associated with congenital heart defects in the United States: trends and racial disparities, 1979–1997. Circulation 2001;**103**:2376–81.

2 **Feltes TF**, Friedman RA. Transesophageal echocardiographic detection of atrial thrombi in patients with nonfibrillation atrial tachyarrhythmias and congenital heart disease. J Am Coll Cardiol 1994;**24**:1365–70.

3 **Gelatt M**, Hamilton RM, McCrindle BW, et al. Arrhythmia and mortality after the Mustard procedure: a 30-year single-center experience. J Am Coll Cardiol 1997;**29**:194–201.
  ▶ A large single centre study of long term outcomes revealed ongoing loss of sinus rhythm and late peaks in the risk of atrial flutter and death in patients with the Mustard procedure.

4 **Nollert G**, Fischlein T, Bouterwek S, et al. Long-term survival in patients with repair of tetralogy of Fallot: 36-year follow-up of 490 survivors of the first year after surgical repair. J Am Coll Cardiol 1997;**30**:1374–83.
  ▶ Long term follow up of patients who have survived repair of TOF reveal risk factors for early demise, and increased mortality in later decades of follow up.

5 **Garson A** Jr, Bink-Boelkens MTE, Hesslein PS, et al. Atrial flutter in the young: a collaborative study in 380 cases. J Am Coll Cardiol 1985;**6**:871–8.
  ▶ This report was the result of a joint effort by the Pediatric Electrophysiology Society and represents the first large scale effort to characterise the natural history of atrial tachycardia in survivors of CHD.

6 **Fishberger SB**, Wernovsky G, Gentles TL, et al. Factors that influence the development of atrial flutter after the Fontan operation. J Thorac Cardiovasc Surg 1997;**113**:80–6.
  ▶ One of three large, single centre follow up studies of Fontan arrhythmia outcomes which documented the progressively increasing risk of IART after Fontans and identified clinical risk factors for its occurrence.

7 **Stamm C**, Triedman JK, Mayer JE, et al. Long-term results of the lateral tunnel Fontan operation. J Thorac Cardiovasc Surg 2001;**121**:28–41.
  ▶ Ten year follow up was obtained in patients who had undergone lateral tunnel creation and total cavopulmonary connection, confirming the impression that Fontans created in this way were less prone to early development of IART.

8 **Shirai LK**, Rosenthal DN, Reitz BA, et al. Arrhythmias and thromboembolic complications after the extracardiac Fontan operation. J Thorac Cardiovasc Surg 1998;**115**:499–505.

9 **Roos-Hesselink J**, Perlroth MG, McGhie J, et al. Atrial arrhythmias in adults after repair of tetralogy of Fallot. Correlations with clinical, exercise, and echocardiographic findings. Circulation 1995;**91**:2214–9.
  ▶ Although prior studies emphasised the importance of ventricular arrhythmias in TOF patients, this group identified atrial arrhythmias as the main source of morbidity, occurring in one third of adult postoperative patients.

10 **Rhodes LA**, Walsh EP, Gamble WJ, et al. Benefits and potential risks of atrial antitachycardia pacing after repair of congenital heart disease. PACE 1995;**18**:1005–16.

11 **Collins KK**, Love BA, Walsh EP, et al. Location of acutely successful radiofrequency catheter ablation of intra-atrial reentrant tachycardia in patients with congenital heart disease. Am J Cardiol 2000;**86**:969–74.
  ▶ Effective catheter ablation sites in patients with biventricular repairs of CHD were most commonly located in the cavotricuspid isthmus, while Fontan patients were more likely to be successfully ablated on the atrial free wall.

12 **Chan DP**, Van Hare GF, Mackall JA, et al. Importance of atrial flutter isthmus in postoperative intra-atrial reentrant tachycardia. Circulation 2000;**102**:1283–9.

13 **Triedman JK**, Bergau DM, Saul JP, et al. Efficacy of radiofrequency ablation for control of intra-atrial reentrant tachycardia in patients with congenital heart disease. J Am Coll Cardiol 1997;**30**:1032–8.
  ▶ Follow up of patients treated for IART with catheter ablation showed that successful ablation reduced the frequency of IART symptoms and need for treatment, but half had at least one IART recurrence within six months.

14 **Marcelletti CF**, Hanley FL, Mavroudis C, et al. Revision of previous Fontan connections to total extracardiac cavopulmonary anastomosis: a multicenter experience. J Thorac Cardiovasc Surg 2000;**119**:340–6.

15 **Deal BJ**, Mavroudis C, Backer CL, et al. Impact of arrhythmia circuit cryoablation during Fontan conversion for refractory atrial tachycardia. Am J Cardiol 1999;**83**:563–8.
  ▶ This is the first case series of significant size that demonstrates that surgical "maze" lesions delivered to the right atrium during Fontan revision procedures can prevent the subsequent recurrence of IART in many patients.

16 **Horton RP**, Canby RC, Kessler DJ, et al. Ablation of ventricular tachycardia associated with tetralogy of Fallot: demonstration of bidirectional block. J Cardiovasc Electrophysiol 1997;**8**:432–5.

17 **Murphy JG**, Gersh BJ, Mair DD, et al. Long-term outcome in patients undergoing surgical repair of tetralogy of Fallot. N Engl J Med 1993;**329**:593–9.

18 **Chandar JS**, Wolff GS, Garson AJ, et al. Ventricular arrhythmias in postoperative tetralogy of Fallot. Am J Cardiol 1990;**65**:655–61.
  ▶ This large, multicentre retrospective study of patients with postoperative TOF investigated the relations between ventricular ectopy discovered by ambulatory monitoring, inducibility of VT at catheterisation, and cardiac outcomes.

19 **Lucron H**, Marcon F, Bosser G, et al. Induction of sustained ventricular tachycardia after surgical repair of tetralogy of Fallot. Am J Cardiol 1999;**83**:1369–73.

20 **Cullen S**, Celermajer DS, Franklin RC, et al. Prognostic significance of ventricular arrhythmia after repair of tetralogy of Fallot: a 12-year prospective study. J Am Coll Cardiol 1994;**23**:1151–5.

21 **Gatzoulis MA**, Till JA, Redington AN. Depolarization-repolarization inhomogeneity after repair of tetralogy of Fallot: the substrate for malignant ventricular tachycardia? Circulation 1997;**95**:401–4.
  ▶ This and earlier reports from the same group associate prolongation and variability in resting ECG intervals with increased risk of ventricular arrhythmia and death, and propose possible pathogenetic mechanisms to link the two.

22 **Alexander ME**, Walsh EP, Saul JP, *et al*. Value of programmed ventricular stimulation in patients with congenital heart disease. *J Cardiovasc Electrophysiol* 1999;**10**:1033–44.
▶ **A single centre retrospective analysis of the utility of programmed stimulation alone and in combination with other clinical factors for risk stratification of cardiac arrest in patients with CHD.**
23 **Gonska BD**, Cao K, Raab J, *et al*. Radiofrequency catheter ablation of right ventricular tachycardia late after repair of congenital heart defects. *Circulation* 1996;**94**:1902–8.
▶ **While other case reports had documented the feasibility of VT ablation in patients with CHD, this article reports the first patient**

series of substantial size and establishes that acute outcomes similar to IART ablation may be expected.
24 **Duster MC**, Bink-Boelkens MT, Wampler D, *et al*. Long-term follow-up of dysrhythmias following the Mustard procedure. *Am Heart J* 1985;**109**:1323–6.
▶ **In long term follow up of patients with the Mustard procedure, sinus node dysfunction is a frequent and progressive problem.**
25 **Vetter VL**, Tanner CS, Horowitz LN. Electrophysiologic consequences of the Mustard repair of d-transposition of the great arteries. *J Am Coll Cardiol* 1987;**10**:1265–73.

16 QUALITY OF LIFE AND PSYCHOLOGICAL FUNCTIONING OF ICD PATIENTS

Samuel F Sears Jr, Jamie B Conti

The use of the implantable cardioverter-defibrillator (ICD) for life threatening ventricular arrhythmias is standard therapy, in large part because clinical trials data have consistently demonstrated its superiority over medical treatment in preventing sudden cardiac death.[1] This success prompts closer examination and refinement of quality of life (QOL) outcomes in ICD patients. Although no universal definition of QOL exists, most researchers agree that "quality of life" is a generic term for a multi-dimensional health outcome in which biological, psychological, and social functioning are interdependent.[2] To date, the clinical trials demonstrating the efficacy of the ICD have focused primarily on mortality differences between the ICD and medical treatment. While the majority of the QOL data from these trials is yet to be published, many small studies are available for review and support the concept that ICD implantation results in desirable QOL for most ICD recipients.[3] In some patients, however, these benefits may be attenuated by symptoms of anxiety and depression when a shock is necessary to accomplish cardioversion or defibrillation. This paper reviews the published literature on QOL and psychological functioning of ICD patients and outlines the clinical and research implications of these findings.

► QUALITY OF LIFE AND THE ICD: PATIENT REPORTS

Definitive conclusions about QOL differences between patients managed with an ICD and those treated with antiarrhythmic drugs are difficult to make in the absence of large, randomised, controlled trials. Available evidence indicates that ICD recipients experience a brief decline in QOL from baseline but improve to pre-implant levels after one year of follow up.[4] The largest clinical trial data published in final form is from the coronary artery bypass graft (CABG) Patch trial which randomised patients to ICD (n = 262) versus no ICD (n = 228) while undergoing CABG surgery.[5] In contrast to May and colleagues,[4] data from this trial indicate that the QOL outcomes (mental and physical) for the ICD patients were significantly worse compared to patients with no ICD. Subanalyses revealed that there was no difference in QOL for *non-shocked ICD* patients versus no ICD patients. These results indicated that the ICD group who had received shocks was responsible for the significantly worse mental and physical QOL outcome scores between the groups. Collectively, these data suggest that the experience of shock may contribute to psychological distress and diminished QOL. Figure 16.1 details the psychological continuum a patient may experience secondary to shock.

Other investigators have examined patients with ICDs and compared them to patients with permanent pacemakers. Very few consistent differences can be demonstrated between these two populations. For example, Duru and colleagues[6] found no differences in QOL score, anxiety or depression when comparing ICD patients with and without shock experience and pacemaker patients. ICD patients with a shock history were more likely to report limitations in leisure activities and anxiety about the ICD, but they also viewed the ICD as a "life extender". Herbst and colleagues[7] recently compared the QOL and psychological distress of four patient groups: ICD only (n = 24) *v* ICD plus antiarrhythmic drug (n = 25) *v* antiarrhythmic drug only (n = 35) *v* a general cardiac sample (n = 73). QOL was assessed using the short form 36 (SF-36) and three supplementary scales examining sleep, marital and family functioning, and sexual problems. Comparisons were made between ICD groups and drug groups. Results indicated that there were no significant differences on the 11 QOL scales, even after controlling for age, sex, disease severity, and duration of treatment. However, significant differences were found in drug groups versus no drug groups, such that the drug treated group consistently reported greater impairment in physical functioning, vitality, emotional, and sleep functioning, as well as psychological distress. Collectively, these results suggest that QOL is maintained in ICD treated groups, while antiarrhythmic drug treatment is associated with diminished QOL and increased psychological distress.

In contrast, others have compared ICD patients to either antiarrhythmic drug treated patients or a cardiac reference group and have not found significant differences between these treated groups. For example, Arteaga and Windle[8] compared three groups: ICD (n = 45), medication (n = 30), and reference group (n = 29) on QOL and psychological distress. No significant differences were

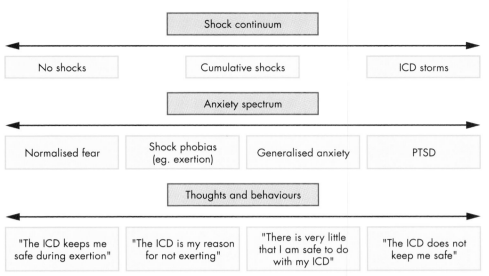

Figure 16.1 Continuum of implantable cardioverter-defibrillator (ICD) shock response. PTSD, post-traumatic stress disorder.

observed on measures of QOL and psychological distress between the treated groups, although psychological distress was associated with lower QOL for all groups. Younger patients and patients with greater cardiac dysfunction reported reduced QOL. Similarly, Carroll and colleagues[9] compared cardiac arrest survivors who received either an ICD or medications and found no significant differences in QOL. Herrmann and associates[10] also compared QOL between a group of ICD and general coronary artery disease (CAD) patients and found no significant differences on measures of QOL. Moreover, ICD patients reported significantly lower levels of anxiety than the CAD reference group.

A US national survey of ICD patients and spouses (NSIRSO) parts 1 and 2[11] examined global QOL and psychosocial issues in 450 patients. Approximately 91% of ICD recipients reported desirable QOL, either better (45%) or the same (46%) following implantation. However, a small group of ICD recipients (approximately 15%) reported significant difficulty in emotional adjustment. Younger patients (50 years of age and under) reported better general health, but worse QOL and emotional functioning than each of the other age groups studied. ICD shock history did not have a significant effect on any of the global outcome ratings. The spouses and partners of these recipients (n = 380) provided convergent validity of the recipients' reports; no significant differences were found between raters on the 10 most common concerns. Of note, frequent ICD shocks, younger age, and being female were associated with increased adjustment difficulty. The results of these two surveys suggest that ICD recipients derive significant health related QOL benefits from ICD therapy, although some (approximately 10–20%) experience difficulty. This percentage is consistent with the expected rates of distress in comparable medical populations.

RETURN TO WORK AS A QOL PROXY

An objective index of QOL is the ability to return to work. ICD recipients have favourable return to work rates in currently available studies. The largest such study (n = 101) indicated that 62% of patients had resumed employment.[12] Those who returned to work were more educated and less likely to have a history of myocardial infarction. No significant differences were found between those who returned to work and those who did not on measures of age, sex, race, functional class,

ejection fraction, extent of CAD, reason for ICD, or concomitant surgery. Similar results were obtained from a sample of young ICD patients in which 10 of the 18 were gainfully employed; eight of those had returned to the same job that they held before implantation.[13] These results suggest that the majority of ICD patients who wish to return to work are capable of doing so.

INCIDENCE AND IMPACT OF PSYCHOLOGICAL ISSUES

The typical ICD recipient must overcome both the stress of experiencing a life threatening arrhythmia and the challenge of adjusting to the ICD. Anxiety is particularly common, with approximately 24–87% of ICD recipients experiencing increased symptoms of anxiety after implantation and diagnostic rates for clinically significant anxiety disorders ranging from 13–38%.[3] The occurrence of ICD shocks is generally faulted for this psychological distress, but its causal influence is confounded by the presence of a life threatening medical condition. Depressive symptoms reported in 24–33% of ICD patients are consistent with other cardiac populations.[3]

ICD related fears are universal and may be the most pervasive psychosocial adjustment challenge ICD patients face. Psychological theory suggests that symptoms of fear and anxiety can result from a classical conditioning paradigm in which certain stimuli or behaviours are coincidentally paired with an ICD shock and are thereby avoided in the future. Because of fear of present and/or future discharges, some patients increasingly limit their range of activities and inadvertently diminish the benefits of the ICD in terms of QOL. Pauli and colleagues[14] examined the anxiety scores of ICD patients and found that anxiety was not related to ICD discharges but was highly related to a set of "catastrophic cognitions". Patients with high anxiety scores tended to interpret bodily symptoms as signs of danger and believed that they had heightened risk of sudden death. In addition, catastrophic cognitions were associated with anxiety scores consistent with the scores of panic disorder patients and different from the scores of the healthy volunteer sample. These results suggest that psychosocial interventions that utilise cognitive–behavioural protocols will likely *prevent and/or reduce* anxiety problems regardless of shock exposure by changing catastrophic thinking and over-interpretation of bodily signs and symptoms. Figure 16.2

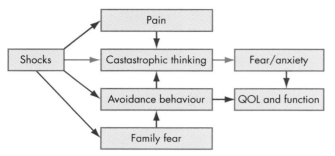

Figure 16.2 Hypothesised interrelationship between shocks, psychological distress, and quality of life (QOL).

illustrates a hypothesised interrelationship between shocks, psychological distress, and QOL based on the available research.

Uncertainty related to illness has been demonstrated to be important and related to QOL and psychological functioning in ICD patients.[9] The uncertainty of life with a potentially life threatening arrhythmia and an ICD may lead patients to resort to a "sickness scoreboard" mentality, by which they view the frequency of ICD shocks as indicative of how healthy they are and as predictive of their future health.[3] In general, outcomes based on the frequency of shocks alone are not a valid indicator of health. ICD shocks can be triggered by both ventricular arrhythmias, for which the device was implanted, and supraventricular arrhythmias, which it was not meant to treat. Shocks for either arrhythmia feel the same to the patient but do not necessarily indicate a decline in health.

EFFECT OF SHOCK ON QOL

Credner and her colleagues defined an "ICD storm" as ≥ 3 shocks in a 24 hour period. She found that approximately 10% of their sample of 136 ICD patients experienced an ICD storm during the first two years following ICD implantation.[15] Moreover, the mean (SD) number of shocks for this group of storm patients was 17 (17) (range 3–50; median 8). The experience of an ICD storm may prompt catastrophic cognitions and feelings of helplessness. These adverse psychological reactions have been linked in initial research as prospective predictors for the occurrence of subsequent arrhythmias and shocks at one, three, six, and nine month intervals, leading the researchers to conclude that "negative emotions were the cause, rather than a consequence, of arrhythmia events".[16] Although additional research focusing on a wide range of potentially identifiable "triggers" of arrhythmias is needed, this initial research indicates that reducing negative emotions and psychological distress may also decrease the chances of receiving a shock.

The literature defines specific risk factors for poor QOL and psychosocial outcomes for ICD patients that include, but extend beyond, simple shock experience. ICD patients who are younger—defined in the literature as < 50 years of age—have increased psychological distress.[17] ICD patients who do not understand their device and their condition often experience difficulties making lifestyle adjustments. Similarly, ICD patients that have the additional stressors such as loss of job or loss of role functioning often experience psychosocial difficulties that warrant additional professional attention and referral. Table 16.1 details additional suspected risk factors from the general cardiac literature that can serve as markers for psychosocial attention.

CLINICAL AND RESEARCH IMPLICATIONS RELATED TO QOL

Psychosocial and QOL interventions for ICD patients

Table 16.2 details each of the studies available that used psychosocial intervention for ICD patients. General methodological problems are consistent across studies. Firstly, the studies report on very limited sample sizes and incur a resulting low statistical power. Secondly, most of the studies were conducted using a support group format, which typically involves a participant led, unstructured approach rather than a professional led, structured approach. Although the participant led approach has some merit, such as a high level of involvement for some members, this approach often does not involve sufficient factual and objective information to produce measurable change. Instead, this approach tends to focus predominantly on the emotional aspects of the illness. In contrast, professional led groups tend to focus more on strategy and skill building rather than simply the expression of emotion. Taken together, the methodologic flaws of most of these interventions limit their utility in gauging the potential of professional led, structured cognitive–behavioural psychosocial intervention.

Support groups are a popular adjunctive treatment for ICD patients because they provide an efficient conduit for patient education spanning the biopsychosocial domains.[2] The active ingredients of support groups probably centre on the universality of many patient concerns and the sharing of information and strategies to deal effectively with these concerns. We suggest that support groups are a valuable but not necessarily sufficient means of providing psychosocial care for all ICD patients. Some patients will need more individualised, tailored cognitive–behavioural or pharmacological interventions to address more completely their psychosocial needs. As noted above, professional led groups are preferable because a systematic presentation of information via selected expert speakers and a broad based curriculum could be designed for maximal benefit for the majority of participants. Certainly patient stories or testimonials can also play a regular role, but that is a process that can occur both formally and informally during the meetings among group members. The majority of the groups are maintained by ICD health professionals with a strong commitment to psychosocial care. There is no formula on how to structure support groups for maximal effectiveness, but they remain important in the care of ICD patients as one of a set of strategies to improve the psychosocial care of ICD patients.

The most significant study of psychosocial interventions for ICD patients involved a randomised controlled methodology to reduce psychological distress.[18] Individual cognitive–behavioural therapy was used to reduce psychological distress in newly implanted ICD patients to determine if such

Table 16.2 Psychosocial intervention studies with ICD recipients

Study	n	Duration of treatment	Summary of results and critique of findings	
Badger and Morris (1989)	12	8 non-structured support group sessions	Purpose: support group intervention v no treatment control group. Results: no significant between group differences. Trends were reported towards improvement in the treatment group	Very small number of patients were studied. No systematic treatment protocol was delivered. This was a patient led methodology
Molchany and Peterson (1994)	11	Not specified	Purpose: support group intervention v no treatment control group. Results: no significant between group differences. Qualitative analyses demonstrated improved ability to cope and increased satisfaction with life in group participants	Very small number of patients were studied. No known systematic treatment protocol was delivered. Duration of treatment is unknown but may not have been sufficient to detect differences
Sneed et al (1997)	34	2 inpatient individual sessions, 2 support group sessions, and 12 telephone contacts over a 16 week period.	Purpose: support group intervention v no treatment control group. Results: no significant between group differences at 4 month follow up. Results indicated that tension/anxiety reduced for both groups	Small number of patients were studied. Systematic treatment protocol was delivered but group format was patient led. Longer duration of treatment was a significant improvement in methodology but the content of the follow up phone contacts was not well specified
Kohn et al (2000)	49	9 sessions (pre-implant, pre-discharge, 7 routine follow up visits)	Purpose: compared individual cognitive–behavioural treatment to usual care. Results: individual treatment group reported less depression, less anxiety, less general distress, (p<0.05), despite receiving a higher level of shocks (p<0.07)	Sufficient sample size. Most comprehensive and well documented treatment protocol study available. Effects were robust enough to detect differences. Used an expensive and time intensive, individual therapy protocol

treatment would also reduce arrhythmic events requiring shocks for termination. These investigators randomised 49 ICD patients to active treatment versus no treatment. The treatment consisted of an individual therapy session at pre-implant, pre-discharge from the hospital, consecutive weeks for four weeks, and then sessions at routine cardiac clinic appointments at one, three, and five months post-implantation. They found that active treatment patients reported less depression, less anxiety, and less general psychological distress than the no treatment group at nine month follow up evaluations. These results suggest that more systematic interventions for new ICD patients would likely produce optimal psychological and QOL outcomes. Although this study did not include information about the cost effectiveness of the intervention, it is reasonable to assume that psychological intervention delivered in this manner would likely be at least cost-neutral if it prevented more expensive hospitalisations, additional medications, and unnecessary accessing of care. Future research on psychosocial interventions should provide further information about the costs of their interventions for closer cost effectiveness analysis.

Clinician readiness for psychosocial interventions

The realistic probability of practising cardiologists and nurses having the time or skills necessary to provide such extensive psychosocial interventions is small. We surveyed physicians and nurses (n = 261) to rate their views of specific ICD patient outcomes, common daily life problems for ICD patients, and their own comfort in managing these concerns.[19] The majority

Table 16.3 Pocket guide to key interview questions for the psychosocial care of ICD patients

Key concept	Sample interview question	Interpretation
Affective functioning depression	Depressed mood question: during the past month, have you often been bothered by feeling down, hopeless, or depressed? Anhedonia question: during the past month, have you felt less interested in or gotten less pleasure from doing the things you typically enjoy?	If either of these questions screen positive, the presence of depression should be pursued via additional interview or referral to a mental health professional. If both of these questions are negative, the patient is unlikely to have major depression
Anxiety	Generalised anxiety: are you generally a nervous person? Specific anxiety: do you have regular and continuous fears of ICD shocks?	A positive response to general anxiety indicates a condition that is unlikely to be responsive to clinic based intervention by a cardiologist and should be referred. Specific anxiety, however, is likely to be improved by a clinic based discussion from a cardiologist. However, referral may still be necessary if education and reassurance related to the specific cardiac concerns are not sufficient
Behavioural functioning avoidance behaviour	Avoidant behaviour: do you avoid doing anything simply because of your fear of shocks?	Confirmed avoidance behaviour increases the probability of a significant anxiety problem and warrants referral for additional work up by a mental health professional
Cognitive functioning attention and memory	Attention and memory change and perceived impact: have you noticed any significant changes in your attention or memory since ICD implantation? Have these changes presented any problems in your daily functioning?	Cognitive changes are a recognised part of significant cardiac illness. Neuropsychological evaluation is indicated if the changes have presented any problems or concerns for the patient or family members

of ICD patients experience desirable QOL, emotional well-being, and family functioning post-implantation, as viewed by health care providers. However, healthcare providers reported that approximately 10–20% of ICD patients were significantly worse in these areas post-implantation. The most common problems for ICD recipients in daily life included driving restrictions/limitations, coping with ICD shocks, and depression. Health care providers generally reported the most comfort handling traditional medical issues (that is, 92% of the sample reported comfort in managing patient adherence concerns), and the least comfort in managing emotional well-being issues (for example, only 39% of the sample reported comfort in managing depression and anxiety symptoms). These results are somewhat disconcerting when we consider that our previous work also showed that ICD patients were equally likely to seek discussion about emotional issues with health care providers (37%) as they were with family and friends (36%).[11] Our survey of health care providers also found that the majority believed that their ICD patients wanted more information to help them cope with or adjust to their ICD (91%) and that they believed that education as an intervention would be effective (83%).

Discomfort while addressing psychosocial issues for cardiology practitioners is not surprising and most likely reflects lack of training and experience in behavioural medicine and psychology. We have suggested the "Four A's checklist" to detect and manage psychosocial issues in ICD clinics: ask, advise, assist, and arrange referral.[17 20] The first step is to *ask* the patient about their ICD related concerns in an effort to define accurately their perceived problem. In table 16.3, we have provided sample diagnostic questions that can assist the clinician and yield sufficient diagnostic precision.[21] Secondly, the healthcare provider can *advise* the ICD patient on the common challenges that lie ahead and how to manage these concerns via supportive communication. The healthcare provider should take care to respect the coping style and adjustment difficulties of each patient. Thirdly, the provider can *assist* the patient by addressing the immediate concerns of the patient, normalising the most common challenges, educating the patient about their device, and provide brief problem solving. Finally, the health care provider should *arrange* a consultation for those recipients who would benefit from speaking with a mental health specialist. ICD recipients should be told that anxiety and depression are common and expected side effects for many medical patients including ICD patients, and for that reason, attending to the psychosocial aspects of adjustment is part of the overall treatment strategy. This rationale of a "stress management" based approach is broadly acceptable to most patients.

CONCLUSIONS

The ICD is the treatment of choice for life threatening arrhythmias. The QOL data from these trials, which focused primarily on mortality, now warrants equal scrutiny. All available data suggest that the ICD will achieve comparable if not better QOL than alternative treatments. Future research must place greater emphasis on ICD specific and arrhythmia specific measures that may be more sensitive to more changes in outcome. Measurement and interventions should focus on patient acceptance of the device. Interdisciplinary studies that include cardiology, psychology, nursing, and cardiac rehabilitation specialists are needed to guide best clinical practice. The reputation of the ICD as a "shock box" is a significant source of anxiety to potential patients. Today, third generation ICDs

QOL and psychological functioning of ICD patients: key points

▶ Incidence of psychological diagnosis
  – anxiety 13–38%
  – depression 34–43%
▶ Risk factors for maladjustment
  – young age
  – frequent shocks
  – women
▶ Four A's
  – ask
  – advise
  – assist
  – arrange
▶ Multidisciplinary care team
  – cardiologist
  – nurse
  – mental health professional
  – rehabilitation

are much improved in their sensing and tiered therapy options to reduce shocks and their resulting distress. Despite improvements in therapy such as antitachycardia pacing, ICD patients are likely always to need some attention to psychological adjustment. We suggest that routine consideration of psychosocial needs be integrated into the clinical care of ICD patients worldwide.

REFERENCES

1 **Glikson M**, Friedman PA. The implantable cardioverter defibrillator. *Lancet* 2001;**357**:1107–17.
▶ This article provides a thorough review of the details of device functioning and clinical trial data for health care professionals.
2 **Engel GE**. The need for a new medical model: a challenge for biomedicine. *Science* 1977;**196**:129–36.
3 **Sears SF**, Todaro JF, Saia TL, *et al.* Examining the psychosocial impact of implantable cardioverter defibrillators: a literature review. *Clin Cardiol* 1999;**22**:481–9.
▶ All psychosocial literature is reviewed and interpreted including specific psychological and behavioural theory posited about the development and manifestation of distress in ICD patients.
4 **May CD**, Smith PR, Murdock CJ, *et al.* The impact of the implantable cardioverter defibrillator on quality of life. *Pacing Clin Electrophysiol* 1995;**18**:1411–8.
5 **Namerow PB**, Firth BR, Heywood GM, *et al.* Quality of life six months after CABG surgery in patients randomized to ICD versus no ICD therapy: findings from the CABG Patch trial. *Pacing Clin Electrophysiol* 1999;**22**:1305–13.
▶ This randomised controlled trial data implicated the specific role of ICD shock in the quality of life outcomes of ICD patients.
6 **Duru F**, Buchi S, Klaghofer R, *et al.* How different from pacemaker patients are recipients of implantable cardioverter-defibrillators with respect to psychosocial adaptation, affective disorders, and quality of life? *Heart* 2001;**85**:375–9.
▶ These authors were the first to use generic quality of life indices to compare implantable device patients on measures of quality of life and adaptation.
7 **Herbst JH**, Goodman M, Feldstein S, *et al.* Health related quality of life assessment of patients with life-threatening ventricular arrhythmias. *Pacing Clin Electrophysiol* 1999;**22**:915–26.
8 **Arteaga WJ**, Windle JR. The quality of life of patients with life threatening arrhythmias. *Arch Intern Med* 1995;**155**:2086–91.
9 **Carroll DL**, Hamilton GA, McGovern BA. Changes in health status and quality of life and the impact of uncertainty in patients who survive life-threatening arrhythmias. *Heart Lung* 1999;**28**:251–60.
10 **Herrmann C**, von zur Muhen F, Schaumann A, *et al.* Standardized assessment of psychological well-being and quality-of-life in patients with implanted defibrillators. *Pacing Clin Electrophysiol* 1997;**20**:95–103.
11 **Sears SF**, Eads A, Marhefka S, *et al.* The U.S. national survey of ICD recipients: examining the global and specific aspects of quality of life [abstract]. *Eur Heart J* 1999;**20**:232.
12 **Kalbfleisch KR**, Lehmann MH, Steinman RT, *et al.* Reemployment following implantation of the automatic cardioverter defibrillator. *Am J Cardiol* 1989;**64**:199–202.
13 **Dubin AM**, Batsford WP, Lewis RJ, *et al.* Quality of life in patients receiving implantable cardioverter defibrillators at or before age 40. *Pacing Clin Electrophysiol* 1996;**19**:1555–9.

14 **Pauli P**, Wiedemann G, Dengler W, *et al.* Anxiety in patients with an automatic implantable cardioverter defibrillator: what differentiates them from panic patients? *Psychosom Med* 1999;**61**:69–76.
▶ **This study provided specific examination of the role of cognitive appraisal processes in the development of psychological distress in ICD patients by comparing their responses to both anxiety populations and healthy same aged populations.**
15 **Credner SC**, Klingenheben T, Mauss O, *et al.* Electrical storm in patients with transvenous implantable cardioverter defibrillators. *J Am Coll Cardiol* 1998;**32**:1909–15.
▶ **These authors defined a criteria for ICD storm and provided data regarding its incidence in a clinical sample of ICD patients.**
16 **Dunbar SB**, Kimble LP, Jenkins LS, *et al.* Association of mood disturbance and arrhythmia events in patients after cardioverter defibrillator implantation. *Depress Anxiety* 1999;**9**:163–8.
▶ **This study provided prospective examination of psychological factors and the incidence of shock that allowed for prediction of shock by psychological distress.**
17 **Sears SF Jr**, Burns JL, Handberg E, *et al.* Young at heart: understanding the unique psychosocial adjustment of young implantable cardioverter defibrillator recipients. *Pacing Clin Electrophysiol* 2001;**24**:1113–7.

18 **Kohn CS**, Petrucci RJ, Baessler C, *et al.* The effect of psychological intervention on patients' long-term adjustment to the ICD: a prospective study. *Pacing Clin Electrophysiol* 2000;**23**:450–6.
▶ **This study was the first randomised controlled trial of a comprehensive psychosocial intervention programme for ICD patients.**
19 **Sears SF**, Todaro JF, Urizar G, *et al.* Assessing the psychosocial impact of the ICD: a national survey of implantable cardioverter defibrillator health care providers. *Pacing Clin Electrophysiol* 2000;**23**:939-45.
▶ **This study provided US physician and nurse data and indicated the specific psychosocial concerns that ICD patients report to health care providers and their degree of comfort managing these concerns.**
20 **Sotile WM**, Sears SF. *You can make a difference: brief psychosocial interventions for ICD patients and their families.* Minneapolis, Minnesota: Medtronic Inc, 1999.
▶ **This book provides a comprehensive review and set of clinical strategies of the common psychosocial challenges for ICD patients and families for nurses and physicians.**
21 **Whooley MA**, Simon GE. Managing depression in medical outpatients. *N Engl J Med* 2000;**343**:1942–50.

17 NOVEL MAPPING TECHNIQUES FOR CARDIAC ELECTROPHYSIOLOGY

Paul A Friedman

Because of its high success rate and low morbidity, radiofrequency (RF) catheter ablation has become first line treatment for many arrhythmias. In this procedure, one or more electrode catheters are advanced percutaneously through the vasculature to contact cardiac tissues. A diagnostic study is performed to define the arrhythmia mechanism, and subsequently an ablation catheter is positioned adjacent to the arrhythmogenic substrate. Radiofrequency energy of up to 50 W is delivered in the form of a continuous unmodulated sinusoidal waveform, typically for 60 seconds. Energy delivery is well tolerated by a mildly sedated patient, and results in a small (5 mm) well circumscribed lesion. Destruction of tissue critical for arrhythmogenesis (such as an accessory pathway) and its subsequent replacement with scar eliminates arrhythmia.

The small size of radiofrequency lesions has led to the greatest success in the treatment of those arrhythmias that have a focal origin or depend on a narrow isthmus for maintenance. Furthermore, since precise lesion placement is required, arrhythmias for which ablation is most effective (accessory pathways, atrioventricular nodal re-entry tachycardia (AVNRT)) have largely anatomically based or directed substrates. Accessory pathways are anomalous epicardial connections between the atria and ventricles, and are located along the mitral or tricuspid valve annulus, reducing the problem of localisation to identification of a point on a line. An electrode catheter in the coronary sinus outlines the mitral annulus fluoroscopically, and is used to guide ablation catheter position. The relative amplitude of the atrial and ventricular components of the bipolar electrogram recorded by the ablation catheter further defines tip position relative to the annulus. Earliest atrial or ventricular activation during pathway conduction identifies pathway location along the annulus. The target for catheter ablation of AVNRT (the AV nodal slow pathway) occurs even more predictably in the posteroseptum. Ablation may be guided entirely by anatomic location relative to His and coronary sinus catheter positions, which serve as fluoroscopic landmarks, or by a combined anatomic and electrogram approach. Detailed discussions of radiofrequency ablation are available elsewhere.[1]

ROLE OF MAPPING SYSTEMS

The high success of catheter ablation in the treatment of AVNRT and accessory pathways, and atrioventricular junction ablation for rate control in atrial fibrillation, has led to interest in application of this therapy to a broad array of arrhythmias. Success in stable arrhythmias with predictable anatomic locations or characteristics identifying endocardial electrograms, such as idiopathic ventricular tachycardia or isthmus dependent atrial flutter, has approached 90%. However, ablation of more complex arrhythmias, including some atrial tachycardias, many forms of intra-atrial re-entry, most ventricular tachycardias, and atrial fibrillation continues to pose a major challenge. This stems in part from the limitations of fluoroscopy and conventional catheter based mapping techniques to localise arrhythmogenic substrates that are removed from fluoroscopic landmarks and lack characteristic electrogram patterns. The inability to associate accurately the intracardiac electrogram with a specific endocardial site also limits the reliability with which the roving catheter tip can be placed at a site that was previously mapped. This results in limitations when the creation of long linear lesions is required to modify the substrate, and when multiple isthmuses or "channels" are present. Additionally, since in conventional endocardial mapping a single localisation is made over several cardiac cycles, the influence of beat-to-beat variability on overall cardiac activation cannot be known. Transient or haemodynamically unstable arrhythmias are also not mappable by conventional techniques. With prolonged procedures, there is increased exposure to ionising radiation, adding risk for both the patient and physician.

New techniques in catheter localisation and arrhythmia mapping have been developed to overcome these limitations and expand the list of arrhythmias amenable to catheter ablation (table 17.1). These include multi-electrode baskets, electroanatomical mapping, and non-contact mapping (table 17.2). The mechanism of operation and clinical experience with these mapping tools will be reviewed.

Table 17.1 Role of advanced mapping systems based on arrhythmia

Limited role for advanced mapping (high conventional success rate)	Advanced mapping shortens procedure, limits fluoroscopy, or enhances success	Advanced mapping extremely helpful or essential
AVNRT	Typical atrial flutter	Macroreentrant atrial arrhythmias after surgical correction of congenital heart disease
Accessory pathway ablation	Idiopathic ventricular tachycardia (RVOT, LVOT, fascicular VT)	Transient/multiple focal atrial tachycardias
AV junction ablation (for rate control in atrial fibrillation)	Repeat ablation after previously failed attempt Haemodynamically stable VT (non-idiopathic)	Haemodynamically unstable VT Atrial fibrillation: linear lesions for atrial compartmentalisation procedures; also useful, but role less defined for encircling pulmonary vein isolation and non-pulmonary vein focus localisation

AVNRT, atriventricular nodal re-entrant tachycardia; LVOT, left ventricular outflow tract; RVOT, right ventricular outflow tract, VT, ventricular tachycardia.

MULTI-ELECTRODE ("BASKET") CATHETER MAPPING

The mapping catheter consists of an open lumen catheter shaft with a collapsible, basket shaped, distal end. Currently basket catheters consist of eight equidistant metallic arms, providing a total of 64 unipolar or 32 bipolar electrodes capable of simultaneously recording electrograms from a cardiac chamber. The catheters are constructed of a superelastic material to allow passive deployment of the array catheter and optimise endocardial contact. The size of the basket catheter used depends on the dimensions of the chamber to be mapped, requiring antecedent evaluation (usually by echocardiogram) to ensure proper size selection. The collapsed catheters are introduced percutaneously into the appropriate chamber where they are expanded.

The mapping system consists of an acquisition module connected to a computer, which is capable of simultaneously processing: (1) 32 bipolar electrograms from the basket catheter; (2) 16 bipolar/unipolar electrograms signals; (3) a 12 lead ECG; and (4) a pressure signal. Colour coded activation maps are reconstructed on-line. The electrograms and activation maps are displayed on a computer monitor and the acquired signals can be stored on optical disk for off-line analysis. Activation marks are generated automatically with either a peak or slope (dV/dt) algorithm, and the activation times are then edited manually as needed.[2]

Clinical experience

Percutaneous endocardial mapping with multi-electrode basket shaped catheter has been shown to be feasible and safe in patients with ventricular tachycardia (VT) in coronary disease. Fragmented early endocardial activation—suggesting a zone of slow conduction that may be a suitable ablation target—is frequently demonstrated. However, the relatively large inter-electrode spacing in available catheters has prevented high resolution reconstruction of the re-entrant circuit in the majority of patients.[3] More recently, a steerable sector basket catheter with improved spatial resolution (±1 cm) to guide ablation procedures in patients with postinfarction VT has been used. This has enabled demonstration of early endocardial activation and localisation of the area of slow conduction during VT.

Basket catheter strengths and limitations

The multi-electrode endocardial mapping system allows simultaneous recording of electrical activation from multiple sites and fast reconstruction of endocardial activation maps. This may limit the time endured in tachycardia compared to single point mapping techniques without the insertion of multiple electrodes and facilitate endocardial mapping of haemodynamically unstable tachycardias.

Because of its poor spatial resolution, the basket catheter in its current iteration has demonstrated only limited clinical

Table 17.2 Mapping system characteristics

	Multi-electrode baskets	Electroanatomical mapping	Non-contact mapping
Parallel data acquisition (shorten procedure time)	Yes	No	Yes
Map resolution	Limited (1 cm)	Medium to High*	High
Non-fluoroscopic catheter navigation	No	Yes	Yes
Transient arrhythmia mapping	Yes	No	Yes
Substrate (bipolar voltage) mapping	No	Yes	No
Catalogue ablation points (guide linear lesion creation)	No	Yes	Yes
Find gap in linear lesion	No	Yes†	Yes

*Function of time spent/number of points collected.
†Time consuming—line must be retraced with mapping catheter.

118

A

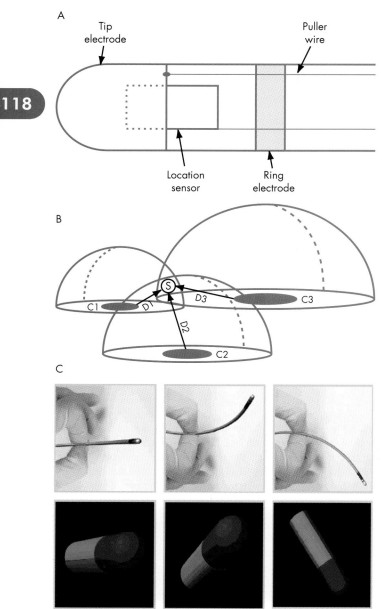

B

C

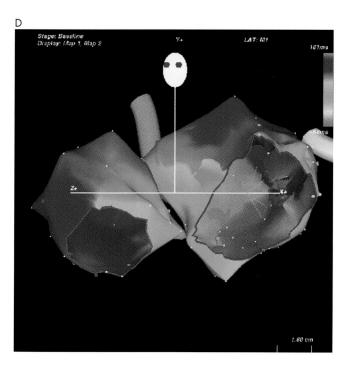

Figure 17.1 Electroanatomic mapping. (A) The catheter is composed of tip and ring electrodes and a location sensor embedded within the catheter. (B) A location pad with three coils (C1, C2, and C3) generates magnetic fields that decay as a function of distance from the coils. The sensor measures the strength of each field, permitting determination of the distance from each coil (D1, D2, D3). The intersection of three theoretical spheres of radii D1, D2, and D3 determines the catheter tip location in space. Reproduced from Gepstein *et al*,[20] with permission. (C) Deflection of the catheter in space (top panels) results in real time display of catheter orientation on the computer screen, to guide non-fluoroscopic manipulation. (D) Activation map from a patient with left atrial figure of eight re-entrant tachycardia. The two atria are shown in the left anterior oblique view, with tricuspid valve and mitral valve cut out. The colour at each anatomic point shows local activation time relative to the reference catheter (scale top right).

utility to guide ablation of re-entrant atrial or ventricular arrhythmias. The spatial resolution (approximately 1 cm along the arms of the catheter and $\geq$ 1 cm between the arms) is generally not sufficient for a catheter based ablation procedure given the small size and precise localisation associated with radiofrequency lesions.[3] The role of multi-electrode basket catheters in mapping smaller structures such as pulmonary veins for the treatment of focal atrial fibrillation (discussed below) may be more promising, but is not known.

ELECTROANATOMIC MAPPING

The CARTO system (Biosense, Diamond Bar, California, USA) correlates electrophysiologic characteristics with endocardial anatomy by continuously recording mapping catheter location. A locator pad placed beneath the operating table generates ultra-low intensity magnetic fields that code the mapping space around the patient's chest with spatial distinguishing characteristics. The pad's three coils each generate a magnetic field that decays in strength as a function of distance from that coil. A sensor embedded in the mapping catheter measures the strength of each magnetic field, enabling determination of the distance from each coil. These distances are the radii of theoretical spheres around each coil; the intersection of the three spheres defines the location of the sensor, and thus the catheter tip, in space (fig 17.1). In addition to catheter location, orientation (roll, pitch, and yaw) is determined.

With this system, a mapping catheter with tip and proximal electrodes to record unipolar and bipolar signals is advanced percutaneously to the chamber of interest. Catheter position is recorded relative to the location of a reference back patch, thus compensating for subject motion within the coils' fields. The mapping procedure involves positioning the mapping catheter at sequential points along the endocardium. Catheter tip location and electrograms are simultaneously acquiring while the catheter remains in stable contact with endocardium. Local activation times are calculated relative to the body surface ECG or a fixed (reference) intracardiac electrode. The system continuously monitors the quality of catheter–tissue contact and local activation time stability to ensure validity and reproducibility of each local measurement. The acquired information is then colour coded and displayed. As each new site is acquired, the reconstruction is updated in real time to progressively create a three dimensional chamber geometry colour encoded with activation time (fig 17.1). In addition to activation time maps, dynamic propagation maps displayed as movies of sequential activation on the computer workstation can be created. Additionally, the collected data can be displayed as voltage maps depicting the magnitude of the local peak voltage in a three dimensional model. These can be useful to define areas scarring and electrically diseased tissue. This system allows precise positioning of the catheter tip at a site of interest that was previously sampled, tagging of regions of interest, and marking positions of veins and valves.

Clinical experience
Atrial tachycardia and flutter

Although catheter ablation of atrial tachycardia guided by standard radiographic imaging has provided effective treatment in some populations, mapping complexity may lead to prolonged procedure and fluoroscopy time. Conventional ablation has been even more challenging in patients with congenital heart disease and previous surgery, as macro-reentrant arrhythmias arise utilising critical channels of slow conduction present within scars, or between scars and anatomic boundaries. Approaches for ablation have included identification of isolated diastolic potentials and entrainment mapping to identify critical circuit components, and creation of linear lesions between atriotomy scar and an anatomic barrier (for example, tricuspid annulus or inferior vena cava) to interrupt the re-entrant circuit. The presence of multiple re-entrant circuits, electrically silent scar zones, fractionated and small potentials, and arrhythmogenic substrate location distant from fluoroscopic landmarks has limited long term procedural success.

Three dimensional non-fluoroscopic electroanatomical mapping has facilitated ablation of this arrhythmia. In patients with focal arrhythmia, detailed, high density mapping of the earliest endocardial activation site during tachycardia can be acquired—assuming the arrhythmia is sustained or frequently recurrent. The system has been highly successful in ablating ectopic atrial tachycardia rapidly and with a small number of RF applications.[4] In the presence of structural heart disease, the system creates useful endocardial three dimensional maps with labelled structures (for example, valves, veins) to guide catheter manipulation. Local bipolar peak voltage maps have been successfully used to identify the complex substrate responsible for arrhythmia in the setting of congenital heart disease with prior corrective surgery. In these patients, multiple isolated channels between scars usually located in the right atrial free wall are responsible macro-reentrant atrial tachycardia. Focal ablation within channels guided by electroanatomical substrate maps eliminates arrhythmia.[5]

Typical human atrial flutter arises from a stable macro-entrant circuit produced utilising the sub-eustachian isthmus between the tricuspid valve annulus and the ostium of the inferior vena cava as its critical zone of slow conduction. Creation of a complete line of conduction block across the sub-eustachian isthmus eliminates counter clockwise (typical) and clockwise atrial flutter. Because of its well defined boundaries, sub-eustachian isthmus dependent flutter is usually easily treated with conventional techniques. Electroanatomical mapping has been used to confirm the anatomic location of the flutter circuit, to guide linear lesion creation, and to decrease fluoroscopy use.[6] Additionally, electroanatomical mapping can identify gaps in the linear lesion in the setting of

Abbreviations

AF: atrial fibrillation
AVNRT: atrioventricular nodal re-entrant tachycardia
MEA: multiple electrode array
RF: radiofrequency
VT: ventricular tachycardia

recurrent flutter after previous ablation, to guide repeat ablation.[7] However, since the technique requires point to point data acquisition, the entire line must be retraced to locate the defect, which can be time consuming.

Atrial fibrillation

Curative non-surgical treatment of atrial fibrillation (AF) still remains a challenge. Currently, two approaches exist to treat AF: elimination or control of rapidly firing foci that trigger AF (mostly commonly from the pulmonary veins), or transcatheter creation of linear lesions to modify the substrate to prevent AF sustenance.[8 9] Since the triggers that initiate AF are often only transiently active or rapidly lead to AF, point to point mapping as employed by the electroanatomical system is of limited utility for localising discharging foci. However, the navigation employed by the system may be useful for returning to sites at which pulmonary vein potentials are recorded. These potentials have been associated with muscle bundles that connect to or give rise to discharging foci; pulmonary vein potential by catheter ablation has resulted in elimination of arrhythmia in some patients. Experience with this use of the system is limited, and requires confirmation. When non-pulmonary vein foci are present, the utility of this system to localise them is quite limited.

Percutaneous linear lesion creation is based upon the surgical maze procedure and aims to compartmentalise the atria into sections too small to support wavefront re-entry. Initial attempts at emulating the surgical approach to treatment of AF in the catheter laboratory have met with limited success. While the three dimensional electroanatomical reconstruction of the targeted atrium and catheter navigation facilitate linear lesion creation by "tagging" ablation sites on the map, catheter "reach" remains challenging. Another technical challenge is assuring the "completeness" of ablation lines, since gaps that permit impulse conduction are often pro-arrhythmic and lead to incisional flutters. Electroanatomical mapping can confirm line integrity, but the entire length of the linear lesion must be retraced with the mapping catheter while pacing from a second site—a time consuming process. Efforts at transcatheter right atrial or biatrial compartmentalisation with this system have resulted in long procedures with highly variable success rates.[9 10] More limited lesion sets to isolate circumferentially the pulmonary veins may hold greater promise.[11]

Ventricular tachycardia

Radiofrequency catheter ablation of VTs in the setting of previous myocardial infarction or other structural heart disease has been challenging because of the frequent presence of multiple re-entry circuits, haemodynamic instability during arrhythmia, frequent changes from one VT to another, and absence of reproducibly inducible VT. The small size of lesions created by RF ablation in the presence of large regions of abnormal substrate further limits treatment.

Electroanatomical activation maps, which must be acquired during tachycardia to define the circuit, are limited to stable arrhythmias amenable to acquisition of multiple sequential points. However, substrate (voltage) maps created during sinus rhythm have been used to define abnormal left ventricular endocardium in patients with drug refractory, monomorphic, unmappable VT and frequent implantable defibrillator shocks.[12] Regions of "dense scar" are defined as those with a bipolar voltage amplitude < 0.5 mV. Placement of a median of four linear lesions with typical length 4 cm in a point by point manner from scar to anatomic boundaries or normal myocardium can effectively control arrhythmia in many patients with otherwise unmappable VT.[12] Success with electroanatomical mapping is greater when at least one critical isthmus for tachycardia can be defined.[13]

Conventional approaches—activation sequence mapping, pace mapping or both—have had great success with ablation of focal VT, and advanced mapping is not usually required. However, electroanatomical mapping has been successfully used to guide ablation of patients with focal tachycardia in order to limit fluoroscopy. Additionally, electroanatomical mapping permits re-navigation of the mapping catheter to previous sites of ablation or mechanically terminated tachycardia locations to further facilitate ablation.

Electroanatomical mapping strengths and limitations

In the setting of stable or frequently repetitive arrhythmia, creation of high spatial resolution (< 1 mm) activation maps and the ability to localise the catheter tip relative to maps facilitates ablation of complex arrhythmias difficult to treat conventionally. Additionally, fluoroscopy time can be reduced via electromagnetic catheter navigation, and the catheter can be accurately guided to positions removed from fluoroscopic markers. In the absence of stable or high frequency arrhythmia, if arrhythmia arises in the setting of cardiac structural abnormalities, voltage maps have been very useful in defining the arrhythmogenic substrate. This technique has been used to guide ablation successfully in patients with re-entrant atrial and ventricular arrhythmias not amenable to conventional ablation treatment.

The sequential data acquisition required for map creation remains very time consuming, particularly if the integrity of long linear lesions is assessed, or if multiple stable arrhythmias require mapping. Since the acquired data are not coherent in time, multiple beats are required for creation of the activation map. Rapidly changing or transient arrhythmias (as seen in the triggers that give rise to focal atrial fibrillation) are not easily recorded, and can only be mapped if significant substrate abnormalities are present.

NON-CONTACT ENDOCARDIAL MAPPING

Non-contact mapping is based on the physical principle that when one three dimensional surface is placed within another, if the electrical potential on one surface is known, the potential on the other can be calculated. To map, a probe with known dimensions is advanced to the cardiac chamber of interest and, once there, expanded. The endocardial surface of the chamber of interest is defined at procedure, and the electrical potential present on the probe's surface recorded, permitting calculation of the endocardial potential. This allows reconstruction of electrograms at endocardial sites in the absence of physical electrode contact at those locations (virtual electrograms), enabling recording of cardiac electrical activity from thousands of points simultaneously.

The non-contact mapping system (EnSite 3000, Endocardial Solutions, Inc, St Paul, Minnesota, USA) consists of catheter mounted multielectrode array (MEA) which serves as the

probe, a custom designed amplifier system, and a computer workstation that is used to display three dimensional maps of cardiac electrical activity. The catheter consists of a 7.5 ml balloon mounted on a 9 French catheter around which is woven a braid of 64 insulated 0.003 mm diameter wires (fig 17.2). Each wire has a 0.025 mm break in insulation that serves as a non-contact unipolar electrode. The raw far-field electrocardiographic data from the MEA are acquired and fed into a multichannel recorder and amplifier system that also has 16 channels for conventional contact catheters, 12 channels for the surface ECG, as well as pressure channels. The unipolar MEA signals are recorded using a ring electrode as a reference, which is located on the shaft of the MEA catheter. An electrically based locator signal is also generated by the system to permit non-fluoroscopic navigation of any standard roving contact catheter used for ablation.

The locator system locates any conventional catheter in space with respect to the MEA (and thus with respect to the cardiac chamber being mapped) by passing a 5.68 kHz, low current "locator" signal between the contact catheter electrode being located and reference electrodes on the non-contact array. This creates a potential gradient across the MEA electrodes used to position the source. This locator signal serves several purposes. Firstly, it is used to construct the three dimensional computer model of the endocardium (virtual endocardium) that is required for the reconstruction of endocardial electrograms and isopotential maps (fig 17.2). This model is acquired by moving a conventional, contact catheter around the cardiac chamber, building up a series of coordinates for the endocardium, and generating a patient specific, anatomically contoured model of its geometry. During geometry creation, only the most distant points visited by the roving catheter are recorded in order to ignore those detected when the catheter is not in contact with the endocardial wall. Geometric points are sampled at the beginning of the study during sinus rhythm, resulting in a contoured model with end diastolic dimensions. Secondly, the locator signal can be used to display and log the position of any catheter (for example, His catheter, coronary sinus catheter, and so on) on the endocardial model. Thirdly, during catheter ablation procedures, the locator system is used in real time to navigate the catheter to sites of interest identified from the isopotential colour maps, to catalogue the position of RF energy applications on the virtual endocardium, and to facilitate re-visitation of sites of interest by the ablation catheter.

The system reconstructs over 3360 electrograms simultaneously over a computer generated model of the chamber of interest ("virtual" endocardium). Because of the high density of data, colour coded isopotential maps are used to depict graphically regions which are depolarised, and wavefront propagation is displayed as a user controlled three dimensional "movie" (fig 17.2). Additionally, unipolar or bipolar virtual electrograms can be displayed by selection of an area of interest, and displayed as if from point, array, or plaque electrodes. The fidelity of virtual unipolar electrograms compared to actual contact electrograms has been confirmed in vitro and in vivo, as has the precision of the catheter navigation system.[14]

Clinical experience

Ectopic atrial tachycardia and atrial flutter

Non-contact mapping has been used to facilitate ectopic tachycardia ablation. As with the electroanatomical system, navigation to regions difficult to pinpoint fluoroscopically is facilitated, pertinent structures (such as the His bundle or

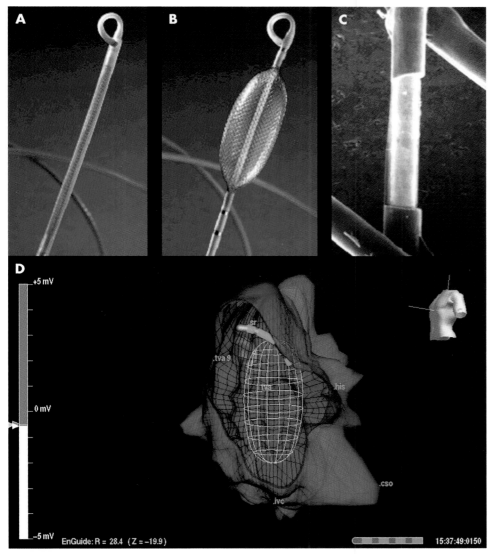

Figure 17.2 Non-contact system multiple electrode array (MEA). (A) In low profile, the MEA is advance through the vasculature to the chamber of interest. (B) After deployment in the chamber of interest, the MEA is expanded to record intracavitary potentials. (C) Photomicrograph of the MEA showing one of the 64 laser etched laser etched unipolar electrodes. (D) Right atrial map in a patient with ectopic tachycardia. Left anterior oblique view is shown. Point of earliest activation is shown (white centre of target). On computer workstation, activation "movie" depicts wavefront propagation. The position of mapping catheter relative to the atrial geometry is shown by means of the locator signal.

valve annuli) can be annotated and localised in three dimensional space, and the ablation catheter can be accurately and repeatedly renavigated to predetermined sites in the cardiac chamber. Additionally, the high density parallel data acquisition permits mapping of arrhythmias seen only transiently in the electrophysiology laboratory, even in the absence of overt abnormalities in cardiac structure to guide substrate localisation. Once the geometry is defined, the origin of multiple arrhythmias can be rapidly determined. This is particularly useful for patients with multiple atrial tachycardia present.

As noted above, typical atrial flutter is usually readily treated using standard ablation techniques. However, non-contact mapping has been used to confirm the anatomic location of the flutter circuit, to reduce fluoroscopy time, and to confirm block in the setting of electrogram degradation subsequent to ablation.[15] Non-contact mapping has also been used to identify and guide RF ablation of the site of residual conduction following incomplete linear lesion at the isthmus. Because of its ability to record from multiple sites simultaneously, the technique can rapidly identify gaps in linear lesions. This is accomplished from analysis of one or more paced complexes originating adjacent to the line being assessed. These global mapping capabilities have also facilitated ablation of atypical flutter. In a study of patients with congenital heart disease and previous Fontan procedure, non-contact mapping

improved recognition of the anatomic and surgical substrate and identified exit sites from zones of slow conduction in all clinical arrhythmias.[16]

Atrial fibrillation

As described above, the two approaches used to treat AF include ablation of focal triggers and creation of linear lesions. Early clinical experience suggests non-contact mapping may play a role in both approaches.

Pulmonary vein foci have been identified as the triggers of paroxysmal and persistent AF.[8] Because of the intermittent and transient nature of pulmonary vein discharges and rapid degeneration to atrial fibrillation, mapping for ablation has been difficult. Using its ability to globally map a single complex, non-contact mapping has been used to identify focal triggers and the bundles of myocardium connecting pulmonary vein to left atrial musculature.[17] Additionally, since up to 30% of triggering foci may emanate from non-pulmonary vein foci (so that anatomical structure cannot readily guide ablation), non-contact mapping may be particularly useful in this setting, although its role is not established. Since focal discharges often occur during the T wave of the preceding ventricular complex, isopotential map interpretation may be challenging, as ventricular repolarisation potentials must be accounted for (or filtered out) in signal interpretation.

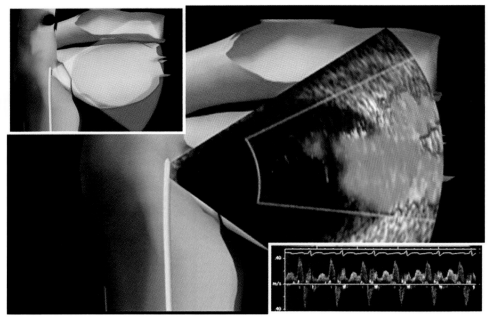

Figure 17.3 Phased array intracardiac echocardiography to image the left sided pulmonary veins with colour flow Doppler. Actual echocardiographic image is superimposed on computer model for orientation. Inset top left: computer graphic to depict ICE catheter position within the right atrium. Inset bottom right: pulse wave Doppler to quantify left superior pulmonary vein flow. This appears to be a sensitive indicator of venous stenosis during ablation. Reproduced from Darbar et al,[2] with permission.

Non-contact mapping has also been used to guide linear lesion creation for the control of atrial fibrillation.[18] The ability to confirm bidirectional block across the entire length of a long ablation line without the need to retrace the line has been very useful, and right atrial lesions have resulted in arrhythmia control with antiarrhythmic medications previously ineffective. However, as noted above, the role of transcatheter right atrial compartmentalisation remains uncertain, and left atrial compartmentalisation is limited in large measure by ablation energy delivery systems.

Ventricular tachycardia

As noted above, catheter ablation of re-entrant VT has been limited by the presence of multiple re-entry circuits, haemodynamic instability during arrhythmia, frequent changes from one VT to another, absence of reproducibly inducible VT, and the time required for sequential endocardial activation mapping.

Because of its ability to record cardiac activation from a single complex, non-contact mapping can facilitate the mapping of hemodynamically unstable rhythms. The multiple electrode array has been advanced to the left ventricle via the retrograde aortic or the transseptal approach. Ventricular tachycardia is induced and immediately terminated after geometry creation. Presystolic critical circuit components and exit sites are readily identified; these localise critical, vulnerable components of the re-entrant circuit.[19] Isolated diastolic potentials, presystolic areas, zones of slow conduction, and exit sites are also identified using virtual electrograms and isopotential maps during VT. Ablation of coronary VT not amenable to conventional ablation has been reported with success rates of approximately 75% at one year.

Non-contact mapping has also been used to guide ablation of idiopathic VT in both the right and left ventricles. Although focal and fascicular VTs are often amenable to conventional ablation approaches, when arrhythmia is non-sustained and infrequently present in the electrophysiology laboratory, conventional mapping may fail. We successfully ablated nine of 10 patients with difficult to treat right ventricular outflow tract VT, of whom seven had failed previous ablation and five had only transient arrhythmia in the electrophysiology

laboratory. After a mean follow up of nine months, 78% of patients remained arrhythmia-free. Similar results have been observed in patients with previously failed ablation of idiopathic left VT.

Non-contact mapping strengths and limitations

Non-contact mapping's high density parallel data acquisition yields high resolution maps of the entire cardiac chamber from a single beat of tachycardia, enabling registration of transient or hypotensive arrhythmias. This also facilitates localisation of gaps in long linear lesions by pacing from both sides of the gap and rapidly remapping. Other useful features include radiation-free catheter navigation, re-visitation of points of interest, and cataloging ablation points on the three dimensional model. In patients with multiple or transient arrhythmias and no overt structural cardiac disease, non-contact mapping is the preferred approach.

Since isopotential maps are predominantly used, ventricular repolarisation must be distinguished from atrial depolarisation and diastolic ventricular activity. Early diastole may be challenging to map. Virtual electrogram quality deteriorates at a distance greater than 4 cm from the MEA, which at times may require MEA repositioning to acquire adequate isopotential maps. Lastly, substrate mapping (based on scar or diseased tissue) is limited with this technology at present.

OTHER ADJUNCTIVE TOOLS TO FACILITATE ABLATION

Catheter navigation systems have been developed that use low energy radiofrequency signals or ultrasound signals to localise catheters. These systems permit identification of points of interest in three dimensional space, cataloging of ablation sites, and re-navigation to sites of interest. However, one system does not create activation or isopotential maps, and does not integrate anatomy with physiology. Compared with the more complete mapping systems described above, its main advantage is reduced cost. Little clinical experience is available for the other system because of its recent introduction.

Cardiac imaging techniques, including intracardiac echocardiography, computed tomographic scanning, and magnetic resonance imaging have been used to plan or guide ablation.

Novel mapping techniques for cardiac electrophysiology: key points

▶ Advanced mapping systems are generally not required for catheter ablation of AVNRT, accessory pathway mediated tachycardia or AV junction ablation for rate control in atrial fibrillation because of the high success rate of conventional ablation approaches

▶ Advanced mapping systems are most useful for guiding ablation in haemodynamically unstable ventricular tachycardia, postsurgical macro-reentrant atrial arrhythmias, and transient arrhythmias.

▶ Advanced mapping systems reduce the need for ionising radiation (fluoroscopy) by means of non-fluoroscopic catheter navigation

▶ Electroanatomic mapping uses ultra low level magnetic fields for catheter localisation, and permits creation of complex three dimensional substrate (bipolar voltage) maps and activation maps for sustained/stable arrhythmias. Transient arrhythmias are not mapped

▶ Non-contact mapping uses low level electric fields for catheter localisation, and permits creation of complex three dimensional activation maps from a single complex, enabling mapping of transient arrhythmias. Substrate maps are not readily generated.

Several practical uses for intracardiac echo have emerged in the setting of electrophysiology procedures (fig 17.3). These include: assessment of catheter contact with cardiac tissues; determination of radiofrequency ablation lesions (by presence of "bubbles" during energy delivery and by tissue characterisation); determination of catheter location relative to cardiac structures (specifically useful in otherwise difficult to localise areas such as pulmonary veins); guidance of transseptal puncture, particularly in the setting of complex or unusual anatomy; facilitation of deployment of mapping or ablation systems such as pulmonary vein encircling devices, non-contact mapping systems, and basket technologies; evaluation of cardiac structures before and after intervention (such as cardiac valves and pulmonary veins); assessment of pulmonary vein anatomy, dimensions, and function via two dimensional anatomic imaging and Doppler physiologic measurements; and assessment of complications (for example, tamponade, electromechanical dissociation, or thrombus formation). Despite its many potential benefits, electrophysiology procedures can be performed in the absence of intracardiac echocardiography, and the role of this imaging modality is not yet defined.

CONCLUSION

Conventional RF ablation has revolutionised the treatment of many supraventricular tachycardias and focal ventricular arrhythmias. As interest has turned to more complex arrhythmias, limitations of conventional treatment are being overcome with the introduction of sophisticated mapping systems that integrate three dimensional catheter localisation with sophisticated complex arrhythmia maps. This has added insight into mechanisms of arrhythmogenesis, and facilitated treatment of complex arrhythmias.

REFERENCES

1 **Calkins H**. Radiofrequency catheter ablation of supraventricular arrhythmias. *Heart* 2001;**85**:594–600.
▶ **Recent comprehensive review of conventional catheter ablation of supraventricular tachycardia.**
2 **Darbar D**, Olgin J, Miller J, *et al*. Localization of the origin of arrhythmias for ablation: from electrocardiography to advanced endocardial mapping systems. *J Cardiovasc Electrophysiol* 2001;**12**:1309–25.
▶ **Recent review of advanced mapping systems and intracardiac imaging.**
3 **Schalij MJ**, van Rugge FP, Siezenga M, *et al*. Endocardial activation mapping of ventricular tachycardia in patients : first application of a 32-site bipolar mapping electrode catheter. *Circulation* 1998;**98**:2168–79.
4 **Kottkamp H**, Hindricks G, Breithardt G, *et al*. Three-dimensional electromagnetic catheter technology: electroanatomical mapping of the right atrium and ablation of ectopic atrial tachycardia. *J Cardiovasc Electrophysiol* 1997;**8**:1332–7.
5 **Nakagawa H**, Shah N, Matsudaira K, *et al*. Characterization of reentrant circuit in macroreentrant right atrial tachycardia after surgical repair of congenital heart disease: isolated channels between scars allow "focal" ablation. *Circulation* 2001;**103**:699–709.
▶ **Elegant paper describing the presence of multiple narrow channels as vulnerable ablation targets in patients with congenital heart disease and previous surgery, and use of electroanatomic mapping to localise them.**
6 **Kottkamp H**, Hügl B, Krauss B, *et al*. Electromagnetic versus fluoroscopic mapping of the inferior isthmus for ablation of typical atrial flutter : a prospective randomized study. *Circulation* 2000;**102**:2082–6.
7 **Shah D**, Haissaguerre M, Jais P, *et al*. High-density mapping of activation through an incomplete isthmus ablation line. *Circulation* 1999;**99**:211–5.
8 **Haïssaguerre M**, Jaïs P, Shah DC, *et al*. Spontaneous initiation of atrial fibrillation by ectopic beats originating in the pulmonary veins. *N Engl J Med* 1998;**339**:659–66.
▶ **Seminal paper describing the focal mechanism for atrial fibrillation, and the use of focal ablation for atrial fibrillation treatment.**
9 **Pappone C**, Oreto G, Lamberti F, *et al*. Catheter ablation of paroxysmal atrial fibrillation using a 3D mapping system. *Circulation* 1999;**100**:1203–8.
10 **Ernst S**, Schluter M, Ouyang F, *et al*. Modification of the substrate for maintenance of idiopathic human atrial fibrillation: efficacy of radiofrequency ablation using nonfluoroscopic catheter guidance. *Circulation* 1999;**100**:2085–92.
11 **Pappone C**, Rosanio S, Oreto G, *et al*. Circumferential radiofrequency ablation of pulmonary vein ostia. A new anatomic approach for curing atrial fibrillation. *Circulation* 2000;**102**:2619–28.
12 **Marchlinski F**, Callans D, Gottlieb C, *et al*. Linear ablation lesions for control of unmappable ventricular tachycardia in patients with ischemic and nonischemic cardiomyopathy. *Circulation* 2000;**101**:1288–96.
▶ **First paper to describe the use of substrate mapping to treat otherwise unmappable ventricular arrhythmias using electroanatomical mapping.**
13 **Soejima K**, Suzuki M, Maisel W, *et al*. Catheter ablation in patients with multiple unstable ventricular tachycardias after myocardial infarction. Short ablation lines guided by reentry circuit isthmuses and sinus rhythm mapping. *Circulation* 2001;**104**:664–9.
14 **Gornick CC**, Adler SW, Pederson B, *et al*. Validation of a new noncontact catheter system for electroanatomic mapping of left ventricular endocardium. *Circulation* 1999;**99**:829–35.
▶ **Early article describing and validating non-contact mapping in a canine model and in vitro. System function described.**
15 **Schneider MA**, Ndrepepa G, Zrenner B, *et al*. Noncontact mapping-guided ablation of atrial flutter and enhanced-density mapping of the inferior vena cava-tricuspid annulus isthmus. *Pacing Clin Electrophysiol* 2001;**24**:1755–64.
16 **Betts T**, Roberts P, Allen S, *et al*. Electrophysiological mapping and ablation of intra-atrial reentry tachycardia after Fontan surgery with the use of a noncontact mapping system. *Circulation* 2000;**102**:2094–9.
17 **Hindricks G**, Kottkamp H. Simultaneous noncontact mapping of left atrium in patients with paroxysmal atrial fibrillation. *Circulation* 2001;**104**:297–303.
18 **Gasparini M**, Mantica M, Coltorti F, *et al*. The use of advanced mapping systems to guide right linear lesions in paroxysmal atrial fibrillation. *Eur Heart J* 2001;3(suppl P):P41–6.
19 **Schilling RJ**, Peters NS, Davies DW. Feasibility of a noncontact catheter for endocardial mapping of human ventricular tachycardia. *Circulation* 1999;**99**:2543–52.
▶ **The first article to describe the use of non-contact mapping for the endocardial mapping of human ventricular tachycardia. Validation of reconstructed electrograms and mapping of exit sites and diastolic components of circuit are described.**
20 **Gepstein L**, Hayam G, Ben-Haim SA. A novel method for nonfluoroscopic catheter-based electroanatomical mapping of the heart. In vitro and in vivo accuracy results. *Circulation* 1997;**95**:1611–22.

123

18 TREATMENT OF ATRIAL FIBRILLATION

Y Blaauw, I C Van Gelder, H J G M Crijns

Atrial fibrillation (AF) is the most common arrhythmia in clinical practice. It may cause symptoms such as palpitations, dyspnoea, fatigue, dizziness or chest discomfort. Mortality risk has been reported to be twice as high when patients are in AF compared to sinus rhythm. As the incidence increases with age and the total number of elderly patients expands, the future clinical burden will be significant.[w1]

▶ ARRHYTHMIA MECHANISMS

Mapping studies in fibrillating atria have confirmed the hypothesis of Moe and colleagues that AF is based on multiple wavelets of re-entry.[w2 w3] The stability of AF is mainly dependent on the number of wavelets that can circulate in the atria. In this respect, this explains why atrial dilatation is a risk factor for AF since the enlarged atria may accommodate more wavelets.[w4] Since the wavelength is determined by the product of refractory period and conduction velocity, a short refractory period or slow conduction facilitate the stability of AF. Interestingly, atrial refractory periods in patients with AF are shorter than in patients with sinus rhythm.[w5]

It has only recently been shown that AF itself causes shortening of the atrial refractory period. In an animal model Wijffels and colleagues demonstrated that repetitive induction of AF by atrial burst pacing led to the development of sustained AF in normal hearts. The hallmark of "AF begets AF" was a shortening of the atrial refractory period (electrical remodelling).[1] Further studies have shown that, in addition to electrical remodelling, structural and contractile remodelling also occurs.[w6 w7] These experimental observations explain why antiarrhythmic drugs (AADs) fail to terminate persistent AF[2] and why paroxysmal AF tends to become persistent or permanent.[w8]

For the induction and maintenance of AF, ectopic beats or rapid focal activity arising from the pulmonary veins play a much greater role than previously appreciated. This has opened up the therapeutic option of catheter ablation of focal AF.[3] In some patients the autonomic nervous system is involved in the genesis of paroxysmal AF. Enhanced sympathetic or parasympathetic tone may both shorten refractoriness and increase dispersion of refractoriness, and sympathetic drive is associated with atrial ectopy. Sympathetic adrenergic AF is relatively rare. It relates to stress and exercise and is frequently associated with coronary artery disease.[w9] Parasympathetic vagal AF occurs more frequently in otherwise normal patients. It predominantly starts during the night or after heavy meals.[w10]

The atrial substrate for AF frequently develops as a result of hypertension, coronary artery disease, or valvar disease, especially if these are complicated by heart failure. The patho-anatomic substrate mostly consists of fibrosis. In turn, fibrosis is associated with arrhythmogenic changes such as slowing and dispersion of conduction and an increase in heterogeneity of refractoriness.[w11] These notions comply with the fact that AF tends to start in the fifth to sixth decade in life, in particular the persistent form of AF. The continued presence of the patho-anatomic substrate explains why both paroxysmal and persistent AF recurs sooner or later in almost all patients.[w12 w13] In this respect, treatment of underlying heart disease is of major importance for long term prevention of AF.

ARRHYTHMIA MANAGEMENT: GENERAL CONSIDERATIONS

Antiarrhythmic treatment of AF can be divided in three strategies: termination of the arrhythmia in paroxysmal and persistent AF, maintenance of sinus rhythm in paroxysmal and persistent AF, and finally control of ventricular rate during paroxysmal, persistent, and permanent AF (table 18.1).

Removal of precipitating factors such as pericarditis, pulmonary embolism, thyrotoxicosis or excessive alcohol intake may result in disappearance of the arrhythmia. For this reason, a thorough diagnostic evaluation and optimal treatment of underlying heart disease should always precede considering a patient for cardioversion or maintenance treatment.

Antiarrhythmic drugs are given to suppress recurrences, but breakthrough arrhythmias may occur. Patients should be informed that a breakthrough arrhythmia does not necessarily mean drug failure. Antiarrhythmic drugs may cause ventricular proarrhythmia, conduction disturbances, and heart failure. Therefore, these patients should be informed about the symptoms associated with these AAD side effects.

Table 18.1 Classification of atrial fibrillation and therapeutic strategies

Type	Duration and character	Therapeutic strategy*
First episode	?	Conversion and prevention either with AAD or electrical cardioversion
Paroxysmal	< 48 hours, mostly spontaneous conversion (self terminating)	Conversion and prevention with VW class IC or III antiarrhythmic drugs. Rate control during arrhythmia
Persistent	>2–7 days, usually requires electrical cardioversion to restore sinus rhythm (non-self terminating)	Electrical cardioversion with/without antiarrhythmic drugs
Permanent	Restoration of sinus rhythm not feasible	Ventricular rate control

*Oral anticoagulation or aspirin as needed on the basis of risk factors (table 18.3) or in case of cardioversion.
AAD, antiarrhythmic drugs; VW, Vaughan Williams

Table 18.2 Clinical conditions and contraindicated antiarrhythmic drug treatment

► Heart failure (VW class I and III*)
► Coronary artery disease (VW class I)
► Left ventricular hypertrophy (VW class III*)
► Long QT interval (VW class I and III)
► Atrial fibrillation and WPW syndrome (verapamil/digoxin)

*Amiodarone is not contraindicated in heart failure and left ventricular hypertrophy.
VW, Vaughan Williams; WPW, Wolf Parkinson White.

In patients considered for AAD treatment pro-arrhythmia risk factors should be evaluated (table 18.2). If heart failure or angina pectoris develops, AADs may become contraindicated and therefore patients put on these agents should be followed regularly.

PHARMACOLOGIC AND ELECTRICAL CARDIOVERSION

Cardioversion of AF should be performed for the following reasons: relief of patient discomfort, prevention of thromboembolic events, and prevention of tachycardiomyopathy. In general, if AF lasts < 48 hours, AADs are highly effective and pericardioversion anticoagulation treatment is not needed. On the other hand, if AF duration is more than 48 hours the likelihood of pharmacological conversion decreases.[w14 w15] In these patients, direct current (DC) cardioversion after adequate anticoaguation treatment is preferred (fig 18.1). Anticoagulation treatment strategies will be discussed below.

Pharmacological conversion

Before considering AAD treatment one should bear in mind that up to 60% of patients with paroxysmal AF spontaneously cardiovert to sinus rhythm within 24 hours. Pharmacological cardioversion is considered in symptomatic patients who are haemodynamically stable. In unstable patients pharmacological cardioversion should be avoided for drug side effects. Electrical cardioversion may be useful but in any case rate controlling drugs should be given. For this purpose amiodarone is useful since it may serve two goals: rate control and cardioversion.

Basically, all AADs can convert short lasting AF to sinus rhythm. However, efficacy differs and the most successful agents are flecainide and propafenone.[w14 w16] Therefore, class IC AADs are first choice for pharmacological cardioversion of AF. However, owing to their negative inotropic effects, these agents should be avoided in patients with compromised ventricular function. In these patients amiodarone can be useful,

although time to conversion is relatively long.[w17 w18] Ibutilide[4] is moderately effective but associated with a significant risk of torsade des pointes. Sotalol is rather ineffective but may reduce heart rate when adopting a wait-and-see approach. These class III agents tend to be much more effective in atrial flutter.[w19 w20] Digitalis, β blockers, and non-dihydropyridine calcium channel antagonists are ineffective for conversion of AF.[w21 w22]

Long term amiodarone pretreatment converts 15–40% of patients to sinus rhythm.[w17 w23]

External and internal DC cardioversion

Since the description of direct current electrical cardioversion of AF by Lown in 1962, this procedure has been widely used for restoration of sinus rhythm.[5] External cardioversion may be applied in the anterolateral or anteroposterior position and is successful in up to 90% of cases. Outcome depends on a carefully performed procedure using firm pressure on appropriately placed paddles and a sufficient amount of energy. Biphasic shocks are more effective than conventional monophasic shocks.[w24] To enhance shock efficacy, pretreatment with ibutilide may be applied.[6] As a last resort, patients with persistent AF unresponsive to external cardioversion may undergo internal catheter cardioversion.[w25]

MAINTENANCE OF SINUS RHYTHM

AF recurs in most patients, despite prophylactic antiarrhythmic treatment, and multiple pharmacological or electrical conversions are needed to maintain sinus rhythm. Risk factors for recurrence of paroxysmal AF include a history of frequent attacks, female sex, and the presence of associated cardiovascular disease.[w12] In patients with persistent AF most recurrences happen in the early post-cardioversion period. The following factors predict an unsuccessful arrhythmia outcome in persistent AF patients cardioverted to sinus rhythm: previous arrhythmia duration (> 1–3 years), age (> 60–65 years), atrial size (> 55 mm on echocardiogram), and rheumatic heart disease.[w13]

It has been questioned whether "rhythm control" is the preferred strategy for the treatment of AF. A recent study (PIAF—pharmacological pacing in atrial fibrillation)[7] showed that rate and rhythm control yielded similar clinical results with respect to symptoms, but exercise tolerance was better with rhythm control. Other studies are ongoing in Canada and the USA (AFFIRM— atrial fibrillation follow-up investigation of rhythm management)[w26] and the Netherlands (RACE—rate control versus electrical cardioversion for persistent AF).[w27]

Antiarrhythmic drugs for maintenance of sinus rhythm

A treatment strategy for the maintenance of sinus rhythm is shown in fig 18.2.

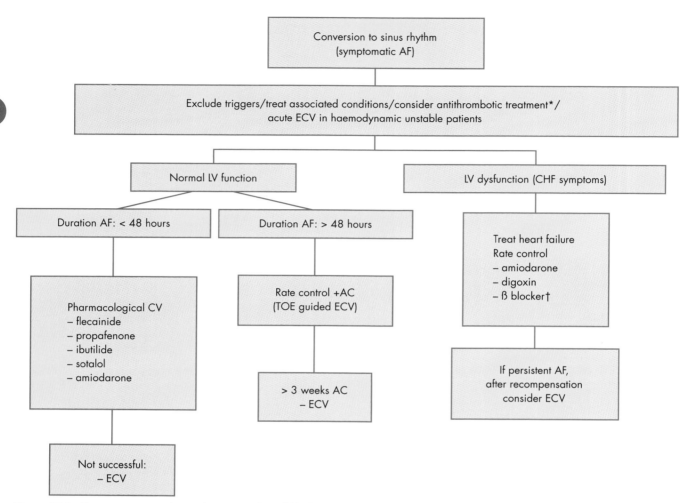

Figure 18.1 Treatment strategy for cardioversion of atrial fibrillation. *See table 18.3. †β Blockade including sotalol should be applied with caution in patients with left ventricular dysfunction to avoid aggravation of heart failure. AC, anticoagulation; AF, atrial fibrillation; CHF, congestive heart failure; ECV, electrical cardioversion; LV, left ventricular; TOE, transoesophageal echocardiogram.

Quinidine has been used most frequently for prevention of recurrences of AF. A meta-analysis showed increased mortality on quinidine compared to control.[8] Most drugs, including flecainide,[w28] propafenone,[w29] or sotalol[8] are equally effective and usually well tolerated. In a recent study, metoprolol appeared moderately effective and in patients with a recurrence, ventricular rate was better controlled by metoprolol than placebo.[w30] Of all available drugs, amiodarone is probably the most effective. In the CTAF (Canadian trial of atrial fibrillation) study patients assigned to amiodarone had a higher maintenance of sinus rhythm than those using sotalol or propafenone (fig 18.3). Adverse events occurred in 18% and 11% of patients using amiodarone and sotalol or propafenone, respectively. Unfortunately, the design of the study could not address the potential side effects associated with long term use of amiodarone.[9] Thus, it may well be that a higher breakthrough attack rate with fewer side effects is preferred above a low attack rate but at the cost of severe amiodarone side effects. This holds true even more since side effects of amiodarone cannot be predicted. Therefore in many patients amiodarone will remain second or last choice.

Recent evidence suggests that verapamil enhances efficacy of prophylactic AAD treatment in patients undergoing electrical cardioversion.[w31] Episodes of AF associated with high vagal activity are usually suppressed by disopyramide or flecainide, but worsened by digoxin or β blockers. Conversely, adrenergic AF should be treated with β blockers.[w10] In sick sinus syndrome, AADs should be avoided unless a pacemaker has been implanted. A pacemaker may even help to reduce the attack rate in these patients.

AF in the setting of chronic heart failure is difficult to treat and most agents are contraindicated under those circumstances. In a subgroup analysis of data from CHF-STAT (congestive heart failure survival trial of antiarrhythmic therapy), amiodarone reduced the incidence of AF over four years from 8% to 4%. Conversion to sinus rhythm occurred in 31% of 51 AF patients on amiodarone versus only 8% on placebo and this was associated with significantly better survival.[10] Similarly, dofetilide, initiated in hospital, was associated with a lower incidence of AF (1.9%, 11 of 556 patients) than placebo (6.6%, 35 of 534 patients) after an average of 18 months. On dofetilide, 25 cases of torsade-de-pointes occurred (three quarters of which occurred within three days after starting treatment). Mortality was equal in both groups (41% and 42%), but dofetilide was associated with a significantly reduced hospital readmission rate for heart failure.[11]

NON-PHARMACOLOGICAL MANAGEMENT OF AF
Surgical treatment

The Maze procedure, introduced in 1987 by Cox, preserves atrial contractility and is the most frequently used of all surgical techniques.[12] The rationale for the Maze procedure is that strategically placed surgical incisions interrupt potential multiple wavelet re-entry circuits, thereby preventing or terminating AF. The latest modification, the Maze III, consists of

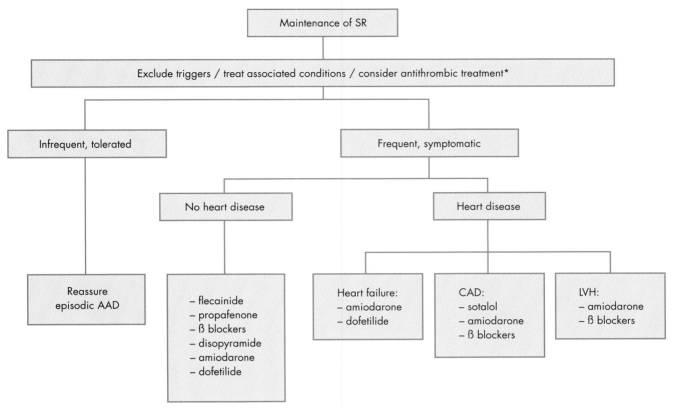

Figure 18.2 Treatment strategy for maintenance of sinus rhythm (SR). *See table 18.3. AAD, antiarrhythmic drugs; CAD, coronary artery disease; LVH, left ventricular hypertrophy.

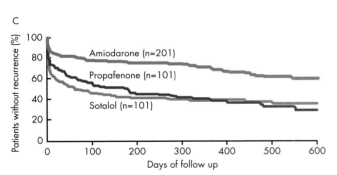

Figure 18.3 Kaplan-Meier curves showing percentage of patients without recurrence of atrial fibrillation who were treated with either amiodarone, propafenone, or sotalol. Reproduced from Roy *et al*,[9] with permission of the Massachusetts Medical Society.

removal of both atrial appendages, isolation of the pulmonary veins, and multiple incisions in both atria. During a 10 year follow up period, Cox and colleagues reported very favourable results in 201 patients[w32] which was confirmed by others.[w33]

New modifications—for example, using radiofrequency catheter ablation techniques—are being evaluated and may contribute to a wider acceptance of this type of treatment of AF.[w34]

In patients with symptomatic AF, who are to undergo surgical correction for coronary artery disease or valvar heart disease, a concomitant Maze should be considered. There are, however, only limited data to support its application and the prolonged procedure time adds to the operative risk.

Radiofrequency catheter ablation of focal AF
Haissaguerre and colleagues described a group of 49 patients with drug refractory AF in whom an ectopic atrial focus or foci

could be identified during a diagnostic electrophysiological study (fig 18.4).[3] Foci were predominantly located within the pulmonary veins. Application of radiofrequency energy to these foci abolished atrial ectopic activity. After a mean (SD) of 8 (6) months of follow up, 62% of patients had no further attacks of AF and all patients use of antiarrhythmic drugs was discontinued.

Ideal candidates for focal AF ablation are young patients with frequent paroxysms of AF initiated by rapid monomorphic atrial tachycardias. Long term complications include pulmonary vein stenosis, pericardial effusion, and cardiac tamponade.[w35] Other techniques like pulmonary vein exclusion and linear ablation are still investigational.[w36]

Pacing strategies to prevent or terminate AF
In several clinical situations atrial pacing has been shown to prevent the development of AF. In patients with sick sinus node disease, AAI pacing proved to be superior to VVI pacing in reducing the incidence of AF.[13 w37] Recent studies also suggest that continuous atrial pacing, especially in combination with β blockers, may prevent postoperative AF. Uncertainty exists about the optimal site and mode (single/multisite) of pacing.[w38 w39] Furthermore, it is not clear whether pacing strategies to prevent AF will also result in a subsequent reduction in thromboembolic events. Atrial pacing for prevention of AF is still an experimental treatment and the results of ongoing trials will determine its clinical value.

Pacing may also be used to terminate AF. Some dual chamber pacemakers are equipped with atrial tachycardia/fibrillation detection and termination algorithms. Results so far demonstrate a reduction in arrhythmia burden in treated patients.[w40 w41] Interestingly, the stored electrograms of AF initiation revealed a relatively high incidence of organised atrial tachycardias. Antitachycardia pacing was most successful in

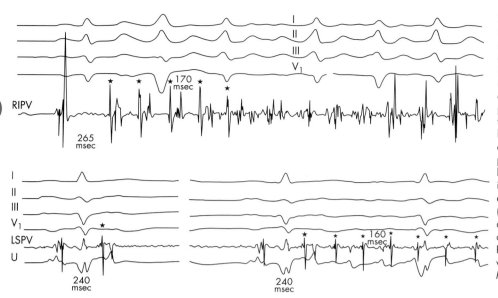

Figure 18.4 Two examples of the onset of atrial fibrillation from foci in a right inferior pulmonary vein (RIVP) and a left superior pulmonary vein (LSVP). In the upper panel, sinus rhythm is followed by a burst of five ectopic beats from the right inferior pulmonary vein, with coarse atrial fibrillation on the surface ECG. In the lower panel, two tracings with ectopic activity from the left superior pulmonary vein are shown. On the left an ectopic beat with a coupling interval of 240 ms does not induce atrial fibrillation. In the same patient (on the right), a train of spike discharges (asterisk) at a cycle length of 160 ms initiates atrial fibrillation. Reproduced from Haissaguerre et al,[3] with permission of the Massachusetts Medical Society.

these types of AF.[w41] In patients with a history of AF and an indication for permanent pacing or implantable cardioverter-defibrillator (ICD) treatment, an antitachycardia pacemaker or a dual chamber ICD with antitachycardia pacing capabilities may be considered, respectively. Optimisation of patient selection criteria (for example, based on initiation pattern) may improve the efficacy.

Atrial implanted cardiac defibrillator

Wellens and colleagues reported the initial experience with the atrial ICD or atrioverter in 51 patients with recurrent episodes of AF who had not responded to antiarrhythmic drugs.[14] During a mean follow up period of 259 (138) days, 96% of 227 episodes of AF were cardioverted successfully. No ventricular pro-arrhythmia events occurred.

The ICD can detect and treat AF early after initiation, which may improve long term arrhythmia outcome. However, important disadvantages exist. First of all, AF is not prevented. Furthermore, the shock is rather painful. Finally, at present, no stand alone atrial ICD is available. Combined atrial and ventricular ICDs are, however, available and may be useful in selected patients, especially in those who need a ventricular ICD and suffer from infrequent but poorly tolerated attacks of AF.

CONTROL OF VENTRICULAR RATE

Control of ventricular rate aims at reducing signs of circulatory insufficiency and prevention of tachycardiomyopathy.[15] This can be achieved by negative chronotropic drugs or atrioventricular node ablation and insertion of a pacemaker. Although the targeted heart rate is unclear, it is reasonable to aim at heart rates under 90 beats/min in resting conditions and below 110 beats/min during light and moderate exercise. Perhaps more importantly, adequate rate control during daily exercise should be assessed using 24 hour Holter recordings.

Most commonly used agents are calcium channel antagonists, β blocking drugs, and digoxin. Historically, digoxin has been the drug of choice. Amiodarone should be avoided for its significant side effects. Surprisingly, only a limited number of studies evaluated the efficacy of these agents. Farshi and colleagues included 12 patients with AF duration of at least one year duration who were randomly assigned to digoxin (0.25 mg), diltiazem (240 mg), atenolol (50 mg), digoxin + diltiazem (0.25 mg + 240 mg), and digoxin + atenolol (0.25 mg + 50 mg). Ventricular rate control was evaluated with 24 hour Holter recordings and exercise testing. Combination therapy of digoxin and atenolol was superior to all other regimens during exercise as well as during daily activities. Digoxin as a single agent proved less effective, especially during exercise testing.[16] Nevertheless digoxin usually suffices if needed at all in the sedentary elderly. In active patients excessive reduction of exercise heart rate is not desirable since it limits exercise capacity. In these patients β blockade with or without digoxin is usually sufficient to control resting heart rate while preserving a reasonable response during daytime exercises. In patients with an accessory atrioventricular pathway (Wolf-Parkinson-White syndrome) paroxysmal AF may be associated with an excessively high heart rate. Use of digoxin, verapamil or a β blocker as rate controlling drugs should be avoided. Intravenous flecainide will reduce heart rate and may provide conversion. In the haemodynamically unstable patient immediate cardioversion is indicated.

Ablate and pace

Patients who remain symptomatic despite adequate negative chronotropic drugs, or those who cannot tolerate these drugs, may undergo atrioventricular node ablation with pacemaker insertion.[15 w42] Prospective data have shown an increase in left ventricular function after atrioventricular node ablation, especially in patients with significant baseline ventricular impairment.[w43 w44] This was parallelled by increased exercise duration, higher quality of life, and reduced health care use.[w45 w46] If AF is paroxysmal DDD(R) pacing mode with mode switch is indicated; in permanent AF a VVI(R) pacemaker suffices.

ANTICOAGULATION IN AF

Long standing non-rheumatic AF is associated with a 5.6 fold increase in risk of thromboembolic complications.[w47] Several predisposing factors for stroke have been identified from pooled data sets: rheumatic heart disease, hypertension, prior strokes or transient ischaemic attacks, diabetes mellitus, recent heart failure, enlarged left atrium, impaired left ventricular function or age > 65 years.[w48 w49] Large trials have been conducted and have convincingly demonstrated the benefit of adequate anticoagulation (international normalised ratio 2–3) in terms of reducing the risk of ischaemic stroke.[w50–57] The above mentioned risk factors should be taken into account irrespective of the rhythm itself (sinus rhythm or

Table 18.3 Antithrombotic treatment in patients with atrial fibrillation

Oral anticoagulation (optimal INR 2–3):
► Rheumatic heart disease (mitral stenosis)
► Prosthetic heart valve
► High risk patients:
   –history of CVA or TIA
   –hypertension
   –diabetes mellitus
   –heart failure
   –age >65 years
   –echocardiogram: LV dysfunction, HCM
   –thyrotoxicosis

Aspirin (75–325 mg/daily):
► "Lone" atrial fibrillation
► No risk factors
► Age <65 years
Contraindication for oral anticoagulation

CVA, cerebrovascular accident; HCM, hypertrophic cardiomyopathy; INR, international normalised ratio; LV, left ventricular; TIA, transient ischemic attack.

AF) and the type of AF (paroxysmal versus persistent versus permanent) (table 18.3).

In both electrical and pharmacological cardioversion the risk of thromboembolic complications surrounding the cardioversion ranges from 1–5.3%.[w58] Therefore, it is now generally accepted that in patients with AF lasting 48 hours or more, adequate anticoagulation should be maintained at least three weeks before and four weeks after cardioversion. Pretreatment before the shock may be avoided after exclusion of intra-atrial thrombi using transoesophageal echocardiography.[17] Post-cardioversion continuation of anticoagulation is necessary since transient mechanical dysfunction of the atria is believed to predispose to the formation of intra-atrial thrombi.

SUMMARY AND PERSPECTIVES

AF often results from underlying heart disease. When AF occurs, electrophysiological, structural, and contractile remodelling promotes its maintenance. Therefore, when treating AF, underlying heart disease should be managed first. Termination of AF can be achieved by using pharmacological or electrical cardioversion. To suppress arrhythmia recurrences or occurrences antiarrhythmic drugs remain the first choice of treatment. New treatment strategies including radiofrequency catheter ablation, surgical techniques, and atrial pacing are of potential value for the treatment of AF. Despite these novel advances AF persists or recurs frequently. Large trials are being conducted to answer the question whether "rhythm" or "rate" control is the optimal treatment for AF. The results of these trials will have important implications for the treatment of AF.

ACKNOWLEDGMENTS

Y Blaauw is supported by grant 920–03–122 from the Netherlands Organisation for Scientific Research.

REFERENCES

1 **Wijffels MC**, Kirchhof CJ, Dorland R, *et al.* Atrial fibrillation begets atrial fibrillation. A study in awake chronically instrumented goats. *Circulation* 1995;**92**:1954–68.
► This elegant experimental study introduced the concept that AF "itself" causes remodelling of the atria, thereby facilitating the maintenance of AF.
2 **Crijns HJ**, van Wijk LM, van Gilst WH, *et al.* Acute conversion of atrial fibrillation to sinus rhythm: clinical efficacy of flecainide acetate. Comparison of two regimens. *Eur Heart J* 1988;**9**:634–8.

► Cardioversion efficacy of flecainide was evaluated in patients with acute (< 24 hours) and chronic (> 24 hours) AF. None of the patients with chronic AF converted compared to 75% of patients with acute AF.
3 **Haissaguerre M**, Jais P, Shah DC, *et al.* Spontaneous initiation of atrial fibrillation by ectopic beats originating in the pulmonary veins. *N Engl J Med* 1998;**339**:659–66.
4 **Stambler BS**, Wood MA, Ellenbogen KA, *et al.* Efficacy and safety of repeated intravenous doses of ibutilide for rapid conversion of atrial flutter or fibrillation. Ibutilide repeat dose study investigators. *Circulation* 1996;**94**:1613–21.
► The cardioversion efficacy of ibutilide was compared to placebo in patients with atrial flutter and AF. Conversion rate was 47% for ibutilide compared to 2% for placebo. Efficacy was higher in patients with atrial flutter than AF (63% v 31%).
5 **Lown B.** Electrical reversion of cardiac arrhythmias. *Br Heart J* 1962;**29**:469–89.
6 **Oral H**, Souza JJ, Michaud GF, *et al.* Facilitating transthoracic cardioversion of atrial fibrillation with ibutilide pretreatment. *N Engl J Med* 1999;**340**:1849–54.
► Patients undergoing electrical cardioversion were randomised to pretreatment with or without ibutilide. All patients on ibutilide could be cardioverted compared to 72% of patients not treated with ibutilide. In all patients with a failed cardioversion AF could be successfully terminated after pretreatment with ibutilide.
7 **Hohnloser SH**, Kuck KH, Lilienthal J. Rhythm or rate control in atrial fibrillation – pharmacological intervention in atrial fibrillation (PIAF): a randomised trial. *Lancet* 2000;**356**:1789–94.
► First study published investigating whether patients with AF should be treated with rate or rhythm control.
8 **Coplen SE**, Antman EM, Berlin JA, *et al.* Efficacy and safety of quinidine therapy for maintenance of sinus rhythm after cardioversion. A meta-analysis of randomized control trials. *Circulation* 1990;**82**:1106–16.
► In this meta-analysis quinidine was more effective than placebo in maintaining sinus rhythm after cardioversion. Quinidine was associated with an increased mortality.
9 **Roy D**, Talajic M, Dorian P, *et al.* Amiodarone to prevent recurrence of atrial fibrillation. Canadian trial of atrial fibrillation investigators. *N Engl J Med* 2000;**342**:913–20.
► This large prospective trial demonstrated superiority of low dose amiodarone over propafenone or sotalol in preventing recurrences of AF. Discontinuation caused by side effects occurred in 18% of patients treated with amiodarone versus 12% of patients assigned to sotalol or propafenone.
10 **Deedwania PC**, Singh BN, Ellenbogen K, *et al.* Spontaneous conversion and maintenance of sinus rhythm by amiodarone in patients with heart failure and atrial fibrillation: observations from the Veterans Affairs congestive heart failure survival trial of antiarrhythmic therapy (CHF-STAT). The Department of Veterans Affairs CHF-STAT investigators. *Circulation* 1998;**98**:2574–9.
11 **Torp-Pedersen C**, Moller M, Bloch-Thomsen PE, *et al.* Dofetilide in patients with congestive heart failure and left ventricular dysfunction. Danish Investigations of arrhythmia and mortality on dofetilide study group. *N Engl J Med* 1999;**341**:857–65.
12 **Cox JL**, Schuessler RB, D'Agostino HJ, Jr, *et al.* The surgical treatment of atrial fibrillation. III. Development of a definitive surgical procedure. *J Thorac Cardiovasc Surg* 1991;**101**:569–83.
► Description of the surgical Maze procedure. Since the publication of this paper the procedure underwent several modifications. The authors have regularly published the follow up results of patients who underwent the procedure.
13 **Andersen HR**, Nielsen JC, Thomsen PE, *et al.* Long-term follow-up of patients from a randomised trial of atrial versus ventricular pacing for sick-sinus syndrome. *Lancet* 1997;**350**:1210–6.
14 **Wellens HJ**, Lau CP, Luderitz B, *et al.* Atrioverter: an implantable device for the treatment of atrial fibrillation. *Circulation* 1998;**98**:1651–6.
► This prospective multicentre study describes the first experience with the atrial defibrillator.
15 **Gallagher JJ**, Svenson RH, Kasell JH, *et al.* Catheter technique for closed-chest ablation of the atrioventricular conduction system. *N Engl J Med* 1982;**306**:194–200.
16 **Farshi R**, Kistner D, Sarma JS, *et al.* Ventricular rate control in chronic atrial fibrillation during daily activity and programmed exercise: a crossover open-label study of five drug regimens. *J Am Coll Cardiol* 1999;**33**:304–10.
17 **Klein AL**, Grimm RA, Murray RD, *et al.* Use of transesophageal echocardiography to guide cardioversion in patients with atrial fibrillation. *N Engl J Med* 2001;**344**:1411–20.
► This study evaluated the safety of transoesophageal echocardiography guided cardioversion in patients with atrial fibrillation (duration > 48 hours). Compared to patients who underwent conventional anticoagulation before cardioversion no difference in thromboembolic events were noted. However, patients who underwent echocardiography guided cardioversion showed a reduced incidence in haemorrhagic events.

Additional references appear on the *Heart* website– www.heartjnl.com

129

19 PATIENTS WITH VENTRICULAR ARRHYTHMIAS: WHO SHOULD BE REFERRED TO AN ELECTROPHYSIOLOGIST?

John M Morgan

Ventricular arrhythmia management can present a difficult clinical challenge. A proportion of the presenting population will be at high risk of sudden cardiac death (SCD). Little or no protection against SCD is afforded by simple prescription of drug treatment.[1] [2] Antiarrhythmic drugs may be proarrhythmic and prescribed without secure understanding of drug effect. Though many ventricular arrhythmias are dangerous, the spectrum of risk ranges from the immediately life threatening to very benign (for example, from ventricular fibrillation through to true right ventricular outflow tract tachycardia). Generating the range of ventricular arrhythmias are diverse disease processes and understanding of the relation between witnessed arrhythmia and underlying disease process is often incomplete. There is debate over whether right ventricular outflow tract tachycardia overlaps with right ventricular cardiomyopathy—the one being a "benign" arrhythmia whose disease process is not understood, the other being a disease process whose principal manifestation is "malignant" arrhythmia.[3] [4]

A parallel management challenge to ventricular arrhythmia control is the prevention of SCD in patients with no previous symptomatic ventricular arrhythmia but who are at high risk. SCD may have non-arrhythmia causes, but evidence strongly suggests that many or even most patients suffering or rescued from SCD have ventricular arrhythmia as the index event.[5] Depending on the clinical scenario, the approach to the management of the phenomenon of SCD includes risk stratification, family screening, genetic analysis, and prophylactic therapeutic strategies in addition to the management of an SCD survivor (fig 19.1).

The electrophysiology specialist has the choice of sophisticated device therapies or interventional ablation techniques, and their combination, for the management of symptomatic ventricular arrhythmias and SCD risk. However, the optimal way to deliver ventricular arrhythmia and SCD management strategies to appropriate patient populations is debatable. There is a tension between the need to make treatments available to appropriate populations, by delegation of clinical services to general cardiologists who express subspecialty interest, and the need to ensure that patients are offered optimal clinical care, which often can only be provided by experts in the field.

Most patients with or at risk of ventricular arrhythmias will benefit from specialist electrophysiological assessment. Generally, SCD prophylaxis, management of SCD syndromes, and management of patients in whom symptomatic ventricular arrhythmias carry a significant burden of morbidity with or without SCD risk is best provided by shared care rather than in electrophysiological exclusivity. Table 19.1 lists those patients who do not require referral to an electrophysiologist, and those who do.

▶ MANAGEMENT OF SUDDEN CARDIAC DEATH RISK

SCD risk may be generated by the presence of a primary disorder of cardiac electrical activity in the absence of any "structural" heart disease (considered here as SCD syndromes), or may be secondary to a cardiac disease process (most often myocardial in origin), which by its legacy of myocardial scarring and dysfunction creates the electrical substrate for sudden lethal arrhythmia, without premonitory symptoms. The evidence base shows that the most effective treatment for SCD prevention is to fit an implantable cardioverter-defibrillator (ICD),[6–8] but the cost, morbidity, and mortality of this must be weighed against SCD risk in an otherwise (arrhythmia) asymptomatic population.

LEFT VENTRICULAR IMPAIRMENT AS A MARKER FOR SCD RISK
The majority of patients at risk of unexpected SCD are those with left ventricular impairment as a consequence of coronary heart disease, a lesser proportion having ventricular impairment as part of another myopathic process. The SCD syndromes are discussed separately. The MADIT (multicenter defibrillator implantation trial) study[6] first offered evidence that primary prophylactic ICD implantation may reduce SCD risk in a high risk population. The complexity of that study design reflected then current electrophysiological practices and focused on antiarrhythmic drug regimens as alternate solutions. Over the past decade there has been a move towards device based

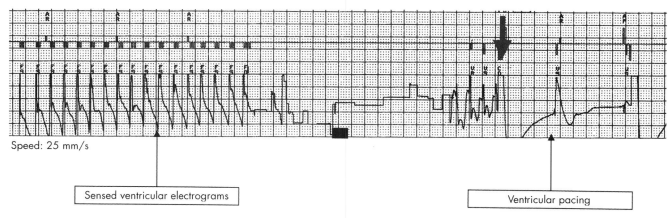

Speed: 25 mm/s

Sensed ventricular electrograms

Ventricular pacing

Figure 19.1 An example of delivery of implantable cardioverter-defibrillator (ICD) shock therapy. The device senses ventricular electrograms. This sensed electrical activity satisfies the criteria of the device's detection algorithm and a 34 J shock is delivered (thick arrow). This returns the patient to (initially) a ventricular paced rhythm with normal sinus rhythm following shortly.

Table 19.1 Ventricular arrhythmias: who to refer and who not to refer to an electrophysiologist

Do not refer:	Do refer:
▶ Patients with mildly symptomatic or asymptomatic ventricular ectopic activity	▶ Patients with highly symptomatic ventricular ectopic activity
▶ Asymptomatic patients with "benign" ventricular tachycardia on or off antiarrhythmic drug treatment	▶ Symptomatic patients with "benign" ventricular tachycardia or controlled only with unacceptable side effects from antiarrhythmic drugs
▶ Patients who are candidates for prophylactic ICD implantation but without symptomatic arrhythmia	▶ Patients who are candidates for prophylactic ICD implantation but with symptomatic arrhythmia
	▶ Any patient with symptomatic ventricular tachycardia with or without prophylactic ICD indication
	▶ Any patient suspected of having a "sudden cardiac death syndrome"
	▶ Any patient in whom arrhythmia mechanism is uncertain

ICD, implantable cardioverter-defibrillator.

---

therapy. Novel antiarrhythmic agents have been long in development, amiodarone continues to offer an unenviable side effect profile and uncertain efficacy, while the newest class III drugs have at best shown neutrality of effect in SCD risk populations.[1][2] The MADIT 2 study[8] recently concluded and demonstrated effective reduction in SCD risk when patients received ICD therapy predicated on left ventricular dysfunction assessment alone.

If the trend to identification of SCD risk based on substrate identification rather than characterisation continues, given the increasing clinical simplicity of ICD implantation technique, it would seem desirable that the therapy diffuses to the recipient population through the general cardiological community. The increased ease of delivery of ICD therapy may enable device implantation to be performed in district general hospitals by cardiologists with training in implant techniques. However, the potential complexity of ICD therapy should not be underestimated. An understanding of the physical principles governing effective ICD therapy is important. Overlap indications for therapy with resynchronisation in devices may make system implantation and overall treatment delivery more complicated again. As many as one fifth of patients who are candidates for prophylactic ICD implantation may benefit from resynchronisation therapy also.[8] Ultimately, well trained physicians and technicians, whose clinical skills are main-

tained and refined by large volume clinical practice, optimally deliver device therapy.

SUDDEN CARDIAC DEATH SYNDROMES

Genetically determined abnormalities of cardiac cell membrane ion transport result in disturbance of myocardial repolarisation or activation. This allows triggering of polymorphic ventricular tachycardia or ventricular fibrillation in the absence of structural damage to ventricular myocardium. Syncope or SCD may follow. The description of clinical signs and symptoms preceded the understanding of the relevant arrhythmia mechanisms and for the time being they continue to be classified by syndrome name rather than by mechanism.

Long QT syndromes

Long QT syndromes comprise a genetically and phenotypically heterogeneous series of abnormal repolarisation syndromes caused by altered potassium and sodium ion transport mechanisms. Multiple gene abnormalities[9][10] with many polymorphisms of those genes have been identified, making simplistic genetic analysis in any individual difficult. However, it is already established that there is a correlation between specific gene defects and SCD risk. A consistent clinical feature in many sufferers is surface ECG QT interval prolongation, from which the syndrome derives its name. A characteristic type of

131

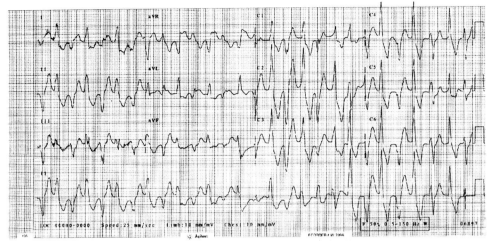

Figure 19.2 An example of the rare arrhythmia termed "catecholamine sensitive polymorphic ventricular tachycardia". This was recorded from a 19 year old white female presenting with syncope and palpitation. Note the alternating QRS morphology said to be a hallmark of the condition.

polymorphic ventricular tachycardia (torsades de pointe) can be generated. There are associations between specific genetic mutations (if identifiable) and risk of SCD.[9] For risk stratification, young age at symptomatic presentation, family history of SCD, and history of cardiac arrest are variably powerful markers of SCD risk but interpretation of ambulatory monitoring, exercise stress testing, and T wave alternans are unproven. There are no currently available electrical provocation tests to aid assessment. β Blockade, other antiarrhythmic drugs, atrial pacing, and ICD implantation may all be indicated.

Brugada syndrome
Patients with Brugada syndrome are predominantly male and in the third to fourth decades of life. Symptomatic presentation is with syncope or cardiac arrest in the absence of structural heart disease. In its most typical form the sufferer's ECG shows a characteristic pattern comprising a right bundle branch-like ECG configuration with ST segment elevation in leads V1 to V3.[11][12] Changes in autonomic tone or intravenous administration of sodium channel blocking drugs (ajmaline, flecainide, procainamide) can unmask ECG features. There is evidence that transmyocardial differential in action potential characteristics, particularly in the right ventricular free wall epicardium, facilitates re-entry during phase 2 of the action potential, resulting in closely coupled cycles of ventricular activation which then precipitate ventricular fibrillation. Death occurs as a result of rapid polymorphic ventricular tachycardia, often initiated during rest or sleep rather than after symptomatic ventricular tachycardia. However, exhibition of these ECG changes may be variable both between and within individuals with time so that intermittent and concealed forms (in terms of ECG manifestation) make diagnosis difficult. There are insufficient data to base risk stratification on ECG analysis or family history. Screening of relatives of index cases should be performed, but there is no agreed approach to management of asymptomatic patients, the only therapy available being ICD implantation. Screening should consist of ECG recording with and without pharmacological challenge with a sodium channel blocker. Investigation of the role of programmed electrical stimulation has suggested that inducibility of ventricular fibrillation is a marker for SCD risk,[13] but the data supporting this observation are insufficient to allow a definitive conclusion.

Polymorphic catecholaminergic ventricular tachycardia
Polymorphic catecholaminergic ventricular tachycardia (fig 19.2) is a rare condition characterised by a bidirectional

pattern of polymorphic ventricular tachycardia.[14] It seems likely that the arrhythmia mechanism is adrenergically mediated and related to intracellular calcium overload. There is no evidence that programmed extrastimulation or non-invasive assessments can guide risk stratification, and the roles of both β blocker treatment and ICD implantation must be decided upon individual assessments of history severity and family history of SCD.

Primary ventricular fibrillation
Survivors of cardiac arrest caused by documented ventricular fibrillation may be found to have no underlying structural heart disease or any of the identifiable primary electrical disorders discussed above.[10][15] In some the ECG is consistently normal, while in others there may be non-specific abnormalities of repolarisation. It is likely that such patients have a forme fruste of the above conditions, but management must be on an individualised basis taking into account clinical and family history.

Summary of genetically determined sudden cardiac death syndrome
Understanding of these conditions is insufficient for algorithm guided management but it is evolving rapidly. Electrophysiologists are likely to be best placed to coordinate a multidisciplinary approach to optimal management of this vulnerable patient group, offer interventions when appropriate in the light of the evolving evidence base, screen relatives, and contribute to national and international databasing and research.

CONTROL OF SYMPTOMATIC ARRHYTHMIA AND MANAGEMENT OF SUDDEN CARDIAC DEATH RISK
Any cardiac disease which has interposition of fibrotic tissue and derangement or destruction of the specialised cardiac conduction system, as part of its effect on disorganisation of ventricular myocardium, has the potential to create the substrate for arrhythmogenesis. While life threatening arrhythmias may occur without premonition, many patients will present with palpitation and haemodynamic compromise and/or syncope. Such circumstances require the use of device or ablation therapies to control symptomatic occurrence as well as protect against SCD risk.

ICD therapy is established as standard of care for secondary prevention of SCD and symptomatic management in patients presenting with ventricular tachycardia or fibrillation.[16][17] It is debatable whether all such patients need to be assessed by an expert electrophysiologist. Shared care with an expert in the field may ensure exposure to ablation therapies and optimal device programming. The weight of patient responsibility may fall more towards the electrophysiologist if cardiac arrhythmia becomes the principal cause of morbidity.

Myocardial scarring secondary to coronary artery disease

The risk of ventricular arrhythmia both near and distant to myocardial infarction is well established. Myocardial re-entry is allowed by the complex interaction of viable myocardium with scarred myocardium in and around infarct territories. These patients represent the majority of patients presenting with ventricular arrhythmias. Antiarrhythmic drug treatment may have a role in suppressing arrhythmia occurrence and thereby reduce the morbidity of such arrhythmias, but the data to support protection from SCD are increasingly weak.[1 2 7 16 17] Most such patients will therefore receive device therapy. However, while ICD therapy may be effective in reducing SCD risk, patients may have an unacceptable morbidity related to either frequency of antitachycardia pacing or delivery of defibrillating shock therapy. In this circumstance adjunctive ablation treatment may reduce this burden. Because such arrhythmias are frequently haemodynamically poorly tolerated, use of novel mapping techniques for rapid data acquisition and characterisation of the arrhythmia circuit may be highly advantageous.[18]

Slow ventricular tachycardia

A subset of patients with "ischaemic heart disease ventricular tachycardia" present with slow rate, haemodynamically well tolerated arrhythmia, which is refractory to drug treatment. Such arrhythmias are often poorly handled by ICD antitachycardia pacing regimens which may fail to terminate the arrhythmia, confuse the arrhythmia with sinus tachycardia, deliver shock therapy to the conscious and uncompromised patient, or successfully terminate the arrhythmia only to see its almost immediate re-initiation. However, the stability of the arrhythmia mechanism and the patients' haemodynamics lend themselves to catheter ablation using conventional techniques[19] (fig 19.3A,B). The end point of the therapy need only be cessation of the target arrhythmia and not an attempt to abolish all inducible arrhythmia circuits. Target ablation may be a highly successful symptomatic strategy although ICD therapy will remain indicated to deal with SCD risk and non-targeted arrhythmias.

Idiopathic dilated cardiomyopathy

Ventricular arrhythmias are a major cause of mortality in this condition and standard electrophysiological techniques are less predictive of SCD risk than in ischaemia related left ventricular dysfunction.[20] Patient prognosis is most closely linked to severity of left ventricular impairment. However, progressive heart failure and SCD are competing causes of death. Therefore, the role of ICD implantation in preventing SCD is uncertain as heart failure death may supervene, with ICD implantation impacting little on patient prognosis. Syncope is reported as a reliable predictor of SCD.[20] Non-sustained ventricular tachycardia is also a sensitive but non-specific marker for SCD risk. Other non-invasive tests have no clear role. Programmed extrastimulation has a low negative predictive accuracy.[20] Catheter ablation is also less effective for arrhythmia control even with modern mapping techniques, in part because of the rapidly evolving nature of the underlying substrate. ICD implantation is often indicated for symptomatic control and prognostic benefit, although adjunctive

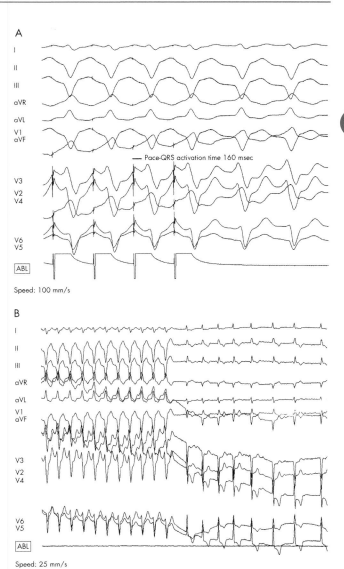

Figure 19.3 (A) Single catheter ventricular ablation technique. Surface ECG pace map during bipolar pacing at a successful ablation site in a patient undergoing emergency ventricular tachycardia circuit ablation for incessant slow ventricular tachycardia. Note the long pace artefact to QRS onset time (160 ms). A mid-diastolic potential with fractionated pre-QRS electrogram was also recorded at this site. (B) Cessation of ventricular tachycardia was achieved after 28 seconds with a single radiofrequency application, power 38 W, end lesion impedance 94 ohms, target temperature 65°C for 60 seconds. No arrhythmia occurrence has been documented over six months follow up.

ablation may be required to reduce the frequency of device therapy. As resynchronisation pacing efficacy becomes established there will be an overlap in indications for device therapy. There is a need for a multidisciplinary approach to the management of the condition.

Idiopathic dilated cardiomyopathy/ischaemic heart disease and bundle branch re-entry tachycardia

Many patients' first presentation with this arrhythmia is syncope or cardiac arrest.[21] More common in dilated cardiomyopathy, it may occur in patients with left ventricular impairment caused by coronary disease. It employs the specialised conduction system as a limb in its re-entry circuit so that targeting and ablation of the right bundle branch may be a "curative" technique.[22]

Hypertrophic cardiomyopathy

At its most threatening, hypertrophic cardiomyopathy may cause unexpected death in asymptomatic young individuals. However, in the majority of patients with the condition the prognosis is relatively benign. The role of the electrophysiologist is to define and manage those patients who are at high risk of SCD but who constitute a small proportion of the total hypertrophic cardiomyopathy population. The literature does allow conclusions to be drawn with respect to risk stratification. Previous cardiac arrest, syncope, a family history of sudden death, extreme left ventricular hypertrophy, a hypotensive blood pressure response to exercise stress testing, and documentation of non-sustained ventricular tachycardia are identified risk factors.[23] In the presence of these observations programmed extrastimulation study does not further refine clinical decisions and in their absence is too non-specific to guide management alone.[24] Assessments of ischaemia, signal averaged ECG, heart rate variability, and T wave alternans are unproven or ineffective as additional risk assessments. Improved genetic understanding will further refine prophylactic device indications.

Right ventricular cardiomyopathy

Fibro-fatty infiltration of right ventricular myocardium characterises this condition.[9 25] Involvement of the septum or left ventricle is uncommon. It may be under-diagnosed at postmortem studies because of the subtleties of histopathological change, both macroscopically and microscopically. Patients most commonly present either with syncope or cardiac arrest, and the condition may be a major cause of sudden death in young (pre-coronary disease) age groups. Most patients will present with ECG abnormalities in the right precordial leads (T wave inversion, increased QRS duration) reflecting right ventricular disease. Necessary investigations include cardiac catheterisation, cross sectional imaging, and the range of non-invasive and invasive electrophysiological assessments. Antiarrhythmic drug treatment, catheter ablation, and ICD implantation all have evidence bases for control of symptoms, but prevention of SCD is probably only achieved by ICD implantation. Right ventricular disarticulation is a highly effective technique in selected patients and with skilled operators. There is an underlying genetic predisposition to the condition so that screening of family members is recommended. However, the role of prophylactic ICD implantation in asymptomatic individuals is undefined.

SYMPTOM CONTROL OF "BENIGN" VENTRICULAR ARRHYTHMIAS

Ventricular ectopic activity

Ventricular ectopy may occur because of myocardial disease causing electrical instability, when it is a marker for that disease rather than a primary electrical disorder, or as part of a specific arrhythmia substrate such as right ventricular outflow tract ventricular tachycardia. Attention should focus on optimum management of underlying heart disease, which may improve patient prognosis and reduce symptom burden. Long term antiarrhythmic drug use should be discouraged. If symptoms are greatly debilitating, catheter ablation, especially using novel mapping techniques, may allow targeting of an arrhythmogenic focus but this approach is rarely employed.

"Benign" ventricular tachycardia

There are a group of conditions which give rise to sustained ventricular tachycardia but, in the absence of any accompanying structural heart disease, are not life threatening. All are amenable to probable curative therapy with catheter ablation.

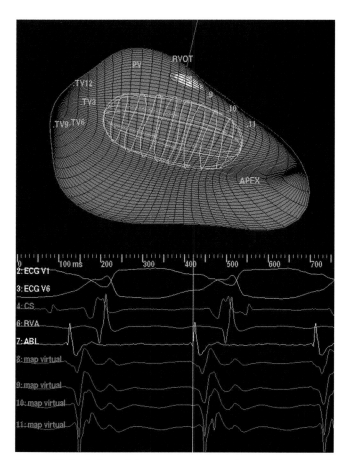

Figure 19.4 Endocardial geometry with superimposed isopotential map recorded using the non-contact mapping system (Endocardial Solutions Inc) in a patient undergoing ablation for right ventricular outflow tract tachycardia. The area coloured white effectively represents the initiation site for the arrhythmia. Note that the "virtual electrograms" demonstrate a characteristic early (relevant to surface ECG) "QS" pattern confirming site of earliest activation.

Right ventricular outflow tract tachycardia

The term right ventricular outflow tract tachycardia is purposefully descriptive. Occasionally the arrhythmia source is in the left ventricular outflow and ECG features do not always allow discrimination. Arrhythmia control may be achieved with drugs, principally β blockers, if ablation is refused. There is at least a presentational overlap between arrhythmogenic right ventricular dysplasia, which should be considered as a possible diagnosis if catheter ablation of the target arrhythmia is unsuccessful, the arrhythmia is recurrent, or there is imaging evidence of right ventricular abnormality.[3] Inducibility of the arrhythmia is variable. Sophisticated mapping tools may aid catheter ablation.[26]

Idiopathic left ventricular tachycardia

Idiopathic left ventricular tachycardia is also of unknown aetiology but is considered to be a focal triggered arrhythmia and commonly emanates from the interventricular septum. It too is optimally managed by catheter ablation in symptomatic individuals[27] (fig 19.4).

Fascicular tachycardia

Fascicular tachycardia is also highly amenable to curative catheter ablation. The tachycardia mechanism involves a re-entrant circuit intimately related to the posterior fascicles of the left conduction system and gives characteristic ECG features of a right bundle branch block, superior access ventricular tachycardia. It may occur in the setting of coronary or other myocardial

---

Ventricular arrhythmias: key points

▶ Not all patients at risk of sudden cardiac death need to be seen by an electrophysiologist

▶ Most patients with symptomatic ventricular arrhythmias should be seen by an electrophysiologist as they may benefit from curative or adjunctive ablation therapy

▶ Patients with "sudden death syndromes" or arrhythmias of uncertain aetiology need to be assessed by an electrophysiologist

---

disease but also occurs as a lone phenomenon. While it is sensitive to antiarrhythmic drug treatment (in particular calcium antagonists) curative ablation is the therapy of choice.[28]

VENTRICULAR ARRHYTHMIAS COMPLICATING CONGENITAL HEART DISEASE

It has been long understood that surgical scars, unavoidably created by palliation of congenital heart anomalies, can contribute to the development of arrhythmia substrate.[29] Catheter mapping and ablation of these arrhythmias can be highly successful,[30] and an electrophysiologist is a necessary part of any adult congenital heart disease management team.

POTENTIAL PITFALLS

A series of supraventricular arrhythmias may generate broad complex tachycardias. Any supraventricular tachycardia may be associated with rate related fatigue of a bundle branch (aberrancy) which gives rise to broad complex tachycardia, then misdiagnosed as ventricular tachycardia. Careful analysis of the ECG usually determines the diagnosis although diagnostic electrophysiology study may be required. In particular, use of flecainide in the management of atrial flutter may result in paradoxical acceleration of the ventricular rate response to a slowed atrial flutter circuit, with bundle branch fatigue related both to rate and the direct effect of flecainide on the specialised conduction system. Other supraventricular tachycardia mechanisms which give rise to broad complex tachycardia include pre-excitation of Wolff-Parkinson-White syndrome with antidromic tachycardia or atrial fibrillation and the characteristic left bundle superior axis of Mahaim tachycardia.

CONCLUSIONS

The increasing breadth of cardiac rhythm management strategies requires greater referral to electrophysiologists for their involvement in the management of patients with ventricular arrhythmias. The extent of that involvement will be determined by arrhythmia mechanism, patient symptoms, co-morbidities, and resource availability.

REFERENCES

1 **Boriani G**, Lubinski A, Capucci A, *et al.* A multicentre, double-blind randomised cross-over comparative study on the efficacy and safety of dofetilide versus sotalol in patients with inducible sustained ventricular tachycardia and ischaemic heart disease. *Eur Heart J* 2001;**22**:2180–91.
  ▶ **Large scale studies of antiarrhythmic drugs, in particular the new generation of "class III" antiarrhythmics, have failed to show significant symptomatic or survival benefits in the management of ventricular arrhythmias.**
2 **Camm AJ**, Pratt CM, Schwartz PJ, *et al.* Azimilide post infarct survival evaluation (ALIVE): azimilide does not affect mortality in post-myocardial infarction patients [abstract]. *Circulation* 2001;**104**:121.
3 **Coggins DL**, Lee RJ, Sweeney J, *et al.* Radiofrequency catheter ablation as a cure for idiopathic ventricular tachycardia of both left and right ventricular origin. *J Am Coll Cardiol* 1994;**23**:1333–41.
  ▶ **Idiopathic ventricular tachycardia can be mapped and curatively ablated in the era of radiofrequency catheter ablation. This should be the standard of care therapy for symptomatic patients with these arrhythmias.**
4 **Corrado D**, Basso C, Nava A, *et al.* Arrhythmogenic right ventricular cardiomyopathy: current diagnostic and management strategies. *Cardiol Rev* 2001;**9**:259–65.

5 **Raitt M**, Dolack GL, Kudenchuk PJ, *et al.* Ventricular arrhythmias detected after transvenous defibrillator implantation in patients with a clinical history of only ventricular fibrillation: implications for implantable defibrillator utilisation. *Circulation* 1995;**91**:1996–2001.
6 **Moss AJ**, Hall WJ, Cannon DS, *et al.* Improved survival with an implanted defibrillator in patients with coronary disease at high risk for ventricular arrhythmia. Multicenter defibrillator implantation trial investigators. *N Engl J Med* 1996;**335**:1933–40.
  ▶ **This study was the first to show survival benefit from the prophylactic use of ICDs in patients with structural heart disease judged to be at high risk of sudden cardiac death. A low use of β blockade, and a protocol design which appeared to favour demonstration of ICD benefit, lead to extensive discussion about general applicability of the study conclusions to clinical practice, but this has now been overtaken by publication of the MADIT II study (see reference 8).**
7 **Buxton AE**, Lee KL, Fisher JD, *et al.* A randomised study of the prevention of sudden death in patients with coronary artery disease. Multicenter unsustained tachycardia trial investigators. *N Engl J Med* 1999;**341**:1882–90.
  ▶ **This study showed the benefit of ICD therapy in improved life expectancy in patients with impaired ventricular function and non-sustained ventricular tachycardia. Electrophysiological study was used to guide therapeutic strategy, but survival benefit was limited to those patients receiving an ICD.**
8 **Moss AJ**, Zareba W, Jackson Hall W, *et al.* Prophylactic implantation of a defibrillator in patients with myocardial infarction and reduced ejection fraction. *N Engl J Med* 2002;**346**:877–83.
  ▶ **This study assessed the benefit in life expectancy for patients with impaired left ventricular function (ejection fraction less than 30%) caused by coronary artery disease. Patients were randomised to ICD therapy or conventional medical treatment (for heart failure). The study outcome is judged to show the efficacy of ICD therapy in prevention of sudden cardiac death in patients with impaired ventricular function, when such patients are selected on the basis of ventricular impairment alone and with no electrophysiological evaluation. This brings application of ICD therapy into the remit of cardiologists with no electrophysiology expertise.**
9 **Roden DM**, Spooner PM. Inherited long QT syndromes: a paradigm for understanding arrhythmogenesis. *J Cardiovasc Electrophysiol* 1999;**10**:1664–83.
  ▶ **This and the following paper are part of the literature which characterises genetic and cellular mechanisms of arrhythmogenesis in certain syndromes. The evolving understanding will aid rational investigation and management of patients with structurally normal hearts but who are at high risk of malignant ventricular arrhythmias.**
10 **Chen Q**, Kirsch GE, Zhang D. Genetic basis and molecular mechanism for idiopathic ventricular fibrillation. *Nature* 1998;**392**:293–6.
11 **Brugada P**, Brugada J. Right bundle branch block, persistent ST segment elevation amd sudden cardiac death: a distinct clinical and electrocardiographic syndrome. A multicenter report. *J Am Coll Cardiol* 1992;**20**:1391–6.
  ▶ **This paper describes the identification of a syndrome which is characterised by sudden death risk and characteristic ECG changes caused by genetically determined abnormalities of transmembrane ionic pump function.**
12 **Brugada J**, Brugada R, Brugada P. Right bundle branch block and ST-segment elevation in leads V1 through V3: a marker for sudden death in patients without demonstrable structural heart. *Circulation* 1998;**97**:457–60.
13 **Brugada J**, Brugada R, Antzelevitch C, *et al.* Long-term follow-up of individuals with the electrocardiographic pattern of right bundle-branch block and ST-segment elevation in precordial leads V1 to V3. *Circulation* 2002;**105**:73–8.
14 **Coumel P**, Fidelle J, Lucet V, *et al.* Catecholaminergic-induced severe ventricular arrhythmias with Adams-Stokes syndrome in children: report of four cases. *Br Heart J* 1978;**40**:28–37.
15 **Priori SG**, Borggrefe M, Camm AJ, on behalf of the UCARE. Role of the implantable defibrillator in patients with idiopathic ventricular fibrillation. Data from the UCARE international registry [abstract]. *Eur Heart J* 1995;**16**:94.
16 **The Antiarrhythmics Versus Implantable Defibrillators (AVID) Investigators**. A comparison of antiarrhythmic drug therapy with implantable defibrillators in patients resuscitated from near fatal ventricular arrhythmias. *N Engl J Med* 1997;**337**:1576–83.
  ▶ **This study demonstrated survival benefit with use of ICDs compared to antiarrhythmic drugs for secondary prevention of sudden cardiac death.**
17 **Connolly SJ**, Hallsrom AP, Cappato R *et al.* Meta-analysis of the implantable cardioverter defibrillator secondary prevention trials. AVID, CASH and CIDS studies. Antiarrhythmics vs implantable defibrillator study. Cardiac arrest study Hamburg. Canadian implantable defibrillator study. *Eur Heart J* 2000;**21**:2071–8.
18 **Strickberger SA**, Knight BP, Michaud GF, *et al.* Mapping and ablation of ventricular tachycardia guided by virtual electrograms using a noncontact, computerized mapping system. *J Am Coll Cardiol* 2000;**35**:414–21.
19 **Stevenson WG**, Khan H, Sager P, *et al.* Identification of reentry circuit sites during catheter mapping and radiofrequency ablation of ventricular tachycardia late after myocardial infarction. *Circulation* 1993;**88**:1647–70.
20 **Brembilla-Perot B**, Donetti J, de la Chaise AT, *et al.* Diagnostic value of ventricular stimulation in patients with idiopathic dilated cardiomyopathy. *Am Heart J* 1991;**121**:1124–31.

21 **Blanck Z**, Dhala A, Deshpande S, *et al*. Bundle branch reentrant ventricular tachycardia: cumulative experience in 48 patients. *J Cardiovasc Electrophysiol* 1993;**4**:253–62.

22 **Cohen TJ**, Chien WW, Lurie KG, *et al*. Radiofrequency catheter ablation for treatment of bundle branch reentrant ventricular tachycardia: results and long term follow up. *J Am Coll Cardiol* 1991;**18**:1767–73.

23 **Fananapazir L**, Chang AC, Epstein SE, *et al*. Prognostic determinants in hypertrophic cardiomyopathy: prognostic evaluation of a therapeutic strategy based on clinical, Holter, hemodynamic and electrophysiologial findings. *Circulation* 1992;**86**:730–40.

24 **Kuck KH**, Kunze KP, Schluter M, *et al*. Programmed electrical stimulation in hypertrophic cardiomyopathy. Results in patients with and without cardiac arrest or syncope. *Eur Heart J* 1988;**9**:177–85.

25 **Richardson P**, McKenna W, Bristow M, *et al*. Report of the 1995 World Health Organization/International Society and Federation of Cardiology task force on the definition and classification of cardiomyopathies. *Circulation* 1996;**93**:841–2.

26 **Betts T**, Roberts P, Allen S, *et al*. Non-contact mapping of right ventricular tachycardia from occult idiopathic right ventricular outflow tract tachycardia from occult arrhythmogenic right ventricular dysplasia. *PACE* 2000;**23**:42.

27 **Betts TR**, Roberts PR, Allen SA, *et al*. Radiofrequency ablation of idiopathic left ventricular tachycardia at the site of earliest activation as determined by non-contact mapping. *J Cardiovascular Electrophysiol* 2000;**11**:973–9.

28 **Crijns HJGM**, Smeets JLRM, Rodrigues LM. Cure of interfascicular reentrant tachycardia by ablation of the anterior fascicle of the left bundle branch. *J Cardiovasc Electrophysiol* 1995;**6**:486–92.

29 **Gillette P**, Yeoman M, Mullins C, *et al*. Sudden death after repair of tetralogy of Fallot. Electrocardiographic and electrophysiologic abnormalities. *Circulation* 1977;**56**:566–70.

30 **Biblo LA**, Carlson MD. Transcatheter radiofrequency ablation of ventricular tachycardia following surgical correction of tetralogy of Fallot. *PACE* 1994;**17**:1556–60.

SECTION VI:
CONGENITAL HEART DISEASE

20 HEART FAILURE IN THE YOUNG

Michael Burch

Heart failure is an enormous clinical burden in adult medicine, largely because of the prevalence of atheromatous coronary disease. In children, where coronary disease is not the leading cause of heart failure, it is less common. It is, however, an important disease, accounting for 10% of paediatric cardiac transplants in children.

Cardiac symptoms in children are usually the result of congenital lesions. Most of these lesions, such as septal defects, are amenable to surgical intervention. It is not appropriate to expand on the management of congenital heart lesions in this review. There is a small subgroup of children that have diastolic failure from cardiomyopathic restriction to flow.

The remaining patients, which will be focused on below, have heart failure that is principally related to poor myocardial function and largely comprise those children with dilated poorly contracting ventricles, which can be related to specific aetiologies in some cases. Particular topics of debate in paediatric heart failure concern:
- the diagnosis and management of myocarditis versus dilated cardiomyopathy
- the most appropriate investigations for new onset heart failure
- cellular responses to heart failure
- the increasing population of anthracycline treated survivors of childhood malignant disease
- treatment strategies.

► DILATED CARDIOMYOPATHY

Indications for transplantation are a guide to the spectrum of causes of severe heart failure. Dilated cardiomyopathy remains the principal indication for cardiac transplantation in children worldwide throughout childhood, apart from infancy when congenital heart disease is a more common indication. The prognosis for dilated cardiomyopathy is around 60% at five years from presentation (fig 20.1), with a high attrition within six months of presentation.[1]

The genetics of dilated cardiomyopathy have been described as a "molecular maze".[w1] Linkage analysis for autosomal dominant dilated cardiomyopathy has proved difficult and direct candidate gene analysis has been used instead, although this is more difficult to use as proof for causation. A variety of lesions have been described including mutations in the cytoskeleton, troponin T,[w2] and other sarcomere protein genes.[2] For the short term molecular genetic analysis is largely a research tool in dilated cardiomyopathy, but it is likely to enter into clinical practice in the foreseeable future. New onset heart failure in children should be investigated for specific causes and these are discussed below. One particular problem is whether the child has myocarditis or cardiomyopathy as this currently alters management in many centres.

MYOCARDITIS

Lymphocytic myocarditis accounts for around 10% of recent onset cardiomyopathy,[w3] and this figure may be higher in children. Survival from myocarditis in children and adults is similar at around 80%.[3] [w4]

Viruses are the main causes in developed countries, coxsackie B and adenovirus accounting for most cases; Chagas disease is the most common cause in Central and South America, and other infectious causes should be considered.[w5] The genetics of the host may determine the outcome.[w6] The majority of infections are insidious, but fulminant infections are well recognised. Perhaps surprisingly, fulminant myocarditis has a better prognosis[4] as these patients are more likely to develop normal cardiac function if they can be supported through the initial illness. Improved techniques of mechanical support, using biventricular assist devices, has allowed recovery from fulminant myocarditis in children[5] with complete recovery of cardiac function in three out of four cases. When a biopsy diagnosis of myocarditis is available for children on an assist device it is likely to influence the intensive care team to await recovery, but they may want to bridge to early transplantation if no lymphocytic infiltration is seen and the diagnosis of dilated cardiomyopathy is inferred. Acute or non-fulminant myocarditis is more likely to result in a progressive course with death or transplantation being required.

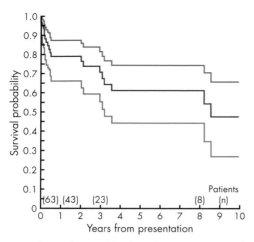

Figure 20.1 Survival curve (blue line) from presentation of 63 children with dilated cardiomyopathy, with 95% confidence intervals (red and green lines). Reproduced from Burch *et al*[1] with permission from the BMJ Publishing Group.

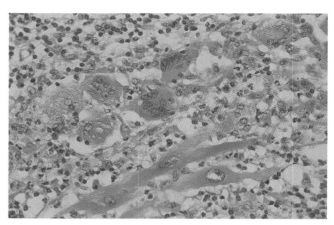

Figure 20.2 Histological sample from an explanted heart of a 15 year old girl who presented with new onset heart failure and required ECMO (extracorporeal membrane oxygenation) bridge to transplant. Histology shows lymphocytic infiltration with giant cell formation— giant cell myocarditis. The patient remains well at follow up. Slide provided by Dr Marian Malone from the pathology department at Great Ormond Street Hospital for Children.

The diagnosis of myocarditis is difficult and has historically rested on endomyocardial biopsy evidence of lymphocytic infiltration, yet biopsy in children is not without risk and changes may be patchy. Other tests may be helpful such as assays for autoimmune markers, cardiac troponin T or I,[w7] and immunocytology may be included in the assessment. Enteroviruses can be looked for using polymerase chain reaction (PCR) from biopsy specimens and from tracheal aspirates.[6] Paired serology and viral culture are helpful, but are not available early in the course. The ECG is rarely normal, but is not specific. Voltages are reduced and arrhythmias are common, ST changes can be seen, and the findings may mimic myocardial infarction. There are many cases of clinically suspected myocarditis where no supporting evidence is seen.

The treatment of heart failure caused by myocarditis in children is supportive and not essentially different from dilated cardiomyopathy, although patients with fulminant myocarditis are more likely to be supported to recovery rather than transplantation. Much has been written on immune suppression and immune globulin therapy. Studies in children and adults showed promise,[7 w8] but myocarditis has a high rate of spontaneous recovery, and when randomised studies have been performed there has been no advantage to treatment with these strategies.[3 8] In paediatrics it is still common practice to treat new onset heart failure with very high dose methylprednisolone and/or immune globulin. Both of these options can result in fluid balance changes that can precipitate worsening failure. Also an improvement in function may not be related to resolution of myocarditis as immune globulins may have a beneficial effect by modulating the effects of cytokines in some cases.[9] Cytokines cause migration of leucocytes and they are up regulated in heart failure, which may cause inflammation and damage in heart muscle (see below). Therefore an early improvement in systolic function during immunoglobulin therapy should not be assumed to be confirmation of the diagnosis of myocarditis, as it is also seen in dilated cardiomyopathy. There was no long term survival benefit for immunoglobulin therapy in a large controlled study.[8] Empirically, there seems little reason for immune modulation to work in children if it does not work in young adults with fulminant myocarditis. At present a blanket policy of immune suppression and/or immune globulin in paediatric practice cannot be justified on the evidence base. Until a randomised study is available in children such treatment is not recommended.

Immune suppression should not be dismissed in all paediatric myocarditis, as there are specific instances where it is indicated. Giant cell myocarditis[10] is a rare disease with a characteristic histological appearance (fig 20.2); these patients appear to benefit from immune suppression. When transplantation is undertaken there is a high risk of recurrence in the transplanted heart, yet it can be effectively treated by increased immune suppression.[w9] Also systemic autoimmune diseases such as systemic lupus erythematosus (SLE) can cause a myocarditis, which will, like the systemic disease, respond to immune suppression. A drug induced/allergic reaction can cause an eosinophilic infiltrate, which may respond to steroids. In addition the role of cellular and humoral immunity in dilated cardiomyopathy has become increasingly implicated in dilated cardiomyopathy. A variety of autoantibodies have been identified, such as those against β receptors[w10] and cardiac myosin heavy chain.[11] Recently, immunoglobulin adsorption and IgG substitution has been shown to improve cardiac function clinical status and reduce oxidative stress in dilated cardiomyopathy[12 w11] and this may be causally related to a reduction in circulating autoantibodies.

INVESTIGATIONS IN NEW ONSET HEART FAILURE IN CHILDREN

Most paediatric cardiac units have extensive investigation sheets for dilated cardiomyopathy/new onset failure, but there is a degree of scepticism about the chance of turning up a positive result and there is a perception that investigations should not be over extensive. While this is not the view of all involved in the field, it is pragmatic, as it is important that the tests are run thoroughly and results followed up. With too many investigations there may be a tendency for results to be mislaid or overlooked. It is probably wise to target the investigations that are considered most likely.

Cardiomyopathy investigations should vary with the type of heart muscle disease—for example, restrictive, hypertrophic, and dilated. Most new onset heart failure in children is caused by congenital heart disease. Clearly this should be excluded at the initial assessment. It is recognised that an anomalous left coronary from the pulmonary artery will present with a dilated left ventricle and this may cause confusion with a dilated cardiomyopathy. Therefore careful assessment of infants with poorly contracting left ventricles should include ECG, echocardiography, and, if there is any doubt, coronary angiography. Metabolic defects should always be considered, as there may be implications for genetic counselling or treatment strategies. Infiltration of the myocardium occurs with inborn errors of metabolism such as glycogen storage diseases, but Fabry's disease, haemochromatosis, and amyloidosis are more common causes of heart failure in adult life, as are damage from toxins such as alcohol, cocaine, and radiation. With infant hypertrophic cardiomyopathy Pompe's disease should be excluded; it can be assessed with initial screening for vacuolated lymphocytes, and confirmed using acid maltase analysis in blood or skin.

Autoimmune diseases are recognised to be associated with cardiomyopathy and these include SLE. It is increasingly recognised that the children of mothers who are anti-Ro positive or anti-La positive may develop cardiomyopathy despite adequate pacing.[13]

Long chain fatty acids supply most of the energy for the heart; they are transported across the plasma membrane and metabolised in the mitochondria. A number of recessive lesions in the proteins required for this have been described. These include carnitine deficiency and medium chain acyl-CoA dehydrogenase deficiency. In general systemic problems such as ammonaemia, acidosis, hypoglycaemia, and coma may be more prominent than cardiomyopathy. Mitochondrial disease typically presents with a hypertrophic and poorly contracting left ventricle. Brain, cardiac, and skeletal muscle function are often affected, as all have a high energy need. Skeletal muscle biopsy shows "ragged red" fibres. Inheritance is through the maternal line. Barth syndrome is an X linked disorder of mitochondrial function related to a lipid remodelling defect; 3-methylglutaconic aciduria is evident and is often associated with neutropenia, hypercholesterolaemia, hypoglycaemia, and lactic acidosis. The mitochondrial dysfunction of Kearns-Sayre disease syndrome is associated with ophthalmoplegia, retinal pigmentation hearing loss, endocrine dysfunction, and cardiomyopathy with conduction defects. Molecular genetic diagnosis is available for a number of these mitochondrial conditions. Mutations in the gene G4.5 cause a variety of severe infant cardiomyopathies including Barth syndrome and isolated left ventricular non-compaction.[w12]

In paediatric practice children with skeletal myopathies such as Duchenne and Becker dystrophy may develop cardiomyopathy, which is initially hypertrophic but becomes dilated. They are suspected clinically before symptomatic cardiomyopathy in the majority of cases. Rarely X linked deficiency of cardiac dystrophin can be seen without skeletal cardiomyopathy.

Some recommended investigations for new onset heart failure are shown in table 20.1, including procedures that could reveal mitochondrial disorders and autoimmune disease. In both instances there may be a strong suspicion from other problems arising. Similarly, some rare causes of cardiomyopathy can be suspected from the history of associated disease and extensive tests should only then be undertaken. Thyroid disease, sarcoid, parathyroid disease, phaeochromocytoma, and severe nutritional deficiencies are rare causes of childhood cardiomyopathy and are not recommended for initial screening unless suspected clinically.

APOPTOSIS, CYTOKINES, AND REGENERATION

The cellular basis of heart failure in children will depend on the cause of ventricular dysfunction, but for most patients apopto-

Table 20.1 Investigations in new onset paediatric failure (dilated left ventricle)

▶ Echocardiography (including check for anomalous coronary)

▶ ECG

▶ Myocarditis: Tracheal aspirate for viral PCR, paired serology (including coxsackie, adenovirus, echo, influenza, parainfluenza, varicella, RSV, rubella, CMV, EBV, HIV, parvovirus, mycoplasma, and endemic infections depending on geography—for example, Chagas' disease, dengue, diphtheria, *Coxiella burnetti*; many organisms cause myocarditis, and this list is not exclusive), troponin T, blood count for lymphocytosis. Myocardial biopsy (see text) for histology and PCR. Consider toxins if suggested by history, and illegal drugs (for example, cocaine)

▶ Autoimmune: Anti-Ro and Anti-La, full SLE screen including antinuclear antibody, double stranded DNA, rheumatoid factor, ESR. Autoantibody screen (availability varies)—for example, anti-mysosin β receptor antibodies

▶ Mitochondrial: Carnitine, acyl carnitine, lactate, glucose, white cell count for neutropenia, urine amino acids for methylglutaconic aciduria, muscle biopsy if clinical suspicion of mitochondrial disease. Molecular genetic diagnosis of Barth syndrome is available in some centres

CMV, cytomegalovirus; EBV, Epstein-Barr virus; ESR, erythrocyte sedimentation rate; HIV, human immunodeficiency virus; PCR, polymerase chain reaction; RSV, respiratory syncytial virus; SLE, systemic lupus erythematosus.

sis is likely to be involved. There is strong histopathological evidence that apoptosis is distinct from necrotic cell death, in that it is genetically programmed and is designed to destroy damaged cells that, for example, could become cancerous. There is controversy over whether apoptosis occurs in myocytes, as they are cells which cannot divide, but it is now accepted that it does occur.[14] Ventricular distension, increased wall stress, and neurohumoral activation upregulate genes such as c-myc, c-fos, and fetal proteins. A fetal metabolic gene profile is seen probably by downregulating adult genes rather than upregulating fetal genes.[w13] Angiotensin II release may stimulate myocyte apoptosis. This leads to release of cytochrome c from mitochondria[w14] and activation of proteolytic capsases, which results in progression of proteolysis. In theory, if the heart is supported the cytoplasmic proteins could recover as the nucleus is initially unaffected. Therefore, left ventricular support is attractive because remodelling, and reversal of neurohumoral abnormalities and wall stress reduction, may lead to cell recovery if the apoptotic process has not become irreversible and damaged the nucleus. Reversal of neurohumoral abnormalities can be achieved with β blockers and angiotensin converting enzyme (ACE) inhibitors.

Surgical procedures may aid remodelling. Clearly closure of a ventricular septal defect allows immediate reduction in left ventricular dimensions. In the setting of dilated cardiomyopathy mitral valve surgery has been successfully used to aid remodelling, although early experience in children in our own centre has not been encouraging. The Batista operation is a partial ventriculectomy,[15] which actively remodels the left ventricle, but it is assumed that the myocytes are functioning well or will recover subsequently. If there is excessive scarring or fibrosis then the outcome of a Batista is less likely to be favourable. There is little experience of the Batista operation in children. The left ventricle can be actively rested by mechanical support, and impeller pumps may allow very long term ambulatory support, although they do involve an incision into the left ventricle.

Cytokines are hormone-like proteins that foster communication between immune cells. Adults with heart failure have

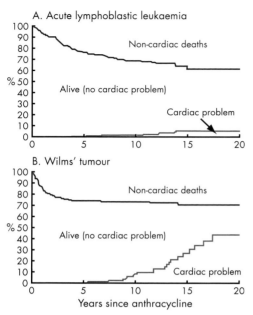

Figure 20.3 Multistate survival curves for 346 consecutive acute lymphoblastic leukaemia and Wilms' tumour patients treated with anthracycline between 1971 and 1990, identifying non-cardiac deaths and cardiac problems (fractional shortening < 25%). Adapted from Sorenson et al.[18]

Heart failure in the young: key points

Myocarditis
- ▶ Coxsackie and adenovirus account for the majority of cases of viral myocarditis
- ▶ Fulminant infections have a better prognosis than non-fulminant infections
- ▶ Children can be bridged to recovery using mechanical support
- ▶ Randomised studies have not shown any benefit from immune suppression
- ▶ Immunoglobulin may reduce cytokines in heart failure and short term echo improvement may be attributable to this, not resolution of myocarditis

Apoptosis, cytokines, and regeneration
- ▶ Apoptosis occurs in myocytes
- ▶ The nucleus is affected later in myocyte apoptosis and this may allow recovery with bridging
- ▶ New myocytes can develop as shown by chimeric studies
- ▶ Circulating cytokines such as tumour necrosis factor α are increased in heart failure

Heart failure treatment in children
- ▶ ACE inhibitors are widely used in children
- ▶ Carvedilol is helpful in stable patients
- ▶ Aspirin may oppose the action of ACE inhibitors and carvedilol

---

raised concentrations of cytokines in the circulation,[w15] and tumour necrosis factor α and interleukin 1 and 6 have been examined. The overexpression of these cytokines may play a role in the pathogenesis of heart failure, perhaps by dysregulation of apoptosis, direct effects on calcium dependent processes, and impaired β adrenergic signal transduction. Systemic administration of tumour necrosis factor causes myocardial depression. Brain natriuretic peptide is a cardiac peptide that is a useful predictor of survival in heart failure.[w16] Cytokines and vasoactive peptides have not been as extensively investigated in children as in adults. It is possible that immunoglobulin infusion may exert its beneficial effect by modulating cytokines.

Myocyte regeneration has been a controversial issue, but a recent study of chimerism after transplantation does appear to demonstrate that it occurs.[16] Furthermore, it has been recently demonstrated that human stem cells can differentiate to a cardiomyocyte phenotype in the adult murine heart.[w17] This suggests that the likely source of the chimeric cells post-transplant is the marrow. All of this gives hope for successful regeneration after prolonged support and may signal the beginning of the age of successful stem cell implantation.

ANTHRACYCLINE CARDIOTOXICITY

About half of all young adults who survive childhood cancer have received anthracyclines, particularly daunorubicin or doxorubicin. The number of young adult patients with potential heart muscle disease is therefore going to be larger than, for example, young adult survivors of tetralogy of Fallot, or transposition. Cardiotoxicity is dose related, and myocyte damage on biopsy has a linear relation with cumulative dose. The myocyte necrosis is irreversible, although echocardiographic improvement in systolic function and recovery from symptomatic heart failure can be seen with treatment in most cases. In children there is progressive, dose related impairment of afterload in asymptomatic individuals.[17] Age at treatment has an inverse relation with end systolic wall stress. The

longer the interval between treatment and assessment the greater the abnormality of wall stress; as most follow up studies do not extend beyond 20 years, there is a potential for a significant increase in the number of patients with overt disease in middle age.

A prospective longitudinal and actuarial assessment of late daunorubicin and doxorubicin cardiotoxicity in 184 survivors of childhood[18] cancer has shown that the most important predictor of worsening cardiac performance was total dose with a cut off of 242 mg/m², above which end systolic wall stress would be expected to deteriorate in a dose related regression. The higher dose used in the Wilms' tumour group was associated with increased cardiac disease at follow up (fig 20.3). It is reassuring that most paediatric acute lymphoblastic leukaemia patients receive less than this dose currently; however, paediatric solid tumours may receive higher doses.

Epirubicin may be less cardiotoxic. Dexrazoxane is used as a cytoprotective agent in metastatic breast cancer patients who have received > 300 mg/m² of doxorubicin. It chelates with iron in the myocytes and prevents the formation of the doxorubicin–iron complex that is thought to be cardiotoxic. Probucol, a strong antioxidant, has also been beneficial in animal studies. Activation of poly-ADP ribose polymerase by oxidant mediated DNA damage has been shown to contribute to the cardiotoxicity of doxorubicin. Inhibitors of this nuclear enzyme may offer cardioprotective effects.[w18]

PAEDIATRIC TREATMENT FOR HEART FAILURE

Heart failure treatment in children is very similar to that of adults. However, because of lack of resources and a reluctance of the pharmaceutical industry to undertake trials, few of the proven treatments in adults are licensed in children and paediatric preparations are not available, leaving parents to grind and dissolve adult tablets. The pharmaceutical industry cannot promote products for indications and age groups outside the licence. The implication of this is that product information outside the licence may be difficult to obtain. A principle of paediatric drug usage is that the therapeutic effect in children is likely to be similar to what it is in adults, but pharmacokinetics are different. On the whole, paediatric cardiologists follow the evidence base in adults, but the thought that drugs work differently or have a different effect in children leaves the potential for individuals to use idiosyncratic treatments and ignore the evidence base. For example, phosphodiesterase III inhibitors have been shown to have a deleterious effect on long term survival, milrinone having a 28% increase in mortality compared to placebo.[w19] Yet oral phosphodiesterase inhibitors such as enoximone are still used by paediatric cardiologists.

ACE inhibitors are widely used in children, but β blockers are less commonly used even though the adult evidence base is strong; carvedilol has been successfully used in New York Heart Association functional class III and IV patients,[19] and it has also been used in children.[20] They should only be introduced in stable patients and the dose increased slowly. β Blockers must be stopped if inotropes are needed. Spironolactone has been shown to be beneficial in heart failure (although careful potassium monitoring is necessary if used with ACE inhibitors) yet amiloride is widely used in paediatrics.[w20] Digoxin use remains controversial in adults and children, and although therapeutic benefits have been seen in adults with a reduced hospitalisation rate, overall mortality is not reduced.[w21] This puts it behind β blockers and ACE inhibitors, which both prolong survival. Digoxin may not be helpful in acute myocarditis. Anticoagulation with warfarin is difficult in children, but those with severe heart failure are at risk of mural thrombus. There is now evidence that aspirin and other non-steroidal anti-inflammatory agents can exacerbate heart failure and may reduce the effect of the diuretics, ACE inhibitors, and β blockers.[w22 w23] The mechanism probably involves the inhibition of prostaglandin synthesis, increasing peripheral resistance and decreasing renal perfusion. Angiotensin II receptor blockers may have a role in replacing ACE inhibitors when there is an unwanted effect such as a severe cough, but they do not convey a survival benefit in adults[w24] and experience of their use in children has been very limited.

There is a small subgroup of patients with diastolic failure from restriction to inflow, such as restrictive cardiomyopathy. They are probably best managed with β blockers and low dose diuretics; anticoagulation may be required as there is a high incidence of embolic disease in this condition.

Ultimately many children with heart failure may deteriorate sufficiently to require mechanical support. For small children extracorporeal membrane oxygenation is used but for older children pneumatic external assists such as the Berlin Heart or the Medos can be used. Both have been used as successful bridges to transplant. The number of paediatric donor organs is closer to the number of children requiring transplantation than is the case in adults, providing bridging is available. This makes long term implantable mechanical support attractive as a bridge to transplant, although it is as yet unclear whether the new impeller pumps can be used in paediatric cardiomyopathy as biventricular pneumatic devices have usually been required. Paediatric transplantation has a five year actuarial survival of approximately 70% overall since 1982 (for 4419 cases,[w25] with infants having a worse outcome of approximately 60%). Our unpublished institutional data show that survival is better when adjusted for era and diagnosis, with a worse outcome for complex congenital heart disease, although this latter difference is becoming less obvious with improvements in surgical technique, intensive care, and mechanical support.

CONCLUSIONS

Paediatric heart failure benefits from the increasing knowledge about the mechanisms of the disease processes. There is potential for significant therapeutic advances in all areas of management in the coming decades.

143

REFERENCES

1 **Burch M**, Siddiqi SA, Celermajer DS, *et al*. Dilated cardiomyopathy in children: determinants of outcome. *Br Heart J* 1994;**72**:246-250.
▶ **This is a review of outcome in dilated cardiomyopathy in children in the UK. The data are useful but are becoming out of date.**
2 **Kamisago M**, Sharma SD, DePalma SR, *et al*. Mutations in sarcomere protein genes as a cause of dilated cardiomyopathy. *N Engl J Med* 2000;**343**:1688-96.
▶ **An interesting genetic paper that shows evidence for mutations causing dilated cardiomyopathy in different sarcomere proteins.**
3 **Mason JW**, O'Connell JB, Herskowitz A, *et al*. A clinical trial of immunosuppressive therapy for myocarditis. The myocarditis treatment trial investigators. *N Engl J Med* 1995;**333**:269-75.
4 **McCarthy RE**, Boehmer JP, Hruban RH, *et al*. Long-term outcome of fulminant myocarditis as compared with acute (nonfulminant) myocarditis. *N Engl J Med* 2000;**342**:690-5.
5 **Stiller B**, Dahnert I, Weng YG, *et al*. Children may survive severe myocarditis with prolonged use of biventricular assist devices. *Heart* 1999;**82**:237-40.
6 **Akhtar N**, Ni J, Stromberg D, *et al*. Tracheal aspirate as a substrate for polymerase chain reaction detection of viral genome in childhood pneumonia and myocarditis. *Circulation* 1999;**99**:2011-18.
7 **Drucker NA**, Colan SD, Lewis AB, *et al*. Gamma-globulin treatment of acute myocarditis in the pediatric population. *Circulation* 1994;**89**:252-7.
8 **McNamara DM**, Holubkov R, Starling RC, *et al*. Controlled trial of intravenous immune globulin in recent-onset dilated cardiomyopathy. *Circulation* 2001;**103**:2254-9.
9 **Damas JK**, Gullestad L, Aass H, *et al*. Enhanced gene expression of chemokines and their corresponding receptors in mononuclear blood cells in chronic heart failure – modulatory effect of intravenous immunoglobulin. *J Am Coll Cardiol* 2001;**38**:187-93.
▶ **An interesting review of the effect of immunoglobulins in heart failure.**
10 **Cooper LTJ**, Berry GJ, Shabetai R. Idiopathic giant-cell myocarditis – natural history and treatment. Multicenter giant cell myocarditis study group investigators. *N Engl J Med* 1997;**336**:1860-6.
▶ **A helpful report of the outcome in a rare condition.**
11 **Caforio AL**, Grazzini M, Mann JM, *et al*. Identification of alpha- and beta-cardiac myosin heavy chain isoforms as major autoantigens in dilated cardiomyopathy. *Circulation* 1992;**85**:1734-42.
12 **Muller J**, Wallukat G, Dandel M, *et al*. Immunoglobulin adsorption in patients with idiopathic dilated cardiomyopathy. *Circulation* 2000;**101**:385-91.
13 **Nield LE**, Silverman ED, Taylor GP, *et al*. Maternal anti-Ro and anti-La antibody-associated endocardial fibroelastosis. *Circulation* 2002;**105**:843-8.
14 **Narula J**, Haider N, Virmani R, *et al*. Apoptosis in myocytes in end-stage heart failure. *N Engl J Med* 1996;**335**:1182-9.
▶ **A landmark paper, documenting apoptosis in the heart.**
15 **Batista RJ**, Santos JL, Takeshita N, *et al*. Partial left ventriculectomy to improve left ventricular function in end-stage heart disease. *J Card Surg* 1996;**11**:96-7.
▶ **A paper that launched a new surgical intervention, although a rigorous assessment of the benefits of the technique was awaited.**
16 **Quaini F**, Urbanek K, Beltrami AP, *et al*. Chimerism of the transplanted heart. *N Engl J Med* 2002;**346**:5-15.
▶ **Elegant proof of cardiac regeneration, using sex mismatched transplants.**
17 **Lipshultz SE**, Colan SD, Gelber RD, *et al*. Late cardiac effects of doxorubicin therapy for acute lymphoblastic leukemia in childhood. *N Engl J Med* 1991;**324**:808-15.
▶ **An important paper that sparked concern in paediatric oncology units.**
18 **Sorensen K**, Levitt G, Bull C, *et al*. Late anthracycline cardiotoxicity after childhood cancer: prospective longitudinal and actuarial assessment. Submitted for publication.
▶ **This paper represents a unique long term follow up of a large number of patients with strong statistics.**
19 **Packer M**, Coats AJ, Fowler MB, *et al*. Effect of carvedilol on survival in severe chronic heart failure. *N Engl J Med* 2001;**344**:1651-8.
▶ **A powerful study showing carvedilol can be used safely in late stage heart failure.**
20 **Bruns LA**, Chrisant MK, Lamour JM, *et al*. Carvedilol as therapy in pediatric heart failure: an initial multicenter experience. *J Pediatr* 2001;**138**:505-11.

Additional references appear on the *Heart* website–
www.heartjnl.com

21 SUDDEN DEATH IN CHILDREN AND ADOLESCENTS

Christopher Wren

Sudden death in childhood is rare. About 10% of paediatric deaths after the first year of life are sudden and population based studies put the individual age related risk at around 1:20 000 to 1:50 000 per year.[1-4 w1-3] About half of these deaths are related to a previously known abnormality, the most common being epilepsy, asthma, and cardiovascular abnormalities. Another third are attributed to an abnormality discovered at necropsy, usually either an infection or a cardiovascular abnormality. At least one sudden death in six remains unexplained, but this is almost certainly an underestimate as some deaths attributed by the coroner's pathologist to epilepsy or respiratory infection are probably more accurately described as being unexplained by findings at necropsy.[4 w4]

▶ MECHANISMS OF SUDDEN DEATH

Although all deaths result in asystole, not all sudden deaths are caused by arrhythmias. The precise mechanism of sudden death depends upon the cause. One report of terminal electrical activity in paediatric patients dying in hospital documented bradycardic arrest in 88% of neonates, 67% of infants, and 64% of children.[5] Ventricular tachycardia or fibrillation was more likely in those with heart disease and in older children. The term "sudden death" should not be confused with non-fatal cardiac arrest.[w5]

Sudden cardiac death in infancy
Sudden death in infancy is usually caused either by infection or by sudden infant death syndrome. A few neonatal or infant deaths are caused by unrecognised congenital cardiovascular malformations, particularly duct dependent abnormalities or obstructive left heart malformations.[w6] Primary arrhythmias are rare causes of death in infancy but fatal ventricular arrhythmias are described.[6] Complete atrioventricular block is usually recognised in utero or soon after birth but may cause death if unrecognised or untreated.[w7]

Sudden death in children with postoperative congenital heart disease
In the 1960s and 1970s sudden cardiac death most often occurred in children with irreversible pulmonary vascular disease associated with unoperated congenital heart disease or in children with unoperated aortic valve stenosis.[w8 w9] In recent years surgical repair has been performed earlier and more effectively so that those most at risk of sudden death now are children with repaired heart disease. In a population based study of late postoperative sudden death, Silka and colleagues identified an average risk of 0.9 per 1000 patient-years follow up for the most common surgically repaired malformations.[7] Those patients with a risk above the average had aortic valve stenosis, transposition of the great arteries, tetralogy of Fallot or coarctation of the aorta. Death was attributed to "arrhythmia" in the majority, based on the history, but in only a few was an arrhythmia identified in life.

Sudden death in adults with congenital heart disease
Among patients in an adult congenital heart follow up clinic in Toronto, not all of whom had undergone surgery, the reported sudden death rate was 5.3 per 1000 patient-years.[8] The most common abnormalities in those who died suddenly were Eisenmenger's syndrome, tetralogy of Fallot, and transposition of the great arteries, but the risk for individual diagnoses could not be assessed for lack of a denominator. In a more recent report from the same unit, 8% of adult patients died during follow up—65% of deaths were cardiovascular and 26% were sudden.[w10] Although numbers for individual diagnoses were small, the highest proportion of deaths were sudden in patients with coarctation of the aorta, Ebstein's anomaly, and congenitally corrected transposition of the great arteries. The highest number of sudden deaths in the clinic population occurred in patients who had undergone repair of tetralogy of Fallot.

Sudden death after repair of tetralogy of Fallot
Of the various problems encountered late after surgical repair of tetralogy of Fallot, sudden death is the most difficult to predict. It usually occurs many years after operation[w11] and thus affects young

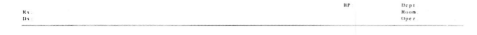

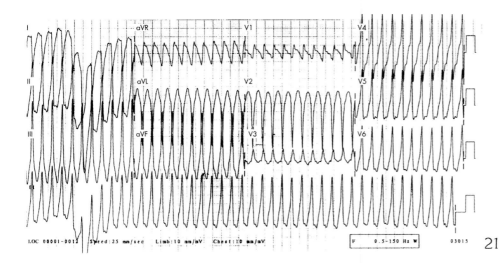

Figure 21.1 Postoperative ventricular tachycardia in a 14 year old boy with a Rastelli repair of complex transposition who presented with syncope. The left bundle branch block pattern and inferior frontal plane vector indicate an origin from the right ventricular outflow. After electrophysiology study he underwent defibrillator implantation.

adults more than children, with an average risk of 1.4 per 1000 patient years, or about 1 in 700 per year.[9] Many risk factors for sudden death have been identified retrospectively, but prospectively, even in combination, they are not useful in predicting risk.[10][w12][w13] Although ventricular tachycardia or fibrillation is thought to be the most common mechanism of sudden death, more minor ventricular arrhythmias are so common as to be unhelpful in predicting risk. An important recent "pseudo-prospective" multicentre study involving six centres in the UK, USA, Canada, and Japan retrospectively identified 793 patients alive in 1985 and "followed" their progress for the next 10 years, yielding more than 7500 patient-years follow up.[11] Thirty three patients developed sustained monomorphic ventricular tachycardia, 29 developed atrial flutter or fibrillation, 16 died suddenly, and 715 remained free from arrhythmia. There were no deaths in those who presented with ventricular tachycardia and there was only one death among patients presenting with atrial arrhythmia. The risk profile for ventricular tachycardia and sudden death was similar, with most of the patients having pulmonary regurgitation and right ventricular dysfunction. The authors suggest that surgical preservation or restoration of pulmonary valve function may reduce the risk of sudden death, but this remains unproven.

Sudden death after atrial repair of transposition of the great arteries

Most major published reports of experience of the Senning and Mustard operations for atrial repair of transposition of the great arteries give a risk of 5–6 per 1000 patient-years or of about 1 in 180 per year.[9] The relation between late sudden death and arrhythmia is not clear. There is a progressive loss of sinus rhythm so that fewer than half of patients have normal rhythm after 10 years.[w14] Junctional rhythm is common but asymptomatic bradycardia does not require treatment. Bradycardia seems not to be a risk factor for sudden death and pacemaker implantation offers no protection against it. One widely accepted theory is that the sudden onset of atrial flutter with 1:1 atrioventricular conduction may lead to sudden

death, particularly if it is associated with impaired right ventricular function or atrial baffle obstruction, but as yet there is only circumstantial evidence for this.[w15] There is a complicated interrelation between arrhythmia, impaired ventricular function, and sudden death, which has yet to be explored fully.[w16] Other possible causes for late death after atrial repair of transposition include ventricular arrhythmias[7] or acute heart failure.

Sudden death after repair of other malformations

Late sudden death after surgical repair of other common cardiovascular malformations is rare, with an incidence of around 0.1 per 1000 patient-years.[7] Surgical repair of some less common cardiac malformations may be associated with a higher risk of late sudden death. In a report of experience with the Rastelli operation for repair of complex transposition of the great arteries from Boston, there were five late sudden deaths in a group of 94 survivors of surgery who were followed for a median of 8.5 years (6.3 deaths per 1000 patient years).[w17] Deaths were thought to be caused by the development of ventricular arrhythmias (fig 21.1) or atrioventricular block. The late postoperative sudden death rate in patients with heart defects characterised by double outlet right ventricle may be even higher.[w18] Among 89 patients the sudden death rate was 26 per 1000 patient years, with 50% of deaths within one year of surgery. Risk factors for late death included perioperative ventricular tachycardia and atrioventricular block. The risk in rare conditions is harder to define but in some, such as pulmonary atresia, it may be significant.[w19]

Sudden death in children with unoperated heart disease

One would hope that most significant cardiovascular malformations would be detected early in life, preferably at an asymptomatic stage. However, despite health screening some significant problems go unrecognised,[w20] and may cause sudden death. Deaths from obstructive left heart malformations are unusual but they do occur.[4] Postoperative deaths in such patients were ascribed to "arrhythmia" in the study by

Silka and colleagues, but syncope in aortic valve stenosis is probably not primarily arrhythmic in origin.[w21] Congenital abnormalities of the coronary arteries are rarely diagnosed in life and prodromal syncope is uncommon. The most frequently recognised abnormalities after sudden death are anomalous origin of the left or right coronary arteries from the contralateral aortic sinus, with a proximal course between the aorta and the main pulmonary artery.[w22] [w23] Although the prevalence of such anomalies is hard to define precisely, the risk of sudden death is probably high enough to warrant surgical treatment.[w24] Sudden death in other specific conditions, such as Williams syndrome, is also reported and may be caused, in some cases at least, by coronary artery stenosis or malformation.[w25]

Sudden death in hypertrophic cardiomyopathy

The risk of sudden death in childhood from hypertrophic cardiomyopathy diagnosed in life is impossible to establish for lack of a denominator. Hypertrophic cardiomyopathy is said to affect as many as 1 in 500 of the adult population, but it is much less common in childhood. The impression given by published reports from specialised referral units is that the risk of sudden death is high whereas evidence from the few population based studies does not support this.[12 w26 w27] "Risk stratification" is encouraged and may identify a few individuals at increased risk.[13 w28] "Risk factors" have been identified but are absent in most children. Risk factors for an increased risk of sudden death in adults include a family history of sudden death from hypertrophic cardiomyopathy, recurrent syncope, non-sustained ventricular tachycardia on an ambulatory ECG, and extreme left ventricular hypertrophy, but their presence does not reliably identify individuals at risk. A recent study of the use of implantable cardioverter-defibrillators (ICDs) in primary and secondary prevention has shown benefit.[w29] Appropriate discharges were triggered by ventricular tachycardia or fibrillation, providing insight into the mechanism of sudden death and an incentive for better risk stratification. However, only eight of 128 patients receiving an ICD were children. In a study of 99 children with hypertrophic cardiomyopathy in Toronto, the reported annual combined risk of sudden death and cardiac arrest was 2.7% between the ages of 8 and 18 years.[w30] In this study syncope did not predict sudden death whereas cardiac arrest did and ventricular tachycardia on ambulatory ECG was a significant risk factor. The risk of sudden death is low for the majority of children, especially in the absence of symptoms. There is no evidence that treatment of asymptomatic patients has any effect on outcome.[w31] Because some sudden deaths occur during or after exercise it is often recommended that affected children should avoid sports or intense physical exertion. While such advice may seem sensible, there is no evidence that this leads to any reduction in risk.[12]

Sudden death from *previously unsuspected* hypertrophic cardiomyopathy is rare—with an age specific risk in apparently normal children or adolescents of less than 1 in 1 000 000 per year.[4 w32] Because hypertrophic cardiomyopathy typically has dominant inheritance, diagnosis at necropsy should lead to screening of other family members. Often no further cases are identified, either because of variable penetrance or because the index case represents a new mutation. Clinical exclusion of the diagnosis is often very difficult as detectable cardiovascular abnormalities may only develop during adolescence.[13] Gene testing is not generally available at present.[14] A non-hypertrophic variant of hypertrophic cardiomyopathy has also been described recently.[w33] Troponin T

Main causes of sudden cardiac death in children

Cardiovascular malformations
- ▶ Atrial repair of transposition of the great arteries (Mustard and Senning operations)
- ▶ Repaired tetralogy of Fallot
- ▶ Aortic valve stenosis
- ▶ Coarctation of the aorta
- ▶ Pulmonary atresia
- ▶ Pulmonary vascular disease (Eisenmenger syndrome)
- ▶ Coronary artery malformations

Other structural heart abnormalities
- ▶ Hypertrophic cardiomyopathy
- ▶ Myocarditis
- ▶ Dilated cardiomyopathy
- ▶ Kawasaki disease
- ▶ Arrhythmogenic right ventricular cardiomyopathy

Primary arrhythmias
- ▶ Long QT syndrome
- ▶ Wolff-Parkinson-White syndrome
- ▶ Atrioventricular block
- ▶ Other ventricular arrhythmia (for example, catecholaminergic ventricular tachycardia, Brugada syndrome, etc)
- ▶ Non-hypertrophic varieties of hypertrophic cardiomyopathy (troponin T mutation)

---

mutations produce characteristic histological myocardial disarray and seem to have a particularly poor prognosis in the few families described but their prevalence is unknown.

Sudden death in other cardiomyopathy

Sudden death in dilated cardiomyopathy is uncommon. A study of 63 children from Houston documented 16% mortality over 10 years, but only one of five deaths was sudden.[w34] In a report from Heidelberg four of 28 children died suddenly during a mean follow up of 4.1 years.[w35] In both studies arrhythmias of various types were present in at least half of the children, but they were unhelpful in risk prediction.

Restrictive cardiomyopathy is a rare diagnosis at any age. There is a high mortality in childhood with a two year survival of only 50%.[w36] Most deaths are sudden. The main predictors of mortality are syncope, chest pain, ischaemic changes on the ECG, and female sex. Cardiac transplantation is the only treatment to offer an improvement in outcome.[w36]

Arrhythmogenic right ventricular cardiomyopathy is a familial disease which usually affects young adult men.[w37] True diagnoses in childhood are exceptional. The disease may present with syncope, or with ventricular tachycardia with left bundle branch block morphology (that is, right ventricular origin). It may cause death in young athletes and seems to be particularly common in Italy.[w37] Risk assessment and therapeutic strategies are not well developed.[15]

The incidence of sudden death in apparently normal children beyond the first year of life is probably around 1–1.5 per 100 000 per year.[4] In addition to the various types of cardiomyopathy and coronary artery abnormalities discussed above, diagnoses first established after death include myocarditis.[4 16 w38] The exact mode of death in myocarditis is uncertain but it is probably caused by an arrhythmia. In other children death may remain unexplained after necropsy, but the circumstances may lead to a retrospective presumed diagnosis of a primary cardiac arrhythmia.

SUDDEN DEATH IN CHILDREN WITH PRIMARY CARDIAC ARRHYTHMIAS

Most sudden cardiac deaths that remain unexplained after necropsy are probably caused by primary cardiac arrhythmias. Arrhythmias which are known to be potentially fatal, and which would leave no trace after death, include polymorphic ventricular tachycardia in congenital long QT syndrome,[17 w39] other primary ventricular arrhythmias such as those described by Brugada[w40 w41] and Coumel,[w42] atrial fibrillation in Wolff-Parkinson-White syndrome,[w43] and congenital complete atrioventricular block. Retrospective confirmation of an arrhythmia is not possible unless a familial condition (such as long QT syndrome) is subsequently recognised in a family member. This group of arrhythmias also comprises the majority of diagnoses made after resuscitation from out of hospital cardiac arrest.[w44 w45]

Sudden death in congenital long QT syndrome

Congenital long QT syndrome is characterised by QT prolongation on the ECG in association with polymorphic ventricular tachycardia, and may affect as many as one child in 7000.[6] It is usually amenable to treatment with a β blocker, but some patients require pacemaker or defibrillator implantation.[w46] It is difficult to establish the overall mortality risk as death may be the first symptom, but 8% of 287 patients reported by the Pediatric Electrophysiology Society died suddenly during a mean follow up of five years.[17] The main predictors of sudden death in that report were extreme QTc prolongation (> 600 ms) and poor compliance with β blocker medication. Congenital long QT syndrome has dominant inheritance. Despite this, in the Pediatric Electrophysiology Society report only 39% of children with a clinical diagnosis had a positive family history of long QT syndrome, probably explained either by variable penetrance or because they represent new mutations. Diagnosis in a child should lead to screening of first degree relatives. However, long QT syndrome can be difficult to diagnose or to exclude because of the overlap of QT intervals in gene carriers and in the normal population. Although several gene defects causing long QT syndrome have been identified, genetic analysis is costly and time consuming and the diagnosis remains clinical in most cases. Because a normal phenotype in the presence of an abnormal genotype is associated with a risk of syncope or death, there may be an indication for genetic investigation of family members with apparently normal or borderline ECGs.[14]

Acquired long QT syndrome is the term sometimes used to describe QT prolongation seen in metabolic disturbances or with use of pharmacological agents. It may also be familial and may cause arrhythmias and sudden death (fig 21.2).[w46]

Sudden death in other ventricular arrhythmias

Catecholaminergic ventricular tachycardia, as described by Coumel, has some similarities with long QT syndrome.[w42] However, the QT interval is normal and polymorphic ventricular tachycardia is preceded by increasingly complex ventricular arrhythmias, including a characteristic bi-directional ventricular tachycardia. The exercise test and ambulatory ECG are often positive and are helpful in making the diagnosis. Treatment with a β blocker is usually effective but poor compliance with medication is associated with a high risk of death.

Brugada syndrome describes the association of polymorphic ventricular tachycardia or ventricular fibrillation with ST segment elevation in right precordial leads on the ECG.[w40 41] It is a familial condition, usually not causing symptoms until

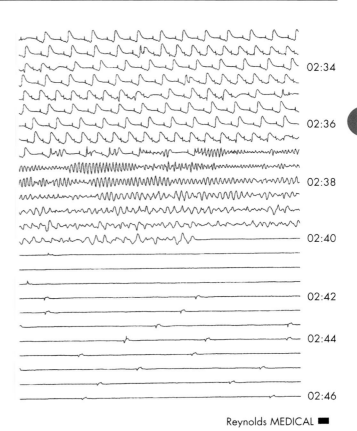

Reynolds MEDICAL ∎

Figure 21.2 Sudden death in acquired QT prolongation. The ambulatory recording shows development of polymorphic ventricular tachycardia which degenerates into ventricular fibrillation and then asystole.

early adult life, and is probably very rare in children. Diagnosis is difficult as the characteristic ECG changes are intermittent and can be very subtle. The only means of preventing sudden death in affected individuals is an implantable defibrillator.

Sudden death in Wolff-Parkinson-White syndrome

Wolff-Parkinson-White syndrome is one of the most common causes of arrhythmias in childhood, but sudden deaths are rare. The overall mortality risk is very difficult to quantify but may be around 1.5 per 1000 patient-years.[w47] Sudden death is probably caused by ventricular fibrillation which, in turn, is precipitated by atrial fibrillation in patients with a very short anterograde accessory pathway refractory period (fig 21.3). Cardiac arrest and sudden death mainly occur in adolescents and young adults and are very rare in younger children.[w48] Resuscitation from cardiac arrest is (perhaps not surprisingly) a strong predictor of risk, but syncope and atrial fibrillation have poor predictive value, although they would be indications for catheter ablation in any case. Although a short anterograde refractory period of the accessory pathway is thought to be the best electrophysiological indicator of risk, the predictive value of such a finding is poor.[w48] Patients with significant symptoms require treatment, irrespective of any associated small risk, but the role of risk stratification by invasive electrophysiology study in children with few or no symptoms remains unclear.

Sudden death in congenital atrioventricular block

Congenital complete atrioventricular block affects around one baby in every 20 000. Not all are recognised at birth, or even in infancy.[w7] The risk of sudden death is probably mainly related

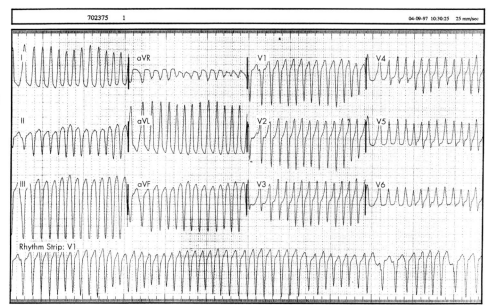

Figure 21.3 Atrial fibrillation in Wolff-Parkinson-White syndrome in a 10 year old girl with a history of recurrent syncope. There is a rapid, irregular, wide QRS tachycardia with a morphology which matched the pre-excitation seen in sinus rhythm. The accessory pathway was ablated.

to the ventricular rate. The development of symptoms is an indication for pacemaker implantation, but absence of symptoms in childhood or adult life does not imply absence of risk of sudden death.[w7] [w49] Risk stratification in asymptomatic patients is imperfect but pacemaker implantation is usually advisable in infants with a resting ventricular rate below 55 per minute, or in children below 50 per minute, especially if there are other arrhythmias or other findings on ambulatory monitoring.[w50]

SUDDEN DEATH IN YOUNG ATHLETES

Deaths during sports attract publicity but they are rare events. Estimates from the USA suggest that 5 per 100 000 young athletes (including children, teenagers, and young adults) have a predisposing condition and that about 10–25 such deaths per year occur in the US population of 260 000 000.[18] The most common structural abnormalities identified at necropsy are hypertrophic cardiomyopathy, coronary artery abnormalities, right ventricular cardiomyopathy, and aortic valve stenosis.[16] "Unexplained" cases may be caused by ventricular arrhythmia or atrial fibrillation in Wolff-Parkinson-White syndrome (as discussed above). Health screening programmes are in place for some young athletes but their efficacy has not been prospectively evaluated.

SYNCOPE IN APPARENTLY NORMAL CHILDREN

Syncope is a frequent problem in childhood. The common causes are benign whereas some rare causes are potentially dangerous.[19] A "simple faint", or vasovagal syncope, is said to occur in up to 15% of the normal population at some time during childhood. Other "vascular" but benign causes of syncope include neurocardiogenic syncope in older children and "pallid syncope" or "reflex asystolic syncope" in younger children. The mechanisms of these may be similar with inappropriate reflex bradycardia and hypotension.[w51] In the former syncope is often postural and in the latter a frequent trigger is surprise, minor hurt or frustration. Children or adults with repaired or unoperated congenital heart disease and children with other known heart disease should already be under review in a specialist follow up clinic. Syncope in such patients may be an indication for urgent reassessment or investigation.

> **Possible ECG abnormalities in children with syncope**
>
> ► QT prolongation
> ► Ventricular pre-excitation
> ► Atrioventricular block
> ► Left ventricular hypertrophy or ST/T abnormalities in hypertrophic cardiomyopathy
> ► ST elevation in V1–V3 in Brugada syndrome

Studies that examine children presenting with syncope rarely identify any diagnoses with a significant risk of death because such problems are rare. However, the spectrum of underlying abnormalities in children resuscitated from cardiac arrest is, not surprisingly, very different and more malignant. Diagnoses include various types of cardiomyopathy and substrates for primary arrhythmias including QT prolongation and ventricular pre-excitation, all discussed above.[w44] [w45]

Investigation of syncope

The history is of paramount importance in the assessment of children with syncope. Common but benign causes such as vasovagal syncope or hyperventilation are usually easily recognised. A history of syncope during or immediately after exertion, syncope preceded by palpitations, or syncope in the presence of a family history of premature sudden death, congenital long QT syndrome or hypertrophic cardiomyopathy should lead to referral for specialist evaluation. Detection of a cardiac murmur (or other abnormal signs on examination) should also lead to specialist referral as it may be a clue to the presence of aortic valve stenosis, coarctation of the aorta or hypertrophic cardiomyopathy.

The ECG is a valuable screening test in children with syncope and may identify QT prolongation, ventricular pre-excitation or atrioventricular block, or may be a clue to the presence of underlying ventricular arrhythmia or cardiomyopathy. Other investigations may include echocardiography, ambulatory or exercise electrocardiography or invasive electrophysiology, but the investigative strategy depends fundamentally on the history.

POPULATION SCREENING FOR UNSUSPECTED HEART DISEASE

The infrequency of prodromal symptoms and the absence of physical signs in children who die suddenly and are found at necropsy to have a cardiac problem may seem to be an indication for screening of the general population. However, there is no evidence that population screening of children for abnormalities such as hypertrophic cardiomyopathy is either feasible or appropriate, and no evidence that either early detection or treatment in the absence of symptoms has any effect on outcome. The only prospective population wide screening programme of normal children has been undertaken in Tokyo.[20] The reported prevalence of hypertrophic cardiomyopathy is around 1 in 15 000 and those children identified seemed to be at particularly low risk.[w52] The programme does also detect children with long QT syndrome, atrioventricular block, and Wolff-Parkinson-White syndrome by routine ECG but these problems are rare. So far it has not been possible to show that screening prevents sudden death.

SUMMARY

Many children who suffer sudden cardiac death are already known to have a heart problem. Many of these have had surgery for congenital heart disease and the risk of sudden death in such patients probably increases with time. The risks for such patients are probably decreasing with better and earlier surgical repair, but prospective identification of individuals at significant risk remains an elusive goal. In some children who die suddenly the necropsy reveals the cause of death. In others, who are apparently normal, the likely cause is a primary cardiac arrhythmia. Only a minority of children who die suddenly have previously experienced syncope.

Most children who experience syncope are not at risk of sudden death. Worrying features which would be an indication for investigation include syncope during or immediately after exercise, collapse in a swimming pool, a family history of premature sudden death or of potentially life-threatening cardiac problems, and abnormalities on clinical examination or ECG.

Several potentially fatal conditions are genetic in origin but unfortunately, at present, many of them are easier to confirm than to exclude. For instance, an echocardiogram during childhood cannot rule out the possibility of later manifestation of hypertrophic cardiomyopathy; some gene carriers of long QT syndrome have normal ECGs and yet 2.5% of normal children have a QT interval above the "upper limit of normal"; and the characteristic ECG appearances of Brugada syndrome are intermittent. For the moment identification of these conditions remains a clinical problem but in the future they will probably be simple genetic diagnoses. Some of the clinical management dilemmas, however, will probably remain.

REFERENCES

1 **Molander N**. Sudden natural death in later childhood and adolescence. *Arch Dis Child* 1982;**57**:572–6.

2 **Driscoll DJ**, Edwards WD. Sudden unexpected death in children and adolescents. *J Am Coll Cardiol* 1985;**5**:118B–21B.

3 **Neuspiel DR**, Kuller LH. Sudden and unexpected natural death in childhood and adolescence. *JAMA* 1985;**254**:1321–5.

4 **Wren C**, O'Sullivan JJ, Wright C. Sudden death in children and adolescents. *Heart* 2000;**83**:410–3.
▶ **A recent population based investigation of sudden death at age 1–20 years, looking at all causes.**

5 **Walsh CK**, Krongrad E. Terminal cardiac electrical activity in pediatric patients. *Am J Cardiol* 1983;**51**:557–61.

6 **Berul CI**. Neonatal long QT syndrome and sudden cardiac death. *Prog Pediatr Cardiol* 2001;**11**:47–54.

7 **Silka MJ**, Hardy BG, Menashe VD, *et al*. A population-based prospective evaluation of risk of sudden cardiac death after operation for common congenital heart defects. *J Am Coll Cardiol* 1998;**32**:245–51.
▶ **An important study identifying the main postoperative diagnoses with an increased risk of late sudden death.**

8 **Harrison DA**, Connelly M, Harris L, *et al*. Sudden cardiac death in the adult with congenital heart disease. *Can J Cardiol* 1996;**12**:1161–3.
▶ **Forty three per cent of deaths not related to surgery in patients in the adult congenital clinic were sudden. Eisenmenger syndrome was common. Very few patients had preceding clinical ventricular arrhythmias.**

9 **Wren C**. Late postoperative arrhythmias. In: Wren C, Campbell RWF, eds. *Paediatric cardiac arrhythmias*. Oxford: Oxford University Press, 1996:238–59.

10 **Saul JP**, Alexander ME. Preventing sudden death after repair of tetralogy of Fallot: complex therapy for complex patients. *J Cardiovasc Electrophysiol* 1999;**10**:1271–87.
▶ **A helpful review of the problems in prediction and prevention of late sudden death late after tetralogy repair.**

11 **Gatzoulis MA**, Balaji S, Webber SA, *et al*. Risk factors for arrhythmia and sudden cardiac death late after repair of tetralogy of Fallot: a multicentre study. *Lancet* 2000;**356**:975–81.

12 **Watkins H**. Sudden death in hypertrophic cardiomyopathy. *N Engl J Med* 2000;**342**:422–4.

13 **McKenna WJ**, Behr ER. Hypertrophic cardiomyopathy: management, risk stratification, and prevention of sudden death. *Heart* 2002;**87**:169–76.
▶ **A review of prediction and prevention, mainly in adult patients.**

14 **Vincent GM**. Role of DNA testing for diagnosis, management, and genetic screening in long QT syndrome, hypertrophic cardiomyopathy, and Marfan syndrome. *Heart* 2001;**86**:12–4.
▶ **A review of the contribution of genetic investigation to the identification of patients with familial, potentially life threatening disorders.**

15 **Corrado D**, Basso C, Thiene G. Arrhythmogenic right ventricular cardiomyopathy: diagnosis, prognosis and treatment. *Heart* 2000;**83**:588–95.

16 **Maron BJ**, Shirani J, Poliac LC, *et al*. Sudden death in young competitive athletes. *JAMA* 1996;**276**:199–204.
▶ **A retrospective series showing that 85% of sudden deaths were cardiovascular and 90% occurred during or immediately after activity. The most common diagnoses were hypertrophic cardiomyopathy and coronary artery anomalies.**

17 **Garson A Jr**, Dick M, Fournier A, *et al*. The long QT syndrome children. An international study of 287 patients. *Circulation* 1993;**87**:1866–72.

18 **Liberthson RR**. Sudden death from cardiac causes in children and young adults. *N Engl J Med* 1996;**334**:1039–44.
▶ **A detailed and authoritative review of sudden cardiac death.**

19 **McLeod KA**. Dizziness and syncope in adolescence. *Heart* 2001;**86**:350–4.
▶ **A comprehensive review of mainly non life-threatening causes of syncope.**

20 **Ino T**, Yabuta K, Yamauchi K. Heart disease screening in Japanese children. *BMJ* 1993;**306**:1128.

Additional references appear on the *Heart* website—www.heartjnl.com

22 PULMONARY HYPERTENSION IN THE YOUNG

Sheila G Haworth

Severe, sustained pulmonary hypertension leads to pulmonary vascular obstructive disease, which is potentially fatal. But recent advances in genetics and cell biology provide insights into the pathogenesis of this disease and new treatments offer an improved quality of life and increased survival. The field is moving rapidly, and it is time to adopt a more positive and aggressive approach to the management of pulmonary hypertension in children. The sustained clinical and haemodynamic improvement seen in many adults with primary pulmonary hypertension treated with continuous prostacyclin, and data from numerous experimental studies indicate that it is possible to arrest and perhaps even reverse the disease process. Potential is likely to be greater in the young in whom the vasculature is still remodelling. However, pulmonary hypertension is frequently unrecognised in early childhood and most children are referred late in the course of the disease, emphasising the need to increase awareness of the condition. This review focuses on the more common forms of pulmonary arterial hypertension in the young— persistent pulmonary hypertension of the newborn (PPHN), primary pulmonary hypertension (PPH), and pulmonary hypertension associated with congenital heart disease. It attempts to represent our current understanding of pulmonary hypertension in childhood, highlighting the key features of the condition, and offers a glimpse into the future.

▶ DIAGNOSTIC DEFINITIONS OF PULMONARY HYPERTENSION

Pulmonary hypertension is defined as a pulmonary arterial pressure > 25 mm Hg at rest or > 30 mm Hg on exercise, although pulmonary hypertension in childhood is usually associated with considerably higher pressures. Pulmonary hypertension can be described as either primary, being of unknown aetiology, or secondary resulting from cardiac or parenchymal lung disease. This description is unsatisfactory, however, since it takes no account of the similarities in pathobiology and response to treatment between primary and certain other types of pulmonary hypertension. It narrows our perspective. A new classification was proposed at a World Health Organization symposium in 1998, based on anatomy, clinical features, and an appreciation of the commonality of at least some of the underlying mechanisms.[1] PPH and pulmonary hypertension related to congenital heart disease, PPHN, connective tissue disease, HIV infection, drugs, and toxins were grouped together as "pulmonary arterial hypertension". This new classification encourages the extension of therapeutic modalities known to be effective in PPH to other forms of hypertension, in both adults and children.

Further clarification is necessary in children with congenital heart disease. In the majority of children pulmonary arterial hypertension is usually caused and driven by a cardiac abnormality which leads to the development of the Eisenmenger syndrome. However, in some children the abnormality is, and always has been, haemodynamically insignificant. Clinically these children behave as though they have PPH, and can be treated as such.

PATHOGENESIS OF PULMONARY VASCULAR DISEASE IN CHILDHOOD

During the past few years we have gained considerable insight into the molecular mechanisms responsible for the development of pulmonary vascular disease. Findings can be related to current treatment strategies and may suggest a new therapeutic approach. Genetic studies have concentrated on familial PPH (FPPH) and the mutations recently identified in FPPH have not yet been sought systematically in other forms of pulmonary hypertension.

Persistent pulmonary hypertension of the newborn

Failure of the pulmonary circulation to adapt normally to extrauterine life causes PPHN, a condition with a high morbidity and mortality despite the advent of inhaled nitric oxide (NO) therapy. PPHN is multifactorial in origin, although commonly associated with congenital and acquired hypoxic lung disease and congenital heart defects. Rarely, it is idiopathic. Irrespective of aetiology, during the first few days of life the intrapulmonary arterial wall structure is similar to that seen in fetal life and neonatal remodelling is impaired[2] (fig 22.1). Functional studies demonstrate impairment of the NO pathway, sometimes a deficiency of the NO substrate L-arginine, increased

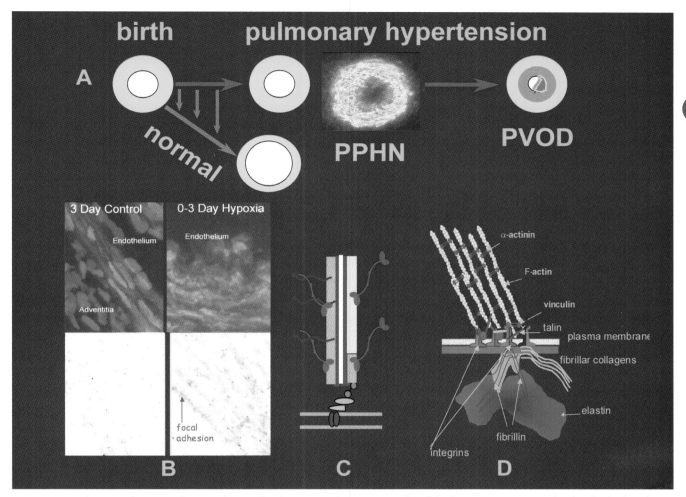

Figure 22.1 The upper figure (A) illustrates the rapid reduction in pulmonary arterial wall thickness occurring immediately after birth in the normal lung. This process is profoundly disturbed in persistent pulmonary hypertension of the newborn (PPHN) and an increase in medial thickness eventually leads to pulmonary vascular obstructive disease (PVOD) if the pressure remains high. Insert shows abnormal, hypertensive human peripheral pulmonary artery at three days, stained for γ actin. Mechanisms are illustrated in B, C, and D. (B) Confocal and transmission electron microscopy shows, in the left hand panel, the normal porcine peripheral pulmonary artery, and in the right hand panel, the pulmonary hypertensive vessel at three days. Normal remodelling entails reorganisation of the smooth muscle cell actin cytoskeleton which undergoes transient disassembly as the cells thin and elongate to spread around an enlarging lumen. In PPHN larger cells are packed with red actin myofilaments (phalloidin stained) while immuno-electron microcopy reveals sheets of actin bundles labelled with gold particles rather than actin being diffusely distributed in the cytosol. (C) Illustration of a myofilament. (D) All aspects of vessel wall remodelling are disturbed in PPHN, from the excessive myofilament assembly within the cell, focal adhesion remodelling at the membrane, and excessive connective tissue deposition in the matrix. Gene expression of tropoelastin and type I procollagen is abnormally high and steady state protein concentrations are increased. Vessels appear to become fixed in an incompletely dilated state. This is the beginning of PVOD in the young if the process cannot be arrested therapeutically.

concentrations of the endogenous inhibitor asymmetric dimethyl arginine, and persistently high circulating endothelin concentrations. Studies on normal animals reveal low NOS activity and relatively poor endothelial dependant relaxation at birth, and these systems fail to mature properly in PPHN.[3] Different relaxation pathways (NO, prostaglandin, endothelium derived hyperpolarising factor) mature at different rates and have different vulnerabilities to insult. Vasoconstrictor endothelin ET-A receptors increase and endothelial vasodilator ET-B receptors decrease. Thus failure to reduce the pulmonary vascular resistance after birth appears to involve a primary structural abnormality, failure of endothelial dependent ± independent relaxation, and an excess of vasoconstrictor activity(s). The rationale for giving NO and phosphodiesterase inhibitors is that there is an absolute or relative lack of the endogenous substance. Oxygenation usually improves and the need for extracorporeal membrane oxygenation is reduced. New strategies directed at antagonising vasoconstriction and

modifying smooth muscle cell cytoskeletal remodelling are indicated. Outcome depends on causality. Some babies who appeared to recover normally were later found to have persistent arterial medial hypertrophy.

The relation between PPHN and PPH is uncertain but children who present with PPH during the first years of life frequently have a history which suggests that they were pulmonary hypertensive from birth. A history of prenatal stress and perinatal morbidity is not uncommon. Occasionally an infant thought to have PPH is found to have a secundum atrial septal defect. This is usually an incidental, though protective abnormality, and should not be closed.

Primary pulmonary hypertension
The number of children diagnosed with PPH and being referred for treatment has increased greatly since it became apparent that even infants could benefit from the treatments given to adult patients with the disease.

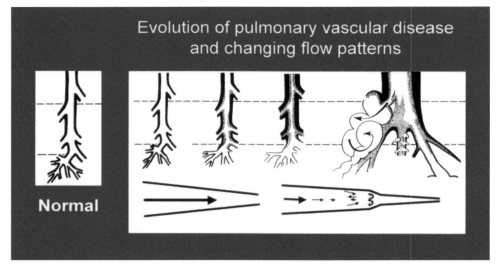

Figure 22.2 Evolution of pulmonary vascular disease in the young showing the early reduction in number of arteries, the increase in muscularity, and development of intimal proliferation. Two classification systems are used to describe these changes, the more recent concentrating on the early structural changes preceding intimal damage in a pulmonary vascular bed which is still developing, the other being the Heath and Edwards classification. A biopsy must be taken at sufficient depth (upper interrupted line) to include some pre-acinar arteries in which intimal proliferation first develops. For a limited time the more peripheral arteries can have a misleading near-normal appearance, a predilatation phase associated with an increase in mortality and morbidity at and after intracardiac repair. Blood flow patterns change from laminar to turbulent with disease progression.

Genetics

Familial PPH

Only 6% of cases of PPH have been reported as familial.

The disease is transmitted as an autosomal dominant trait, with incomplete penetrance. The chance of a person carrying a gene for FPPH developing the disease is higher in females (0.30) than males (0.15), and a female predominance is present from early childhood. FPPH shows gene anticipation, the disease frequently presenting at an earlier age in successive generations.

The FPPH locus maps to chromosome 2q31-32 and germline mutations have been identified in the bone morphogenetic protein receptor -II (BMPR2).[4] The BMPs form the largest group within the transforming growth factor β (TGF-β) family of cytokines. The PPH disease associated mutations identified would be expected to disrupt signalling pathways mediated by BMPR2, thereby removing a mechanism for keeping vascular remodelling in check and facilitating abnormal proliferation of pulmonary vascular cells.

Mutation in another TGF-β family member, the type I receptor gene, activin receptor-like kinase (ALK1) has been implicated in hereditary haemorrhagic telangectasia associated pulmonary hypertension.[5]

It is likely that other PPH genes remain to be identified. BMPR2 mutations have not been identified in some 60% of FPPH cases, and most sporadic cases do not appear to harbour BMPR2 mutations. There are also families in whom pulmonary hypertension is associated with haemoglobinopathies and platelet storage defects.

Sporadic PPH

BMPR2 defects have been described in 26% of sporadic cases of PPH, in some cases arising as "de novo" or spontaneous mutations.[6] Sporadic and familial PPH have the same pathological features and the patients can be treated in the same manner.

Pathobiology

At necropsy, most adults have advanced pulmonary vascular obstructive disease with plexiform lesions (fig 22.2). This picture is also common in older children and can be seen before three years of age. Particularly in young children, however, the cellular changes can be restricted to severe pulmonary arterial medial hypertrophy with pronounced intimal proliferation, lesions which are more likely to be potentially reversible. The instigators of this process are uncertain. Loss of one normal BMPR2 allele does not, in itself, produce the phenotype. It is now thought that PPH affects those with a genetic predisposition to respond adversely to a variety of stimuli, and that the clinical and structural findings represent the final common pathway. The following are thought important in the pathogenesis.

Endothelial dysfunction

Concentrations of circulating endothelin, a powerful vasoconstrictor and mitogen, are raised and expression of endothelin converting enzyme is increased. Prostacyclin and NO, vasodilators with antiproliferative and antimigratory properties, are reduced. Chronic treatment with prostacyclin or one of its analogues is a proven, effective treatment[7] while inhaled NO, NO donors and the phosphodiesterase 5/6 inhibitor sildenafil are as yet unproven alternatives/adjuncts in terms of both efficacy and safety. Endothelin receptor antagonists have proved safe and effective in small trials, mostly in adult patients, and are being trialled in younger patients.[8]

Intense vasoconstriction

Intense vasoconstriction is thought to be an early, common response to injury. Although pulmonary vascular disease is usually well advanced at presentation, the pulmonary vascular resistance falls in many patients on acute vasodilator testing, more often in children (50–60%) than in adults (20%). Calcium channel blockers are an accepted, conventional treatment, known to prolong survival in adults. Both hypoxia and anorexic agents which can cause pulmonary hypertension inhibit potassium currents in pulmonary artery smooth muscle cells causing membrane depolarisation, which promotes an increase in intracellular calcium concentration and hence vasoconstriction.[9] Moreover, finding dysfunctional voltage gated potassium channels in primary but not secondary

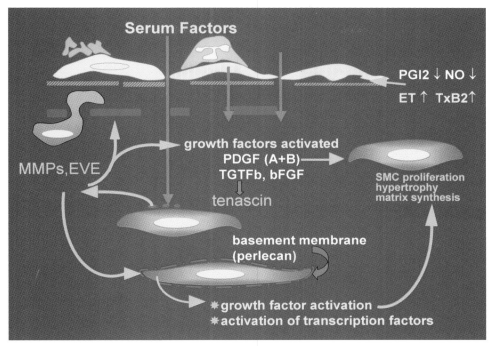

Figure 22.3 Factors driving the evolution of pulmonary vascular obstructive disease. Endothelial dysfunction reduces release of prostacyclin and nitric oxide (NO), causes adherence of activated platelets and leucocytes, enhanced release of thromboxane and endothelin, and loss of barrier function with leakage of serum factor into the subendothelium. This last action is thought to heighten activity of metalloproteinases (MMPs), including the proteolytic enzyme endogenous vascular elastase (EVE)[14 21] released from smooth muscle cells, to help induce structural remodelling, cause smooth muscle cell activation, disruption of the internal elastic lamina, and facilitate smooth muscle cell migration. MMPs also activate growth factors normally sequestered in the matrix in an inactive form. Increased tenascin expression is associated with cell proliferation, its downregulation with apoptosis. Tenascin amplifies the proliferative response to epidermal growth factor and fibroblast growth factor (FGF)-2 in vitro. Expression of fibronectin is widespread and this glycoprotein can facilitate smooth muscle migration. The innermost smooth muscle cells cease to express many smooth muscle specific contractile and cytoskeletal proteins before migrating through gaps in the internal elastic lamina. Changes in phenotype are widespread.

pulmonary hypertension suggests that potassium channels may play a significant role in the pathogenesis of PPH. Indeed, there is a general downregulation of potassium channel function in proliferating human pulmonary arterial smooth muscle cells.[10] In terms of potential treatment, ATP sensitive potassium channel openers probably offer the greatest promise since these agents are potent dilators of the pulmonary circulation and are still able to promote membrane hyperpolarisation in proliferating smooth muscle cells. However, the recent evidence that non-voltage dependent calcium entry pathways (transient receptor potential channels) are upregulated during pulmonary vascular cell growth, could point to other novel targets in the treatment of this disease.

Platelet function
There is an excess of thromboxane in relation to prostacyclin, predisposing to vasoconstriction and platelet aggregation. The role of serotonin in the pathogenesis of PPH is still uncertain, but raised plasma concentrations and impaired platelet storage of serotonin can occur. Serotonin transporters are overexpressed on pulmonary arterial smooth muscle cells.[11] Raised fibrinopeptide A concentrations and pathological studies indicate thrombosis in situ, and there is evidence of impaired local fibrinolysis. Anticoagulation increases survival in adults and is used routinely in children.

Dysfunction of the immune system
PPH appears to be autoimmune in some children, and pulmonary hypertension is a component of several autoimmune disorders, particularly scleroderma.

Whatever the nature of the initiating stimulus, the onset of pulmonary vascular disease is characterised by abnormal proliferation of endothelial and smooth muscle cells and fibroblasts (fig 22.3). Identifying a mutation in the BMPR2 receptor implicating defective control of vascular remodelling puts the structural abnormalities back in the forefront of research interest as being a/the prime mover in the pathogenesis, rather than being viewed always as the inevitable consequence of endothelial injury. Monoclonal cell expansion is thought to lead to the production of plexiform lesions in a subset of adult patients with PPH.

Congenital heart disease
Intrauterine pulmonary vascular disease is unusual, and the disease generally starts at birth.[12] The rate of change depends on the type of intracardiac abnormality, but some exceptional children appear to be genetically predisposed to develop an accelerated form of the disease. Endothelial cell damage, medial smooth muscle cell hyperplasia, hypertrophy, and site specific changes in cell phenotype are well described in early infancy[12] (fig 22.2). Respiratory unit arteries, about half of which normally form after birth, are reduced in size and number. This is the morphological substrate of pulmonary hypertensive crises, which most often occur in the presence of potentially reversible structural abnormalities. Endothelial dysfunction is present early. In potentially operable children the relaxation response to acetylcholine is impaired, basal NO production may be raised initially but then decreases, and the ratio of thromboxane to prostacyclin is raised, tipping the balance in favour of vasoconstriction and platelet aggregation. Impaired endothelial dependant relaxation occurs later in association with elevation in resistance and more advanced structural disease (fig 22.3). Dilatation and plexiform lesions contain abundant vascular endothelial growth factor (VEGF)

Abbreviations

ALK1: activin receptor-like kinase
BMPR2: bone morphogenetic protein receptor-II
FPPH: familial primary pulmonary hypertension
NO: nitric oxide
PPH: primary pulmonary hypertension
PPHN: persistent pulmonary hypertension of the newborn
PVOD: pulmonary vascular obstructive disease
TGF-β: transforming growth factor β
VEGF: vascular endothelial growth factor

which co-localises with TGFβ1. VEGF induces endothelium dependent relaxation, which may help ensure continued perfusion of the capillary bed. But it is also a potent angiogenic factor, and TGFβ upregulates its angiogenic activity in vitro. The VEGF in the plexiform lesions could in theory stimulate angiogenesis. As intimal obstruction develops, flow becomes more turbulent (fig 22.2) and in vitro studies suggest that this is likely to have an unfavourable influence on gene transcription. Laminar flow is associated with activation of genes such as eNOS and cyclo-oxygenase COX2 but turbulent flow is associated with the localised upregulation of VCAM-1 and ICAM-1, encouraging leucocyte recruitment and activation.[13] Changes in mechanical stress also alter expression of specific genes in the smooth muscle cell, such as platelet drived growth factor.

Postoperative pulmonary hypertension

The patient with repaired congenital heart disease has effectively been turned into a patient with PPH, with the added problem of a compromised myocardium. Survival is significantly worse in the untreated patient with PPH than in most patients with Eisenmenger syndrome. Assuming that these patients cannot be helped by further surgery, they should generally be treated as though they had PPH, and without delay.

Pulmonary hypertension and portal hypertension

An increased pulmonary arterial pressure can sometimes complicate the question of liver transplantation and necessitate careful haemodynamic assessment. The pathological features can resemble those found in hypertensive congenital heart disease, possibly caused by vasoconstriction because the damaged liver cannot degrade circulating vasoconstrictor mediator(s). But generalised pulmonary arterial dilatation can also occur. Pulmonary hypertension is not usually a contraindication to liver transplantation.

Pathobiology: a comment

Clinical and experimental studies have identified potentially important structural and functional abnormalities, but whether these are a cause or a consequence of the disease remains to be determined. Experimental models of PPHN have demonstrated that the term "endothelial dysfunction" does not apply to all aspects of endothelial function, but to specific signal transduction pathways in certain segments/regions of the pulmonary vascular bed. Functioning pathways should be identified and exploited. Strategies shown to be effective in attenuating the hypertensive response to hypoxia and monocrotaline in rats include endothelin receptor blockers, modulating potassium channels, inhibition of 5-lipoxygenase activating protein, serine elastase inhibitors,[14] inhaled NO, and inhibition of 3'5'guanosinemonophosphate specific phosphodiesterase. In vitro studies indicate that there will be a role for smooth muscle growth

inhibitors. The approach to gene therapy has concentrated on the overexpression of vasodilator genes, principally NO and prostaglandin I synthase, and results are encouraging.[15 16]

Tackling the different facets of angiogenesis is problematic. Growth of new vessels is a priority in the young who have developed pulmonary hypertension before the lung fulfilled its growth potential. Intratracheal (VGEF) 165 gene injection attenuated hypoxic pulmonary hypertension in rats, but the mechanism is uncertain. VEGF may not stimulate growth of normal vessels and in man it is abundant in plexiform lesions, which some have described as a form of uncontrolled angiogenesis. Evidence that advanced disease can be arrested has come from clinical experience with continuous intravenous prostacyclin therapy in PPH.[17] Prostacyclin appears to be acting primarily by structurally remodelling the pulmonary vasculature rather than acting solely as a pulmonary vasodilator. New treatments will preferentially target the long term control of vascular remodelling rather than vasoconstriction. In young people, the aim must be to act as quickly and as effectively as possible to re-track pulmonary arterial remodelling along the normal pathway.

DIAGNOSIS AND CLINICAL INVESTIGATION OF PPH

In PPH, symptoms vary and are age related. Infants and young children may fail to thrive, tire easily, have exertional dyspnoea, and occasionally have chest pain. Symptoms suggestive of pulmonary hypertensive crises as well as syncope can occur at any age. In patients treated with chronic vasodilator therapy the most important determinants of survival are: (1) age—a 5 year survival of 88% in children of less than 6 years of age, as compared with 25% for older children; and (2) the acute response to prostacyclin—the 5 year survival being 86% as compared with 33% for non-responders. In congenital heart disease, symptoms and signs reflect the natural history of pulmonary vascular disease with and without surgery in the different anomalies.

The accepted approach to evaluating a child who has, or is suspected of having pulmonary hypertension is well described[18]. The following tests are crucial:

► Cross sectional echocardiography clarifies intracardiac anatomy and an atrial communication is sought, particularly in the presence of an anatomically normal heart. Estimation of the pulmonary arterial pressure, right atrial and ventricular cavity size, and ventricular function is essential, and posterior bowing of the interventricular septum is sought in the presence of normal intracardiac anatomy.

At this point children should be referred to a specialist centre for further evaluation and treatment.

► Exercise test, a six minute walk test or surrogate according to age and capacity, to measure the degree of functional impairment. In PPH exercise capacity correlates with right atrial pressure, pulmonary arterial pressure, and cardiac index. Pronounced limitation (< 10% predicted) is associated with increased risk at cardiac catheterisation.

► Pulmonary function tests, which reflect clinical severity and haemodynamic status.

► Oxygen saturation measurements, including a sleep assessment.

All the above tests are also used to monitor progress and the response to treatment. Tests carried out primarily to detect chronic thromboembolic disease are rarely indicated in childhood.

Cardiac catheterisation

Adequate sedation and meticulous attention to acid base status and blood loss is essential in children. Following a conventional study, acute vasodilator testing is carried out using 100% oxygen and short acting vasodilators such as inhaled NO, intravenous epoprostenol, and intravenous adenosine. Patients are perhaps best studied under light general anaesthesia, with respiratory gas analysis. Using measured oxygen consumption together with arteriovenous oxygen difference (bound and dissolved) cardiac output is calculated and pulmonary vascular resistance determined. In children who are extremely ill, cardiac catheterisation should not be unduly prolonged but testing with at least 100% oxygen and inhaled NO is mandatory in all cases because long term treatment is based on the response. A positive response to acute vasodilator testing is defined as $\geq 20\%$ fall in pulmonary arterial pressure in the presence of an unchanged or increased cardiac output. Atrial septostomy/septectomy should be considered at the time of diagnostic catheterisation in severely ill children (particularly if there is a history of drop attacks) whose anatomy is such that there is no opportunity for right to left shunting to acutely decompress the right heart and improve systemic output.

An open lung biopsy may be indicated in complex congenital heart disease, suspected veno-occlusive disease, and vasculitis. Assessment includes quantitative morphometry to determine vascular development and a description of the pathological abnormalities. When evaluating an individual lung biopsy it is wiser to describe all the abnormalities present rather than to try to classify them, and relate the structural findings to the clinical and haemodynamic data. In young children with congenital heart disease the Heath and Edwards classification can underestimate the risk of surgery when severe medial hypertrophy (grade I) and/or exuberant cellular intimal proliferation (grade II) can be associated with pulmonary hypertensive crises and a high resistance.

MANAGEMENT OF THE PULMONARY HYPERTENSIVE CHILD
Lessons learnt in the management of children with PPH are now being applied to other forms of pulmonary hypertension in childhood.

Primary pulmonary hypertension
Treatment for PPH is treatment for life. The therapeutic regimen has to be tailored to meet the needs of each individual and adjusted as and when required according to changes in clinical and haemodynamic status. Children need close monitoring of the clinical course to ensure that a satisfactory response to treatment is sustained, with recatheterisation if necessary. Optimising the management of these patients greatly improves quality of life and survival.

Children with a positive response to acute vasodilator testing are given calcium channel blockers, usually nifedipine. Actuarial survival increased in adults treated with this drug. However, the magnitude of response which predicts long term survival is unknown in the young and clinical deterioration demands urgent revision of treatment.

Children unresponsive to acute vasodilator testing are not treated with calcium channel blockers which can have adverse effects and precipitate or worsen right heart failure. Older, compliant children in New York Heart Association functional class II can take nebulised iloprost which has a similar molecular structure to epoprostenol. But regular, effective dosing (6–12 times a day) is difficult in young children. The dual endothelin receptor antagonist Tracleer (bosentan), efficacious in adults, is now being trialled in children. The oral prostacyclin analogue beraprost sodium is efficacious in adults, but recommended only for those with less severe pulmonary hypertension and is largely untried in children. The subcutaneous analogue of prostacyclin treponistil (UT-15) is too painful for use in children. The phosphodiesterase inhibitor sildenafil is untrialled, its effect appears to be relatively short lived in sick children, and there is a risk of irreversible retinal damage linked to phosphodiesterase VI inhibition. The proven treatment of choice for the very sick child is chronic intravenous epoprostenol (prostacyclin) therapy. The dose is titrated according to clinical response, subjective and objective. Children generally need much higher doses of prostacyclin than adults and can become very tolerant of the drug, requiring constant, aggressive, upward adjustment of their dosage. Despite the obvious logistical problems, infants and young children can be managed satisfactorily. Training of two family carers by experienced nursing staff and a network of local support is essential. The side effects of the drug experienced by children are similar to those seen in adults. Clinical and haemodynamic improvement is generally sustained.

Other management strategies include:
- supplemental domiciliary oxygen—this provides symptomatic improvement for those with systemic arterial desaturation
- anticoagulation—warfarin rather than aspirin or dipyridamole is recommended to prevent thrombosis in situ, although aspirin is more tolerable in early infancy
- supportive medical therapy—diuretics are indicated to control the fluid retention of right heart failure, but fluid can also appear with the onset of medical therapy; there is no good evidence that digoxin is helpful in the treatment of right heart failure in children
- atrial septostomy/septectomy, if indicated
- organisation of care in the community and contact with patients' support groups is essential.

Screening and genetic testing
Parents almost invariably request screening of siblings and genetic counselling. All first degree relatives are screened in FPPH. It is thought that an individual in a family with FPPH has a 5–10% lifetime risk of developing PPH. Genetic testing is still not routine. DNA sequencing is necessary because mutations in the BMPR-2 gene appear to be "private" to each family.

Congenital heart disease
Correlating the physiological findings with structural observations in different types intracardiac abnormality has improved the accuracy with which immediate and long term outcome can be predicted with and without corrective surgery.[19] However, prediction is still more difficult in young than in older children. Severe medial hypertrophy, although potentially reversible, increases the risk of postoperative pulmonary hypertensive crises. The most crucial factor in determining late outcome is the age at which repair is carried out. Most children operated upon by 9 months of age have a normal pulmonary vascular resistance one year after repair. After 2 years of age resistance may fall, but not to a normal level. These observations indicate vessel wall remodelling towards normality, continued growth, and a demonstrable improvement in endothelial function. Repairing an intracardiac abnormality in the presence of established disease accelerates the progression of disease and the onset of right ventricular failure and death. The effect of associated lesions, such as coarctation of the aorta, must also be taken into account, even when repaired earlier. If there is doubt about the likely outcome of surgical repair, then an open lung biopsy should clarify the position.

For patients with the Eisenmenger syndrome treatment is still largely empirical and includes:

- long term oxygen treatment at home which gives subjective improvement and can increase survival
- dipyridomole to reduce platelet aggregation, but it may also have a beneficial vasodilatory effect as a phosphodiesterase inhibitor
- anticoagulation
- venesection with plasma dilution in those with a high haematocrit is not used routinely but may afford symptomatic relief to some patients; frequent venesections causing iron deficiency can increase the risk of cerebrovascular accidents.

Treatment with prostacyclin is tempting, but its efficacy is not yet proven in patients with the classical Eisenmenger syndrome. Given intravenously this non-selective vasodilator can cause systemic hypotension in the presence of a pulmonary–systemic communication. Inhalation of a stable analogue would be more appropriate. Patients with advanced pulmonary vascular obstructive disease may, like those with PPH, be unable to increase their NO production on exercise. Chronic administration of L-arginine might be helpful if it could be shown conclusively that these patients have a relative substrate deficiency of NO production.

Calcium channel blockers are not used.

Scleroderma and other connective tissue disorders

Chronic intravenous epoprostenol treatment has improved exercise capacity and haemodynamics in adults,[20] and children are treated in a similar fashion. Those with inflammatory disease are also given immunosuppressive drugs.

Finally, the only effective treatment for the very sick patient with pulmonary vascular disease of any aetiology who has failed medical treatment is lung transplantation. This is not usually an option in young children, but some older patients with PPH being treated as a bridge to transplantation have improved to such an extent that they are being treated medically long term rather than being transplanted. Since the results of transplantation are less than optimal, transplantation should only be considered when the expected survival time is less than the expected survival after transplantation. In future, we can hope that prompt early referral and effective treatment with the new and emerging therapies will postpone the need for transplantation indefinitely in many young people.

PERSPECTIVES ON FUTURE MANAGEMENT

There is an urgency to:

- educate the medical professions to ensure earlier diagnosis and referral
- improve non-invasive evaluation of disease severity, progression, and response to treatment in children
- maximise the effect of current treatment, by selective, trialled combinations of drugs for use at different stages of disease
- elucidate the role of endothelin receptor antagonists—the extent to which they can replace/be used with intravenous prostacyclin and the different analogues
- develop new, stable prostacyclin analogues with a longer half life for oral and inhalational use and specific phosphodiesterase V inhibitors
- explore novel treatments such as elastase inhibitors, gene therapy, and treatments based on exploitation of key signalling pathways identified by BMPR2 mutations in FPPH

- stimulate growth of new, normal vessels, particularly in the young who have developed pulmonary hypertension before the lung fulfilled its growth potential and in whom growth potential is greater.

REFERENCES

1 **Rich S**. Primary pulmonary hypertension: executive summary from the world symposium on primary pulmonary hypertension 1998, Evian, France, 6–10 September 1998. Rich S, 2002.
- **Recent WHO consensus classification of pulmonary hypertension.**
2 **Haworth SG**. Pathobiology of pulmonary hypertension in infants and children. *Prog Ped Card* 2001;**12**:249–69.
- **Useful review.**
3 **Tulloh RMR**, Hislop AA, Boels PJ, *et al.* Chronic hypoxia inhibits postnatal maturation of porcine intrapulmonary artery relaxation. *Am J Physiol* 1997;**272**:H2436–45.
4 **The International PPH Consortium**, Lane KB, Machado RD, Pauciulo MW, *et al.* Heterozygous germline mutations in a TGF-β receptor, BMPR2, are the cause of familial primary pulmonary hypertension. *Genetics* 2000;**26**:81–4.
- **The first paper reporting germline mutations in the BMPR2 gene in FPPH.**
5 **Johnson DW**, Berg JN, Baldwin MA, *et al.* Mutations in the activin receptor-like kinase 1 gene in hereditary haemorrhagic telangiectasia type 2. *Nat Genet* 1996;**13**:189–95.
6 **Thompson JR**, Machado RD, Pauciulo MW. Sporadic primary pulmonary hypertension is associated with germline mutations of the gene encoding BMPR-II, a receptor member of the TGF-β family. *J Med Genet* 2000;**37**:741–5.
- **The first paper reporting mutations in the BMPR2 gene in 26% of sporadic cases of PPH.**
7 **Barst RJ**, Rubin LJ, Long WA, *et al.* A comparison of continuous intravenous epoprostenol (prostacyclin) with conventional treatment for primary pulmonary hypertension. *N Engl J Med* 1996;**334**:296–301.
- **Definitive paper showing that this treatment improves quality of life and survival.**
8 **Rubin LJ**, Badesch DB, Barst RJ, *et al.* Bosentan therapy for pulmonary arterial hypertension. *N Engl J Med* 2002;**346**:896–903.
- **Definitive study demonstrating efficacy of bosentan.**
9 **Weir EK**, Reeve HL, Huang JM, *et al.* Anorexic agents aminorex, fenfluramine, and dexfenfluramine inhibit potassium current in rat pulmonary vascular smooth muscle and cause pulmonary vasoconstriction. *Circulation* 1996;**94**:2216–20.
10 **Cui Y**, Tran S, Tinker A, *et al.* The molecular composition of K(ATP) channels in human pulmonary artery smooth muscle cells and their modulation by growth. *Am J Respir Cell Mol Biol* 2002;**26**:135–43.
11 **Eddahibi S**, Humbert M, Fadel E, *et al.* Serotonin transporter overexpression is responsible for pulmonary artery smooth muscle hyperplasia in primary pulmonary hypertension. *J Clin Invest* 2001;**108**:1141–50.
12 **Hall SM**, Haworth SG. Onset and evolution of pulmonary vascular disease in young children: abnormal postnatal remodelling studied in lung biopsies. *J Pathol* 1992;**166**:183–94.
- **Clinico-pathological studies describing onset and evolution of pulmonary vascular disease in children with congenital heart disease.**
13 **Resnick N**, Gimbrone MA Jr. Hemodynamic forces are complex regulators of endothelial gene expression. *FASEB J* 1995;**9**:874–82.
- **Describes the impact of patterns of flow on gene expression.**
14 **Cowan KN**, Heilbut A, Humpl T, *et al.* Complete reversal of fatal pulmonary hypertension in rats by a serine elastase inhibitor. *Nat Med* 2000;**6**:698–702.
- **Indicates potential role of elastase inhibitors in treatment of pulmonary vascular disease.**
15 **Geraci MW**, Gao B, Shepherd DC, *et al.* Pulmonary prostacyclin synthase overexpression in transgenic mice protects against development of hypoxic pulmonary hypertension. *J Clin Invest* 1999;**103**:1509–15.
16 **Nagaya N**, Yokoyama C, Kyotani S, *et al.* Gene transfer of human prostacyclin synthase ameliorates monocrotaline-induced pulmonary hypertension in rats. *Circulation* 2000;**102**:2005–10.
- **Interesting study indicating potential for gene therapy while helping clarify rationale for treating pulmonary hypertensive patients with prostacyclin.**
17 **Ziesche R**, Petkov V, Wittmann K, *et al.* Treatment with epoprostenol reverts nitric oxide non-responsiveness in patients with primary pulmonary hypertension. *Heart* 2000;**83**:406–9.
18 **Barst RJ**. Primary pulmonary hypertension in children. In: Rubin LJ, Rich S, eds. *Primary pulmonary hypertension*. New York: Marcel Dekker, 1997:179–225.
19 **Haworth SG**. Pulmonary hypertension. In: Moller JH, Hoffman JIE, eds. *Paediatric cardiovascular medicine*. Philiadelphia: Churchill Livingstone, 1998.
20 **Badesch DB**, Tapson VF, McGoon MD, *et al.* Continuous intravenous epoprostenol for pulmonary hypertension due to the scleroderma spectrum of disease. A randomized, controlled trial. *Ann Intern Med* 2000;**132**:425–34.
21 **Rabinovitch M**. Pathobiology of pulmonary hypertension: impact on clinical management. *Semin Thorac Cardiovasc Surg Pediatr Card Surg Annu* 2000;**3**:63–81.

SECTION VII: IMAGING TECHNIQUES

23 UNDERSTANDING CORONARY ARTERY DISEASE: TOMOGRAPHIC IMAGING WITH INTRAVASCULAR ULTRASOUND

Paul Schoenhagen, Steven Nissen

In 1856 the pathologist Virchow published his now classic observations on atherothrombosis based on the examination of postmortem tomographic artery sections. The Virchow triad describes three components contributing to the atherothrombotic disease process: the vessel wall, the blood constituents, and blood flow.

In vivo coronary imaging techniques became available more than 100 years later with the introduction of selective coronary angiography in 1958 by Mason Sones. Selective coronary angiography has allowed the identification of significantly stenotic, advanced coronary lesions and narrowed the clinical interest of cardiologists on luminal dimensions. This singular focus on angiographic stenosis has resulted in a proliferation of surgical and catheter based revascularisation techniques allowing mechanical treatment of focal coronary artery disease (CAD). Expressions like "fixing rusty pipes" and "plumbing", used by cardiologist to describe atherosclerosis and its treatment, reflect a mechanistic view of CAD, based on the enormous success of these myocardial revascularisation techniques.

However, Virschow's observations and more contemporary models of atherosclerotic disease have led to an understanding of CAD as a systemic disease of a complex organ system (the vessel wall) and its environment (the blood components and flow phenomena). Importantly, the complex atherosclerotic disease process is frequently not reflected in the luminal silhouette because most lesions have silently developed over a long time before they obstruct the lumen.

Therefore direct imaging of the vessel wall has become a new goal in the assessment of CAD progression and prevention. Intravascular ultrasound (IVUS) represents the first clinical imaging technique enabling routine tomographic imaging of coronary arteries. Comprehensive technical and clinical reviews of IVUS have recently been published.[1 2] In this article we will give a brief summary of IVUS techniques and then describe the role of tomographic coronary imaging for a contemporary understanding of CAD using examples from past and present experience with IVUS.

▶ TECHNICAL CONSIDERATIONS

IVUS is performed during cardiac catheterisation using miniature ultrasound probes mounted on the tip of a coronary catheter. The IVUS probe emits high ultrasound frequencies, typically centred at 20–50 MHz. The ultrasound signal reflected from arterial wall structures is used to generate a grey scale image. Using a 30 MHz probe, corresponding to a wavelength of 50 µm, axial and lateral resolution is approximately 150 and 250 µm, respectively. The probe is placed beyond the target lesion site and the ultrasound catheter is then withdrawn during continuous imaging, resulting in a series of tomographic images of the vessel wall (fig 23.1).

Ultrasound is strongly reflected at the interface of different tissue structures. In coronary arteries these are the blood–intimal border and the external elastic membrane (EEM). Manual or computer aided planimetry of these two borders allows precise measurements of the lumen area, intima–media area, and EEM.[1] In addition, the ultrasound signal backscattered from the arterial wall allows the various tissue components to be differentiated, including the atherosclerotic plaque. The visual appearance of IVUS images of atheroma describe a continuum from echodense (bright echo signal) to echolucent (faint echo signal).[2] However, recent approaches using advanced image processing of the raw IVUS data such as radiofrequency analysis have improved characterisation of vessel wall characteristics.

Using IVUS, some morphologic features of atherosclerotic coronary plaques can be readily recognised. The reliability of ultrasound imaging in predicting the composition of atherosclerotic plaque components has been demonstrated in comparative studies of histology. Lipid laden lesions appear as hypoechoic, "soft" areas and fibrous or calcified tissues are recognised as bright echoes. In lipid laden lesions with prominent overlying fibrous "caps", a more reflective structure separating the soft echoes from the lumen is identified on the corresponding images (fig 23.2). The integration of information from adjacent images in a coronary segment allows three dimensional reconstruction and the calculation of atheroma volume (fig 23.1).

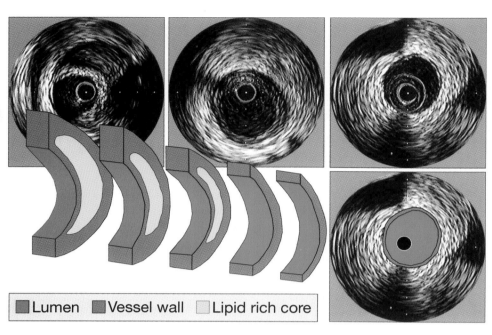

Figure 23.1 Principle of IVUS transducer pullback. The transducer pullback through a vessel segment allows the assessment of adjacent image slices and the three dimensional reconstruction. Importantly, tomographic imaging with IVUS allows the assessment of the coronary arterial lumen and vessel wall. Therefore the atherosclerotic plaque can be directly visualised. The first IVUS panel (top left) shows a crescent of severe atheroma extending for most of the vessel circumference from the 10 o'clock position to the 7 o'clock position. This lesion has a faint (lucent) echo signal of a lipid rich core of atheroma with a more echogenic fibrous cap.

NATIVE ATHEROSCLEROTIC LESIONS AND THE VESSEL WALL

Selective coronary angiography depicts coronary arteries as a planar silhouette of the contrast filled lumen. Lesions are defined angiographically by the focal narrowing of the luminal silhouette. However, severe atherosclerosis may not lead to an apparent luminal stenosis if the atheroma affects the entire vessel segment (diffuse disease). Furthermore, as originally described by Glagov and colleagues, atheromatous disease may result in focal expansion of the vessel size (enlargement of the EEM), a process known as arterial remodelling.[3] IVUS has been extraordinarily useful in confirming these two phenomena (diffuse disease and remodelling) in vivo (figs 23.1 and 23.2).

Diffuse disease

The experience with transplant vasculopathy is a particularly striking demonstration of the angiographic underestimation of diffuse disease. Coronary transplant vasculopathy represents the major cause of death in the first year after transplantation. However, because the heart is denervated, post-transplant coronary obstruction does not lead to angina pectoris. Therefore annual surveillance angiography, with and without IVUS, is commonly performed in patients after cardiac transplantation. Comparative IVUS studies have demonstrated the insensitivity of angiography in detecting transplant vasculopathy. Angiographic disease is present in only 10–20% of patients at one year and in 50% by five years, while the prevalence of arteriopathy detected by ultrasound is much higher, with abnormal intimal thickening seen by IVUS in 50% of patients by one year.[4] The diffuse involvement of entire coronary segments, which is characteristic for transplant vasculopathy, explains why this disease process does not lead to focal luminal narrowing and therefore is frequently not detected by angiography.

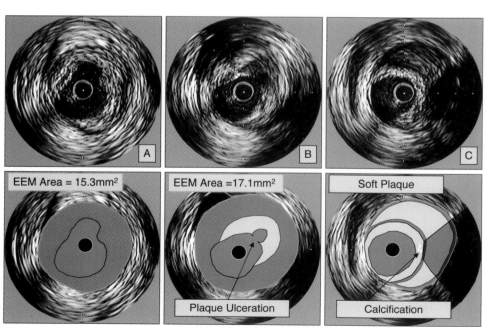

Figure 23.2 Examples of adjacent IVUS images showing different plaque composition. In panel A, there is mainly fibrous composition to the plaque. In panel B, there are both fibrous and soft components to the plaque, with associated plaque ulceration and expansion of the vessel EEM, indicating positive remodelling at the site of severe narrowing. Panel C shows a large area of soft plaque with some calcification of the fibrous cap, indicated by the presence of acoustic shadowing of the image behind the calcification.

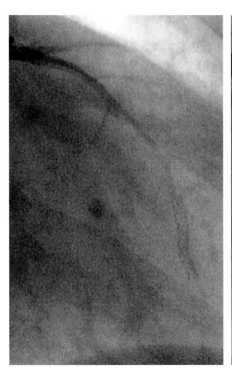
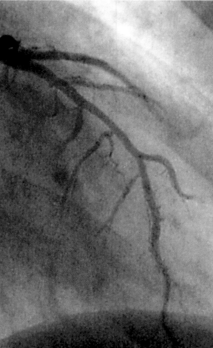
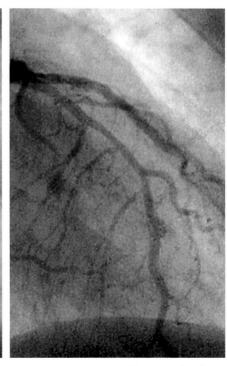

Figure 23.3 Clinical application of IVUS. Figures 3–5 show images obtained from a 26 year old patient, who presented three months after stent deployment in the LAD for severe CAD. This fig shows the selective coronary angiogram of the previously stented LAD lesion. A focal expansion of the lumen at the proximal stent edge is visible. The silhouette of the angiogram does not define the anatomy of such non-obstructive lesions.

A similar process may go unrecognised in typical native vessel atherosclerosis. Several IVUS studies have shown that angiographically "normal reference sites" are frequently affected by atherosclerosis.[5] The angiographic finding of "small vessels"—for example, in diabetic patients—represents another extreme example of diffuse plaque accumulation without focal narrowing.

Arterial remodelling
Another important observation has evolved from IVUS examination of transplanted hearts. In some transplant centres, a baseline angiographic and IVUS examination of one or more coronary vessels has been performed routinely. This is typically performed within a few weeks following transplantation and thus reflects the state of the vessel at the time of donor death. Most transplant donors are young in age, typically succumbing to trauma from motor vehicle accidents. Despite the young age of these donors, significant atherosclerosis is frequently detected by IVUS in donor coronary arteries. In one published study, more than half of donors at a mean age of 32 years had at least one site with an intimal thickness exceeding 0.5 mm.[6] Strikingly, nearly all of these subjects had completely normal angiograms.

The finding of diffuse or focal lesions without angiographic stenosis perplexed cardiologists who viewed diseased coronary arteries as "rusty pipes". In a solid pipe, accumulation of debris should always lead to a decreased luminal diameter. However, it seems clear that this paradigm is not appropriate in coronary arteries. In 1987 the pathologist Seymour Glagov described a crucial observation about early atherosclerotic lesion development.[3] Based on previous examinations in postmortem and animal models, Glagov described a positive correlation between EEM area and atheroma area in necropsy specimens of human postmortem arteries. The author hypothesised that focal disease is often not evident as luminal obstruction because of "compensatory" expansion of the vessel wall (arterial remodelling). Specifically, lesions with a stenosis < 40% were counterbalanced by an increase in arterial size that "compensated" for plaque accumulation, maintaining lumen area. In advanced lesions, remodelling was less evident and lumen size was reduced.

IVUS has allowed the in vivo study of remodelling. Ultrasound studies confirmed the correlation between EEM and plaque area and compensatory vessel enlargement or "positive remodelling" in early disease.[7] Subsequent IVUS studies have demonstrated a new dimension to arterial remodelling, negative remodelling or arterial shrinkage.[8] At diseased sites, the EEM may actually shrink in size, contributing to luminal stenosis. Initially described in restenotic lesions after coronary intervention, negative remodelling can also be found in mildly stenotic lesions of native coronary arteries.

Our understanding of the central role of remodelling in the pathophysiology of CAD is evolving. Initially positive remodelling was seen as merely compensatory, and therefore a welcome "positive" process. However, recent IVUS studies examining the relation between remodelling and clinical presentation in patients with CAD suggest a more complex role. In unstable patients, both EEM and plaque areas were significantly larger than the corresponding measurements in stable patients. In other words, positive remodelling is significantly more prevalent in the unstable patients and negative remodelling more prevalent in the stable patients.[9] Lesion development and, in particular, lesion stability appear to be related to the direction of arterial remodeling.

The initial experience with IVUS showed that the simultaneous assessment of lumen and vessel wall could provide important insights into lesion development and significance. It was soon discovered that these principles also apply to lesion response during coronary interventions (figs 23.3, 23.4, and 23.5).

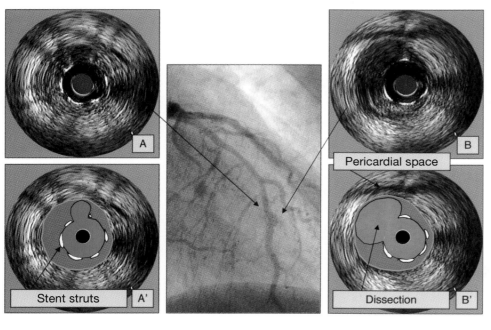

Figure 23.4 An IVUS interrogation of this segment shows a dissection of the vessel wall extending beyond the stent struts. In the video sequences flow was evident in the dissection cavities. The close proximity to the epicardium is obvious and influenced the decision to intervene.

Pericardial space

Stent struts   A'

Dissection   B'

PERCUTANEOUS CORONARY INTERVENTIONS
Restenosis

IVUS has shaped our understanding of restenosis after coronary percutaneous intervention. Initially, investigators believed that the predominant mechanism of restenosis after balloon angioplasty was intimal proliferation. However, ultrasound studies in peripheral vessels provided evidence that negative remodelling, or localised shrinkage of the vessel, was a major mechanism of late lumen loss.[8] Mintz and colleagues studied 212 native coronary arteries in patients undergoing repeat catheterisation after coronary interventions. At follow up, there was a decrease in EEM area and an increase in plaque area at the target lesion.[10] Interestingly, more than 70% of lumen loss was attributable to the decrease in EEM area, whereas the neointimal growth accounted for only 23%. Moreover, the change in lumen area correlated more strongly with the change in EEM area than with the change in plaque area. Lesions with an increase in EEM area at follow up (47% of segments studied) showed no change or an actual gain in lumen area and a reduction in angiographic restenosis (26% v

62%, p < 0.0001). These and other studies have established the role of negative remodelling in restenosis after mechanical intervention and explained the success of the concept of additional stenting in an attempt to prevent negative remodelling.

Stenting

IVUS has provided key insights into the reduction of restenosis rate observed with coronary stenting in comparison to balloon angioplasty. In serial IVUS studies of stented coronary segments, no significant change occurred in the area bound by stent struts, indicating that stents can resist the arterial remodelling process and that stent restenosis is primarily caused by neointimal proliferation. The prevention of negative remodelling, combined with the greater initial lumen expansion with stenting, results in a lower net restenosis rate.

However, during the initial clinical experience with stent implantation, acute stent thrombosis limited application to a relatively narrow subset of patients and required routine use of warfarin. Here, again, IVUS imaging played a pivotal role in optimising clinical results. The pioneering observations of

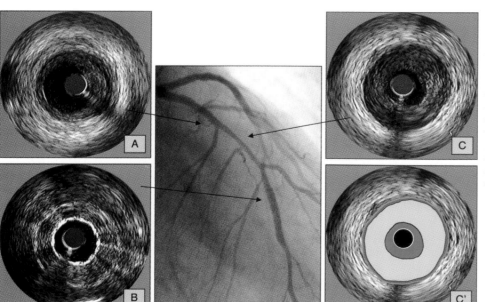

Figure 23.5 In panel A, the left anterior descending (LAD) artery appears normal on the angiogram, yet on IVUS there is a clear crescent of soft atheromatous plaque. Similarly in panels C and C' there is a severe concentric plaque indicating significant luminal narrowing. On angiography, at this point, there is a tubular narrowing as seen by IVUS. In panel B, the presence of the covered stent is seen with good and uniform stent expansion and a good angiographic result.

Colombo and colleagues, based upon IVUS, dramatically changed clinical practice.[11] These and other investigators showed that stent deployment with conventional balloon pressures resulted in a high incidence of incomplete stent expansion and poor apposition. In a pivotal series, Colombo and colleagues used IVUS imaging to guide high pressure dilatation, achieving full expansion and complete stent apposition in 96% of 359 consecutive, but non-randomised, patients. Patients with optimal expansion received antiplatelet treatment using aspirin and ticlopidine, but not warfarin. These technical modifications resulted in outstanding clinical outcomes. The incidence of acute and subacute stent thrombosis was less than 1%, and target vessel revascularisation for symptomatic restenosis at six months was 13%.

Thereafter, the concept of high pressure stent deployment disseminated rapidly, and larger trials demonstrated the safety of stent implantation using high pressures and antiplatelet treatment alone (without IVUS guidance). Consistent with these later trials, IVUS is no longer routinely used for stent optimisation. However, as newer interventional approaches are developed, IVUS imaging is routinely applied early in the life cycle of these innovations, often providing crucial insights into the mechanisms of benefit or complications. Accordingly, IVUS imaging is currently playing an important role in understanding the effects of radiation therapy for in-stent restenosis (brachytherapy), and the effects of drug eluting stents.

ATHEROMA BURDEN AND VULNERABILITY

It is not uncommon to see a young, previously healthy patient present with a massive myocardial infarction as the first manifestation of CAD. Despite great advances in the acute and chronic management of such patients, these cases demonstrate our failure to make the diagnosis of CAD in time to prevent serious complications. Traditional angiographic methods for assessing atherosclerotic disease rely exclusively upon the identification of significant luminal stenoses as a marker for disease burden. However, IVUS and histological studies show that "significant" stenoses represent only a small fraction of the total atheroma burden in patients with CAD (fig 23.5).[12] Presumably, patients with major, unheralded coronary events lack sufficient luminal narrowing to result in exertion ischaemia. In this setting, the acute event originates from rupture of a non-stenotic, clinically "silent" atheroma. Epidemiological data strongly support this model—several angiographic studies have documented that the majority of patients with acute myocardial infarction previously had only low grade stenoses at the culprit lesion site.

Because most acute coronary events are initiated from unheralded rupture of such subclinical "vulnerable" plaques, it is not surprising that angiography provides limited predictive value in identifying the risk of subsequent coronary events.[13] Currently, the best predictors of future events are established clinical and biochemical risk factors including age, sex, history of diabetes mellitus, hyperlipidemia, family history, and inflammatory markers. However, intracoronary ultrasound offers significant potential as a means to identify and characterise "non-stenotic" coronary atheroma burden, and plaque vulnerability. This approach may allow development of new strategies for interventions (medical or mechanical) by targeting atheromas at risk of rupture. Two strategies are being actively pursued: the assessment of focal plaque vulnerability and quantification of diffuse overall atheroma burden.

Focal plaque vulnerability
Plaque vulnerability describes the tendency of atherosclerotic lesions to cause atherothrombotic complications. It is well

163

established that most acute coronary syndromes are caused by the sudden rupture or superficial erosion of an atherosclerotic plaque.[12] The histology of these unstable plaques often reveals a lipid laden atheroma with a thin fibrous cap. A cascade of inflammatory processes probably plays a central role in the development and rupture of these lesions.[12 13] IVUS can demonstrate certain morphologic characteristics associated with plaque instability, including the necrotic, lipid rich core, the fibrous cap, and plaque rupture (fig 23.2).[14 15]

More recently, studies have demonstrated a strong association between positive remodelling (enlargement of the EEM) and an unstable clinical presentation (acute myocardial infarction or unstable angina). We examined 85 patients with unstable and 46 patients with stable coronary syndromes using IVUS and found positive remodelling significantly more frequent in unstable than in stable lesions (51.8% v 19.6%), while negative remodelling was more frequent in stable lesions (56.5% v 31.8%) (p = 0.001).[9] It is an attractive hypothesis that atheroma inflammation associated with lipid deposition, characteristic of unstable lesions, causes both plaque rupture and vessel expansion. A fibrotic response associated with plaque healing may be associated with negative remodeling.[16]

Diffuse overall plaque burden
Recent studies demonstrate that plaque vulnerability, plaque rupture, and subsequent plaque stabilisation are highly dynamic and widespread processes.[17] Subclinical plaque rupture and subsequent healing frequently occur during the development of atherosclerotic lesions and may be a common mode of disease progression. It is therefore an attractive hypothesis that the total plaque burden may be related to the propensity to develop morbid complications of CAD. This is supported by the experience with calcium quantification using computed tomography. Although calcium scoring only quantitates the calcified component of the overall plaque burden, a correlation between the calcium score and clinical events has been consistently demonstrated. In addition, pharmacological studies have suggested a decreased rate of calcium score progression during lipid lowering treatment.[18]

IVUS has great potential as a means to quantify the overall extent of atherosclerotic disease burden. IVUS imaging in patients with limited angiographic CAD typically demonstrates a large disease burden, often showing atherosclerosis in every cross section. Results from a serial IVUS study with measurements of plaque burden as the primary efficacy parameter have recently been reported.[19] Large serial IVUS

164

studies are currently underway examining the effects of different lipid lowering regimens and alternative antihypertensive agents on plaque burden. The results from these studies may further define the role of IVUS in the assessment of CAD progression or regression and the observation of the transition from stable "silent" disease to acute coronary syndromes.

IVUS represents the first tomographic coronary image technique allowing the assessment of the intramural structures of the vessel wall. However, non-invasive imaging modalities, in particular multi-slice computed tomography and magnetic resonance imaging, are under development for clinical coronary artery imaging.[20] These non-invasive techniques have particular appeal in a setting of prevention, where the invasive nature of IVUS is a distinct disadvantage. The future cardiologist will use a broadened diagnostic armamentarium to identify a wide range of obstructive and non-obstructive forms of CAD. In addition to the identification and treatment of highly stenotic lesions, which already cause clinical disease, new emphasis will be placed on the identification of "silent" non-obstructive lesions in accordance with the Virschow triad. The systemic and local treatment of these developing lesions has the potential to prevent CAD progression and avoid morbid complications such as acute coronary syndromes.

CONCLUSION

The above discussion shows that tomographic imaging of coronary arteries with IVUS has significantly influenced our understanding of the pathophysiology and treatment of CAD. The comparison to angiography explains the complementary role of tomographic imaging of lumen and vessel wall and is exemplified in figs 23.3, 23.4, and 23.5. In this young patient with precocious CAD, IVUS guided the therapeutic, interventional approach of the non-obstructive left anterior descending artery lesion. On the other hand IVUS allowed surprising insights into the disease process by showing extensive, diffuse disease in an angiographically relatively unsuspicious coronary segment.

We believe that tomographic coronary imaging with IVUS and emerging non-invasive modalities can contribute to an early diagnosis of subclinical CAD. It is an attractive hypothesis that this information could lead to improved preventive strategies.

REFERENCES

1 **Mintz GS**, Nissen SE, Anderson WD, *et al*. American College of Cardiology clinical expert consensus document on standards for acquisition, measurement and reporting of intravascular ultrasound studies (IVUS). *J Am Coll Cardiol* 2001;**37**:1478–92.
   ▶ **This ACC/AHA guideline paper gives a complete overview over procedural details of IVUS.**
2 **Nissen SE**, Yock P. Intravascular ultrasound: novel pathophysiological insights and current clinical applications. *Circulation* 2001;**103**:604–16.
3 **Glagov S**, Weisenberg E, Zarins C, *et al*. Compensatory enlargement of human atherosclerotic coronary arteries. *N Engl J Med* 1987;**316**:1371–5.
   ▶ **This seminal article describing arterial remodelling in human coronary arteries has changed our understanding of CAD.**
4 **Tuzcu EM**, Kapadia SR, Tutar E, *et al*. High prevalence of coronary atherosclerosis in asymptomatic teenagers and young adults: evidence from intravascular ultrasound. *Circulation* 2001;**103**:2705–10.
   ▶ **This article describes the frequent presence of atherosclerotic lesions in young persons who died from non-cardiovascular causes.**
5 **Mintz GS**, Painter JA, Pichard AD, *et al*. Atherosclerosis in angiographically "normal" coronary artery reference segments: an intravascular ultrasound study with clinical correlations. *J Am Coll Cardiol* 1995;**25**:1479–85.
6 **Tuzcu EM**, Hobbs RE, Rincon G, *et al*. Occult and frequent transmission of atherosclerotic coronary disease with cardiac transplantation: insights from intravascular ultrasound. *Circulation* 1995;**91**:1706–13.
7 **Losordo DW**, Rosenfield K, Kaufman J, *et al*. Focal compensatory enlargement of human arteries in response to progressive atherosclerosis: in vivo documentation using intravascular ultrasound. *Circulation* 1994;**89**:2570–7.
8 **Pasterkamp G**, Wensing PJ, Post MJ, *et al*. Paradoxical arterial wall shrinkage may contribute to luminal narrowing of human atherosclerotic femoral arteries. *Circulation* 1995;**91**:1444–9.
9 **Schoenhagen P**, Ziada K, Kapadia SR, *et al*. Extent and direction of arterial remodeling in stable versus unstable coronary syndromes: an intravascular ultrasound study. *Circulation* 2000;**101**:598–603.
   ▶ **One of the first articles describing the association between direction of remodelling and clinical presentation.**
10 **Mintz GS**, Kent KM, Pichard AD, *et al*. Contribution of inadequate arterial remodeling to the development of focal coronary artery stenoses: an intravascular ultrasound study. *Circulation* 1997;**95**:1791–8.
11 **Colombo A**, Hall P, Nakamura S, *et al*. Intracoronary stenting without anticoagulation accomplished with intravascular ultrasound guidance. *Circulation* 1995;**91**:1676–88.
   ▶ **This clinical series influenced the contemporary practice of stenting.**
12 **Ross R**. The pathogenesis of atherosclerosis: a perspective for the 1990's. *Nature* 1993;**362**:801–9.
   ▶ **Classical review of CAD which changed the concept of this disease.**
13 **Libby P**. Current concepts of the pathogenesis of the acute coronary syndromes. *Circulation* 2001;**104**:365–72.
   ▶ **A concise review of current concepts about acute coronary syndromes.**
14 **Yamagishi M**, Terashima M, Awano K, *et al*. Morphology of vulnerable coronary plaque: insights from follow-up of patients examined by intravascular ultrasound before an acute coronary syndrome. *J Am Coll Cardiol* 2000;**35**:106–11.
   ▶ **The first prospective IVUS study defining characteristics of mildly stenotic lesions which subsequently cause acute coronary syndromes.**
15 **von Birgelen C**, Klinkhart W, Mintz GS, *et al*. Size of emptied plaque cavity following spontaneous rupture is related to coronary dimensions, not to the degree of lumen narrowing. A study with intravascular ultrasound in vivo. *Heart* 2000;**84**:483–8.
16 **Burke AP**, Kolodgie FD, Farb A, *et al*. Morphological predictors of arterial remodeling in coronary atherosclerosis. *Circulation* 2002;**105**:297–303.
17 **Goldstein JA**, Demetriou D, Grines CL, *et al*. Multiple complex coronary plaques in patients with acute myocardial infarction. *N Engl J Med* 2000;**343**:915–22.
   ▶ **This article describes the frequent finding of additional complex angiographic lesions distant from the culprit lesions in patients presenting with acute myocardial infarction.**
18 **Callister TQ**, Raggi P, Cooil B, *et al*. Effect of HMG-CoA reductase inhibitors on coronary artery disease by electron-beam computed tomography. *N Engl J Med* 1998;**339**:1972–8.
19 **Schartl M**, Bocksch W, Koschyk DH, *et al*. Use of intravascular ultrasound to compare effects of different strategies of lipid-lowering therapy on plaque volume and composition in patients with coronary artery disease. *Circulation* 2001;**104**:387–92.
20 **Schroeder S**, Kopp AF, Baumbach A, *et al*. Non-invasive characterization of coronary lesion morphology by multi-slice computed tomography: a promising new technology for risk stratification of patients with coronary artery disease. *Heart* 2001;**85**:576–7.

24 ROLE OF ECHOCARDIOGRAPHY IN ACUTE CORONARY SYNDROMES

Sally C Greaves

The term "acute coronary syndrome" covers a spectrum of presentations, from unstable angina through to ST segment elevation myocardial infarction. There have been remarkable changes in the management of these conditions in the past two decades. With increasing emphasis on early reperfusion and prevention of left ventricular remodelling, echocardiography is assuming a prominent role in this area. It is non-invasive and relatively cheap, and is an ideal portable imaging technique. Newer imaging modalities, including myocardial contrast echo for the assessment of perfusion, hold great promise.

▶ TECHNICAL ASPECTS

The first cardiac ultrasound machines displayed an ultrasound pulse versus depth on an oscilloscope screen. Incorporation of time as a dimension in the late 1960s converted this to a single line M mode display. M mode echocardiography is still in use, but has largely been supplanted by two dimensional (2D) echocardiography,[1] which was developed in the 1970s. In the 1980s, spectral and colour Doppler were developed. The Doppler principle allows determination of the velocity and direction of blood flow, enabling assessment of valvar disease, shunts, and diastolic function. Transoesophageal echocardiography (TOE) was also introduced in the 1980s; initial probes were uniplane but multiplane probes are now routinely used, and there has been progressive transducer miniaturisation. TOE is very safe, with a mortality of less than 1/10 000,[2] but not completely risk free (table 24.1) and should be performed by experienced physicians. It is relatively contraindicated in patients with oesophageal disease—for example, varices, stricture, oesophagitis, scleroderma—and may be hazardous in patients with severe coagulopathy or poor respiratory function; it is essential that the performing physician be aware of such conditions. Transthoracic echocardiography (TTE) and TOE are complementary techniques. While TOE avoids image degradation related to the chest wall and lungs, TTE may visualise anterior structures and the cardiac apex better. More windows for Doppler interrogation are available from TTE, and it is easier to make standard measurements. Both TTE and TOE are technically demanding procedures, and meticulous attention is required to ensure optimal images are obtained.

One of the most important recent technological achievements has been the development of harmonic imaging, which greatly improves endocardial definition.[1] In conventional echocardiography, images are derived from ultrasound waves returned at the same frequency as the transmitted waves. However harmonic frequencies are also produced by the transmitted wave; in harmonic imaging, the machine uses the returning second harmonic to construct images. This improves image quality because there is less distortion of returned ultrasound waves (they are generated in the heart and only have to pass through tissue once), and few harmonics are produced close to the chest wall where many artefacts arise.

Digital echocardiography is an important advance[3] of particular relevance to the coronary care unit. This is a process by which cardiac cycles are recorded in digital format rather than on videotape. It has huge practical advantages and is ideal for the temporal monitoring of left ventricular (LV) function as it enables side by side high quality images to be quickly available at multiple stations.

COMPLICATIONS OF ACUTE MYOCARDIAL INFARCTION
Echocardiography is the mainstay of diagnosis of mechanical complications of myocardial infarction (MI),[4] and patients with unexplained haemodynamic deterioration should be immediately evaluated. It is important to recognise that TTE and TOE are complementary, and that TTE performed by an experienced echocardiographer may make an immediate diagnosis. In critically ill patients, image acquisition may be difficult; in these circumstances, TOE is extremely helpful.

Cardiac rupture
Many LV ruptures cause sudden death. However rupture may be subacute, allowing time for intervention. Direct visualisation of the rupture is often difficult as it may be only a "slit" in the myocardium and the location of pericardial fluid may not correlate with the area of rupture. However,

Table 24.1 Potential complications of
transoesophageal echocardiography

- ▶ Respiratory depression
- ▶ Hypotension
- ▶ Arrhythmias
- ▶ Laryngospasm/bronchospasm
- ▶ Dental trauma
- ▶ Pharyngeal/oesophageal/gastric trauma and perforation
- ▶ Aspiration
- ▶ Displacement of ET/nasogastric tubes
- ▶ Death

ET, endotracheal.

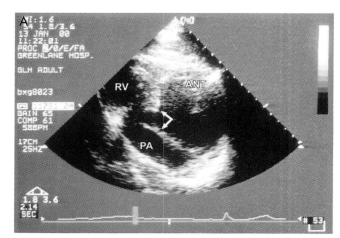

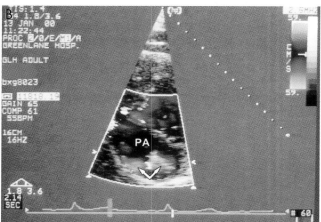

Figure 24.2 (A) Parasternal short axis transthoracic image showing a pseudoaneurysm of the inferior wall. The arrows show the characteristic abrupt disruption of the inferior wall and a narrow neck leading to the pseudoaneurysm. (B) Parasternal short axis transthoracic image (same patient as in A) showing bidirectional flow (arrows) from colour Doppler. Ant, anterior left ventricular wall, RV, right ventricle. PA, pseudoaneurysm.

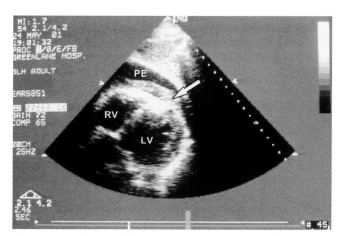

Figure 24.1 Subcostal long axis transthoracic image showing a pericardial effusion (PE) and intrapericardial thrombus (arrow) in a patient with left ventricular rupture post-infarction. LV, left ventricle; RV, right ventricle.

intrapericardial thrombus is often present (fig 24.1) and is very characteristic. It is rare to show flow into the pericardium. When caused by abrupt intrapericardial haemorrhage, the characteristic echocardiographic signs of tamponade may be absent, and diagnosis may rest on the volume of fluid and the clinical context. An LV pseudoaneurysm forms when the rupture is contained, so that a cavity outside the LV develops lined by pericardium and often thrombus. This can be distinguished from a true aneurysm by an abrupt interruption in the LV wall (as opposed to the smooth curve of a true aneurysm), a narrow neck, and low velocity bidirectional flow (fig 24.2A, B).

Ventricular septal rupture

Septal rupture may be difficult to distinguish clinically from mitral regurgitation (MR). From 2D echocardiography a discrete defect may be visible, but there may also be multiple serpiginous channels in the necrotic myocardium. The diagnosis can usually be made by TTE; experience is essential as the most useful views depend on the location of defect. Subcostal views are particularly useful in the critically ill, supine patient with inferior infarction (fig 24.3A). Small defects may not be visible but colour Doppler is very sensitive (fig 24.3B). Because these defects are often not discrete the degree of shunting may be difficult to evaluate. A large left–right shunt is characterised by hypercontractility of non-infarcted LV segments with a low LV stroke volume, high pulmonary artery flow velocities, and pulmonary hypertension. Posterior septal ruptures in particular tend to be complex and often associated with right ventricular infarction, which has an adverse prognosis.

Papillary muscle rupture

Papillary muscle rupture is the most serious mechanism of MR in acute infarction. It usually involves the posteromedial muscle which is perfused from the posterior descending artery, whereas the anterolateral muscle has blood supply from both diagonal and circumflex arteries. Rupture of a papillary muscle head causes severe MR; rupture of the entire trunk is generally fatal. Transthoracic echocardiography is often suboptimal in evaluation—views of the papillary muscles are often limited, the MR jet is eccentric, and colour Doppler is influenced by the low LV/LA gradient in acute severe MR. TOE is a particularly suitable imaging modality[4] and should be performed immediately if this diagnosis is suspected—it provides high resolution images of the papillary muscles (fig 24.4A) and accurate assessment of MR.

Rarely, multiple catastrophic mechanical complications of MI may occur in the same patient (figs 24.3A and 24.4A, B).

Aneurysm formation and left ventricular thrombus

True aneurysms complicate transmural infarction and are caused by dilatation of an area of scar (fig 24.5). An aneurysm is defined as deformation of both the diastolic and systolic LV contours with dyskinesis in systole. TTE is a sensitive tool for the diagnosis but occasional false negatives occur, usually when the aneurysm involves a small part of the apex or the

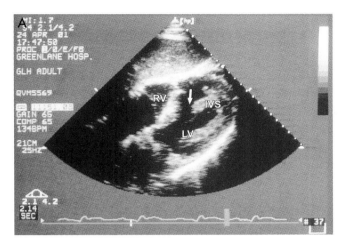

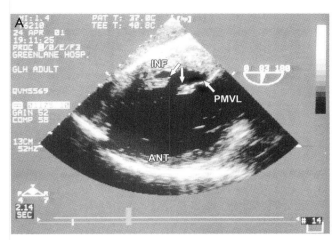

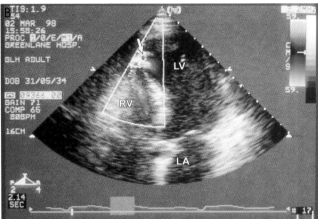

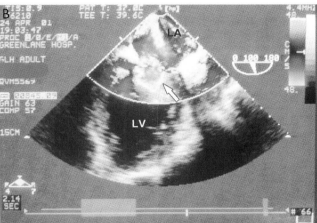

Figure 24.3 (A) Subcostal long axis transthoracic image showing a large post-infarction rupture (arrow) in the mid inferior ventricular septum (IVS). (B) Apical four chamber transthoracic image showing colour Doppler flow (arrow) through a postinfarction apical ventricular septal defect. LA, left atrium; LV, left ventricle; RV, right ventricle.

Figure 24.4 (A) Transgastric image showing rupture of the posteromedial papillary muscle postinfarction. The arrows point to the separated portions of the trunk of the papillary muscle. (B) Transoesophageal image (same patient as in A) showing pronounced flow convergence from colour Doppler (arrow) as flow accelerates towards a regurgitant orifice; this is characteristic of severe mitral regurgitation. PMVL, posterior mitral valve leaflet; INF, inferior LV wall; ANT, anterior LV wall; LV, left ventricle; LA, left atrium.

basal anterolateral wall. Aneurysm formation is a poor prognostic sign and is associated with congestive cardiac failure, arrhythmias, and thrombus formation. Left ventricular thrombi form in regions of stasis; they most commonly occur in the apex (fig 24.5) but may also be seen in lateral and inferior aneurysms. Certain echocardiographic characteristics (pedunculated and mobile thrombi) are associated with higher risk of embolisation.[5] TOE may not visualise the apex as well as TTE.

Pericarditis

Echocardiography is a sensitive technique for the diagnosis of pericardial effusion; however the absence of fluid does not exclude pericarditis. In patients who are anticoagulated, intrapericardial thrombus may be recognised. Echocardiography can identify a site for percutaneous drainage if required and be used to monitor the procedure.

Right ventricular infarction

Recognition of right ventricular (RV) infarction is important, as it requires specific haemodynamic management. This syndrome occurs in more than 30% of patients with inferior MI but is rare in anterior infarction and in isolation. Many right coronary artery occlusions do not result in significant RV infarction due to the lower RV oxygen demand, higher oxygen extraction ration, greater systolic/diastolic flow ratio, and collateral supply. Right ventricular infarction may be diagnosed

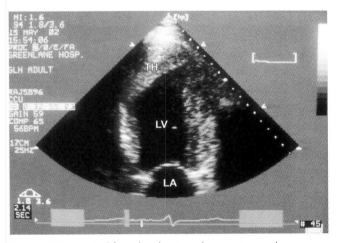

Figure 24.5 Apical four chamber transthoracic image showing extensive thrombus in an apical aneurysm. TH, thrombus; LV, left ventricle; LA, left atrium.

clinically and from right sided ECG leads, but echocardiography provides better assessment of the extent and severity.[6] Right ventricular dysfunction may be global or regional; the

RV outflow tract and apex are often spared, and hypercontractility in these regions may be a diagnostic clue. Echocardiography can evaluate complications of RV infarction. Functional tricuspid regurgitation is common; rarer complications are papillary muscle rupture and hypoxaemia from shunting through a patent foramen ovale caused by raised RA pressure.

RISK STRATIFICATION IN THE CORONARY CARE UNIT

Echocardiography is of tremendous value in risk stratification in MI and unstable angina. In general, it is helpful for these patients to have assessment of LV function before angiography. Echocardiography can provide a non-invasive biplane assessment, identify unsuspected valvar abnormalities, and evaluate right heart function. Left ventricular angiography may not be appropriate in critically ill patients and it is easier to obtain accurate information before invasive testing.

Patients with unstable angina and non-ST segment elevation MI are a heterogeneous group. Risk stratification is particularly relevant if conservative management is planned. Those patients with persistent wall motion abnormalities have more severe, chronic ischaemia and are at higher risk of adverse events.[7] All patients with acute MI should ideally have early echocardiography. In some patients it may assist in diagnosis; it may also assist decision making if the appropriateness of reperfusion is uncertain, by demonstrating the localisation and extent of wall motion abnormality. Echocardiography is particularly important in those patients who are not obviously high risk; many patients without clinical evidence of LV dysfunction will have significant wall motion abnormalities.[7] Patients with extensive regional abnormalities should have follow up echocardiography—this may detect early LV remodelling and other complications, and affect subsequent medical management.

Multiple indices of LV systolic and diastolic function have predictive value post-MI. Left ventricular wall motion score index (WMSI) is obtained by grading the motion of myocardial segments based on a standard model (table 24.2). It is particularly appealing, as while significant experience is required to interpret wall motion, it is highly reproducible. It reflects LV ejection fraction, but not LV size, so that quantitative measurements are also helpful. Left ventricular ejection fraction,[7] end systolic volume,[7] WMSI,[8] and the presence of even mild MR[9] are all early predictors of adverse outcome. Severe LV diastolic dysfunction tends to be associated with large infarctions, but a restrictive pattern is also independently associated with poor outcome.[10] Although there are numerous factors which can alter filling patterns, Doppler echocardiography is very repeatable. The Doppler myocardial performance index is a more recently developed measurement combining indices of systolic and diastolic function.[11] Repeated echocardiographic measurements have particular value,[12] as they reflect LV remodelling, characterised by alterations in LV size, shape, and wall thickness. Remodelling may initially be compensatory in that it helps maintain LV stroke volume, but it progressively leads to increased LV wall stress, further dilatation, and eventually deleterious effects. Early remodelling and LV aneurysm formation is a particularly poor prognostic sign. Three dimensional echocardiography is more accurate than 2D echocardiography in the assessment of LV size and shape and may have a particular role in the evaluation of LV remodelling. It is a gold standard in research and is now coming into more routine clinical use, although the work involved in data acquisition and image reconstruction remains significant.

Table 24.2 Qualitative scale for derivation of the echocardiographic wall motion score index

Score*	Wall motion	Definition
0	Hyperkinetic	Increased endocardial inward movement and systolic wall thickening
1	Normal	Normal endocardial inward movement and systolic wall thickening
2	Hypokinetic	Reduced endocardial inward movement and systolic wall thickening
3	Akinetic	Absence of endocardial inward movement; no systolic wall thickening
4	Dyskinetic	Outward wall movement in systole with absent wall thickening; often associated with myocardial thinning and fibrosis

*The score for each segment is divided by the number of segments visualised to obtain the wall motion score index.

There are many newer techniques that can be utilised for evaluation of LV function and ischaemia, including tissue Doppler imaging, strain rate imaging, and tissue characterisation; the discussion of these is beyond the scope of this review.

Stress echocardiography has an important role post-MI. Although some centres use a stress imaging modality routinely post-MI, standard treadmill testing is adequate for many patients. Exercise echocardiography is appropriate for patients who can walk on a treadmill. Pharmacological stress echo is indicated primarily in patients unable to exercise adequately for non-cardiac reasons and for assessment of viability.

ECHOCARDIOGRAPHY IN THE EMERGENCY ROOM AND CHEST PAIN UNIT

The potential use of echocardiography for diagnosis of MI is based on observations of the effects of interruption of coronary flow. Left ventricular diastolic dysfunction occurs before systolic dysfunction; ECG abnormalities and chest pain are relatively late events. Segmental wall motion abnormalities seen by echocardiography correspond closely with coronary artery territories, although there is some variation depending on dominance of the right coronary artery and circumflex arteries and extent of "watershed" areas.

Optimal use of any diagnostic technique needs review of its cost effectiveness and impact on decision making, and use should always depend on the availability of resource and expertise. Sensitivity and specificity are inversely related; which is most important depends on the implications of missing the diagnosis versus making an incorrect diagnosis. Sensitivity and specificity are influenced by the pretest likelihood of disease (Bayes theorem). These are important considerations in examining the role of echocardiography in the emergency room as this is a much less selected patient group than in the coronary care unit. The problem is both economic and medico-legal. Many patients admitted with chest pain do not have an acute coronary syndrome whereas 5–10% of those who do are discharged. The challenge is to identify low risk patients without compromising the care of higher risk patients; the latter consideration is particularly relevant given the importance of early reperfusion. Chest pain units linked to the emergency room are an important approach to improving the quality and efficiency of care for these patients, with emphasis not only on reducing costs but on improving early diagnosis and triage to effective management.

There are many studies of echocardiography for MI diagnosis.[13 14] Some are in small, highly selected groups but most have found similar diagnostic sensitivity (approximately

90–95%). The negative predictive value is high (approximately 95%), but the positive predictive value is much lower and more variable.[14] This may partly relate to interpretation difficulties in the presence of prior infarction, and aggressive interpretation of minor abnormalities by physicians anxious to avoid false negatives. From these studies, echocardiography appears more sensitive than standard criteria for the diagnosis of infarction; it is also sensitive for the diagnosis of myocardial ischaemia, but only if performed during pain. Echocardiography provides incremental prognostic information in the identification of patients at risk of cardiac events. However, if echocardiography is used alone, a small number of patients with subendocardial infarction will be discharged.

The study by Trippi and colleagues[15] is an example of how echocardiography might be aggressively used in the emergency room. These authors enrolled 163 patients with no evidence of MI on initial cardiac markers or ECG, who were recommended for admission. If rest echocardiographic images were normal, dobutamine stress echocardiography was performed, initially supervised by a cardiologist and, in later stages, by a trained nurse. Echocardiographic images were transmitted by tele-echocardiography and interpreted off-site. In the first three stages, all patients were admitted. In the final stage, patients were discharged if the stress echocardiogram was negative. Average length of stay was only 5.4 hours. In the third and fourth stages recruitment was less selective, so that in the final phase mild residual chest pain, a non-diagnostic rather than normal ECG, and mild elevation of initial creatine kinase (CK) with normal CK-MB were permitted. The negative predictive value of dobutamine stress echocardiography was 98.5% based on final diagnosis, which was largely based on clinical follow up. There were two false negative results—one in a patient who was admitted in the third stage but discharged without a clinical diagnosis, and one in a patient who was discharged following a normal stress echocardiogram. The study is interesting because of the aggressive approach to achieving discharges, the use of tele-echocardiography and nursing supervision to avoid having a cardiologist on-site, and the choice of pharmacological stress to avoid the noise of a treadmill and the requirement for patient cooperation with exercise. However, most authors would argue that MI should be fully excluded by serial markers and ECGs, and that there be complete resolution of chest pain before stress testing.

In summary, echocardiography in the emergency room may facilitate early diagnosis and management in those patients with a high clinical suspicion of MI but a non-diagnostic ECG. It may also diagnose unstable angina if performed during pain. Aggressive use of rest and stress echocardiography can reduce admissions, but some false negatives will occur and

Echocardiography in acute coronary syndromes: key points

► Transthoracic and transoesophageal echocardiography are complementary techniques with different strengths
► Transoesophageal echocardiography is very safe, but does have potential complications and should be performed by experienced physicians
► Hand held cardiac ultrasound devices are likely to be increasingly used in both the emergency room and coronary care unit but remain controversial
► Echocardiography for diagnosis of myocardial infarction is most helpful in patients with a high clinical suspicion but a normal or non-diagnostic ECG
► Patients with unexplained haemodynamic deterioration postinfarction should be referred immediately for echocardiography
► Echocardiographic indices of left ventricular systolic and diastolic function provide prognostic information in unstable angina and myocardial infarction
► Contrast echocardiography for left ventricular opacification may be helpful in the evaluation of cardiac function in "technically difficult" subjects
► Myocardial contrast echocardiography can evaluate the success of reperfusion and assess myocardial viability
► Intravenous myocardial contrast echocardiography is likely to become a routine clinical tool

small subendocardial infarctions may not be detected. These patients may be at a lower risk of complications but data on this are limited. False positives will also occur and differentiation of ischaemia from old infarction may be difficult; this is not of major importance, given that these patients are likely to be admitted. The chief logistical difficulty is the necessity for experienced staff and expensive equipment on a 24 hour basis.

Hand held, battery powered echocardiographic devices are now available.[16] In many emergency rooms these devices are routinely used (a popular option as it avoids having to call the echocardiography laboratory); they are also used on ward rounds as "ultrasound stethoscopes" and for teaching. Studies show that they are more accurate than physical examination. However, they have limitations that can result in significant errors; Doppler functions on these devices are substantially inferior to the 2D imaging, although the quality will undoubtedly continue to improve. The optimal use of these devices and the implications for training and medicolegal issues remain controversial.

CONTRAST ECHOCARDIOGRAPHY

First generation contrast agents such as agitated saline have been available for many years and are still useful for detection of intracardiac shunts. However these agents do not opacify the LV, as the bubbles cannot survive passage through the lungs. Second generation contrast agents[17] incorporate high molecular weight gases which are more stable and can traverse pulmonary capillaries. Microbubble properties depend on bubble size, shell composition, and the gas used.

When harmonic imaging is used, contrast agents achieve RV and LV opacification with improved image quality and reviewer confidence,[17] and are of particular value in technically challenging subjects. They can also be used to enhance spectral Doppler signals; in patients with acute MI, they can occasionally be of value in other situations—for example, detection of myocardial rupture and LV thrombus.

Abbrevations

CK: creatine kinase
2D: two dimensional
LV: left ventricular
MCE: myocardial contrast echocardiography
MI: myocardial infarction
MR: mitral regurgitation
RV: right ventricular
TIMI: thrombolysis in myocardial infarction
TOE: transoesophageal echocardiography
TTE: transthoracic echocardiography
WMSI: wall motion score index

Myocardial contrast echocardiography

After many years of research, the assessment of coronary perfusion using myocardial contrast echocardiography (MCE) is starting to become a clinical reality. Visual assessment of myocardial perfusion from grey scale images is limited by the poor signal to noise ratio and the limited ability of the human eye to distinguish different shades of grey. Innovative ultrasound methods using harmonic imaging have been developed to exploit the interaction between microbubbles and ultrasound and enable assessment of perfusion. The use of contrast agents for LV opacification is very safe; the safety of MCE may depend on the type of contrast agent and mode of administration, and needs study in larger populations.

Myocardial perfusion has been extensively investigated by intracoronary injection, although no agents are specifically approved for intracoronary use. It is a reproducible and reliable technique for evaluation of the risk area after coronary occlusion, regional coronary flow reserve, myocardial viability, and the outcome of reperfusion.[18]

Intravenous MCE is an emerging technology,[19] particularly in the assessment of reperfusion. The no-reflow phenomenon is a continuing challenge in cardiology. Angiographic TIMI (thrombolysis in myocardial infarction) flow grades provide prognostic information following reperfusion—TIMI 0–II flow is associated with poor recovery of contractile function, while TIMI III flow is associated with good recovery. However, up to 30% of segments with TIMI III flow have no reperfusion at microvascular level and in these regions there is myocardial necrosis. Multiple mechanisms, including microvascular disruption, endothelial and myocardial oedema, neutrophilic infiltration, and obstruction by thromboembolic debris may be involved. MCE is potentially ideal for assessment of reperfusion because the microbubbles stay largely in the capillaries, and 90% of the myocardial microvasculature is capillaries. Preserved microvascular integrity by MCE does not always translate into recovery, but absent perfusion has a high predictive value for lack of recovery and may identify patients requiring further management. Treatment options are limited at present but this is an area of active research.

There are limited data on MCE in acute MI, but it is being used in some centres.[20] There are important technical questions that remain, but MCE could potentially become routine within the next five years. As with any new technique, clinical outcome and economic implications are important; indeed the proliferation of new technologies is a major factor in the rising costs of health care. Undoubtedly this technology will enter the coronary care and emergency room arenas. It could potentially be used to make the diagnosis of acute MI, define the area at risk, and then assess the results of reperfusion. There are exciting additional possibilities in the world of microbubbles; this is because they can be destroyed by ultrasound, and they can also serve as a vehicle for drug delivery to specific tissues, raising the possibility of ultrasound enhanced thrombolysis.

In summary, echocardiography is a critical modality in the diagnosis and management of patients with acute coronary syndromes. With the development of MCE it is anticipated that the routine use of echocardiography will extend into the cardiac catheterisation laboratory and operating room.

REFERENCES

1 **Premawardhana U**, Celermajer DS. Advances in echocardiography. *Aust NZ J Med* 2000;**30**:360–6.

▶ This is a basic, very readable review of some of the more recent advances in echocardiography imaging techniques and provides a good background for readers not familiar with the technology.

2 **Daniel WG**, Erbel R, Kasper W, et al. Safety of transesophageal echocardiography. A multicenter survey of 10,419 examinations. *Circulation* 1991;**83**:817–21.

3 **Thomas JD**. Digital storage and retrieval: the future in echocardiography. *Heart* 1997;**78**(suppl I):19–22.

4 **Kishon Y**, Iqbal A, Oh JK, et al. Evolution of echocardiographic modalities in detection of post myocardial infarction ventricular septal defect and papillary muscle rupture: study of 62 patients. *Am Heart J* 1993;**126**(3 Pt 1):667–75.

▶ This study reports a large series of patients with septal and papillary muscle rupture postmyocardial infarction. It demonstrates the high sensitivity of transthoracic echocardiography for the detection of septal rupture and illustrates the use of transesophageal echocardiography.

5 **Jugdutt BI**, Sivaram CA. Prospective two-dimensional echocardiographic evaluation of LV thrombus and embolism after acute myocardial infarction. *J Am Coll Cardiol* 1989;**13**:554–64.

6 **Goldberger JJ**, Himelman RB, Wolfe CL, et al. Right ventricular infarction: recognition and assessment of its hemodynamic significance by two-dimensional echocardiography. *J Am Soc Echocardiogr* 1991;**4**:140–6.

7 **Romano S**, Dagianti A, Penco M, et al. Usefulness of echocardiography in the prognostic evaluation of non-Q-wave myocardial infarction. *Am J Cardiol* 2000;**86**(suppl 4A):43G–5G.

8 **Peels KH**, Visser CA, Dambrink JHE, et al on behalf of the CATS Investigators Group. Left ventricular wall motion score as an early predictor of left ventricular dilation and mortality after first anterior infarction treated with thrombolysis. The CATS investigators group. *Am J Cardiol* 1996;**77**:1149–54.

9 **Feinberg MS**, Schwammenthal E, Shlizerman L, et al. Prognostic significance of mild mitral regurgitation by color Doppler echocardiography in acute myocardial infarction. *Am J Cardiol* 2000;**86**:903–7.

10 **Cerisano G**, Bolognese L, Carrabba N, et al. Doppler-derived mitral deceleration time. An early strong predictor of LV remodeling after reperfused anterior acute myocardial infarction. *Circulation* 1999;**99**:230–6.

▶ This is the first prospective study to correlate serial changes in LV volumes with changes in filling patterns and to show that a simple, early measurement of LV diastolic function can predict late left ventricular dilatation.

11 **Moller JE**, Sondergaard E, Poulsen SH, et al. The Doppler echocardiographic myocardial performance index predicts left-ventricular dilation and cardiac death after myocardial infarction. *Cardiology* 2001;**95**:105–11.

12 **Korup E**, Kober L, Torp-Pedersen C, et al on behalf of the TRACE Study Group. Prognostic usefulness of repeated echocardiographic evaluation after acute myocardial infarction. *Am J Cardiol* 1999;**83**:1559–62.

▶ This is a prospective study showing the value of serial echocardiographic measurements postinfarction. It is a relatively selected patient group but is of particular value in that patients with reinfarction were excluded. The wall motion index used in the study is derived in a different fashion from the more standard wall motion score index.

13 **Ioannidis JPA**, Salem D, Chew PW, et al. Accuracy of imaging technologies in the diagnosis of acute cardiac ischemia in the emergency department: a meta-analysis. *Ann Emerg Med* 2001;**37**:471–7.

▶ This is a meta-analysis of rest and stress echocardiography and nuclear studies from studies conducted between 1966 and 1998; although only three rest echocardiography studies are considered to meet the criteria specified, others are included in the sensitivity analyses.

14 **Zabalgoitia M**, Ismaeil M. Diagnostic and prognostic use of stress echocardiography in acute coronary syndromes including emergency department imaging. *Echocardiography* 2000;**17**:479–93.

▶ This is an excellent review of the use of both rest and stress echocardiography in the emergency room. It also has a good general review of the different modalities of stress echocardiographic testing and the relevant advances in imaging technology.

15 **Trippi JA**, Lee KS, Kopp G, et al. Dobutamine stress tele-echocardiography for evaluation of emergency department patients with chest pain. *J Am Coll Cardiol* 1997;**30**:627–32.

▶ This is a prospective, well designed study illustrating a possible, aggressive approach to using echocardiography to discharge patients early from the emergency room. It indicates methods by which some of the logistical difficulties might be overcome. It should be noted, however, that many authors would not be comfortable with the very early use of dobutamine stress echocardiography in some of these patients.

16 **Seward JB**, Douglas PS, Erbel R, et al. Hand-carried cardiac ultrasound (HCU) device: recommendations regarding new technology. A report from the echocardiography task force on new technology of the nomenclature and standards committee of the American Society of Echocardiography. *J Am Soc Echocardiogr* 2002;**15**:369–73.

▶ This article contains recommendations from the American Society of Echocardiography regarding use of hand held cardiac ultrasound devices. It gives some general background, but concentrates primarily on clinical/legal issues. Physicians should become familiar with the issues involved; this paper also provides insight into considerations arising with the introduction of other forms of cardiovascular technology.

17 **Mulvagh SL**, DeMaria AN, Feinstein SB, *et al.* Contrast echocardiography: current and future applications. *J Am Soc Echocardiogr* 2000;**13**:331–42.

▶ **This is an American Society of Echocardiography position paper. It reviews contrast agents available and relevant imaging advances, concentrating on the clinical uses of these agents.**

18 **Czitrom D**, Karila-Cohen D, Brochet E, *et al.* Acute assessment of microvascular perfusion patterns by myocardial contrast echocardiography during myocardial infarction: relation to timing and extent of functional recovery. *Heart* 1999;**81**:12–16.

19 **Lepper W**, Hoffmann R, Kamp O, *et al.* Assessment of myocardial reperfusion by intravenous myocardial contrast echocardiography and coronary flow reserve after primary percutaneous transluminal coronary angioplasty in patients with acute myocardial infarction. *Circulation* 2000;**101**:2368–74.

20 **Kaul S**. Myocardial contrast echocardiography in acute myocardial infarction: time to test for routine clinical use? *Heart* 1999;**81**:2–5.

▶ **This is an editorial linked to a study of intracoronary myocardial contrast echocardiography. However, it is written by an international expert in this field, and provides an insightful view into the possible use of myocardial contrast echocardiography in the management of acute myocardial infarction.**

25 DOPPLER ECHOCARDIOGRAPHIC ASSESSMENT OF VALVAR REGURGITATION

James D Thomas

Improvements in outcomes for heart valve surgery, in particular mitral valve repair, have dictated a need for better assessment of valvar regurgitation. Whereas in the past surgery was delayed until the patient's symptomatic status required intervention, patients today are often sent to the operating room while still asymptomatic or minimally symptomatic. Before committing an asymptomatic patient to open heart surgery, however, it is essential that the severity of valvar regurgitation be quantified to ensure the surgery is actually required. Doppler echocardiography has emerged as the premier way of assessing valvar regurgitation, as it allows characterisation of valve morphology, severity of regurgitation, and secondary effects, such as left ventricular dysfunction, left atrial enlargement, and pulmonary hypertension. This review will outline current methods available to the echocardiographer in assessing valvar regurgitation, focusing on simple practical ways that true quantitative information can be obtained in a clinical laboratory. Techniques that are generally applicable in all forms of valve regurgitation will be introduced first, followed by specific techniques for mitral and aortic regurgitation.

► COLOUR JET AREA METHOD

The most common way of assessing the severity of valvar regurgitation is to inspect the area of the colour Doppler jet in the downstream chamber.[1] The advantage of this approach is that it is fast, easy, and also provides information on the mechanism of regurgitation, as the jet is generally directed away from the most severely affected leaflet. However, jet area alone is impacted by many factors other than regurgitant flow rate, and an understanding of these will aid in its utilisation.

Determinants of colour jet Doppler area

The physical parameter that is most predictive of the size of a regurgitant jet by colour Doppler is jet momentum, given by the product of regurgitant flow rate multiplied by velocity.[2] Since jet velocity is directly related to the driving pressure across a regurgitant orifice (by the Bernoulli equation), the patient's blood pressure will have an important impact on jet size and so should be recorded at the time of the echo examination. Chamber constraint is the second major factor determining jet size. Obviously a jet, which is directed centrally into the left atrium, cannot extend further than the superior wall of the atrium, but chamber constraint is even more important for eccentrically directed jets that hug the chamber wall. In general, such a wall jet will appear much smaller (as much as 60% smaller) than the equivalent centrally directed jet because it is flattened against the wall and cannot recruit stagnant flow into the jet from all sides the way a centrally directed jet can.[3] The final factor impacting colour jet area size is the instrumentation set-up of the echocardiograph.[4] Increasing either the transmitted power of the instrument or the receiver gain will result in a larger jet, as weaker echoes on the periphery of the jet are detected. In general, colour gain should be increased until random colour pixels begin to appear in the tissue and then the gain reduced just slightly. The scale of the colour Doppler display (determined by the pulse repetition frequency) can have a profound effect on jet size as low velocity motion at the periphery of the jet will be encoded at low scales. Figure 25.1 shows how reducing the scale or Nyquist limit from 69 cm to 39 cm to 17 cm per second results in a dramatic increase in jet size.

For most purposes, the scale should be set at the highest limit allowed by the combination of imaging depth and interrogation frequency (and usually selected automatically by the instrument). Transducer frequency can have a dual effect on jet size. Because the Doppler shift is more profound at higher interrogating frequencies, jets tend to appear larger with higher frequency imaging. However, higher imaging frequencies are also prone to greater tissue attenuation and so the jets may appear smaller. In general, for transoesophageal imaging the Doppler enhancing effect of the higher imaging frequency dominates while for transthoracic imaging the attenuation factor predominates, causing jets to appear smaller at higher interrogating frequencies. Increasing the wall filter of the instrument will decrease the size of jets, by excluding velocities below a certain cutoff value, while increasing the ensemble length (sometimes referred to as the quality of the Doppler map) will yield a larger jet as lower velocities can be displayed by the finer colour maps.

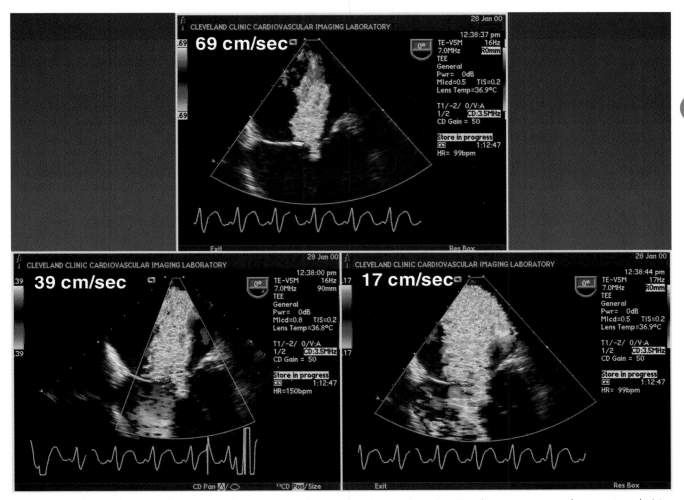

Figure 25.1 Impact of scale (pulse repetition frequency) on colour jet size. Because the colour Doppler processor records approximately 16 levels of red and 16 levels of blue, the lowest velocity encoded is approximately 1/16 of the maximal velocity. Thus the minimal velocities recorded in the above images are approximately 4 cm/s, 2 cm/s, and 1 cm/s as the scale is reduced from 69 to 39 to 17 cm/s.

The best rule of thumb is to standardise the instrument set-up within a given laboratory and leave these constant for all examinations. Unfortunately, regardless of the care that is taken in assessing the colour jet area, this method can only yield a semiquantitative assessment of regurgitant severity, with perhaps 4–6 distinct grades of severity detectable. Modern assessment of valvar regurgitation requires a more quantitative approach.

QUANTITATIVE TECHNIQUES

A variety of techniques have been described for the echo Doppler quantification of valvar regurgitation. Among the key parameters to be determined by these methods are the following:

▶ regurgitant volume, the amount of blood leaking through the valve in each cardiac cycle (given in ml)

▶ regurgitant flow rate, the maximal rate of leakage through the valve (given in ml/s)

▶ regurgitant fraction, the percentage of left ventricular stroke volume that leaks back through the valve

▶ regurgitant orifice area, the actual anatomic area of the regurgitant lesion and perhaps the best physical descriptor of valve disruption.

Volumetric approach to quantification

In general the approach to regurgitant quantification can be divided into two broad areas—volumetric assessment and direct assessment. The volumetric assessment relies on measuring stroke volume in two regions of the heart, one of which includes the regurgitant volume, the other of which includes only the systemic stroke volume.[5] The difference between these two stroke volumes is the regurgitant volume through the valve (fig 25.2). For example, in the case of mitral regurgitation, measuring stroke volume across the mitral annulus and left ventricular outflow tract and subtracting the latter from the former will yield the mitral regurgitant stroke volume. The stroke volumes can be obtained in a variety of fashions. Flow through the left ventricular outflow tract can be calculated by multiplying the area of the left ventricular outflow tract ($\pi D^2/4$, where D is the diameter of the left ventricular outflow tract measured just below the aortic valve in the parasternal long axis view) by the time velocity integral of the pulsed Doppler velocity measurement obtained in the same location. A similar approach can be used for measuring flow across the mitral annulus, by measuring the mitral annular area and multiplying this by the time velocity integral of the velocity obtained at that location. Alternatively, stroke volume can be obtained from two dimensional echocardiography by subtracting left ventricular end systolic volume from end diastolic volume, calculated by using Simpson's rule or the area–length formula from the left ventricular apex. It is also possible to obtain stroke volume in an automated fashion, by integrating colour Doppler velocities across the left ventricular outflow tract or mitral annulus throughout space

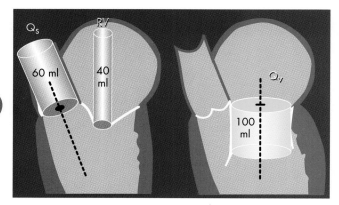

Figure 25.2 The principle of the volumetric assessment of valvar regurgitation. By measuring stroke volume in two areas of the heart, it is possible to use the difference between these to estimate regurgitant volume. Qs, systemic stroke volume; Qv, stroke volume across regurgitant valve; RV, regurgitant volume.

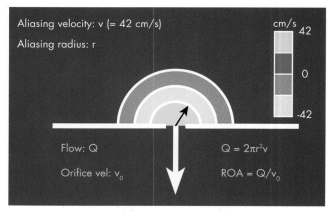

Figure 25.3 The proximal convergence method. By using the aliasing velocity of the colour Doppler display, it is possible to measure the radius to an isovelocity shell as blood converges on the regurgitant orifice. Assuming a hemispheric shape to the shell, flow rate is given as $Q = 2\pi r^2 v$. Dividing this flow rate by the maximal velocity through the orifice (given by continuous wave Doppler) yields an estimation for the regurgitant orifice area (ROA).

and time.[6][7] Such an approach, unfortunately, is only available on one manufacturer's instrument at the current time.

While these volumetric methods are theoretically sound and have been well validated in many carefully performed trials, they have not achieved widespread use within the clinical echocardiographic community for a variety of reasons. First, they are time consuming to implement, requiring multiple measurements from a variety of echocardiographic imaging windows and multistage calculations. Furthermore, they are exquisitely sensitive to the error in the primary measurements, and an error in any of these will be propagated throughout all the calculations. This is compounded by the need to subtract two fairly large numbers from each other to obtain a much smaller number at the end of the process. The absolute value of the uncertainty in the measurement rises as the square root of the sum of the squares of the component uncertainties, but the relative uncertainty rises even more, since the denominator (the regurgitant volume) is so much smaller. For example, if we assume that mitral and aortic stroke volume can be measured with approximately 15% accuracy (not a bad accuracy), we might obtain the following sample calculations: aortic stroke volume, 70 (10) ml; mitral stroke volume, 100 (15) ml; mitral regurgitant volume, 30 (18) ml, indicating that the 95% confidence intervals for regurgitant volume (2 standard deviations) extend from −6 ml to 66 ml, a range which is simply too great to be clinically useful. For these reasons, echocardiographic clinicians have turned with great enthusiasm to more direct methods, in particular the proximal convergence method.

Proximal convergence method

The proximal convergence method is a more direct approach to the quantification of valvar regurgitation. As blood rushes into a regurgitant orifice, it forms concentric shells of increasing blood velocity and decreasing surface area. Since blood is incompressible, if we could measure flow through any one of the shells, that would yield the instantaneous flow through the regurgitant orifice itself.[8] Fortunately, there is a straightforward way to estimate flow through one of the shells. Fluid dynamics theory demonstrates that for a small orifice in a flat plate, these isovelocity shells are hemispheric in shape, with an area of $2\pi r^2$, where r is the distance of the shell from the regurgitant orifice. Multiplying this area by the velocity v of the isovelocity shell will yield the flow rate. This radius and velocity can most easily be obtained by using the aliasing of the colour Doppler display, as blood rushes into the orifice. As shown schematically in fig 25.3, as blood velocity increases, there is an abrupt change from yellow to blue at which point we know the blood is moving at 42 cm/s and where we can easily measure the radius from the regurgitant orifice. Once flow rate is obtained as $Q = 2\pi r^2 v$, then the regurgitant orifice area (ROA) is obtained by dividing this by the maximal velocity through the valve measured with continuous wave Doppler: $ROA = Q/v_{max}$. This approach has been well validated in a number of experimental and clinical studies.[9] It has advantages over the volumetric approach in that all measurements are obtained from a single imaging window, typically one of the apical windows, and the flow rate is measured directly, not requiring subtraction of two large quantities from each other as in the volumetric approach. Nevertheless, there are some limitations to the proximal convergence method, also known as the PISA (proximal isovelocity surface area) method, which the reader should be aware of. Additionally, there is an important simplification to this method that will greatly aid in its clinical application.

Limitations to the proximal convergence method

There are four important limitations to the proximal convergence method: flattening of the contours near the orifice, constraint of the flow by proximal structures, uncertainty in localising the regurgitant orifice, and variability in the regurgitant orifice throughout cardiac cycle. These will be dealt with in turn.

Contour flattening of the orifice

Since the regurgitant orifice is in fact not infinitely small, the hemispheric shape of the isovelocity contours is not maintained all the way into the orifice; rather, they flatten out on approach to the orifice, and if flow were calculated using the standard formula, flow underestimation would ensue. An in vitro and computational study has shown that this underestimation is closely related to the aliasing velocity used in calculating the flow rate.[10] For example, if an aliasing velocity (v_a) that is 10% of the orifice velocity is used, then approximately 10% of the flow will be missed with the standard formula. This underestimation can be corrected by multiplying the calculated flow rate by the quantity $v_{max}/(v_{max} - v_a)$. Fortunately, for

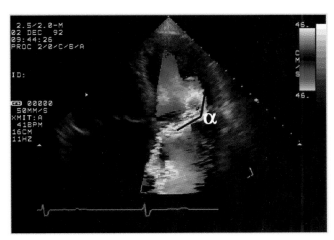

Figure 25.4 The influence of proximal flow constraint. In this patient with a flail posterior leaflet, the proximal convergence zone is constrained by the posterolateral wall, pushing the contours outward. This can be corrected by calculating flow rate in the usual manner and then multiplying by $\alpha/180$.

left sided lesions (aortic and mitral regurgitation), this correction factor is rarely needed, since the aliasing velocity usually is less than 10% of the orifice velocity. The correction may be necessary for tricuspid regurgitation, where the aliasing velocity is a larger proportion of the orifice velocity and the underestimation of flow would be more significant.

Flow constraint by proximal structures

A more important limitation is the distortion in the isovelocity contours caused by encroachment of proximal structures on the flow field. For example, fig 25.4 shows mitral regurgitation caused by a flail posterior leaflet, where the convergence zone is immediately adjacent to the posterolateral wall. It is clear that the proximal convergence zone cannot form full hemispheric contours, and thus is pushed outward from the orifice. Applying the standard formula in this case would lead to significant flow overestimation, but again a simple solution to this exists. By simply excluding from the calculations an amount of flow approximately equal to the geometric reduction in the orifice shape from a hemisphere, most of this overestimation can be eliminated.[11] Ideally, a full three dimensional analysis of the flow field would allow refinement of the method, but until such methods are widely available, the simple "eyeball" approach works reasonably well. As shown in fig 25.4, simply multiplying the calculated flow rate by the ratio $\alpha/180$ will permit estimation of the true flow rate.

Where's the orifice?

While it is generally quite easy to see where the colour Doppler display changes from blue to red, it is often not so easy to see exactly where the centre of the regurgitant orifice is located. This is an important issue, as the radius is defined on the basis of that orifice location; and since the radius is squared in the proximal convergence formula, a 10% error in radius measurement will cause more than 20% error in flow rate and regurgitant orifice area calculations. When the images are being obtained live on the echo machine, it is possible to freeze the image and toggle colour display on and off, improving the anatomical delineation of the regurgitant orifice. Once the images are stored off either digitally or on videotape, however, the colour generally is a fixed overlay on the black and white anatomy and cannot be removed. While some automated methods have been proposed to localise the orifice automatically from the full velocity field,[12] these have not reached clinical use yet. Another alternative is to look not at the first aliasing radius but rather to look at the separation between the first

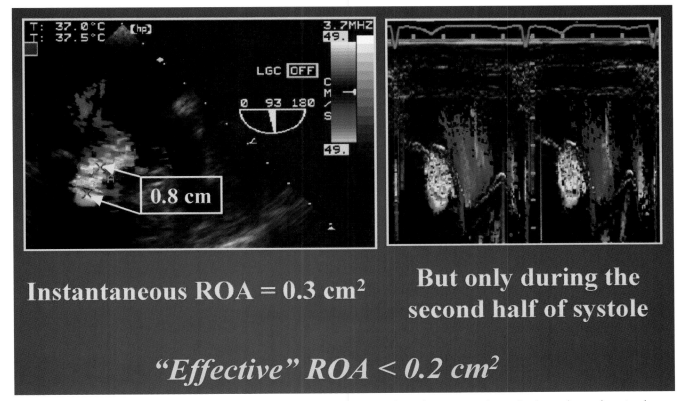

Figure 25.5 Variability of the regurgitant orifice area throughout the cardiac cycle. In this patient with mitral valve prolapse, there is a large regurgitant orifice area at peak regurgitation (0.3 cm²), but as shown on the colour M mode to the right, this significant regurgitation only occurs in the latter half of systole, so that the effective regurgitant orifice area is less than 0.2 cm².

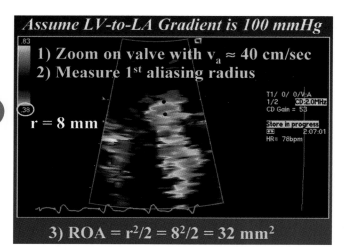

Figure 25.6 Simplification of the proximal convergence method. By assuming that the left ventricle (LV) to left atrium (LA) pressure difference is 100 mm Hg and setting the aliasing velocity to approximately 40 cm/s, the regurgitant orifice area can be calculated simply as ROA = r²/2.

and second aliasing contours.[13] Clinical experience with this interaliasing distance method is limited, but it may prove helpful, particularly for moderate to severe mitral regurgitation where a second aliasing contour is visible.

Variable regurgitant orifice

In many patients the degree of regurgitation is not constant throughout systole (or diastole in the case of aortic regurgitation), and categorising the regurgitant severity on the basis of the maximal regurgitant orifice area may give a misleading overestimation of the haemodynamic impact of the regurgitation. For example, in cases of classic mitral valve prolapse, the severe regurgitation is often confined to the latter half of systole. Conversely, it has been shown in some cases of functional mitral regurgitation in dilated cardiomyopathy that the most significant regurgitation occurs early in systole and then again during isovolumic relaxation with relatively little flow in mid systole, as ventricular pressure is sufficient to keep the valve closed.[14] One way of addressing this issue is to image the

proximal convergence zone with colour Doppler M mode echocardiography, which shows a temporal display of the velocity through the valve throughout cardiac cycle. Figure 25.5 shows a patient with mitral valve prolapse in whom significant regurgitation occurs only at the end of systole. While methods have been proposed for using the colour M mode display in a quantitative fashion,[15] it is often possible to use it in a semiquantitative fashion simply to adjust the clinical judgment of the severity of regurgitation based on the duration of the leakage.

Simplified proximal convergence method

While the proximal convergence method is considerably simpler then the previous volumetric methods, it is still considered by some to be too complex for routine clinical application. To address this issue, we have devised a simplification to the proximal convergence method that allows the mitral regurgitant orifice area to be estimated with only one measurement.[16] Underlying this simplification is an assumption that the driving pressure between the left ventricle and the left atrium is 100 mm Hg (which would yield a 5 m/s mitral regurgitant jet). With this assumption, if the aliasing velocity is set to approximately 40 cm/s and the radius of the first aliasing contour obtained, then the regurgitant orifice area is stated quite simply as: ROA = r²/2. Figure 25.6 shows an application of this method in a patient with moderately severe mitral regurgitation from an inferoposterior infarction. After zooming on the proximal convergence zone and baseline shifting to an aliasing velocity of 38 cm/s (close enough to 40 for this application), the aliasing contour is noted 8 mm from the regurgitant orifice, yielding a regurgitant orifice area of 32 mm². A recent validation study has shown that this simplified method yields results that are almost the same as the more complete proximal convergence method. Naturally, to the extent that the left ventricle to left atrium pressure difference differs from 100 mm Hg, there will be some intrinsic error in the calculations, but over a pressure range between 64–144 mm Hg, this error should not exceed 20% or 25%. Using the simplified method, it is possible to add quantitation to the assessment of mitral regurgitation with only a minute or two of extra imaging and calculation.

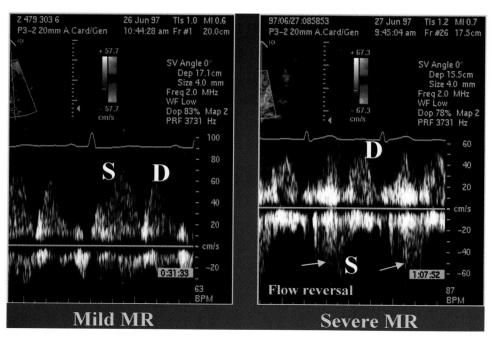

Figure 25.7 Impact of mitral regurgitation on pulmonary venous flow. With mild mitral regurgitation the pulmonary venous S wave is larger than the D wave (left panel), while with severe mitral regurgitation the S wave becomes frankly reversed.

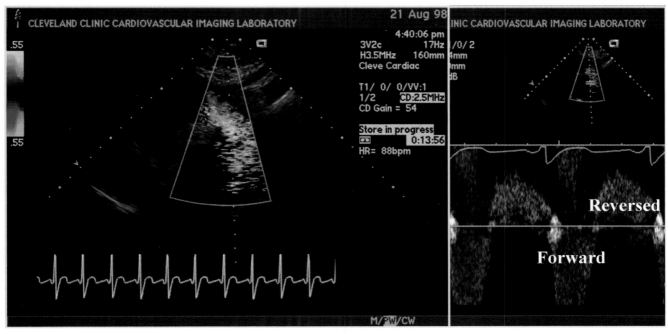

Figure 25.8   Aortic flow reversal indicates haemodynamically significant aortic regurgitation. By positioning a pulsed Doppler sample volume in the distal aortic arch (left panel), the ratio of the forward versus reversed velocity time integrals gives a rough estimate of the regurgitant fraction (right panel).

Vena contracta method

Another direct approach to quantifying the regurgitant orifice area is by direct visualisation of the vena contracta, the narrowest portion of the regurgitant jet just behind the leaking valve. This has long had a role in the assessment of aortic regurgitation[17] and has recently been proposed for mitral regurgitation.[18] While this approach is theoretically sound, it is limited by the lateral resolution of colour Doppler echocardiography, which frequently is inadequate to distinguish minor variations in the width of the vena contracta.

METHOD SPECIFIC TO INDIVIDUAL VALVES

In addition to these general quantitative and colour jet area techniques, there are several parameters that are useful for only the mitral or aortic valve.

Mitral valve

Assessment of pulmonary venous flow is a useful adjunct in the characterisation of mitral regurgitation.[19] Normally the S wave (during ventricular systole) is larger than the D wave. With progressive degrees of mitral regurgitation, however, the maximal velocity of the S wave is reduced, becoming frankly reversed when mitral regurgitation is severe. Figure 25.7 shows an example of normal versus reversed pulmonary venous flow. Unfortunately, the intermediate pattern, where the S wave is merely blunted (smaller than the D wave but not reversed) is very non-specific. It may be an indicator of moderately severe mitral regurgitation, but it also occurs in situations of left ventricular dysfunction and atrial fibrillation.[20] Another useful adjunct in assessing mitral regurgitant severity is inspection of the transmitral flow pattern. It is almost impossible to have haemodynamically significant mitral regurgitation without having an elevated E wave through the mitral valve.

Aortic valve

For the aortic valve there are two special indices that are useful in characterising regurgitation: the aortic pressure half-time, and flow reversal in the aorta. The aortic pressure half-time is obtained from the continuous wave Doppler recording of reversed flow across the aortic valve in diastole.[21] By measuring the time required for the aorta-to-left ventricle pressure difference to fall by half, one gets an indication of the severity of regurgitation, with values less than 250 ms typically indicating haemodynamically significant regurgitation. However, the pressure half-time depends critically on the chronicity of the regurgitation, with acute aortic regurgitation leading to much shorter values than longstanding leakage, in which case the ventricle has dilated with increased compliance. In addition, the half-time also varies with systemic vascular resistance, such that patients who are treated with vasodilators may shorten their half-time even as the aortic regurgitant fraction improves, in contrast to the usual expectation of this parameter.[22]

When aortic regurgitation is haemodynamically significant, flow reversal may be visualised in the aortic arch and descending aorta.[23] As shown in figure 25.8, the ratio of the reversed flow to the forward flow velocity time integral may be taken as an estimate of the aortic regurgitant fraction. Indeed, if I were to be given only one piece of data upon which to decide whether aortic regurgitation was haemodynamically significant or not, a pulsed Doppler recording in the distal aortic arch would probably be the best one.

CONCLUSIONS

Careful quantification of valvar regurgitation is critical for deciding on the need and success of medical management as well as determining the timing of surgery. The colour Doppler jet area method, despite its many limitations, is still useful for separating regurgitation into several broad degrees of severity. However, any patient with a significant degree of regurgitation should undergo a formal quantification study, which in general can most easily and accurately be done using the proximal convergence method. Combining this with observations of chamber size and function, pulmonary artery pressure, and adjunct parameters such as pulmonary venous flow and aortic flow, will give the echocardiographer much improved confidence in the proper assessment about the regurgitation.

REFERENCES

1 **Helmcke F**, Nanda NC, Hsiung MC, *et al.* Color Doppler assessment of mitral regurgitation with orthogonal planes. *Circulation* 1987;**75**:175–83.
   ▶ **This early paper outlined the use of colour jet area in the assessment of mitral regurgitation, particularly as a proportion of left atrial area. Although it has many limitations, this method is still frequently used.**
2 **Thomas JD**, Liu CM, Flachskampf FA, *et al.* Quantification of jet flow by momentum analysis. An in vitro color Doppler flow study. *Circulation* 1990;**81**:247–59.
   ▶ **An exposition on the physical and instrumentation determinants of colour jet area, demonstrating the importance of jet momentum (flow rate × velocity).**
3 **Chen CG**, Thomas JD, Anconina J, *et al.* Impact of impinging wall jet on color Doppler quantification of mitral regurgitation. *Circulation* 1991;**84**:712–20.
   ▶ **A study demonstrating that wall jets are less than half the size of centrally directed jets for the same degree of regurgitation.**
4 **Simpson IA**, Sahn DJ. Quantification of valvular regurgitation by Doppler echocardiography. *Circulation* 1991;**84**(3 suppl):I188–92.
   ▶ **An excellent summary of instrumentation issues in visualisation of colour Doppler jets.**
5 **Enriquez-Sarano M**, Bailey KR, Seward JB, *et al.* Quantitative Doppler assessment of valvular regurgitation. *Circulation* 1993;**87**:841–8.
   ▶ **Summary and validation of the use of volumetric analysis in the quantification of valvar regurgitation.**
6 **Sun JP**, Pu M, Fouad FM, *et al.* Automated cardiac output measurement by spatiotemporal integration of color Doppler data. In vitro and clinical validation. *Circulation* 1997;**95**:932–9.
   ▶ **A validation study demonstrating that colour Doppler velocities can be integrated across the left ventricular outflow tract throughout space and time to yield stroke volume.**
7 **Sun JP**, Yang XS, Qin JX, *et al.* Quantification of mitral regurgitation by automated cardiac output measurement: experimental and clinical validation. *J Am Coll Cardiol* 1998;**32**:1074–82.
   ▶ **Application of the automated cardiac output method to quantify mitral regurgitation.**
8 **Bargiggia GS**, Tronconi L, Sahn DJ, *et al.* A new method for quantitation of mitral regurgitation based on color flow Doppler imaging of flow convergence proximal to regurgitant orifice. *Circulation* 1991;**84**:1481–9.
   ▶ **Initial description of the proximal convergence method.**
9 **Vandervoort PM**, Rivera JM, Mele D, *et al.* Application of color Doppler flow mapping to calculate effective regurgitant orifice area. An in vitro study and initial clinical observations. *Circulation* 1993;**88**:1150–6.
   ▶ **Application of the proximal convergence method for calculation of the regurgitant orifice area.**
10 **Rodriguez L**, Anconina J, Flachskampf FA, *et al.* Impact of finite orifice size on proximal flow convergence. Implications for Doppler quantification of valvular regurgitation. *Circulation Res* 1992;**70**:923–30.
   ▶ **Analysis of flow underestimation due to contour flattening near the orifice and a simple method for correcting this.**
11 **Pu M**, Vandervoort PM, Griffin BP, *et al.* Quantification of mitral regurgitation by the proximal convergence method using transesophageal echocardiography. Clinical validation of a geometric correction for proximal flow constraint. *Circulation* 1995;**92**:2169–77.
   ▶ **Analysis of flow overestimation due to constraint by proximal structures and a simple method for correcting this.**
12 **Vandervoort PM**, Thoreau DH, Rivera JM, *et al.* Automated flow rate calculations based on digital analysis of flow convergence proximal to regurgitant orifices. *J Am Coll Cardiol* 1993;**22**:535–41.
   ▶ **Description of a computational method for analysing the full proximal flow field to automatically localise the regurgitant orifice and calculate the peak flow rate.**
13 **Sitges M**, Jones M, Shiota T, *et al.* Interaliasing distance of the flow convergence surface for determining mitral regurgitant volume: a validation study in a chronic animal model. *J Am Coll Cardiol* 2001;**38**:1195–202.
   ▶ **A new method for avoiding the problem of localising the regurgitant orifice by measuring the distance between the first two aliasing contours.**
14 **Schwammenthal E**, Chen C, Benning F, *et al.* Dynamics of mitral regurgitant flow and orifice area. Physiologic application of the proximal flow convergence method: clinical data and experimental testing. *Circulation* 1994;**90**:307–22.
   ▶ **An interesting study demonstrating dramatic variability in regurgitant orifice area throughout the cardiac cycle and methods for recognising this by colour M mode Doppler recording.**
15 **Schwammenthal E**, Chen C, Giesler M, *et al.* New method for accurate calculation of regurgitant flow rate based on analysis of Doppler color flow maps of the proximal flow field. Validation in a canine model of mitral regurgitation with initial application in patients. *J Am Coll Cardiol* 1996;**27**:161–72.
   ▶ **A proposed method to analyse the velocities along a colour M mode acquisition of the proximal convergence zone to adjust for variable regurgitant orifice areas.**
16 **Pu M**, Prior DL, Fan X, *et al.* Calculation of mitral regurgitant orifice area with use of a simplified proximal convergence method: initial clinical application. *J Am Soc Echocardiogr* 2001;**14**:180–5.
   ▶ **Description and validation of a simplified method for applying the proximal convergence approach.**
17 **Perry GJ**, Helmcke F, Nanda NC, *et al.* Evaluation of aortic insufficiency by Doppler color flow mapping. *J Am Coll Cardiol* 1987;**9**:952–9.
   ▶ **Initial description of the jet area within the left ventricular outflow tract as a measure of aortic regurgitant severity.**
18 **Hall SA**, Brickner ME, Willett DL, *et al.* Assessment of mitral regurgitation severity by Doppler color flow mapping of the vena contracta. *Circulation* 1997;**95**:636–42.
   ▶ **Validation of the vena contracta method for assessing the severity of mitral regurgitation.**
19 **Castello R**, Pearson AC, Lenzen P, *et al.* Effect of mitral regurgitation on pulmonary venous velocities derived from transesophageal echocardiography color-guided pulsed Doppler imaging. *J Am Coll Cardiol* 1991;**17**:1499–506.
   ▶ **Early description of the utility of pulmonary venous flow reversal in identifying severe mitral regurgitation.**
20 **Pu M**, Griffin BP, Vandervoort PM, *et al.* The value of assessing pulmonary venous flow velocity for predicting severity of mitral regurgitation: a quantitative assessment integrating left ventricular function. *J Am Soc Echocardiogr* 1999;**12**:736–43.
   ▶ **A critical appraisal of the pulmonary venous approach to assessing valvar regurgitation, demonstrating that the blunted S wave is non-specific with regards to regurgitant severity.**
21 **Teague SM**, Heinsimer JA, Anderson JL, *et al.* Quantification of aortic regurgitation utilizing continuous wave Doppler ultrasound. *J Am Coll Cardiol* 1986;**8**:592–9.
   ▶ **Early description of the aortic pressure half-time method for assessing aortic regurgitant severity.**
22 **Griffin BP**, Flachskampf FA, Reimold SC, *et al.* Relationship of aortic regurgitant velocity slope and pressure half-time to severity of aortic regurgitation under changing haemodynamic conditions. *Eur Heart J* 1994;**15**:681–5.
   ▶ **An animal study demonstrating the sensitivity of the aortic pressure half-time to changes in systemic vascular resistance. This limits its utility in following patients receiving vasodilator therapy.**
23 **Reimold SC**, Maier SE, Aggarwal K, *et al.* Aortic flow velocity patterns in chronic aortic regurgitation: implications for Doppler echocardiography. *J Am Soc Echocardiogr* 1996;**9**:675–83.
   ▶ **Demonstration of the utility of aortic flow reversal in identifying patients with haemodynamically significant aortic regurgitation.**

SECTION VIII: HYPERTENSION

26 CARDIOVASCULAR AND CORONARY RISK ESTIMATION IN HYPERTENSION MANAGEMENT

Erica J Wallis, Lawrence E Ramsay, Peter R Jackson

For many years decisions to treat or not treat hypertension with drugs were made considering the level of blood pressure alone. There was vigorous debate over whether patients should be treated at diastolic pressures of 110, 100, 90 mm Hg or some other threshold. However, epidemiological studies show that the risk of cardiovascular complications such as stroke or myocardial infarction is not determined by blood pressure alone, but is strongly influenced by other major risk factors such as age, sex, smoking habit, lipid concentrations, diabetes, target organ damage such as left ventricular hypertrophy (LVH), and established vascular disease such as angina or myocardial infarction.[1] Furthermore clinical trials have shown that the absolute risk of cardiovascular disease (CVD) determines the chance of benefit from antihypertensive treatment.[2] In 1995 a New Zealand guideline development group turned this knowledge into practice and recommended that treatment of hypertension should be determined by absolute cardiovascular disease risk and not blood pressure thresholds alone.[3] Since then most international and national guidelines have embraced the principle of targeting antihypertensive drug treatment at absolute CVD risk, although the details and methods of estimating CVD risk differ greatly between guidelines. In the UK the British Hypertension Society and Joint British Societies (which include cardiology, lipid, hypertension, and diabetes specialist groups) have developed guidelines for the management of uncomplicated mild hypertension according to estimated absolute coronary heart disease (CHD) risk.[4][5] This means that hypertension guidelines and guidelines for statins and aspirin in primary prevention cannot be implemented without a working knowledge of the estimation of absolute CHD or CVD risk. This article discusses the principle and practice of using absolute CVD or CHD risk for decisions on antihypertensive treatment.

▶ IMPORTANCE OF ABSOLUTE RISK IN HYPERTENSION

Hypertension is consistently associated with an increased risk of cardiovascular complications, including stroke, myocardial infarction, heart failure, and renal failure. Antihypertensive treatment decreases the risk of all cardiovascular complications by about 25%, largely through reducing stroke by 38% and coronary events by 16%.[6] A key point is that the relative risk reduction, 25%, is approximately constant across all groups of patients,[2] meaning that it is similar in men and women, young and old, smokers and non-smokers, and so on. When antihypertensive treatment was targeted only at a predetermined blood pressure threshold, the assumption was that the 25% relative risk reduction translated into a worthwhile chance of benefit for all patients. This assumption was incorrect. The *relative* risk reduction tells us nothing about the chance of an individual benefiting from treatment by avoiding a cardiovascular complication.[7] The chance of benefit is determined by the *absolute* reduction in risk of cardiovascular complications, which is a product of the relative risk reduction and the absolute risk of developing a cardiovascular complication. Figure 26.1 shows the absolute reductions in cardiovascular events (or absolute benefit) from antihypertensive treatment plotted against the absolute CVD event rate observed in the placebo treated groups in randomised controlled trials of antihypertensive treatment. Because the relative risk reduction for CVD events was similar in all trials at around 25% there is a linear relation between absolute risk and benefit from treatment. Thus the absolute CVD risk and not the level of blood pressure per se determines the probability of benefit when treating hypertension.

Table 26.1 shows data for two patients with the same average blood pressure, 150/96 mm Hg, which illustrate the key role of estimation of absolute risk in determining the chance of benefit from treatment. Patient A has very low CVD risk (2.5% over 10 years) because her other risk factors are favourable, and her chance of benefit from treatment is only 0.6% over 10 years. Patient B has a much higher CVD risk (51% over 10 years) because of his age, sex, smoking habit, and lipid profile, and his chance of benefit is nearly 13% over 10 years. The absolute benefit is succinctly described as the "number needed to treat" or "NNT",[8] which is the number of similar patients who have to be treated for a specified time period (usually five years) to prevent a CVD complication in one. Thus the five year NNT for patient A in table 26.1 is 321, and the five year NNT for patient B is 16. Although the two patients have the same blood pressure, 150/96 mm Hg, patient B has a

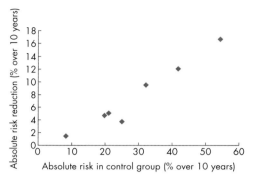

Figure 26.1 Absolute cardiovascular disease (CVD) risk reductions observed in selected randomised controlled trials of antihypertensive treatments plotted against the absolute CVD risk in the placebo groups. Note the linear relation between absolute risk and absolute risk reduction. Data from Collins and Peto[6] and the Syst-Eur trial (see website for reference).

Table 26.1 Two patients with identical blood pressures (150/96 mm Hg) but pronounced differences in other major risk factors, illustrating a 20-fold difference in absolute cardiovascular risk and in chance of benefit from treatment between patients with "mild hypertension"

	Patient A	Patient B
Blood pressure (mm Hg)	150/96	150/96
Sex	Female	Male
Age (years)	35	65
Total cholesterol (mmol/l)	5.0	7.0
HDL cholesterol (mmol/l)	1.4	1.0
Smoking	No	Yes
Diabetes	No	No
Left ventricular hypertrophy	No	No
Absolute CVD risk (% over 10 years)	2.5	51.0
Relative risk reduction (%)	25	25
Absolute benefit (% over 10 years)	0.6	12.8
NNT (5 years)	321	16

much higher absolute risk of cardiovascular disease and is far more likely to benefit from treatment. When compared to other treatments in general use, the benefit from treatment for patient B (NNT 16) would be considered very worthwhile whereas the merits of treatment for patient A (NNT 321) might be debated. Informed people may decline treatment with such a small chance of benefit, and it is also possible that "harm" from treatment might outweigh any benefit.

POSSIBLE HARM FROM TREATING LOW RISK PATIENTS

Harm from treatment can take several forms. Serious adverse reactions to modern antihypertensive drugs, such as fatal airways obstruction with β blockers or renal failure with angiotensin converting enzyme (ACE) inhibitors, are probably very rare. However, the chance of an adverse reaction is generally unrelated to the CVD risk, and therefore similar in low risk and high risk patients.[9] Below some level of CVD risk the chance of harm from treatment will outweigh benefit. Hoes and colleagues suggested that the risk from antihypertensive treatment may exceed benefit when the pretreatment risk of all cause mortality was below 6% over 10 years,[10] although their analysis has been criticised. Antihypertensive drugs can also cause subjective side effects (for example, cold extremities

with β blockers, flushing with calcium channel blockers, cough with ACE inhibitors) which may be harmful, although the treatment withdrawal rates in unbiased studies are very low, and quality of life is not influenced adversely when compared with placebo treatment. However the "labelling" effect of treating hypertension can itself cause perceived ill health and psychological morbidity. People do not like taking tablets and may develop "side effects" that impair quality of life. These disadvantages of treatment are of little concern when treating high risk patients who have a high probability of benefiting from treatment, but they may outweigh the benefits of treatment in very low risk patients.

Patients with high CVD risk who will get worthwhile benefit from treatment need to be identified and offered treatment, whereas very low risk patients may choose observation rather than drug treatment. Estimation of the absolute CHD or CVD risk is essential to separate those who require treatment from those who may not.

HIGH RISK HYPERTENSIVE PATIENTS

Some patient groups have such high CVD risk and chance of benefit that they require antihypertensive treatment even for mild hypertension (≥ 140/90 mm Hg) without formal calculation of absolute risk. Patients with any form of symptomatic atherosclerotic vascular disease, including previous myocardial infarction, bypass graft surgery, angina, stroke or transient ischaemic attack, peripheral vascular disease or atherosclerotic renovascular disease need treatment of even very mild hypertension (≥ 140/90 mm Hg) for *secondary prevention*. Indeed there is mounting evidence that secondary prevention patients with "normal" blood pressure (< 140/90 mm Hg) benefit from blood pressure reduction. This is similar in principle to reducing normal or even "low" cholesterol with statins. Patients with target organ damage such as LVH, heart failure, proteinuria or renal impairment also have high CVD risk and need treatment of even very mild hypertension. Older patients (> 60 years) have high CHD risk by virtue of their age alone, and benefit from treatment of even mild hypertension (≥ 140/90 mm Hg). Patients with *long term* average blood pressure ≥ 160/100 mm Hg have high CVD risk because of the steep association between blood pressure and risk of stroke. The risk of developing cardiovascular complications increases dramatically with the long term average diastolic blood pressure ≥ 100 mm Hg.[11] Formal risk calculation will underestimate true CVD risk for reasons discussed later, and all patients with blood pressure ≥ 160/100 mm Hg after prolonged observation and despite lifestyle advice should be treated.

Patients with type II diabetes also have high CVD risk, but in addition gain extra benefit from antihypertensive treatment because it prevents microvascular complications (for example, nephropathy, retinopathy) as well as large vessel complications. All patients with type II diabetes and mild hypertension (≥ 140/90 mm Hg) should be treated regardless of their absolute CVD risk. Patients with type I diabetes and mild hypertension (≥ 140/90 mm Hg) generally have diabetic nephropathy and should be treated.

These high risk groups all require drug treatment for hypertension and it follows that formal risk assessment is only necessary for decisions on antihypertensive treatment in patients below age 60 with *uncomplicated* mild hypertension (long term average blood pressure 140–159/90–99 mm Hg). However, because of the distribution of blood pressure levels in the population, a large majority of hypertensive patients do have uncomplicated mild hypertension, and do require formal risk calculation.

ESTIMATING ABSOLUTE RISK
Single risk factors such as blood pressure or serum cholesterol are very poor predictors of absolute risk. Counting the number of risk factors present improves accuracy, but the most accurate method of absolute risk estimation is to count and weight appropriately all the major risk factors for CVD.[12] This is done using risk equations which are derived from large prospective epidemiological studies such as the Framingham study and use age, sex, systolic blood pressure, total cholesterol, high density lipoprotein (HDL) cholesterol, smoking history, and presence or absence of diabetes and LVH to compute CVD or CHD risk.[1] Computer programs and paper based risk assessment tables or charts based on the Framingham risk function have been developed to enable doctors to calculate absolute risk easily and with reasonable accuracy.[3 5 13 14] Figure 26.2 illustrates how a paper based risk assessment method based on the Framingham risk function can identify patients at high or low CVD risk much more accurately than methods based on counting risk factors or a single threshold for blood pressure. Thus, the risk assessment methods based on Framingham recommended by the British,[5] New Zealand,[2] and European[14] guidelines all estimate absolute risk much more accurately than the methods based on counting risk factors recommended in the World Health Organization-International Society of Hypertension (WHO-ISH) and Joint National Committee (JNC) VI guidelines. The WHO-ISH and JNC-VI methods do not differentiate patients at high risk from those at low risk with acceptable accuracy.

ACCURACY OF FRAMINGHAM RISK ESTIMATES
Framingham risk estimates are acceptably accurate in North American, UK, and northern European populations, but underestimate absolute risk in populations with much lower rates of cardiovascular disease than North America—for example, some Far Eastern and Mediterranean populations. Framingham may not be accurate in individuals from certain ethnic groups such as British Asians. The Framingham function incorporates the most powerful predictors of cardiovascular disease and omitted family history because its independent effect on risk was less than the other risk factors that were included. A family history of CHD death in a first degree relative before age 65 increases absolute CHD risk by a factor of 1.4, and this can be approximated simply by adding six years to age when calculating risk.

The Framingham risk function may seriously underestimate risk in those with persistent extreme values of blood pressure or total cholesterol:HDL ratio because it was derived from single measurements rather than long term averages as

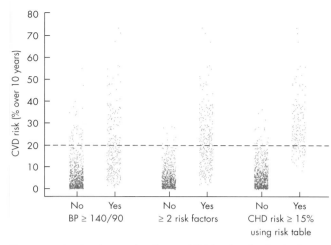

Figure 26.2 Cardiovascular disease (CVD) risks of individuals identified ("Yes"' columns) or not identified ("No" columns) as "high risk" using a single risk factor threshold (systolic blood pressure ≥ 140 mm Hg); counting risk factors (two or more risk factors for CVD); or a Framingham based method (the Sheffield table) to identify individuals with CVD risk ≥ 20% over 10 years. Note that use of a single risk factor gives very poor discrimination between people at low and high CHD risk. Counting risk factors improves the targeting of treatments but leads to identification for treatment of many low risk people. Framingham based methods such as the Sheffield table are more accurate in ensuring identification of those at high risk while avoiding treatment of those at low risk.

discussed previously. Patients with long term average blood pressure ≥ 160/100 mm Hg (or total cholesterol:HDL ratio ≥ 8.0) probably have considerably higher risk than is estimated by Framingham and should be treated.

There are also difficulties in estimating CHD/CVD risk in patients with treated hypertension. Use of the "on treatment" blood pressure underestimates risk because antihypertensive treatment does not completely reverse the increased CHD risk associated with hypertension. Conversely use of the pretreatment blood pressure will overestimate risk because risk is reduced by treatment. Overestimation of risk is preferable to underestimation, and pretreatment blood pressure should be used when possible. "Controlled" hypertension should be regarded as having CHD/CVD risk equivalent to that of untreated mild hypertension—for example, with systolic blood pressure of 160 mm Hg.

Absolute CHD/CVD risk increase with age and risk assessment is not therefore once only. Patients with uncomplicated mild hypertension and very low risk may be observed rather than treated, but they also need advice on lifestyle measures to reduce blood pressure. Blood pressure should be followed up and CHD risk should be reassessed periodically. Around 10% of patients with mild hypertension will progress to levels needing treatment (≥ 160/100 mm Hg) within 5–6 years.[2] Furthermore, advancing age increases absolute CHD risk and most risk assessment methods can be used to "look forward" in time and predict when the CHD risk threshold needing treatment will be reached.

CHD OR CVD RISK?
The Framingham risk function can calculate the absolute risk of any cardiovascular event (CVD risk) or only coronary events (CHD risk). The guidelines from New Zealand which first targeted antihypertensive treatment at absolute risk logically

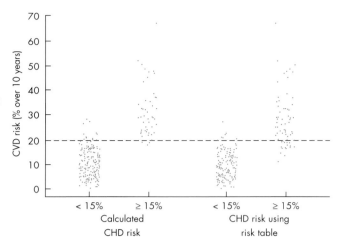

Figure 26.3 Accuracy of CHD risk ≥ 15% over 10 years calculated from the full Framingham equation (shown on the left) or estimated using the Sheffield table (on the right) for predicting CVD risk ≥20% over 10 years in 202 patients with mild uncomplicated hypertension. Reproduced with permission from Wallis et al.[15]

Table 26.2 Accuracy (with 95% confidence intervals) of the New Zealand chart, Sheffield table, and Joint British Societies chart for predicting cardiovascular disease risk ≥ 20% over 10 years in 202 patients with uncomplicated mild hypertension

	New Zealand chart	Sheffield table	Joint Societies chart
Sensitivity (%)	75 (64 to 86)	81 (71 to 91)	63 (51 to 75)
Specificity (%)	96 (92 to 99)	96 (92 to 99)	98 (95 to 100)
PPV (%)	88 (79 to 97)	89 (81 to 97)	93 (85 to 100)
NPV (%)	90 (85 to 95)	92 (87 to 96)	86 (80 to 91)

NPV, negative predictive value; PPV, positive predictive value.

used absolute CVD rather than CHD risk because antihypertensive treatment prevents CHD events and strokes.[3] Treatment of mild hypertension was recommended at CVD risk ≥ 20% over 10 years. However, decisions about statins and aspirin often have to be made in the same patient and these are aimed logically at CHD risk, not CVD risk, because they prevent myocardial infarction but have not been shown to prevent stroke in primary prevention. British guidelines recommend CHD risk assessment for all three preventative treatments[4 5] to avoid confusion. CHD and CVD risks are not numerically equivalent but correlate highly with a ratio of 4:3.[15] British guidelines recommend antihypertensive treatment at CHD risk ≥ 15% over 10 years and this is equivalent to CVD risk of 20% over 10 years. The accuracy of CHD risk 15% for targeting CVD risk 20% is acceptable and is shown on the left hand side of fig 26.3.

ACCURACY OF RISK ESTIMATION METHODS

Computer programs based on the Framingham risk function are available and are slightly more accurate than paper based methods, and may be valuable if the program can be linked to the risk factor database. However, when data have to be entered to calculate risk, computers are considerably slower than paper based methods. Also computers are not available in every clinical setting. Precise risk calculation is of doubtful value when guidelines target only two risk thresholds that can be identified accurately by paper based methods (see below). Some of the computer programs available are over-elaborate and misleading. Some give CHD risk and stroke risk separately, which is unnecessary given their high correlation. Some give relative risk in addition to absolute risk. Relative risk may have a role in motivating patients towards dietary or lifestyle change but has no role in drug treatment decisions. Some computer programs incorporate "risk factors" that are not independent predictors of CHD risk for patient motivation or political correctness (for example, obesity and exercise levels). Finally some programs purport to show the effect of treatment on absolute risk but use inaccurate estimates of relative risk reduction.

Paper based risk estimation methods such as the Joint British Societies chart,[5] the Sheffield table,[13] and the New Zealand chart[3] are used widely in the UK. These use all of the major

risk factors in the Framingham function except for LVH, and use the total cholesterol:HDL cholesterol ratio rather than total cholesterol alone, unlike the European Task Force guidelines chart.[14] The Joint British Societies chart and Sheffield table estimate 10 year risk of CHD events, whereas the New Zealand chart estimates five year risk of CVD events.

The accuracy of these methods for antihypertensive treatment decisions is determined by the proportion of patients with uncomplicated mild hypertension (140–159/90–99 mm Hg) classified correctly as having CVD risk over 10 years above or below the 20% threshold. High sensitivity is essential because the CHD risk threshold recommended in British guidelines is relatively conservative—high risk patients should not be left untreated. Specificity, meaning the proportion of low risk people identified correctly as *not* requiring treatment, is less important than the sensitivity—provided that people with *very* low risk are not identified for treatment. The accuracy of these methods for predicting CVD risk ≥ 20% over 10 years in patients with uncomplicated mild hypertension is shown in table 26.2 and illustrated for the Sheffield table on the right hand side of fig 26.3. The New Zealand chart was surprisingly inaccurate, despite using CVD risk, as it failed to identify 25% of patients with CVD risk ≥ 20%. The Sheffield table had higher sensitivity (81% v 75% for the New Zealand chart), but similar specificity (96% for both charts) even though it targets CVD risk indirectly through CHD risk. The Joint British Societies chart has unacceptably low sensitivity (63%) and fails to treat 37% of patients with mild hypertension who have high CVD risk (≥ 20% over 10 years). None of these methods identified any very low risk patients for treatment.

ADDITIONAL METHODS OF RISK ESTIMATION
Ambulatory blood pressure measurement

There has been considerable interest and debate over whether accurate blood pressure measurement by ambulatory blood pressure monitoring (ABPM) improves CVD risk prediction. ABPM does predict CVD risk, and the benefit from treatment, better than a limited number of clinic or surgery measurements, and there is some evidence that it may even be superior to the long term average of numerous clinic or surgery measurements.[16] However blood pressure itself makes only a relatively small contribution to absolute risk, and improvements in accuracy of measurement will therefore alter absolute risk estimates little. ABPM is not needed routinely for decisions to start antihypertensive treatment. It is valuable for treatment decisions in patients who have uncomplicated moderate–severe hypertension (≥ 160/100 mm Hg) in clinic but low absolute CHD risk (< 15% over 10 years). In such patients the blood pressure level is the only indication for

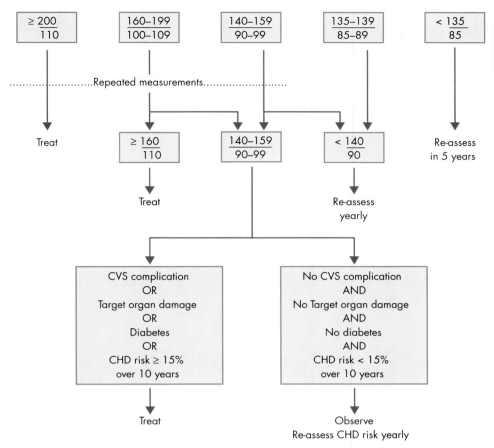

Figure 26.4 Summary of recommendations in the British Hypertension Society guidelines for targeting of antihypertensive treatment.[4]

treatment and it is important to ensure accuracy. ABPM is also useful if there is unusual variability in blood pressure, if there are symptoms of hypotension with normal clinic measurements, or in resistant hypertension. ABPM is remarkably variable on repeated measurements and should be repeated when it influences treatment decisions. The average of the two results should be used. Blood pressure thresholds and targets for treatment should be adjusted downwards for ABPM readings by a factor of around 10/5 mm Hg. Thus in a low risk patient with no indications for treatment of mild hypertension, antihypertensive treatment should be started if the average daytime ABPM blood pressure is ≥ 150/95 mm Hg.

Echocardiography
LVH on ECG, defined as increased voltage plus T wave abnormality, doubles CHD risk. However, LVH with T wave abnormality is uncommon in hypertensive patients. Echocardiography is more "sensitive" for detecting LVH in patients with hypertension. Many doctors equate higher sensitivity with more powerful risk prediction and believe that echocardiography is superior to the ECG for CHD risk estimation. This is incorrect. Because echocardiographic LVH is more prevalent it is a much less powerful predictor of risk than LVH detected on an ECG. Quantitative measurement of left ventricular mass by echocardiography has been shown to add to the accuracy of risk prediction using the ECG, but the very small gain in accuracy is irrelevant for clinical decisions.[17] There are also major problems with the accuracy of left ventricular mass measurement and test–retest variability, and disagreement over the definition of echo LVH and the thresholds of normality. Of course, when echocardiographic LVH is detected this represents end organ damage and so even mild hypertension should be treated regardless of the absolute risk

estimate. Echocardiography should not be done routinely in hypertensive patients. It should be reserved for patients with "voltage criteria" LVH on ECG but no T wave abnormality in whom echocardiography often *disproves* the presence of true LVH, and in patients with other indications for echocardiography such as a heart murmur or symptoms suggestive of heart failure.

AT WHAT LEVEL OF CVD RISK IS TREATMENT JUSTIFIED?
British guidelines recommend treatment for those with CHD risk ≥ 15% over 10 years,[4][5] and this is equivalent to the CVD risk threshold of ≥ 20% over 10 years recommended in the New Zealand guidelines.[3] Around 25% of patients with uncomplicated mild hypertension have CHD risk ≥ 15% over 10 years.[15] The relative risk reduction by treatment is 25%, and the absolute risk reduction with treatment at this level of risk is 5% over 10 years. This equates to a five year NNT of 40 to prevent one major cardiovascular complication. The WHO-ISH and JNC-VI guidelines advocate risk assessment but are not explicit on the level of risk to be treated. However, their risk assessment methods lead to treatment of very low risk patients and to a much larger NNT. The minimum acceptable level of absolute benefit from antihypertensive treatment can be debated but really needs to be studied. Antihypertensive treatment targeted at the level of risk recommended in British guidelines is undoubtedly safe, meaning that benefit clearly outweighs any serious harm. Cost effectiveness is also well within generally accepted limits. However, the level of absolute benefit at which treatment becomes *worthwhile* is extremely difficult to assess. The chance of a cardiovascular complication being prevented, and the value of this, must be

weighed against possible harm, discomfort, and inconvenience of long term tablet taking. Doctors can debate this endlessly, but the correct answers can only come from formal study of the choices of fully informed patients or potential patients. Little research has been done to determine what benefit (or NNT) is generally acceptable to patients. One study suggested that most would opt to take preventative treatment for an NNT of 40, while another suggested they would not. It is doubtful whether fully informed people would choose to take treatment for the extremely low chance of benefit (or high NNT) that follows from the WHO-ISH or JNC-VI guidelines.

PROBLEMS WITH TARGETING ABSOLUTE RISK

The principle of targeting treatment at high absolute CHD risk rather than high cholesterol is now accepted for statin treatment, but the similar policy for antihypertensive treatment is less widely known and practised. Antihypertensive treatment was targeted at defined blood pressure thresholds for decades, and the idea that treatment to lower blood pressure should not be targeted at blood pressure but at CHD risk is difficult for some to grasp. This difficulty is compounded by the intense interest in more precise measurement of blood pressure using ABPM, and ever more detailed analyses of ABPM patterns.

The overwhelming influence of age on CHD risk leads to treatment of mild hypertension in older people while most younger people are observed rather than treated.[18] European guidelines for CHD prevention suggest that CHD risk should be projected to age 60 to target treatment.[14] This may be better than using blood pressure thresholds alone, but in essence it identifies those at high *relative risk* rather than high absolute risk. Many of those treated will have extremely low absolute risk and may be disadvantaged by treatment. One reason for this recommendation may be concern that failure to treat mild hypertension in young people may allow development of LVH or other target organ damage. Once established, target organ damage confers a bad prognosis that cannot be completely reversed by treatment. However, the risk of developing LVH in patients with uncomplicated mild hypertension is remote.[2] Concern has been expressed that absolute risk reduction may not be the best measure of benefit because it assumes that the prevention of a CVD event has equal worth in all people regardless of age.[18] Prevention of death in a younger person may save more years of extra life than prevention of death in an older person, and similarly prevention of a non-fatal complication may attain more quality adjusted life-years. Therefore prevention of a cardiovascular complication may be more valuable in younger patients. If so, applying a uniform absolute risk threshold for treatment regardless of age would disadvantage the young.

Methods of targeting treatment at total life-years gained, total quality adjusted life-years gained, or life-years gained per year of treatment have been examined.[19] The latter method makes surprisingly little difference to the age of introducing treatment when compared to the use of a single absolute risk threshold.[20] Furthermore there will always be a trade off in these methods. Any reduction in the level of absolute risk treated or absolute benefit sought will narrow the margin between benefit and harm from treatment. Younger people may value benefit more highly, but will they take more kindly to rare but serious side effects, subjective side effects, inconvenience, and the need to take tablets? One suspects not.

Key points

- The absolute risk of cardiovascular disease dictates the absolute benefit from antihypertensive treatment. Absolute risk assessment is essential to ensure high risk patients are treated while avoiding treatment of low risk patients
- In certain patients formal risk assessment is unnecessary because certain risk factors always place patients at high risk
- Where formal risk assessment is necessary, methods based on the Framingham risk function are preferable and a number of computer programs and simple paper based risk assessment methods are available
- CHD risk multiplied by 4/3 is an acceptable surrogate for CVD risk.
- Additional refinements in risk factor measurement such as ambulatory blood pressure measurement or echocardiography usually add little information to formal risk estimates
- The threshold of CVD risk at which treatment is justified is a matter for continued research and debate

Our own view is that the question of whether the risk threshold should differ with age, and how, is unlikely to be resolved by any mechanistic method. Fully informed patients should decide what benefit they require from treatment, not their doctors, and there is a need to develop better methods to study patient choice. Only then will we know whether older people feel that they have had a "good innings" and do not wish treatment, or whether they have attended many funerals and wish to postpone their own. Are young people keen to take treatment to prevent complications 20–40 years in the future or are their priorities elsewhere?

CONCLUSION

There is a consensus in the UK that antihypertensive treatment should be targeted at absolute risk rather than at any single blood pressure threshold. A summary of the recommendations for targeting of antihypertensive treatment by the British Hypertension Society[4] is shown in fig 26.4.

REFERENCES

1 **Anderson KM**, Odel PM, Wilson PWF, *et al.* Cardiovascular disease risk profiles. *Am Heart J* 1991;**121**:293–8.
- ▶ This paper contains the Framingham risk functions.
2 **Ramsay LE**. The hypertension detection and follow-up program 17 years on. *JAMA* 1997;**277**:167–70.
- ▶ A discussion outlining how absolute benefit is predicted by absolute risk and the implications of this for antihypertensive treatment guidelines.
3 **New Zealand Ministry of Health**. *Guidelines for the management of mildly raised blood pressure in New Zealand.* Wellington: Core Services Committee, Ministry of Health, 1995.
- ▶ These were the first guidelines to advocate the use of absolute risk in antihypertensive treatment decisions.
4 **Ramsay LE**, Williams B, Johnston GD, *et al.* British Hypertension Society guidelines for hypertension management 1999: summary. *BMJ* 1999;**319**:630–5.
- ▶ Summary version of British Hypertension Society guidelines.
5 **Wood D**, Durrington P, Poulter N, *et al* on behalf of the British Cardiac Society, British Hyperlipidaemia Association, British Hypertension Society and endorsed by the British Diabetic Association. Joint British recommendations on prevention of coronary heart disease in clinical practice. *Heart* 1998;**80**(suppl 2):S1–29.
- ▶ Guidelines containing the Joint British Societies chart.
6 **Collins R**, Peto R. Antihypertensive drug therapy: effects on stroke and coronary heart disease. In: Swales JD, ed. *Textbook of hypertension.* Oxford: Blackwell Scientific, 1992:1156–64.
7 **Madhavan S**, Alderman MH. The potential effect of blood pressure reduction on cardiovascular disease. *Arch Intern Med* 1981;**141**:1583–6.
8 **Cook RJ**, Sackett DL. The number needed to treat: a clinically useful measure of treatment effect. *BMJ* 1995;**310**:452–4.
9 **Glasziou PP**, Irwig LM. An evidence based approach to individualising patient treatment. *BMJ* 1995;**311**:1356–9.

10 **Hoes AW**, Grobbee DE, Lubson J. Does drug treatment improve survival? Reconciling the trials in mild to moderate hypertension. *J Hypertens* 1995;**13**:805–11.
► **This paper attempts to quantify the risk of serious harm from antihypertensive treatment. It has methodological weaknesses outlined in an accompanying editorial by Eggar.**
11 **Ramsay LE**. Mild hypertension: treat patients, not populations. *J Hypertens* 1985;**3**:449–55.
12 **Grover SA**, Coupal L, Hu X-P. Identifying adults at increased risk of coronary disease. How well do the current cholesterol guidelines work? *JAMA* 1995;**274**:801–6.
13 **Wallis EJ**, Ramsay LE, Haq IU, *et al*. Coronary and cardiovascular risk estimation for primary prevention: validation of a new Sheffield table in the 1995 Scottish health survey population. *BMJ* 2000;**320**:671–6.
► **This paper contains a colour version of the updated Sheffield table, a detailed assessment of its accuracy, and a critical assessment of the use of absolute risk in primary prevention.**
14 **Wood D**, De Backer G, Faergeman O, *et al* with members of the Task Force. Prevention of coronary heart disease in clinical practice. Recommendations of the second joint task force of European and other societies on coronary prevention. *Eur Heart J* 1998;**19**:1434–503.
15 **Wallis EJ**, Ramsay LE, Haq IU, *et al*. Is coronary risk an accurate surrogate for cardiovascular risk for treatment decisions in mild hypertension? A population validation. *J Hypertens* 2001;**19**:691–6.
► **This paper examines the relation between coronary and cardiovascular risk in patients with mild hypertension in detail.**

16 **Staessen JA**, Thijs L, Fagard R, *et al*. Predicting cardiovascular risk using conventional vs ambulatory blood pressure in older patients with systolic hypertension. Systolic hypertension in Europe trial investigators. *JAMA* 2000;**282**:539–46.
17 **Levy D**, Garrison RJ, Savage MS, *et al*. Prognostic implications of echocardiographically determined left ventricular mass in the Framingham heart study. *N Engl J Med* 1990;**322**:1561–6.
18 **Simpson FO**. Guidelines for antihypertensive therapy: problems with a strategy based on absolute cardiovascular risk. *J Hypertens* 1996;**14**:683–9.
► **This editorial gives a full discussion of the problems with targeting treatment at absolute risk relating to patient age.**
19 **Ulrich S**, Hingorani AD, Martin J, *et al*. What is the optimal age for starting lipid lowering treatment? A mathematical model. *BMJ* 2000;**320**:1134–40.
► **One of the first articles to show how preventative treatments could be targeted at life-years gained rather than absolute risk, although it has methodological weaknesses.**
20 **Jackson PR**, Wallis EJ, Ramsay LE. Optimal age for starting lipid lowering treatment. Adjusted data do not justify a lower optimal age. *BMJ* 2000;**34**:637.

Additional references appear on the *Heart* website–
www.heartjnl.com

SECTION IX: GENERAL CARDIOLOGY

27 ANAESTHESIA AND THE CARDIAC PATIENT: THE PATIENT VERSUS THE PROCEDURE

James B Froehlich, Kim A Eagle

For patients undergoing elective surgery, the most common cause of significant morbidity and mortality is occurrence of complications related to cardiac disease.[1] It is estimated that approximately one million patients undergoing surgery each year in the USA suffer a perioperative myocardial infarction.[1] This is particularly true for those with previous coronary disease and those facing higher risk surgery. Because of this fact, a great deal of research has focused on assessing cardiac risk before elective surgery. Less attention has been paid to methods of modifying the risk of cardiac complications attending surgery through medication use or other strategies. The risk of cardiac complications engenders a sense of conflict in that the patient perceives surgery as a threatening foe to be overcome: the patient versus the procedure. We would like to change that paradigm, and encourage an appreciation for the risk inherent to the patient, rather than to the procedure itself. That is, preoperative evaluation of the patient's risk, versus the procedure's risk.

During the past 10–20 years, the assessment of cardiac risk before surgery evolved a great deal. Initially, the focus was on appropriate identification of surgical procedures that carried high risk. The focus then shifted to identifying those patient factors associated with increased risk of cardiac complications during surgery. Several technical advances were made during this time, including the introduction of imaging stress tests to assess cardiac ischaemia, such as dobutamine echocardiogram, dobutamine thallium, and adenosine or dipyridamole thallium testing. All of these modalities have been shown to identify patients at increased risk for cardiac complications of surgery. Cardiac catheterisation has also been used as a screening modality before elective surgery, though this has not been shown to be cost effective, especially given the low overall incidence of severe coronary artery disease. Studies performed during this time period also delineated the clinical factors that identify patients at increased risk of cardiac complications. More recently, efforts have been made to combine both clinical evaluation and testing in the most efficient and appropriate manner to identify patients at risk of cardiac complications. Finally, recent studies have addressed the effectiveness of medications or interventions to decrease risk in high risk patients.

Preoperative cardiac evaluation has several goals:

- evaluate and assess perioperative cardiac risk, and provide this information to both patient and surgeon for decision making purposes
- optimise appropriateness of preoperative testing and/or intervention
- to the extent possible, adjust care in order to decrease operative risk
- given the prevalence of coronary disease and its complications, assess and intervene to modify long term risks for cardiovascular disease.

We discuss below the current state of preoperative cardiac evaluation and interventions to decrease perioperative cardiac risk, and offer an approach to the preoperative assessment and perioperative care of patients with cardiac disease, focusing on risk reduction.

▶ CLINICAL EVALUATION

Historically, the preoperative assessment of patients before elective surgery was based almost entirely on the clinical evaluation and examination. The American Society of Anesthesiology has used the ASA physical status classification system (1963) to grade perioperative risk. This classification could identify those at extremely high risk of complications from surgery, but did not offer much sensitivity in assessing patients' risk. The patients in level IV or V were at extremely elevated risk, but patients categorised in level III constituted a very wide spectrum of risk and comorbid disease. Furthermore, the ASA classification system does not focus on cardiac risk per se. It offers no consideration for the presence or absence of serious coronary disease in otherwise asymptomatic or undiagnosed patients.

Lee Goldman, then a resident at Massachusetts General Hospital, conducted a study that identified clinical factors conferring elevated risk of surgical complications.[2] By performing a multivariate logistic regression analysis of a wide range of clinical parameters on 1000 consecutive patients undergoing elective surgery at the Massachusetts General Hospital, Goldman and his

192

colleagues identified clinical markers of increased risk, and appropriately weighted them based on the epidemiological risk they conferred. The Goldman grading system allowed an estimate of the weighted risk of perioperative cardiac complications based on the presence or absence of clinical factors including the history of recent myocardial infarction, presence of congestive heart failure, critical aortic stenosis, significant non-cardiac organ failure or disease, urgency of surgery, and advanced age. The presence of these factors, particularly when added together, correlated with elevated risk. However, the majority of patients studied did not have markers of high risk and the index proved to be insensitive for discriminating risk in patients who would be considered intermediate in risk. The Goldman index did not include evaluation by objective stress testing, nor does it allow one to infer a plan for appropriate further steps in the evaluation process.

Several other studies have confirmed the utility of clinical evaluation in identifying patients at increased risk of significant coronary disease. L'Italien and others reviewed the clinical risk factors of patients undergoing elective vascular surgery at Massachusetts General Hospital, University of Massachusetts Medical Center, and the University of Vermont Medical Center, and analysed these clinical risk assessments with the results of thallium functional testing, also done before surgery.[3] This group initially identified a small list of clinical factors that conferred risk based on multivariate logistic regression analysis. These clinical factors are advanced age, a history of diabetes, myocardial infarction, angina, or congestive heart failure. This group's findings, corroborated by other groups, revealed that the absence of any of these clinical markers of risk conferred a very low risk of complications of surgery (3% in this study). Likewise, the presence of one or two of these factors conferred a moderately increased risk (8%) and the presence of three or more a high risk of death or myocardial infarction during vascular surgery (18% in this study).

Paul and colleagues reviewed an extensive database of cardiac catheterisation results on 878 consecutive patients undergoing elective vascular surgery at the Cleveland Clinic.[4] They reviewed these same five clinical markers of risk, and observed that the presence of three or more of these clinical markers was coincident with a high likelihood of three vessel or left main coronary artery disease. Similarly, the absence of any of these markers of risk was coincident with a very low likelihood of having severe coronary artery disease on catheterisation. Taken together, these studies of clinical markers of cardiac risk suggest that patients who are properly evaluated, and have none of these clinical markers of risk, have a very low likelihood of suffering cardiac complications of surgery. This finding has recently been corroborated in clinical trials of the effect of perioperative β blockade on cardiac complications.

NON-INVASIVE TESTING

The introduction of sensitive non-invasive tests for coronary artery disease, particularly pharmacologic stress tests that require no treadmill exercise, has greatly influenced the preoperative assessment of cardiac risk. Several early studies demonstrated a very high sensitivity of these tests for identifying patients at increased risk of perioperative cardiac complications. Most impressively, these results have been repeatedly duplicated by a large number of investigators. In an important work on the subject, Boucher and others demonstrated that thallium testing before elective vascular surgery accurately identified those patients who suffered cardiac complications of surgery.[5] Furthermore, those patients with a normal thallium study had a very low incidence of cardiac complications. This was followed by several other studies, which demonstrated essentially similar results. Taken together, the clinical studies of thallium testing before vascular surgery have shown strikingly consistent results. These are a very high sensitivity (between 85–100%), but a fairly low specificity for the identification of patients who suffer cardiac complications of surgery. For this reason, the negative predictive value of thallium is quite high, better than 95%, even combining all current clinical studies. The positive predictive value, however, is quite low because of the low specificity (a problem of false positive tests in lower risk patients). This makes thallium stress testing a reassuring test when negative, but clinically confusing when positive. Such results highlight the fact that thallium testing is inappropriate as a uniform screening test, particularly when applied to "low risk" individuals.

Fewer studies have examined dobutamine echocardiogram as a preoperative screening modality; however, the results are quite similar to those found with thallium testing. There is similar sensitivity with the same problem of relatively low specificity. At institutions that have established proficiency at dobutamine echocardiogram testing, the results are considered interchangeable with thallium testing. Dobutamine echocardiography has the advantage of providing information regarding valvar structure and function.

Exercise tolerance testing, without cardiac imaging, also has an important role in screening for cardiac risk. Exercise tolerance, combined with electrocardiographic interpretation (assuming a normal baseline ECG), has great prognostic power for the patient with known or suspected coronary disease. Similarly, the ability to achieve maximum predicted heart rate without ECG confers a low risk for cardiac complications of elective surgery. Because it evaluates exercise tolerance and gives an idea of the level of stress that may induce inducible ischaemia, exercise testing is generally preferable to pharmacologic testing, particularly for long term prognostication.

Because of the relatively non-specific nature of functional testing, it is best employed as a component of an organised programme for cardiac risk evaluation. Proper clinical assessment of pre-test probability of significant coronary disease will allow more prudent use and interpretation of ischaemia testing.

Invasive testing has been proposed as a screening modality for patients undergoing high risk surgery—for example, peripheral vascular reconstructions. Hertzer and colleagues reported from the Cleveland Clinic on the use of routine catheterisation on 1000 consecutive patients scheduled for vascular surgery.[6] Although they reported a high incidence of patients with severe coronary disease, requiring coronary bypass grafting, subsequent review of the data suggests that most of those patients with coronary disease sufficiently severe to warrant revascularisation could be identified on clinical grounds. This, and the expense and risk of routine catheterisation, have led most to consider clinical and functional assessment as initial screening for cardiac risk.

METHODS FOR LOWERING PERIOPERATIVE CARDIAC RISK

Coronary bypass surgery

Recently, attention has turned to evaluating the effectiveness of methods for intervening to lower risk of cardiac complications during elective surgery. Coronary revascularisation is one such intervention. A retrospective review by Eagle and colleagues of the CASS (coronary artery surgery study) registry data supports such a protective effect.[7] These data demonstrate that patients undergoing elective vascular surgery, who had previously undergone coronary artery bypass grafting, did better than control patients who had similar amounts of coronary disease, but no surgical coronary revascularisation. This type of analysis does not take into consideration the cumulative risk of both coronary and peripheral revascularisation, and so does not necessarily argue for prophylactic surgical coronary revascularisation before elective peripheral vascular surgery. But it does suggest a protective effect of prior coronary bypass surgery. Data from the Cleveland Clinic showed similar findings—that patients with a history of coronary artery bypass grafting, regardless of clinical risk factors, had lower perioperative cardiac complication rates surrounding vascular surgery than patients with coronary disease managed medically. These studies argue that a history of successful coronary artery bypass surgery confers a lower risk of cardiac complications surrounding elective surgery.

Percutaneous coronary intervention

The discovery of ischaemia on functional testing frequently leads to consideration of percutaneous revascularisation before elective vascular surgery. This practice has not been subjected to randomised controlled trials to assess its efficacy. Trials are currently underway for this purpose. Previous randomised studies comparing medical treatment with angioplasty in patients with stable coronary disease of limited severity have demonstrated an increased event rate in those patients undergoing angioplasty. The bulk of this increase came in the form of periprocedural complications. Retrospective studies reporting the rates of perioperative cardiac complications in patients who underwent previous preoperative angioplasty and/or coronary stent placement have shown very mixed results. Posner and colleagues reported a lower rate of cardiac complications among patients who underwent angioplasty before surgery compared with a group of patients with coronary artery disease managed medically.[8] This study is uncontrolled for severity of disease or medical management, however. Massie and associates performed a case–control study comparing patients with abnormal thallium studies who did and did not undergo angiography before vascular surgery, and found no difference in event rates.[9] Hassan and colleagues found similarly low rates of cardiac complications after non-cardiac surgery among patients in the BARI (bypass angioplasty revascularization investigation) study.[10] This was equally true for patients who had undergone multivessel percutaneous coronary intervention, as for those who underwent coronary bypass surgery. Finally, Kaluza and colleagues reported a very high incidence of stent thrombosis, death, and myocardial infarction in patients undergoing non-cardiac surgery within two weeks of coronary stent placement.[11] These data raise concern that the strategy of prophylactic, percutaneous coronary revascularisation before elective surgery may result in destabilisation of previously stable coronary disease which offsets the potential advantage of improving ischaemic thresholds of the heart by reducing severe, fixed coronary stenoses.

Perioperative medical treatment

Several recent studies have suggested that β blockers decrease risk of perioperative complications. A randomised study by Mangano and colleagues evaluated brief courses of perioperative β blockade in patients undergoing a variety of surgical procedures.[12] The study was small, and demonstrated no difference in perioperative complication rate. However, over the succeeding two years, the patients who received this brief course of perioperative β blockade had a lower incidence of cardiac events. This study did not control for medications between the two groups, but at least raises the question of a protective effect of perioperative β blockade. A more recent study by Poldermans and associates randomised only clinically high risk patients undergoing elective, major vascular surgery, to the β blocker bucindolol or placebo.[13] This study demonstrated a significant reduction in perioperative cardiac events, both fatal and non-fatal, with the use of a β blocker. These patients were given β blocker treatment days or weeks before surgery. The β blocker was titrated to a target dose of 10 mg per day, so long as the heart rate remained above 60 beats per minute. These studies, combined with previous investigations that show a protective effect of β blockers for both ambulatory and perioperative ischaemia, support the hypothesis that perioperative β blockade decreases cardiac risk among high risk patients.

Finally, several recent studies evaluated the effect of α receptor agonists in the perioperative period on the incidence of cardiac events. In a large randomised controlled trial of intravenous α_2 agonist mivazerol during surgery, Oliver and colleagues compared outcomes during surgery in patients who had either a history of coronary artery disease, or the presence of significant risk factors.[14] They found no significant effect in the patients undergoing non-cardiac surgery in general, but a significant reduction in both cardiac events and death in the subset of patients undergoing vascular surgery. Mangano and colleagues reported the results of a randomised trial of the same agent in 300 patients undergoing non-cardiac surgery, and found no significant effect on cardiac events.[15] These and other studies at least raise the possibility that intraoperative α agonists may reduce perioperative cardiac events.

These reports certainly raise hope for therapeutic intervention to lower perioperative risk of cardiac events. The initial β blocker study of Poldermans and colleagues demonstrated benefit in a high risk cohort of patients undergoing vascular surgery.[13] More recent data from the same group suggests benefit from β blockade across all risk groups. This requires prospective trial validation. Currently, it seems quite reasonable to use the American College of Cardiology/American Heart Association (ACC/AHA) guidelines to assess risk,[16] and consider β blockade in any patients at increased risk not already taking them. The role of α agonists is less clear. The above mentioned studies suggest some benefit from their use in patients undergoing vascular surgery, but little is known about these patients, and what the indications for use of this agent would be.

PUTTING IT ALL TOGETHER

The past two decades have answered many questions about perioperative cardiac complications, and who is at increased risk for them. As discussed above, we have a good understanding of what constitutes a high risk patient, and what tests are useful in further defining risk. The ACC/AHA preoperative evaluation guidelines describe a method of integrating these data into an efficient, evidence based approach to evaluating cardiac risk.[16] This approach incorporates three

194

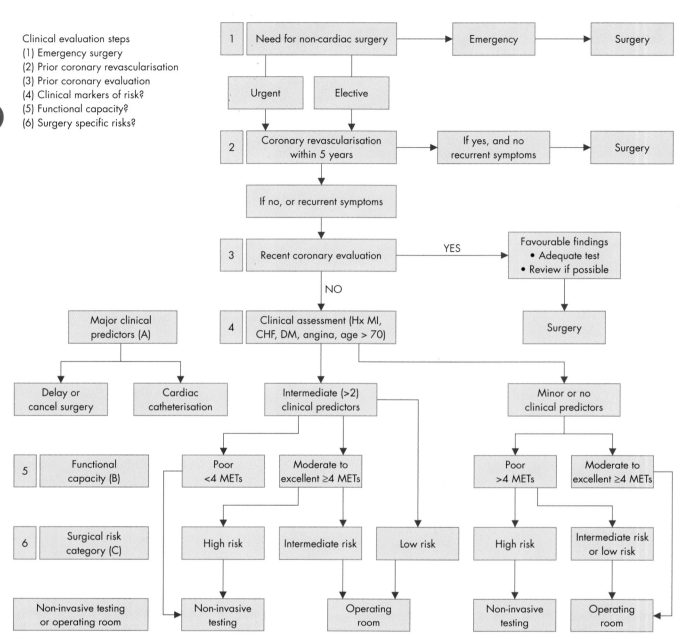

Clinical evaluation steps
(1) Emergency surgery
(2) Prior coronary revascularisation
(3) Prior coronary evaluation
(4) Clinical markers of risk?
(5) Functional capacity?
(6) Surgery specific risks?

Figure 27.1 Algorithm for cardiac risk assessment before non-cardiac surgery. Hx MI, history of myocardial infarction; CHF, congestive heart failure; DM, diabetes mellitus.

steps: first, a clinical evaluation to determine the patient's likelihood of significant coronary disease, and perioperative cardiac event risk; second, selective use of non-invasive testing to further refine risk assessment; and third, intervention to further assess and/or modify cardiac risk. This approach should be taken with the patient's lifetime risk of cardiac disease manifestations as the end point, not just the perioperative period. The following algorithm outlines this approach (fig 27.1).

The first step in this algorithm is to determine urgency of the planned surgery. Obviously, emergent surgery should proceed without the delay of cardiac evaluation. Any surgical procedures not felt to be emergent allow for more thorough evaluation of cardiac risk. For patients who have undergone coronary revascularisation within the previous five years, without any recurrent symptoms of cardiac disease, further evaluation is probably unnecessary (step 2). If previous, recent, (within two years) adequate cardiac evaluation has taken place, without any change in clinical status, then there is usually no need to repeat

A. Major clinical predictors of increased cardiovascular risk

- ▶ Unstable coronary syndromes
- ▶ Recent myocardial infarction with evidence of important ischaemic risk by clinical symptoms or non-invasive study
- ▶ Unstable or severe angina (Canadian Cardiovascular Society class III or IV)
- ▶ Decompensated heart failure
- ▶ Significant arrhythmias
- ▶ High grade ventricular arrhythmias in the presence of underlying heart disease
- ▶ Supraventricular arrhythmias with uncontrolled ventricular rate
- ▶ Severe valvar disease

before surgery, if the results indicated low risk (step 3). Finally, a thorough clinical evaluation should be undertaken to determine if major markers of risk are present (for which

B. Estimated functional capacity, based on daily activities

1 MET

▸ Can you take care of yourself?
▸ Eat, dress or use the toilet?
▸ Walk indoors around the house?
▸ Walk a block or two on level ground at 2–3 mph or 3.2–4.8 km/h?
▸ Do light work around the house like dusting or washing dishes?
↓
4 METs
4 METs

▸ Climb a flight of stairs or walk up a hill?
▸ Walk on level ground at 4 mph or 6.4 km/h?
▸ Run a short distance?
▸ Do heavy work around the house like scrubbing floors or lifting or moving heavy furniture?
▸ Participate in moderate recreational activities like golf, bowling, dancing, doubles tennis, or throwing a baseball or football?
▸ Participate in strenuous sports like swimming, singles tennis, football, basketball, or skiing?
↓
>10 METs

METs, metabolic equivalents

C. Risk stratification for non-cardiac surgical procedures

Major (reported cardiac risk often > 5%)
▸ Emergent major operations, particularly in the elderly
▸ Aortic and other major vascular
▸ Peripheral vascular
▸ Anticipated prolonged surgical procedures associated with large fluid shifts and/or blood loss

Intermediate (reported cardiac risk 1–5%)
▸ Carotid endarterectomy
▸ Head and neck
▸ Intraperitoneal and intrathoracic
▸ Orthopaedic
▸ Prostate

Low* (reported cardiac risk generally < 1%)
▸ Endoscopic procedures
▸ Superficial procedure
▸ Cataract
▸ Breast

*Do not generally require further preoperative cardiac testing

cardiac catheterisation should be considered), or if any of the five clinical markers of risk are present (history of myocardial infarction, diabetes mellitus, congestive heart failure, angina, age > 70 years). A decision about stress testing is based on the clinical markers of risk present, the patient's functional capacity by history, and the expected cardiovascular stress posed by non-cardiac surgery (fig 27.1).

In this way, a systematic approach, based on the current literature and validated prediction tools, can guide the assessment of risk, and the prudent use of further diagnostic testing of cardiac risk before non-cardiac surgery. As stated above, this systematic approach does not rely on testing, but incorporates clinical evaluation with objective testing to define cardiac risk of non-cardiac surgery optimally.

Key points

● Exploit opportunity of preoperative evaluation to assess and intervene upon reversible cardiovascular risk factors
● Evaluation based on cardiac risk, not pending surgery.
● Utilise history, physical, and ECG findings to stratify clinical risk
● Further evaluation (for example, stress testing, catheterisation), based on clinical evaluation, and probability of disease
● Use stress testing to modify, not co-opt, pre-testing likelihood of disease
● Decision regarding stress testing, cardiac catheterisation, or revascularisation, based on algorithm
● β Blockade indicated for higher risk patients undergoing vascular surgery.

REFERENCES

1 **Mangano DT**, Goldman L. Preoperative assessment of patients with known or suspected coronary disease. N Engl J Med 1995;**333**:1750–6.
▸ **Excellent review of the topic.**
2 **Goldman L**, Caldera DL, Nussbaum SR, et al. Multifactorial index of cardiac risk in non-cardiac surgical procedures. N Engl J Med 1977;**297**:845–50.
▸ **Seminal work, identifying for the first time the magnitude and nature of the impact on perioperative cardiac risk of several important clinical findings.**
3 **L'Italien GJ**, Paul SD, Hendel RC, et al. Development and validation of a Bayesian model for perioperative cardiac risk assessment in a cohort of 1,081 vascular surgical candidates. J Am Coll Cardiol 1996;**27**:779–86.
▸ **This study shows the relative roles of clinical and radiological evaluation of patients before vascular surgery, and the value of combining the two to improve accuracy and decrease testing.**
4 **Paul SD**, Eagle KA, Kuntz KM, et al. Concordance of preoperative clinical risk with angiographic severity of coronary artery disease in patients undergoing vascular surgery Circulation 1996;**94**:1561–6.
▸ **Confirmatory study, documenting the power of clinical risk factors to predict severity of coronary disease.**
5 **Boucher CA**, Brewster DC, Darling RC, et al. Determination of cardiac risk by dipyridamole-thallium imaging before peripheral vascular surgery. N Engl J Med 1985;**312**:389–94.
6 **Hertzer NR**, Beven EG, Young JR, et al. Coronary artery disease in peripheral vascular patients: a classification of 1000 coronary angiograms and results of surgical management. Ann Surg 1984;**199**:223–32.
▸ **Early, single centre report of findings on routine cardiac catheterisation in patients undergoing vascular surgery.**
7 **Eagle KA**, Rihal CS, Mickel MC, et al. Cardiac risk of noncardiac surgery: influence of coronary disease and type of surgery in 3368 operations. CASS Investigators and University of Michigan Heart Care Program. Coronary artery surgery study. Circulation 1997; **96**:1882–7.
8 **Posner KL**, Van Norman GA, Chan V. Adverse cardiac outcomes after noncardiac surgery in patients with prior percutaneous transluminal coronary angioplasty. Anesth Analg 1999;**89**:553–60.
9 **Massie MT**, Rohrer MJ, Leppo JA, et al. Is coronary angiography necessary for vascular surgery patients who have positive results of dipyridamole thallium scans. J Vasc Surg 1997;**25**:975–82; discussion 982–3.
10 **Hassan SA**, Hlatky MA, Boothroyd D, et al. Outcomes of non-cardiac surgery after coronary bypass surgery or coronary angioplasty in the bypass angioplasty revascularization investigation (BARI). Am J Med (in press).
▸ **BARI study data suggesting low rates of cardiac events after either coronary bypass surgery or multi-vessel coronary angioplasty before non-cardiac surgery.**
11 **Kaluza GL**, Joseph J, Lee JR, et al. Catastrophic outcomes of non-cardiac surgery soon after coronary stenting. J Am Coll Cardiol 2000;**35**:1288–94.
▸ **One of few observations about the important question of timing of surgery after percutaneous coronary intervention (PCI). This study suggests significant risk associated with stopping antiplatelet agents within 2–4 weeks of PCI.**
12 **Mangano DT**, Layug EL, Wallace A, et al. Effect of atenolol on mortality and cardiovascular morbidity after noncardiac surgery. Multicenter study of perioperative ischemia research group. N Engl J Med 1996;**335**:1713–20.

13 **Poldermans D**, Boersma E, Bax JJ, *et al*. The effect of bisoprolol on perioperative mortality and myocardial infarction in high-risk patients undergoing vascular surgery. Dutch echocardiographic cardiac risk evaluation applying stress echocardiography study group. *N Engl J Med* 1999;**341**:1789–94.

14 **Oliver MF**, Goldman L, Julian DG, *et al*. Effect of mivazerol on perioperative cardiac complications during non-cardiac surgery in patients with coronary heart disease. The European mivazerol trial (EMIT). *Anesthesiology* 1999;**91**:951–61.

15 **Anon**. Perioperative sympatholysis. Beneficial effects of the alpha 2-adrenoceptor agonist mivazerol on hemodynamic stability and myocardial ischemia, MeSPI –Europe research group. *Anesthesiology* 1997;**86**:346–63.

16 **Eagle KA**, Brundage BH, Chaitman BR, *et al*. Guidelines for perioperative cardiovascular evaluation for non-cardiac surgery. *Circulation*. 1996;**93**:1278–317.
▶ **Current ACC/AHA guidelines for cardiac evaluation prior to non-cardiac surgery. Contains a very thorough review of the entire English language literature.**

28 MYOCARDIAL MOLECULAR BIOLOGY: AN INTRODUCTION

Nigel J Brand, Paul J R Barton

The recent publication of draft copies of the human genome sequence from both public and private sector consortia has fuelled anticipation that eventually, once all genes have been identified, we will be able to ascertain which of them are involved in human diseases, including those affecting the cardiovascular system. Understanding the molecular biology behind both inherited and acquired disorders is now viewed as essential to provide a full picture of the aetiology and progression of disease. Within the past decade considerable advances have been made in identifying the genetic basis of myocardial disorders such as familial hypertrophic cardiomyopathy and dilated cardiomyopathy, as well as the molecular signalling pathways and gene regulatory events that characterise acquired disease such as pressure overload induced cardiac hypertrophy. Furthermore, by defining the molecular processes underlying normal development we may be able to manipulate immature cell phenotypes such as those of embryonic stem cells or skeletal myoblasts to replace damaged, terminally differentiated cells such as cardiac myocytes. In this review we outline the basic principals of gene expression, the different mechanisms by which expression is regulated and how these can be examined experimentally.

▶ DNA MAKES RNA MAKES PROTEIN

The blueprint for any organism is contained within its genome in the form of chromosomes and is written in the universal four "base" language of adenine (A), guanine (G), cytosine (C), and thymine (T). Chromosomes are built of **chromatin**, double stranded DNA wrapped around a multi-protein complex core comprised of **histone** proteins. This DNA contains the language (DNA or **nucleotide** sequence) that can be read and translated into proteins, and these areas of DNA are called **genes**.[1,2] In higher organisms, ranging from yeast to plants and man, practically all genes are interrupted, with sequences coding for protein (coding **exons**) separated by regions of non-coding DNA called **introns**. The beginning and ends of genes are usually marked by exons that do not code for parts of the protein, the so called non-coding exons. Within coding exons, contiguous groups of three bases (**codons**), form the genetic code. The 64 (4^3) individual codons specify for the 20 amino acids from which proteins are made, or signal the start (initiator methionine codon) or end (stop codon) of translation. It is therefore the contiguous order of the codons within a gene that delineate the linear amino acid sequence of the protein produced.

In general, **gene expression** describes the production of RNA and, subsequently, protein from a gene. This process can be split into three major parts: **transcription** of the gene in the nucleus to make primary RNA, splicing of the primary transcript to form the mature **messenger RNA** (**mRNA**) and **translation** of mRNA in the cytoplasm to produce the protein for which the gene codes (fig 28.1). Transcription is carried out by an enzyme called RNA polymerase II (RNA pol II) under the direction of specialised basal transcription factors that form a multi-protein complex with RNA pol II on the gene **promoter**.[1] The promoter contains the start site of transcription, usually designated +1, which marks the beginning of the first exon of the gene and hence corresponds to the first nucleotide of the mRNA. Binding sites for various **transcription factors**, which are DNA binding proteins with highly specific affinities for particular DNA sequences, sequester transcription factors to the gene where they participate in boosting (or, in some cases, repressing) the level of transcription. Transcription factors may bind within the promoter or lie within areas called **enhancers** that are located distally—usually upstream, but occasionally downstream, of the promoter. Considerable effort has focused on identifying promoter and enhancer sequences responsible for directing gene transcription and the identification of the factors that act on them.[3] Once bound to their cognate DNA sequences, transcription factors help drive the rate at which RNA pol II initiates fresh rounds of transcription. The polymerase moves along the gene making a primary RNA copy of one strand of the DNA duplex, copying both exonic and intronic sequences. This primary RNA transcript is subsequently processed to remove the intron derived sequences and the

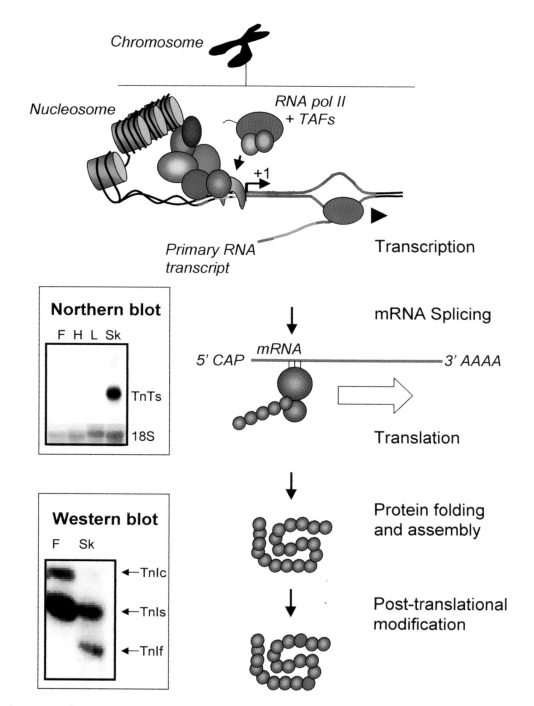

Figure 28.1 The process of gene expression. Chromosomes are scaffolds of DNA organised around protein (histones) in units called nucleosomes. DNA is unwound from histones before transcription of a gene by RNA polymerase II and transcription factors (coloured). The primary RNA transcript, which is a copy of both exonic (red) and intronic (blue) DNA sequences, is processed subsequently to remove intronic sequences (mRNA splicing). The resulting mRNA is then exported to the cytoplasm for translation and subsequent post-translational modification such as methylation, glycosylation or phosphorylation. Detection of mRNA by northern blot is illustrated: the blot shows that mRNA for the slow skeletal isoform of troponin T (TnTs) is expressed only in adult skeletal muscle (Sk) and not in fetal (F) or adult (H) heart or liver (L). Rehybridisation of the blot with a probe to 18S rRNA (18S) shows presence of RNA in each lane. Protein expression is analysed by western blotting: in the example shown, a universal antibody recognising all three troponin I (TnI) isoforms shows distribution of fast skeletal (f), slow skeletal (s) and cardiac (c) isoforms in adult skeletal muscle (Sk) and fetal heart (F). Figure courtesy of KA Dellow.

exons joined together (**RNA splicing**). Following some 5′ and 3′ modifications, such as the addition of a 3′ poly-adenylic acid tract (polyA tail), the final mRNA product is exported from the nucleus to the cytoplasm, where it serves as a template for the production of protein by the ribosomes. Subsequent post-translational modifications such as cleaving off any propeptide or leader sequences which direct the protein to its ultimate destination in the cell or the attachment of phosphate or

acetyl groups to specific amino acid residues may be necessary to produce the final functional form of the protein.

CONTROL POINTS FOR GENE EXPRESSION

All of the stages of gene expression are points at which regulation can be exerted. However, the primary point of control is at the level of transcription. Many promoters and enhancers of myocardial genes have been cloned and transcription factors

Table 28.1 Some examples of key transcription factors expressed in the heart

Factor	Gene family	DNA binding site	Expression pattern	Examples of gene regulated
MEF-2 A, B, C, D[4]	MADS box family	CTA(A/T)$_4$TAG	Widely expressed	TnIc CK-M
SRF[5]	MADS box family	CC(A/T)$_6$GG ("AcrG box")	Widely expressed	α-cardiac actin, SM22, c-fos
Myocardin[6]	SAP domain family	Does not bind directly to DNA, but binds to SRF as co-factor	Heart	SM 22, ANF
GATA-4, 5, 6[7]	GATA family	$^A/_T$GATA$^A/_g$	Myocardium, endoderm	α-MHC, cardiac TnC, TnIc
Nkx-2.5[8]	Homeobox	TNNAGTG (high affinity) C($^A/_T$)TTAATTN (low affinity)	Cardiac mesoderm	MLC2v, ANF, cardiac α-actin
HIF-1[9]	bHLH	α/β heterodimers bind CANNTG	Ubiquitous; HIF-1β constitutively expressed, changes in levels of active HIF-1α induced by hypoxia	MLC2v, ANF, cardiac α-actin

α-MHC, cardiac α myosin heavy chain; ANF, atrial natriuretic factor; bHLH, basic helix-loop-helix; CK-M, muscle creatine kinase; HIF-1, hypoxia inducible factor-1; MEF-2, myocyte enhancer factor-2; MLC2v, ventricular myosin light chain 2; SM22, smooth muscle 22; SRF, serum response factor; TnIc, cardiac troponin I; TnC, troponin C.

active in heart and belonging to a variety of gene families have been identified in recent years (table 28.1).[4–9] The overwhelming observation that can be drawn is that expression of individual genes is regulated (1) through the coordinate binding of different types of transcription factors, (2) by interactions between factors and with ancillary co-factors such as histone acetylases (HATs) or deacetylases (HDACs), which do not necessarily bind to DNA themselves, and (3) through signal transduction pathways which influence their activity by, for example, phosphorylation.[3] Most transcription factors are modular in structure, containing separable protein domains that carry out a particular function such as DNA binding, dimerisation with other family members (for example, the related bHLH proteins HIF-1α and β, products of separate genes[9]) or serving as transcriptional activation domains (**TAD**s) to promote high level transcription. Ultimately, once bound to DNA transcription factors interact with other bound proteins and act to increase the rate of RNA synthesis. TAD activity, which is often measured by introducing cloned transcription factors into cells grown in culture (see below) may be intrinsic or may reflect the binding of a co-activator or co-factor protein which itself possesses significant activation properties. For example, myocardin is a recently identified heart restricted co-factor for the ubiquitously expressed serum response factor (SRF).[6] SRF binds to the promoters of several genes expressed in heart, including cardiac α actin, and has been shown to interact with many factors including the **homeobox** factor Nkx-2.5 and the zinc finger factor **GATA**-4 to regulate expression. In contrast to Nkx-2.5 and GATA-4, which are transcriptional activators in their own right, myocardin does not bind to DNA but complexes with bound SRF and serves as an extremely potent co-factor for transcription, promoting up to a thousand-fold activation in combination with SRF.

Transcription factors may be expressed in a highly tissue restricted manner or at particular developmental stages, in turn regulating the expression of their target genes. For example, GATA factors are expressed from the earliest detectable stages of cardiogenesis and may play a role in gene regulation at this stage.[10] Later, Nkx2.5 shows regional variation in expression and may play a specific role in the developing myocardial conduction system. Most transcription factors can be grouped into gene families on the basis of sequence similarity in regions of functional importance, such as a DNA binding domain or a protein dimerisation interface. Such a high degree of sequence homology allows new family members to be discovered by searching DNA or protein sequence databases across diverse phyla. In this way Nkx-2.5 was identified as the

mammalian homologue of a Drosophila gene called tinman, (named after one of the characters in The Wizard of Oz) originally identified as a mutation that resulted in lack of development of the heart equivalent in the fly, the dorsal vessel.[8] In humans, mutations in the Nkx-2.5 gene have been correlated with a variety of cardiac anomalies including tetralogy of Fallot and idiopathic atrioventricular block.[11]

Currently, there is renewed interest in the role that chromatin structure plays in regulating gene expression.[12] It has long been known that when DNA is wrapped around histones in the form of chromatin, gene activity is silenced, and that the localised unwinding of the DNA from chromatin, accompanied with histone displacement, is vital to allow gene expression to progress. Central to recent studies has been the identification and biochemical characterisation of proteins that possess HAT or HDAC activity, adding or removing, respectively, acetyl groups from exposed lysine residues on histones. HAT activity correlates with activation of gene expression, while HDAC activity results in repression.[13] In several cases the functions of these proteins have been shown to be intimately linked to the state of transcription factors binding to target genes. For example, the active heterodimeric form of the basic helix-loop-helix transcription factor HIF-1 (table 28.1) senses changes in partial pressure of oxygen and thus acts as a hypoxia sensor in several systems, including angiogenesis and vascular remodelling.[9] Once bound to the DNA of target genes for regulation, C terminal TADs in the HIF heterodimer interact with transcriptional co-activators such as the CREB-binding protein, CBP. (In cardiac muscle, the most likely co-activator is the related protein p300). These large proteins possess intrinsic chromatin remodelling activity by recruiting to the DNA still more proteins which allow chromatin to unwind. Probably the best understood system is currently that involving retinoid and steroid hormone receptors such as thyroid hormone receptor α1 (TRα1) that, once it has bound its cognate ligand T3, activates expression of genes such as cardiac α myosin heavy chain.[2] The binding of T3 to the hormone binding domain of TRα1 results in a conformational change in the proteins' structure, allowing the receptor to interact with co-activators. The net result is that HAT activity promotes localised unwinding of chromatin, allowing access of RNA pol II and basal transcription factors to the DNA. In the absence of T3, the nuclear receptor still binds to DNA but interacts instead with co-repressors such as N-CoR and SMRT, which then recruit HDACs to the DNA, leading to chromatin condensation and repression of gene expression.[14]

The activation of transcription factors by phosphorylation is a focal point for transducing extracellular stimuli through

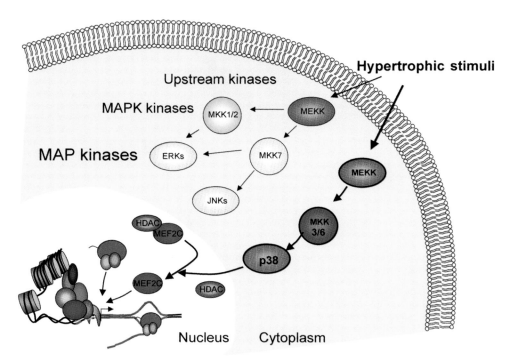

Figure 28.2 Linking MEF2 to hypertrophy. Hypertrophic stimuli activate intracellular signalling pathways. Upstream protein kinases (for example, MEKKs) activate MAP kinase family members (MKKs) which in turn phosphorylate the three MAP kinases p38-MAPK, JNKs, and ERKs. MAP kinases have been linked to the phosphorylation of certain transcription factors, for example, p38-MAPK has been shown to activate MEF2 family members (see text for details). This implicates MEF2 proteins as direct transducers of intracellular signalling pathways to bring about some, or all, of the changes in gene expression associated with hypertrophy. Figure courtesy of KA Dellow.

MAP kinase signal transduction pathways. For example, CBP associates only with the phosphorylated form of the CREB protein, a transcription factor that binds the cyclic AMP response element found in many gene promoters. Once bound to CREB, CBP forms protein–protein interactions with the basal transcription factor TFIIB, allowing transcription by RNA pol II to progress. Members of the myocyte enhancer factor-2 (MEF-2) family of transcription factors (table 28.1), which are widely expressed but appear to be enriched and have particular roles in skeletal and cardiac muscle, may regulate changes in gene expression arising from a hypertrophic stimulus. MEF-2 proteins have been implicated as responders to MAP kinases activated by hypertrophic stimuli in cardiac myocytes.[15] The hypertrophic agonists endothelin-1 and phenylepherine activate p38 MAPKs in cultured rat neonatal cardiac myocytes[16], and in vivo p38 activity increases in aortic banded mice which go on to develop pressure overloaded hypertrophy (Wang and colleagues 1998, cited in Han and Molkentin[15]). In rat, a similarly induced hypertrophy results in an increase in DNA binding activity of MEF-2.[17] As development of hypertrophy is associated with changes in transcription of various myocardial genes which require MEF-2, this suggests that MEF-2 may be a direct target for MAP kinase signalling (fig 28.2).

A second point at which gene expression can be controlled is at the level of mRNA splicing. The primary RNA transcript of many genes may be alternatively spliced in that certain exons may be excluded or included from the transcript to produce the final mRNA. In this way, multiple proteins may be generated from a single gene according to the combination of exon derived RNA segments that are spliced together. The vertebrate tropomyosin (TM) genes are examples of genes expressed in both cardiac and skeletal muscle that are subject to complex patterns of alternative mRNA splicing. For example, two isoforms of the α-TM gene in *Xenopus*, differ in their inclusion of alternative 3′untranslated region exons and show restricted expression in the embryo.[18] The XTMα7 isoform is found in the somites, from which the skeletal muscle develops, whereas the XTMα2 isoform is expressed in both somites and embryonic heart. In the adult, XTMα2, but not XTMα7, is selectively expressed in striated muscle and heart.

Following translation of the mRNA into polypeptide, production of mature active protein may require several steps, each of which is open to regulation. This is well illustrated by the matrix metallproteinases (MMPs) which are believed to play a key role in myocardial remodelling.[19] MMPs are produced in an inactive form (as a zymogen) which requires cleavage to produce active enzyme and are further regulated by specific inhibitory molecules (tissue inhibitors of metalloproteinases or TIMPs). Examining MMP gene expression at the level of RNA is of importance to understanding gene regulation, but may not therefore be a good indicator of MMP enzyme activity. Clearly, it is important to understand the biological system in question before deciding which is the most relevant level of regulation. For the purposes of this review we will be focusing on the initial stage of gene expression, namely transcription, and the methods of examining this as well as monitoring RNA content.

DISSECTING PROMOTER FUNCTION

In order to understand how genes are regulated in the heart, many gene promoters have been isolated and characterised with regard to the key regulatory DNA sequences they harbour and the transcription factors that bind them. A widely used method of measuring promoter function is to insert (**clone**) the promoter and various lengths of upstream sequence into an artificial plasmid-based construct in front of a **reporter gene** whose expression can be easily monitored. Typically the firefly gene luciferase or the bacterial genes chloramphenicol acetyl transferase (*CAT*) and β-galactosidase (*LacZ*) are used for this purpose. Constructs can be introduced into cells in culture by a variety of **transfection** techniques, or into whole animals using **transgenic** approaches. By careful choice of expression constructs containing progressively smaller deletions, the positions of DNA sequences responsible for high level transcription, tissue specificity or specific responses to stimuli (for example, stretch or agonist induced hypertrophy) can be found. The binding sites for candidate transcription factors can then be pinpointed accurately through mutagenesis of individual nucleotides to test the validity of those sequences. In this way, we and others have dissected the promoter of the cardiac troponin I gene, which is only ever expressed in cardiac muscle.

Deletion analysis of the human gene promoter and upstream sequences has revealed several important transcription factor binding sites within 100 nucleotides upstream of +1 (the conventional notation for promoter sequence is negative numbering running upstream from the transcription start site). Among these is an A/T rich element centred around −30 that binds the TATA-box factor, TBP, the octamer protein Oct-1, and several MEF2 proteins. There are two binding sites in the human TnIc gene for GATA-4 and a C-rich sequence around −95 that encompasses both binding sites for the zinc finger factor Sp1 and a CACC-box with the sequence CCCACCCC.[20] Mutation of each site in TnIc promoter-*CAT* reporter constructs results in a 50–95% reduction in transcriptional activity when transfected into cultured cardiac myocytes, suggesting that each site serves to bind proteins involved in maximal transcriptional activity. The identity of these proteins was characterised using the electrophoretic mobility shift assay (EMSA), also known as band shift assay. In this assay, a radiolabelled double stranded DNA fragment containing a putative binding site for a transcription factor (usually referred to as a cassette and generated by annealing short synthetic oligonucleotides corresponding to the two complementary strands of DNA) is mixed with an extract of nuclear proteins prepared from cells or tissue. If a protein binds the cassette, it will retard its migration compared to unbound cassette when subjected to electrophoresis through a non-denaturing polyacrylamide gel on account of the added mass of the protein.

Mutagenesis of individual nucleotides in the cassette or titration of unlabelled competitor cassettes in molar excess enable us to analyse the specificity of interaction between factor and DNA. By incubating the protein–DNA complex with antibody to putative factors, a "supershift" complex can be obtained (due to the added mass of the antibody) and the identity of bound proteins thereby confirmed (fig 28.3). Furthermore, by using nuclear extracts from different cells, an indication of the distribution of the factor can be determined. For example, our group has recently found shown that of four proteins binding the human TnIc CACC-box, two are members of the widely expressed Sp family of zinc finger factors while the other two appear to be expressed only in cardiac myocytes.[21] These experiments therefore identify the regions involved and the factors they bind. Similar experiments in mouse have been taken further by showing that only 230bp of the mouse TnIc promoter are necessary to drive cardiac restricted expression of a *LacZ* reporter gene in transgenic mice.[22]

The role of specific factors in regulating a promoter can be assessed by simultaneous introduction (co-transfection) of suitable promoter-reporter constructs with an expression construct encoding the factor(s) in question. For example, the role of GATA-4 in regulating cardiac specific expression has been examined in a number of contexts. In an elegant experi-

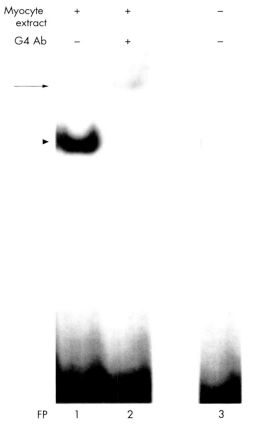

Figure 28.3 Visualising DNA–protein interaction by electrophoretic mobility shift assay (EMSA). A double stranded oligonucleotide cassette containing a consensus binding site for GATA factors (A/TGATAA/G) was radiolabelled and incubated with nuclear protein extracts from neonatal cardiac myocytes. Lane 1: A specific GATA-4-DNA complex is formed (solid arrowhead) which migrates behind (hence mobility shift) the free probe (FP). Lane 2: The identity of the bound protein is confirmed by addition of a specific antibody which results in a DNA/protein/antibody complex (supershift) (arrow). Specificity of binding can be demonstrated by mutation of the oligonucleotide sequence which results in loss of GATA-4 binding—not shown (see Dellow and colleagues[21]).

ment a reporter construct containing the promoter and upstream sequences of the α-MHC gene, which contains two binding sites for GATA-4, was barely active when injected into skeletal muscle, which lacks endogenous GATA-4.[23] However, expression could be boosted fourfold by co-injection of an expression vector for GATA-4 (fig 28.4). In contrast, a mutant reporter construct in which both GATA-4 binding sites had been mutated exhibited only 12% of the activity of the wild-type construct.

METHODS FOR MEASURING GENE EXPRESSION
Many techniques have been established for studying gene structure and expression. In particular, a variety of methods for measuring mRNA have been developed that allow abundance, tissue specificity, and developmental expression to be followed. The relative advantages and disadvantages of the major techniques are shown in table 28.2.

Southerns, northerns, and westerns
Electrophoresis of DNA or RNA molecules through an agarose or polyacrylamide gel matrix form the backbone of some key molecular biology techniques as the speed and distance that molecules migrate is in direct proportion to their size. Hence,

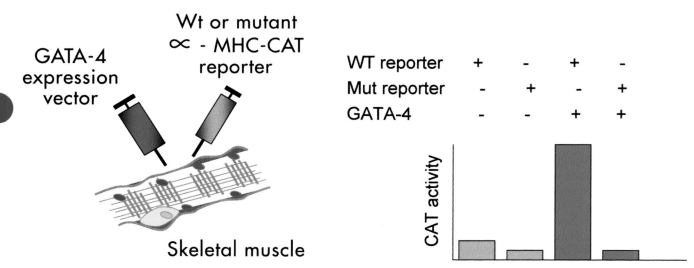

Figure 28.4 GATA-4 directs expression of an α-MHC-CAT reporter when co-injected into skeletal muscle, which lacks endogenous GATA-4. Neither GATA-4 nor the cardiac α-MHC gene, which contains GATA-4 binding sites in its promoter, are normally expressed in skeletal muscle. Co-injection of a promoter-reporter construct gene containing a CAT gene under control of the wild type (WT) α-MHC promoter together with a GATA-4 expression vector results in a fourfold increase in reporter activity compared to in the absence of GATA-4. Mutation of the GATA-4 binding sites (*mut*) abrogates activation by the transcription factor (see Molkentin and colleagues[23]).

DNA or RNA fragments can be easily separated according to size.[2] Denaturing and transferring DNA fragments out of gel onto a membrane of similar dimensions to the gel is known as **Southern blotting**, so called in deference to its inventor, Ed Southern. The blot preserves the spatial distribution of the separated fragments and fixes them permanently on the membrane. Thus, we can separate out individual molecules from a complex starting mixture such as total genomic DNA digested with restriction enzymes and look at specific DNA sequences by hybridising the resulting Southern blot with gene specific probes. Often, the high degree of conservation between the same gene from different species can be exploited

Table 28.2	Comparison of some commonly used methods for RNA detection		
Method	**Protocol**	**Advantages**	**Disadvantages**
Northern blot	▶ Separate RNA on gel ▶ Transfer (blot) to filter ▶ Hybridise to probe Autoradiography or phosphoimaging to detect probe signal	▶ Reliable ▶ Quantitative ▶ Reusable (limited number of times)	▶ Usually involves radioactivity ▶ Requires large amount of RNA ▶ Sensitive to degradation
RPA (RNase protection assay)	▶ Hybridise radiolabelled RNA probe with RNA ▶ Digest un-hybridised probe with ribonuclease (RNase) ▶ Separate protected probe on gel ▶ Detect signal by autoradiography or phosphoimaging	▶ Highly sensitive ▶ Quantitative ▶ Reliably distinguish similar sequences and splice variants	▶ Labour intensive ▶ Non-reusable
Polymerase chain reaction (PCR) methods	▶ Make cDNA of mRNA by reverse transcription (RT) ▶ Amplify specific cDNA target by PCR cycling ▶ Visualise PCR products on gel and by Southern blot, if necessary	▶ Highly sensitive ▶ Requires minimal RNA input	▶ Largely non-quantitative (with exception of competitive PCR methods which require labour intensive construction and prior quantification of a competitor target molecule)
Real time PCR	▶ Convert RNA to cDNA by RT ▶ Amplify specific cDNA target by PCR ▶ Detect product using internal fluorescent probe (e.g. TaqMan) or by fluorescent dye (e.g. SYBR green)	▶ Highly sensitive ▶ Quantitative ▶ Product is monitored each PCR cycle (hence "real time") ▶ Requires minimal RNA input	▶ Requires expensive real time fluorescence detection hardware
Gridded array filters	▶ DNA copies of specific genes spotted in gridded array on filters ▶ Probe array with labelled cDNA made by RT of RNA from a particular source ▶ Visualise hybridised spots (signal is proportional to abundance of RNA corresponding to each spotted gene)	▶ Allows analysis of several hundred genes simultaneously ▶ Many commercial companies offer pre-gridded filters (e.g. cytokine array) ▶ Can custom make arrays	▶ Requires large input of RNA ▶ Relatively insensitive ▶ Semiquantitative (individual results require verification)
Microarrays, (cDNA arrays, Gene Chip)	▶ DNA copies of genes (or oligonucleotides) are spotted onto high density grid on glass slide ▶ Hybridisation with labelled cDNA prepared by RT of source RNA. (Typically, dual hybridisation protocols with fluorescent probes are used to look for global differences between two or more RNA sources)	▶ Allows simultaneous analysis of thousands of genes	▶ Requires expensive hardware/software or commercial service costs

to use a probe to **hybridise** across species on a Southern blot. For example, a new gene from heart may be identified in mouse and we would wish to analyse the gene structure of its counterpart in man. As many genes belong to extensive gene families related in terms of DNA or protein sequence (**homology**), this can be exploited to use one gene to identify a related family member, as in the earlier cited example of using the fly gene *tinman* to isolate its vertebrate homologue *Nkx-2.5*.[24]

The majority of techniques for studying the expression of a gene take messenger RNA as the starting material. As with DNA analysis by Southern blotting, RNA can be studied by **northern blotting** (fig 28.1). In Northern blotting, RNA molecules are resolved on agarose gels and a DNA probe for the gene of interest is then used to identify expression of the gene and to gauge the size of the transcript. By including RNA samples from various human tissues on a blot it is possible to determine in which tissues in the body a particular gene is expressed. Various methods of measuring RNA are described in table 28.2.

The expression profile of proteins can be determined in a similar way by resolving a protein mixture by electrophoresis on a polyacrylamide gel matrix under denaturing conditions (to ensure proteins migrate according to their molecular mass). A modified blot procedure (**western blotting**) is used to transfer the proteins to a membrane, the proteins are then renatured and target protein(s) identified using specific antibodies (fig 28.1). Analysis of protein expression is an important aspect to understanding the constituents and function of the cell, and modern techniques of analysis, referred to generically as proteomics, have been reviewed elsewhere.[25]

Polymerase chain reaction

One of the most useful innovations in molecular biology in the last few decades has been the development and continued refinement of the polymerase chain reaction (PCR). This technique is an enzymatic reaction which allows the exponential amplification of specific DNA sequences from vanishingly small amounts of starting material, often leading to an amplification of a million-fold or more.[26] PCR amplification works by successive rounds of thermal denaturation at temperatures above 90°C to separate the two strands of the DNA template, cooling to allow annealing of oligonucleotide primers with their target sequences, and elongation by a thermostable DNA polymerase at 72°C (whereby new DNA is synthesised by extension of the annealed primers), thereby making two copies of the original target. Each round of PCR results in a doubling of the target DNA.

The amplification process of PCR makes it well suited to identifying gene expression in RNA, particularly prepared from biopsies or similar limiting sources of material. RNA is prepared and then converted to cDNA (**reverse transcription**) to provide the initial DNA template for PCR amplification. Small, chemically synthesised DNA molecules specific to the gene under investigation (**oligonucleotide primers**) are used to define the two ends of the region to be amplified, leading to the accumulation of a product of defined size which can later be resolved by gel electrophoresis and, if necessary, transferred to filter by Southern blotting for downstream analysis. PCR has been demonstrated to have many uses in the clinical environment, including: rapid and efficient amplification of bacterial or viral DNA gene sequences for detection of infection, blood typing, and identification of single base changes or other **polymorphisms** characteristic of genetic variation or a disease phenotype.[26]

While powerful in terms of detection, PCR methods are in general difficult to quantify with any real accuracy. Thus, while reverse transcriptase PCR (RT-PCR) is widely used to detect RNA in tissue or cell extracts, such data are often presented as "semi-quantitative". To overcome these limitations, "real time" quantitative PCR was developed. This is based on the principle that quantitative detection of the PCR product at each round of the PCR cycle allows the investigator to plot a complete amplification curve for each reaction and thereby select the part of the PCR process where exponential amplification is being achieved. TaqMan is widely used for product detection. TaqMan uses a third oligonucleotide primer in the reaction mix which corresponds to sequence located between the two amplifying primers. This oligonucleotide carries a fluorescence tag at one end and a quenching tag at the other. During each PCR cycle the TaqMan probe anneals with the target sequence and is degraded as the DNA polymerase passes the annealed TaqMan probe thereby releasing the fluorescent tag which can be monitored. As well as offering considerably improved quantitation, automation of the detection process and the use of 96 well plate technology allows TaqMan real time PCR to be adapted to high throughput analysis which makes it especially useful for a clinical environment.

Fishing with chips: the rise of microarrays

Increased use of robotics in molecular biology has led to ways of planting far more genetic information in the form of cDNA or oligonucleotide sequences onto solid matrices than achievable before. Indeed, a complete cDNA library can now be gridded onto a single filter (called a gene array), rather than the dozen or so we might have expected to use five years ago. The move to miniaturisation is exemplified by the development of **DNA microarrays,** where DNAs or oligonucleotides are printed onto glass slides, allowing the simultaneous screening of many thousands of sequences in a single sample.[27] This is an exciting development as in the last year a working draft of the human genome has been published which indicates that there are no more that 40 000 human genes making this a manageable figure. Microarray technology, variously referred to as microarrays, cDNA arrays, gene expression arrays, and gene chips, can usually detect changes in gene expression of twofold and above and can highlight single or global changes in gene expression arising from a pathological event or a developmental change. For example, Aitman and colleagues used microarrays as part of a strategy to identify genes implicated in human insulin resistance syndromes such as type 2 diabetes, combined hyperlipidaemia, and essential hypertension. Using a rat model for these diseases, the insulin resistant spontaneously hypertensive rat (SHR), a gene on rat chromosome 4 was identified encoding a fatty acid translocase which appears to underlie defects in fatty acid metabolism and hypertriglyceridaemia.[28]

DNA arrays work by the hybridisation of labelled DNA or RNA in solution to unique and specific DNA molecules gridded in an ordered pattern on a solid matrix such as a glass filter (microarray) or nylon membrane. When fluorescent labelled RNAs used the output can be read as a false colour trace using computer imaging software. With several different fluorescent groups available, it is possible to label RNA pools representing different developmental points, or compare a pathological state with the normal one, and then hybridise these to a common array. The outputs can then be digitally superimposed and changes in the expression of individual genes recorded (fig 28.5). The gridded sequences are usually

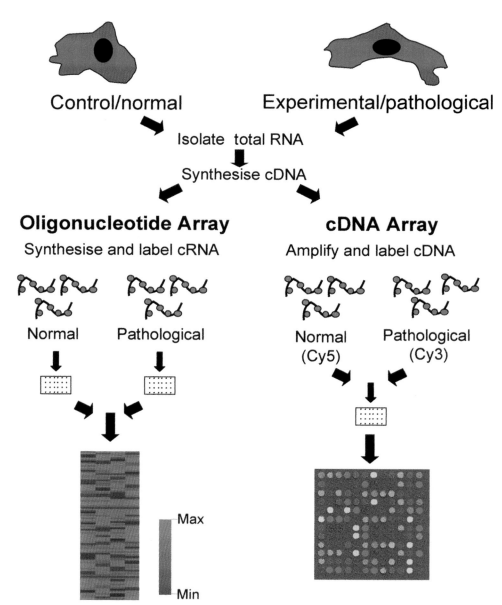

Figure 28.5 Schematic illustrating the stages involved in using DNA microarrays, highlighting the differences between oligonucleotide and cDNA arrays. In both procedures, total RNA is extracted from control and test samples (for example, normal and pathological) and converted to cDNA. For oligonucleotide microarrays the cDNA is then used as a template to generate fluorescently labelled complementary RNA (cRNA) by in vitro transcription. Control and experimental cRNA pools, labelled with the same dye, are hybridised to separate microarrays. After washing the arrays are scanned in order to create a quantitative fluorescence image where the signal intensity at each "gene probe" is proportional to the number of molecules attached (and hence abundance of that sequence in the original sample). Data from control and experimental samples are then compared, resulting in a cluster diagram where each column represents a single experiment and each row a single gene. Ratios of gene expression are shown relative to the control sample (illustrated): the scale ranges from red (maximal expression) to black (minimal expression). With cDNA arrays, the synthesised cDNA is first amplified and labelled through multiple rounds of cDNA synthesis and in vitro transcription, the two pools being labelled with different dyes—for example, Cy3 (green) and Cy5 (red). Equal quantities of each sample are mixed and hybridised to the same cDNA microarray, which is then scanned at two different wavelengths giving the relative abundance of Cy3 and Cy5 transcripts in each sample. The images are then overlaid (illustrated) and spots visualised as ratios of red and green (in this illustration a red spot indicates a gene more highly expressed in normal than pathological tissue) with yellow indicating equal expression.

derived from the 3′ non-coding regions of genes, cDNA and ESTs. There are now a number of commercially available platforms of "affinity matrix" systems available, including high density oligonucleotide arrays (GeneChips), representing up to 12 000 characterised genes and using glass as matrix and fluorescence for detection. In this system, in order to improve the noise-to-signal ratio and thereby improve RNA quantification, each gene is represented by 20 oligonucleotides (25–75 nt) of different sequence designed to hybridise to multiple regions of the same RNA molecule. Glass slide arrays are also

available with PCR-amplified cDNAs (300–1000bp) attached. Nylon membranes, which use autoradiography for detection, are also used for the spotting of cDNA as probe but usually at a much lower density than that permissible on glass slides.

For all DNA array analyses high quality RNA is essential, although the quantities required can range between 50 μg to 50 ng depending on the array used. Plentiful quantities of RNA can be easily extracted from in vitro cell culture systems or from large tissue samples. However, where cell numbers or tissue yield is limited—for example, if using clinical biopsies or cells obtained by laser capture microdissection—mRNA amplification is required. A major application for the use of arrays is the monitoring of gene expression (mRNA abundance). The collection of genes transcribed, sometimes referred to as the expression profile, within a given cell determines its cellular phenotype and function. Differences in gene expression profiles are responsible for both morphological and phenotypic differences and can be indicative of cellular responses to environmental stimuli. Knowing when, where, and to what extent a gene is expressed is pivotal to understanding the biological role of its encoded protein. A fundamental advantage of using arrays containing probes for thousands of different genes is that it provides a less biased view of cellular responses than a hypothesis based on the role of an isolated gene.

DNA arrays should not be viewed as replacements for the established techniques used for gene expression quantification such as northern blots or RT-PCR. Indeed, it is essential that individual results of array experiments are verified and apparent differences more accurately quantified using, for example, real time RT-PCR. Although constantly improving, there are still several limitations to their widespread use that need to be overcome, such as the cost of microarrays (most are single use) and data handling software, the number of genes identified and gridded, and the limited number of species for which arrays are available. Many of the filter based arrays and microarrays available "off-the-shelf" contain a plethora of well characterised genes from a variety of cell types. For investigators only interested in a particular tissue or cell type, such arrays are of limited use. For this reason companies are now offering custom made arrays containing specific sets of genes. Needless to say, these are not cheap. The more experienced laboratories are now producing their own custom made cDNA arrays. For example, in order to obtain a global picture of gene expression in the failing heart, Barrans and colleagues amplified by PCR 10 368 redundant sequenced expressed sequences from a number of human heart and artery cDNA libraries representing 4777 sequence verified transcripts from known genes, human EST database entries, and novel cardiac ESTs.[29] The importance of monitoring a large number of genes has been illustrated by the molecular classification of cancer. Through the analysis of samples obtained from individuals with and without acute leukaemia or diffuse large B cell lymphoma, it was apparent that reliable tumour classification predictions could not be made on the basis of any single gene, but that predictions based on the expression levels of 50 genes (selected from the more than 6000 monitored on the arrays) were highly accurate.[30]

SUMMARY

Understanding the molecular mechanisms underlying how genes in the heart are expressed and how their expression may be modulated in response to external stimuli is now recognised as being an essential part of understanding how the heart develops, functions, and responds to pathological events. Such knowledge will lead to improved or new strategies for treating heart disease. Whereas the last decade has seen considerable advances in examining individual gene expression patterns, the new technologies now offer the ability to analyse global patterns of expression of many hundreds of genes. This will serve both as a methodology for identifying new genes involved in disease processes and in categorising global shifts in expression and hence general regulatory networks

Myocardial molecular biology: key points

► Transcription (RNA synthesis) plays a significant role in regulating gene expression
► Interactions between transcription factors bound to DNA directs cardiac specific gene expression
► RNA splicing increases the diversity of proteins that can be produced from a single gene
► A variety of techniques are available for monitoring RNA and protein expression
► Some techniques allow quantification—for example, real time polymerase chain reaction
► Modern techniques are aimed at identifying global patterns of expression involved in disease (for example, gene chip analysis) rather than studying individual genes

ACKNOWLEDGEMENTS

PJRB is a Senior Research Fellow of the British Heart Foundation. We are grateful to our colleagues Dr Kim Dellow and Dr Pank Bhavsar for their support and comments during the preparation of this manuscript.

GLOSSARY

Chromatin: DNA wrapped around a histone protein core at periodic intervals; the basic structure of the chromosome.

Clone: (*noun*), descriptive term in recombinant DNA terminology for any individual DNA sequence obtained through the process of cloning. (*verb*), to isolate a particular gene sequence of interest (genomic DNA or cDNA copy of mRNA) and to insert it, for example, into an artificial plasmid vector which can be introduced into bacterial cells where it will replicate within the bacterial cell, allowing unlimited amounts of the isolated sequence to be propagated from cells harbouring the plasmid. Other types of vector allow propagation and expression in yeast or mammalian cells.

Codon: Group of three nucleotides, whose sequence specifies a particular amino acid. The order in a continuous mRNA sequence reproduced from the gene thereby dictates the correct order of amino acids in the protein.

Complementary DNA (cDNA): A DNA copy of an RNA sequence, produced by the action of the enzyme reverse transcriptase.

Chromatin: DNA wrapped around a histone protein core at periodic intervals; the basic structure of the chromosome.

Cloning: various meanings include (1) inserting a DNA fragment of interest into a vector molecule, thereby generating a recombinant DNA molecule, which allows one to propagate that DNA fragment in bacteria; (2) isolating a new organism from a single somatic cell (for example, "Dolly" the cloned sheep).

Enhancer: DNA sequence capable of conferring a significant increase in gene transcription through its ability to bind cognate transcription factors. Enhancers are *cis*-acting but can function at distance from the gene promoter and are position and orientation independent.

Exons: Regions of a gene that are represented in the final mRNA molecule. Most, but not all, exons of a gene code for the protein.

GATA: Family of transcription factors utilising a zinc chelating protein "finger" structure to recognise and bind with high affinity to specific DNA sequences.

Gene expression: The process by which a gene is transcribed in the nucleus to give mRNA (transcription), from which protein is later produced in the cytoplasm by translation.

Homeobox: DNA binding motif comprised of three α helices, two of which are separated by a short, mobile peptide linker. Found in all homeodomain proteins, many of which are implicated in activating patterns of gene expression associated with patterning and other early development events.

Homology: Similarity resulting from being derived from a common ancestral gene. Often used (incorrectly) to refer simply to sequence similarity.

Hybridise: To use a (usually) radioactively labelled DNA or RNA single stranded molecule specific for one strand of a particular gene as a probe to find and bind to its immobilised, single stranded complement strand (usually presented within a pool of many unrelated sequences) in a liquid environment in which salt molarity and temperature direct the efficiency of the hybridisation process.

Introns: Regions of a gene that lie between exons and, unlike exons, are excluded from the final mRNA by the process of mRNA splicing.

MAP kinase: Mitogen activated protein kinase. Enzymes which modify proteins, especially transcription factors, by adding a phosphate group, resulting in altered activity. Three major MAPK subgroups have been identified: the extracellular signal regulated kinases (ERKs), the c-Jun N-terminal kinases/stress-activated protein kinases (JNK/SAPKs), and the p38 MAP kinases. Together with their upstream regulators (fig 2), MAP kinases represent one of the major signal systems used by eukaryotic cells to transduce extracellular signals into cellular responses.

Messenger RNA (mRNA): Produced by the process of transcription, mRNA is exported to the cytoplasm where protein is produced from it at the ribosome (translation).

Microarray: A solid matrix on which minute amounts of DNA sequences are imprinted robotically for analysis of differential gene expression using fluorescently labelled RNA probes.

Northern blot: Method of analysing mRNA expression using a nylon or nitrocellulose blot on which are immobilised electrophoretically separated RNA mixtures.

Nucleotide: Basic unit of nucleic acid consisting of one of four bases (adenine (A), guanine (G), cytosine (C) and thymine (T)—the four letter alphabet of DNA) coupled to sugar and phosphate groups.

Oligonucleotide: Short (for example 18–24 nucleotides) chemically synthesised single stranded DNA molecules. Used in PCR reactions and, when radiolabelled, as probes for Southern blots.

PCR: Polymerase chain reaction. Enzymatic method of synthesising multiple copies of a particular gene sequence by repeated cycles of thermal DNA denaturation and extension of gene specific oligonucleotide primers.

PolyA tail: A tract of adenylic acid residues attached post-splicing to the 3′ end of all messenger RNAs. Useful for purifying mature mRNA by hybridising to solid matrices bearing poly-T tracts, or for serving as template for annealing of polyT primers before cDNA synthesis by reverse transcriptase.

Primer: Short single stranded DNA molecules, used to prime DNA synthesis from RNA (by reverse transcription) or DNA templates.

Probe: Generic term for a DNA or RNA molecule used to detect the presence of specific genes or their RNA products, whether by northern blot or hybridisation in situ.

Promoter: Region of DNA just upstream of the gene which is responsible for binding transcription factors and RNA polymerase in order to initiate gene transcription.

Reporter gene: Generic term for a vector containing a biologically measurable marker (for example, the *Escherichia coli* β-galactosidase gene *LacZ* or the firefly luciferase gene). By inserting an isolated promoter sequence in front of the reporter gene, the activity of that promoter can be followed once the vector has been introduced into cultured cells or a transgenic animal.

Reverse transcription: Process of making a cDNA copy of an RNA molecule; carried out by the retroviral enzyme reverse transcriptase.

RNA splicing: The process of removing intron-derived RNA sequences from the primary transcript to give mRNA.

Southern blot: Named after its inventor, a technique for transferring DNA to a solid membrane which can then be analysed by hybridisation with labelled probes specific to particular genes.

TAD: Transcription activation domain. A region of a transcription factor that has been experimentally determined to be essential for contributing to high levels of gene transcription once brought in close proximity to RNA polymerase by virtue of the factor binding to DNA.

Transgenic: Refers to the transference of foreign DNA into the germline of a host (transgenic) animal.

Transcription: The production of a primary RNA transcript by RNA polymerase from a gene.

Transcription factors: DNA-binding proteins which bind to gene promoters or enhancers and interact with RNA polymerase to alter the overall rate of gene transcription.

Translation: The production of protein from a mRNA template at the ribosome.

Western blot: Electrophoretic method of transferring proteins, separated by molecular weight on a polyacrylamide gel matrix, to a solid filter. Filters are then probed with a specific antibody to detect proteins under investigation.

REFERENCES

1 **Lewin B**. *Genes VII*. Oxford: Oxford University Press, 2000.
  ▶ A comprehensive primer for understanding the biochemistry and molecular basis of gene expression and regulation.
2 **Chien KR**, ed. *Molecular basis of cardiovascular disease*. Philadelphia: WB Saunders, 1999. 637 pages.
  ▶ This book includes detailed sections of basic molecular biology in the context of cardiovascular disease. In addition, it describes in detail the basics of many key molecular biology procedures and gives a good synopsis of transgenic techniques in cardiovascular research.
3 **Latchman DS**. *Eukaryotic transcription factors*, 3rd ed. San Diego: Academic Press 1999:1–52.

  ▶ This gives a comprehensive and up-to-date description of gene expression and the key factors involved in relation to chromatin structure.
4 **Black BL**, Olson EN. Transcriptional control of muscle development by myocyte enhancer factor-2 (MEF2) proteins. *Annu Rev Cell Dev Biol* 1998;**14**:167–96.
5 **Price MA**, Hill C, Treisman R. Integration of growth factor signals at the c-fos serum response element. *Philos Trans R Soc Lond B Biol Sci* 1996;**351**:551–9.
6 **Wang D**, Chang PS, Wang Z, et al. Activation of cardiac gene expression by myocardin, a transcriptional cofactor for serum response factor. *Cell* 2001;**105**:851–62.
  ▶ A good example of a "basic science" paper, this describes the various strands of evidence brought together to identify myocardin as a new and important transcriptional regulator of cardiac gene regulation.
7 **Laverriere AC**, MacNeill C, Mueller C, et al. GATA-4/5/6, a subfamily of three transcription factors transcribed in developing heart and gut. *J Biol Chem* 1994;**269**:23177–84.
8 **Harvey RP**. NK-2 Homeobox genes and heart development. *Dev Biol* 1996;**178**:203–16.
9 **Semenza GL**. Hypoxia-inducible factor 1: oxygen homeostasis and disease pathophysiology. *Trends in Molecular Medicine* 2001;**7**:345–50.
10 **Parmacek MS** , Leiden JM. GATA transcription factors and cardiac development. In: Harvey RP, Rosthental N, eds. *Heart development*. Academic Press, 1999:291–306.
  ▶ While this chapter focuses specifically on the GATA factors, the whole book is worth reading for comprehensive reviews of cardiac development, cardiac cell cycle, and human cardiac developmental abnormalities.
11 **Benson DW**, Silberbach GM, Kavanaugh-McHugh A, et al. *J Clin Invest* 1999;**104**:1567–73.
12 **Huang WY**, Liew CC. Chromatin structure and cardiac gene expression. *J Mol Cell Cardiol* 1998;**30**:1673–81.
13 **Collingwood TN**, Urnov FD, Wolffe AP. Nuclear receptors: coactivators, corepressors and chromatin remodeling in the control of transcription. *J Mol Endocrinol* 1999;**23**:255–75.
14 **Hu X**, Lazar MA. Transcriptional repression by nuclear hormone receptors. *Trends Endocrinol Metab* 2000;**11**:6–10.
15 **Han J**, Molkentin JD. Regulation of MEF2 by p38 MAPK and its implication in cardiomyocyte biology. *Trends Cardiovasc Med* 2000;**10**:19–22.
16 **Sugden PH**, Clerk A. Cellular mechanisms of cardiac hypertrophy. *J Mol Med* 1998;**76**:725–46.
17 **Molkentin JD**, Markham BE. Myocyte-specific enhancer-binding factor (MEF-2) regulates α-cardiac myosin heavy chain gene expression *in vitro* and *in vivo*. *J Biol Chem* 1993;**268**:19512–20.
18 **Hardy S**, Hamon S, Cooper B, et al. Two skeletal α-tropomyosin transcripts with distinct 3′UTR have different temporal and spatial patterns of expression in the striated muscle lineages of Xenopus laevis. *Mech Develop* 1999;**87**:199–202.
19 **Spinale FG**, Cocker ML, Bond BR, et al. Myocardial matrix degradation and metalloproteinase activity in the failing heart: a potential therapeutic target. *Cardiovasc Res* 2000;**46**:225–38.
20 **Bhavsar PK**, Dellow KA, Yacoub MH, et al. Identification of cis-acting DNA elements required for expression of the human cardiac troponin I gene promoter. *J Mol Cell Cardiol* 2000;**32**:95–108.
21 **Dellow KA**, Bhavsar PK, Brand NJ, et al. Identification of novel, cardiac-restricted transcription factors binding to a CACC-box within the human cardiac Troponin I promoter. *Cardiovasc Res* 2001;**50**:24–33.
22 **Di Lisi R**, Millino C, Calabria E, et al. Combinatorial cis-acting elements control tissue-specific activation of the cardiac troponin I gene in vitro and in vivo. *J Biol Chem* 1998;**273**:25371–80.
23 **Molkentin JD**, Kalvakolanu DV, Markham BE. Transcription factor GATA-4 regulates cardiac muscle-specific expression of the α-myosin heavy-chain gene. *Mol Cell Biol* 1994;**14**:4947–57.
24 **Lints TJ**, Parsons LM, Hartley L, et al. Nkx-2.5: a novel murine homeobox gene expressed in early heart progenitor cells and their myogenic descendants. *Development* 1993;**119**:419–31.
25 **Macri J**, Rupundalo ST. Application of proteomics to the study of cardiovascular biology. *Trends Cardiovasc Med* 2001;**11**:66–75.
26 **Latchman DS**, ed. *PCR applications in pathology: principles and practice*. Oxford: Oxford University Press, 1995:269 pages.
  ▶ A good starting point for understanding the basics of PCR and its many and diverse applications in the clinical environment.
27 **Stanton LW**. Methods to profile gene expression. *Trends Cardiovasc Med* 2001;**11**:49–54.
28 **Aitman TJ**, Glazier AM, Wallace CA, et al. Identification of Cd36 (Fat) as an insulin-resistance gene causing defective fatty acid and glucose metabolism in hypertensive rats. *Nat Genet* 1999;**21**:76–83.
  ▶ An early example of the use of microarray technology in unravelling the genetic background to a complex, multigenic syndrome.
29 **Hwang DM**, Dempsey AA, Wang RX, et al. A genome-based resource for molecular cardiovascular medicine: toward a compendium of cardiovascular genes. *Circulation* 1997;**96**:4146–203.
30 **Golub TR**, Slonim DK, Tamayo P, et al. Molecular classification of cancer: class discovery and class prediction by gene expression monitoring. *Science* 1999;**286**:531–7.

29 HEART DISEASE, GUIDELINES, REGULATIONS, AND THE LAW

M C Petch

The practice of cardiology is increasingly constrained by guidelines, regulations, and legal considerations. Cardiologists, like any other group of doctors, have a primary duty of care to individual patients, but also have wider responsibilities to society in general, to their institution, and to their colleagues. In the UK these duties and responsibilities have been defined by the General Medical Council and have been described in a series of publications which have been sent to every doctor; these contain the answers to questions about good medical practice, the role of doctors in the management of health care, confidentiality and other issues.

▶ THE DEMISE OF CLINICAL FREEDOM

Clinical freedom died around 1983.[1] A number of factors sounded the death knell. Among the more important were, first, the incontrovertible results of randomised controlled trials. Many of these were in the cardiovascular field—for example, coronary artery bypass grafting for patients with angina and severe disease, thrombolysis and β blockade for myocardial infarction, and aspirin for the acute coronary syndromes. These, together with earlier trials demonstrating the efficacy of antihypertensive treatment, and subsequent trials showing the benefits of statins and angiotensin converting enzyme inhibitors, have fundamentally altered the practice of medicine. Physicians have to have good reasons for denying patients the potential benefits of these treatments.

Financial constraints were a second factor that killed off clinical freedom. These became apparent in the British National Health Service (NHS) somewhat before other countries and have led to the universal recognition that third party payers of health care should not be expected to fund treatments simply on the assertions of a doctor, however distinguished. Evidence of benefit is mandatory.

A third factor has been the gradual realisation by the public that doctors are not always to be trusted. Some have fallen off their pedestals rather publicly, so that nowadays doctors not only have to keep up to date but must also be able to demonstrate their continuing competency. Although continuing medical education (CME) is deemed compulsory, methods of enforcement have yet to be agreed for specialists in the UK. In other countries this obligation is ensured by linking CME to remuneration. A similar development here seems inevitable.

Managers and doctors nowadays share the responsibility for providing a clinical service. The term "clinical governance" describes an institution's method of assuring that individual doctors and groups of doctors provide a competent clinical service.

SAFE PRACTICE OF CARDIOLOGY

In the NHS ultimate responsibility for the safe practice of cardiology rests with the hospital trust board. Accountable managers are required to ensure that doctors maintain their skills through continuing professional development, audit, and appraisal. While demonstration of continuing competence is primarily a prerequisite for a doctor's employing authority, cardiology, like any other specialty, has to be subject to national scrutiny. The British Cardiac Society's peer review scheme, the annual publication of interventional cardiological practice and similar databases, and the production of national guidelines are all designed to enable institutions and their doctors to compare their practice with others and to ensure uniformity of standards within the NHS.

In the UK every doctor has to comply with the provisions of the Medical Act 1983 and appear on the medical register. A specialist register was established under the European Specialist Medical Qualifications Order 1995. This includes cardiovascular disease among the specialties. Cardiologists who held substantive posts in NHS hospitals on 31 December 1996 were automatically entered into the specialist register. Only those whose names appear on the register can legally practise the specialty in the UK and be employed as a consultant cardiologist in an NHS hospital. Entry to the register is either through completion of the six year training programme and award of the appropriate certificate, or via direct entry. The latter demands that the training and experience be at least equivalent to that required by the specialist advisory committee in cardiology; it is very rarely granted.

208

Physicians who wish to practise cardiology and who have been denied entry onto the specialist register have had the right of appeal to the statutory training authority. They were entitled to a hearing which was held before a barrister. This right was exercised by specialists, many of whom had been employed in subconsultant grades before 1996; the right to this method of entry expired in 2001. But others, notably those who qualified overseas, may be allowed entry onto the register, if they can demonstrate that their training and experience is equivalent or superior. The appointment of a senior academic cardiologist from another country would be an example. The register does allow those physicians who have a CCST in general internal medicine to practise some cardiology, but to what extent is ill-defined. At the moment general medicine is largely acute medicine, hence coronary care is certainly within the remit of the generalist. In future, however, the dissemination of data showing that patients cared for by cardiologists have better outcomes will add to the pressure from patients and their relatives who want all those suspected of suffering from heart disease to be seen by a cardiologist.

Cardiologists also belong to a wider international community. The major European and US meetings and journals are a rich source of CME. Management protocols for specific cardiac problems have unsurprising similarities, regardless of their country of origin. There is free movement of labour throughout the European Community, in theory at least. Every member of a national cardiac society in Europe is automatically a member of the European Society of Cardiology (ESC). Increasingly, therefore, cardiologists will have to heed developments in other countries. Two are of current interest in Europe.

The first development is the "European cardiologist". This is a diploma that recognises clinical skills and is granted on completion of basic training in the specialty comprising two years of a common trunk of medicine, three years of cardiology, and one flexible year spent in a related discipline. Currently applicants are also acceptable if they can demonstrate that their training and experience are equivalent to that set out in the recommendations.[2] Most of the many hundreds of diplomas awarded so far have been to cardiologists in countries in southern and eastern Europe. The legal status of the diploma has yet to be tested but under European law a holder can apply for a post in any EU country and his/her application has to receive due consideration. Any country, however, has the right to impose higher standards as a condition of employment in their healthcare system, as would almost certainly be the case in the UK at present. The second European venture is the creation of a European Board for Accreditation in Cardiology (EBAC). This board, like that which grants the diploma—the European Board for the Specialty of Cardiology (EBSC)—is an offspring of two parent bodies, the ESC and the cardiology section of the European Union of Monospecialists (UEMS), which is the cardiologists' official channel of communication with Brussels. EBAC became operational in September 2001 and provides a European umbrella for the approval of postgraduate meetings and courses.

Guidelines, regulations, and legal considerations may be locally driven, or emanate from national authorities, and an increasing number will stem from Europe. All have to be given due consideration; only the law has to be obeyed.

GUIDELINES

Guidelines are what they say they are, no more and no less. They may be defined as "systematically developed statements to assist practitioner and patient decisions about appropriate health care for specific clinical circumstances".[3] The concept of medical practice according to guidelines was recognised by Plato who considered it debasing because the emphasis is on the average patient not the particular, and because guidelines produced by others "are not rooted in the mental processes of clinicians".[4] Plato foresaw the likelihood of governmental insistence on guidelines and the potential legal consequences. Nowadays we suffer from an excess of guidelines. They may be inconsistent[5] and lack quality.[6] So where does the practising cardiologist stand?

Randomised trials

Most current guidelines are based on the analysis of randomised controlled trials. Cardiologists should remind themselves that such trials recruit a minority of eligible patients. In the stroke prevention in atrial fibrillation trials only a small fraction of patients screened were finally randomised to receive warfarin or placebo. In the statin trials 20–30% of those screened were randomised. In the thrombolytic trials recruitment was better, as might be expected from the captive population, but the best—GISSI 2—only recruited 60% of those eligible. Many of the earlier trials do not state the size of the screening programme.

A further weakness of guidelines based on randomised trials is that the participants are usually a highly selected subgroup of patients. Those with other pathologies are excluded. There may be an upper age limit—for example, 70 years in most of the statin trials. Yet the patients encountered in clinical practice are often elderly and have other diseases. Anyone who agrees to participate in a trial is likely to comply with medical advice. Even those in the placebo limb of a trial fare better than those who are not recruited.

Traditionally the practice of medicine was based on experience, not "evidence". From the outset it was evident that coronary angioplasty and bypass surgery could reliably abolish angina. A trial was never undertaken. Our advice to symptomatic patients to have a heart valve replaced or a permanent pacemaker inserted is likewise based on experience. Guidelines for the management of many cardiovascular disorders are thus drawn up by panels of experts without the benefit of an "evidence base". These are termed "consensus statements". There is a danger that such groups of experts may contain enthusiasts whose influence may lead to recommendations that go beyond the evidence. The pacemaker prescription in the British Pacing and Electrophysiology guidelines, for example, strongly favours dual chamber devices which seems perfectly reasonable in view of their physiological performance. The advice would be more compelling, however, if supported by the results of randomised trials which are currently being undertaken.

In the UK, guidelines also now emanate from the National Institute for Clinical Excellence (NICE). The encouraging recommendations for the more widespread use of intracoronary stents, implantable cardioverter-defibrillators, and platelet glycoprotein IIb/IIIa receptor antagonists have been very welcome, but may again reflect the views of advocates for these forms of treatment. There is a nagging doubt in some minds that the strength of some of the recommendations is not entirely supported by the evidence, and not equal to the authority of other guidelines, on the use of statins, for example.

Problems of guidelines

Implementing guidelines produces three problems: cost, complications, and the fact that a majority of patients are going to receive a treatment that they do not need. No nation can afford universal healthcare. Some form of rationing is therefore inevitable, and this is of course a major reason for the development of guidelines. In those states and countries where criteria for treatments have been drawn up—for example, Oregon in the USA, and New Zealand in the case of coronary artery bypass grafting—the experience has not been a happy one. In theory guidelines for expensive treatments ought to provide equitable access based on clinical need. This is what every government desires of the profession. In practice each patient presents a unique set of problems and many if not most do not conform to the agreed indications for the treatment, especially when they become emergencies. Where rationing is achieved by waiting, as in the UK, the apparently random distribution of scant resources is not demonstrably less unfair. Implementing guidelines in a country such as the UK where the provision of cardiac services lags far behind most developed countries is going to be hugely expensive. The cost of the NICE recommendations, for example, cannot be met by the purchasers of healthcare.

The side effects of treatment recommended by guidelines is the second reason for caution in their interpretation. On balance, thrombolysis in myocardial infarction and use of warfarin in atrial fibrillation save lives. But both may result in catastrophic bleeding. This is particularly sad for those who were previously active and asymptomatic and whose infarct or arrhythmia was not particularly symptomatic. The complications of treatment instituted on the active recommendation of a physician also engender more heart searching than those that occur naturally. While the physician is less often blamed for the sins of omission, he is nevertheless just as guilty if he fails to recommend a treatment which has been shown to confer benefit overall. Junior medical staff in particular must pay careful attention to the exclusion criteria.

The third problem with guidelines is that many patients receive a treatment in order that a few may benefit. Most trials demonstrating benefit in the treatment of cardiovascular conditions report an absolute reduction in major adverse events of a few per cent per annum, although the results are often reported as a relative reduction in order to amplify the potential gain in the public mind. We cannot yet identify which patients will benefit from which drugs and hence the victim of a heart attack will be recommended to take aspirin, a statin, a β blocker, and an angiotensin converting enzyme inhibitor, in addition to other drugs for diabetes, hypertension, etc. No wonder the cupboards of the elderly are full of pills.

The analogy has been drawn with anaemia; a randomised trial of the use of iron supplements in all cases of anaemia would demonstrate that a percentage would benefit. So all cases would be treated, until we learned to select those whose anaemia was caused by iron deficiency. In our current state of knowledge we are overtreating patients with cardiovascular disorders and are encouraged to do so by well intentioned guidelines. The general practitioner often bears the blame, and the cost, of this polypharmacy, and seldom challenges the advice of panels of experts. Cardiologists have the authority and the knowledge to provide intelligent interpretation of guidelines and should do so more often in order to reduce the drug burden in the elderly.

Physicians should remember and teach their junior staff that our job is to advise, not insist. Any decision about treatment should be discussed with the patient and his or her relatives, wherever possible. Interestingly many older patients decline the offer of anticoagulation for atrial fibrillation. The existence of guidelines, however, means that we must record

our discussion and the reasons for our decision. We should remember that many guidelines are available on the internet so that patients will be aware of what our peers have recommended. Guidelines then should inform the practice of cardiology and can never replace the individual advice to a patient, taking into account his or her particular circumstances. The authors of guidelines will be reassured to know that none has yet been held liable for harm resulting from the application of a recommendation, although this is a possibility and a disclaimer might be advisable.[3]

REGULATIONS

Regulations carry greater authority than guidelines, but lack the force of the law. Many are devised by organisations allied to government—for example, the Army. Others are imposed by institutions on their workforce in order to ensure safe practices. Regulations for the management of medical conditions are called protocols and have the same authority; they may be imposed by managers. Regulations are intended to provide written, reasoned, and prospective policies for employees. In many industries where the incapacity of an individual compromises the safety of others, regulations relating to cardiovascular fitness are imposed. Compliance with regulations is guaranteed when the perpetrator of the regulations is also the employer, or is acting on behalf of a group of employers such as the airlines. The Civil Aviation Authority has set fitness standards for pilots of commercial aircraft which are now agreed internationally by the Joint Aviation Authority. Therefore, throughout the world pilots who have or are suspected of having heart disease are subject to similar regulations.

Workers with heart disease are treated more fairly nowadays, although many employers still discriminate against those with heart disease, mainly because of the risk of sudden incapacity, and death. This risk can be assessed and if the risk is judged unacceptable then permanent sickness benefit may be available. In some industries, a diagnosis of heart disease with its perceived increased risk of incapacity makes employment unacceptable. Tanker drivers are one current example. Others include drivers of main line railway trains and seafarers in UK registered vessels, although this last group is undergoing reappraisal and in the near future may be permitted to return to sea subject to the precise nature of their responsibilities and heart condition.

What level of risk is acceptable for such workers? The answer depends on the industry in question. The cardiology advisors to the aviation industry were the first to develop the concept of acceptable risk. They proposed that the pilot could be likened to a part of the airframe. Engineers accept a risk of component failure of one per billion flying hours. Making a number of assumptions about the time the pilot spends in the air, and in particular during the critical phases of the flight—taking off and landing—then it can be calculated that this equates to an annual risk of incapacity of 1% per annum. A pilot may therefore be allowed to fly if his risk of a cardiovascular event is less than this. This happens to be the annual risk of a heart attack (myocardial infarction or sudden cardiac death) in healthy men aged 45–64 years based on data derived from the cardiovascular literature. Hence the 1% "rule" is tantamount to recommending that the pilot should continue at work provided he is at no increased risk as compared with his peers.[7]

Regulations governing drivers

Among the most widely used regulations in cardiological practice in the UK are those governing drivers with heart disease. They have been generally welcomed as striking a reasonable balance between the liberty of the individual and his or her potential to cause harm to others; hence they are widely used in other industries.

The regulations are drawn up by an honorary medical advisory panel currently comprising six cardiologists, one cardiac surgeon, representatives from the medical branch of the Drivers and Vehicle Licensing Authority (DVLA), the chief medical officer at the Department of Transport (currently linked with Local Government and Regions), and others. Following the Phillip's report into the BSE (bovine spongiform encephalophy, or "mad cow disease") outbreak, government concern over the wisdom of the advice that it was receiving from expert scientific committees resulted in the recruitment of lay members to the medical panels—an initiative that was implemented in the cardiac panel in November 2001.

Other panels with similar constitutions and tasks are concerned with neurological disorders, diabetes, eyesight, psychiatric disorders, drugs, and alcohol. A panel's duty is to advise the secretary of state who formulates policy in conjunction with ministerial colleagues; DVLA is the agency responsible for implementing his policies. The UK is unusual in that the regulations do have their origin in law—the Road Traffic Act (1986). The relevant sentences for the cardiologist state that drivers must not suffer from "Sudden attacks of disabling giddiness or faintness", nor "Severe physical or mental handicap". The wording of both may be quaint but the intention of the first is clear and has been so since first promulgated in the 1930s.

Any driver who suffers from a disorder which might render him or her liable to such attacks is said to have a "prospective disability", and should stop driving until the risk has been assessed medically. Examples for the ordinary driver would include epilepsy, recent heart attack, or the implantable cardioverter-defibrillator.

The regulations governing drivers are the panel's interpretation of the law. Sudden incapacity, caused for example by a Stokes-Adams attack, obviously falls within the meaning of the Act and is a bar to driving. There are many more disorders in which the faintness is not so sudden or the mental handicap not so severe or merely transient. Neurocardiogenic syncope in the older driver, the onset of an arrhythmia, or severe cardiac pain are three common examples. The essential issue in each case is whether the disorder is sufficient to cause the driver to lose control of his or her vehicle. The term "cognitive distraction" nicely describes the effect that the disorder has on the driver and is the currently favoured wording. It is always a matter for individual judgment whether the prospective disability is sufficient to warrant suspension of driving. The regulations may on occasion be overridden if the cardiologist can show that there are very good reasons why that particular patient does not conform to the regulations formulated by the panel. One example might be a shortening of time off driving after a heart attack for someone who was at demonstrably low risk as compared with the average victim. In the event of an accident as a result of incapacity, however, the cardiologist would be required to defend his or her position.

The consequences of driver incapacity are much greater for vocational (group 2) drivers as compared with ordinary (group 1) drivers. The former include drivers of large goods and passenger carrying vehicles (LGV and PCV) and, in some traffic areas, others who drive for a living—for example, taxi drivers.

Taylor showed that the case fatality rates for accidents involving these vehicles, using the definitions in force at the time, were 3–4 times greater than those involving ordinary private motor cars.[8] Vocational drivers also have longer occupational exposure. Hence more stringent criteria are justified.

Acceptable level of risk

In an ideal world the risk of driver incapacity would be subject to objective appraisal, using data from the medical literature, as in aviation. Medical advisors can then define the risk for an individual. Society—that is, politicians—can independently decide what level of risk is acceptable. The medical profession is then absolved from deciding about that level. But the world is far from ideal and the medical literature, while helpful for some conditions such coronary heart disease, does not generally provide sufficiently accurate data for individual decisions. Hence medical advice does tend to be based on the distilled wisdom of groups of specialists. And in seeking to define an acceptable level of risk, this should obviously be comparable whether the prospective disability be cardiovascular or neurological. A major difficulty in providing an objective basis for assessing the risk of incapacity at the wheel from a cardiovascular cause is that the risk of incapacity does not necessarily equate with the cardiovascular event rate, as described in the literature. The classic cardiovascular end point, namely death, may be sudden in epidemiological terms, yet may allow time for the driver to pull over safely to the side of the road. Conversely neurocardiogenic syncope may be sudden and incapacitating, but is not an event that would appear as an end point in the cardiovascular literature. A reasonable assumption that has been made is that the cardiovascular mortality rate is similar to the incapacity rate. This is tantamount to suggesting that for every cardiac death on the road that does not cause incapacity there is another survivor of a cardiac event who was transiently incapacitated by a non-fatal arrhythmia or hypotensive episode.

Society already accepts that drivers in their late 70s may hold a vocational licence by which age their annual death rate from coronary disease exceeds 2%. This is very similar to the recurrence rate agreed for the epilepsy guidelines which are a risk of recurrence of 2% per annum or less for vocational (group 2) drivers. This is, however, double the risk accepted by the Civil Aviation Authority for commercial pilots, The latter, more stringent figure is justified on the basis of the greater consequences resulting from pilot incapacity. Also pilots are required to retire at the age of 65 years; therefore, regulations do not have to accommodate the elderly pilot. For ordinary drivers suffering from cardiovascular disorders a greater risk of incapacity is acceptable.

A figure of 20% annual risk of an event has been arrived at by consultation, and has been accepted by neurologists for those drivers who have had a seizure. This sort of event rate is rarely encountered in cardiovascular disorders, except in those who had continuing symptoms of heart failure or a major heart attack less than one month ago—in keeping with the current guidelines. There is again no irrefutable logic behind this figure, but society places no restrictions on a young man who has recently passed his driving test, and whose annual risk of an accident is of this order.

The level of acceptable risk for driver incapacity is thus an event rate at or below 20% per annum for ordinary licences and 2% for vocational licences. Vocational (group 2) drivers with coronary heart disease, for example, may thus resume driving six weeks after a coronary event provided that they are asymptomatic and can satisfactorily complete three stages of the Bruce treadmill test. This test does contain useful prognostic information but it tells us nothing about the ulcerated atheromatous plaque which was the cause of the event. The cardiologist therefore has to ask himself supplementary questions such as whether the plaque has had time to heal, and is the patient taking aspirin, and also satisfy himself that the risk of further thrombosis is minimal. Often the patient's own cardiologist is not the right person to do this because he will tend to act as his patient's advocate. An independent opinion may be advisable.

Regulations change

The guidance material published in *At a glance medical aspects of fitness to drive* is the panel's interpretation of those disorders which constitute a prospective disability. They are inevitably imperfect and may lag behind clinical practice. Regulations that affect medical practice change, for three good reasons. Firstly, our knowledge of the disease process and understanding of the natural history gets better; secondly, new diagnostic tools are introduced; and thirdly, new treatments improve the prognosis. Examples of each include our recognition of the benign nature of some cases of hypertrophic cardiomyopathy, tilt testing for the investigation of syncope, and the demonstrable benefits of implantable cardioverter-defibrillators. Officially any change in guidelines is effective from the moment of the panel's decision. Informing the profession and public remains a problem which has been partly resolved by the introduction of the DVLA website (www.dvla.gov.uk). Regulations necessarily lag behind changes in clinical practice because the regulators have to have a sufficient body of evidence to demonstrate that a change, generally a relaxation, is justified. The implantable cardioverter-defibrillator is a good current example. Treatments delivered by the early devices were potentially incapacitating. This is no longer so likely. So recommended times off driving have shortened. But there remain longer term anxieties about lead malfunction so the recommendations remain cautious, much to the frustration of some cardiologists.

Individual cases may sometimes appear unfair and drivers may feel aggrieved at the loss of their licence, which in the case of some group 2 drivers may mean the loss of their livelihood. They do, however, have the right of appeal. If the licence is not restored then they can pursue their claim through the courts. This has not happened in cardiology in the past decade, which may indicate that regulations are seen to strike a correct balance between the rights of the individual and the safety of others. Some drivers ignore medical advice. In this situation the doctor should first make sure of his reasons for giving the advice. An example might be a driver with blackouts, thought to be caused by an arrhythmia. The doctor should repeat the advice and make careful notes. He or she may seek a second opinion, and consult a defence organisation. If the driver persists then the doctor should tell the patient in writing that he is informing the medical branch at DVLA, who can then take any necessary action. If the doctor does not do this and the driver causes an accident then the doctor shares the responsibility. The patient may lodge a complaint against the doctor but when this has happened hitherto the ombudsman has found in favour of the doctor.

Regulations, even the Queen's regulations, may be challenged in law. There are instances where well intentioned regulations have contravened the more basic rights, relating to employment and discrimination, for example. This is a further reason why regulations have to change; in cardiology, however, the various sets of regulations governing the medical fitness of drivers, aircraft pilots, offshore workers, railwaymen, and many others in industry have not needed to be changed as a result of litigation—yet.

Cardiologists are also commonly asked to give advice about fitness to work. If the individual's job is subject to regulations, such as those outlined above, then clearly the cardiologist should acquaint himself with these. If not, then the cardiologist would still be well advised to obtain a job description and propose that the question of continuing employment should also be referred to an expert—that is, an occupational health physician. Cardiologists and cardiac surgeons who assert that their patient is now cured and can return to full employment are liable to end up in conflict with the employer's representatives and may find themselves and their patient disadvantaged.

THE LAW
General Medical Council (GMC)

This statutory body is responsible for ensuring that the standards of professional conduct are maintained. Disciplinary powers were conferred on the GMC by the Medical Act of 1858, which also established the register. A doctor's name may be struck off the register if he is found guilty of "serious professional misconduct". Long before that ultimate sanction, members of the profession are required to comply with the standards set by the GMC whose advice (protecting patients, guiding doctors) is contained in a series of publications and on their website (www.gmc-uk.org).

The booklets which are of particular relevance to the cardiologist include those on *Training* (1997), *Good medical practice and maintaining good medical practice* (1998), *Seeking patient's consent: the ethical considerations* (1998), *Management in health care: the role of doctors* (1999), *Confidentiality: protecting and providing information* (2000), and the *Annual review of the work of the GMC*. Additional publications which cover some of the same ground are available from the Royal Colleges and medical defence organisations. In all these publications practical advice on daily problems may be found. Some issues are necessarily devolved to others, such as clinical governance which is a function of the cardiologist's institution.

All cardiologists and trainees must be very aware of the duties and responsibilities of a doctor. Issues such as informed consent, confidentiality, death certification, living wills, etc, are generic and not specific to cardiology. For further reading the aforementioned texts are recommended. The issue of what constitutes informed consent has also been discussed recently in this journal.[9] Cardiologists need to remember that truly informed consent can only be obtained by a doctor or a nurse who is fully familiar with the procedure and that nowadays any risk should be brought into the open; in practice a complication rate in excess of one in several hundred must be noted, as should the rarer but very important complications of cardiac catheterisation such as stroke. Although a patient's consent for clinical and non-invasive examinations is being discussed in some specialties, this is unlikely to be necessary in cardiology. A potential defence in the event of a complaint is that attendance for a predefined purpose implies consent.

Medical negligence

No cardiologist or indeed cardiac surgeon is above the law, and sooner or later a letter will arrive threatening legal action as a result of a patient's perceived misfortune. Such is the climate in which we live. No longer is free healthcare a privilege. People have been led to believe that they have a right to perfect health and if this is not achieved then someone has to take the blame and compensate the victim.

Governments and guidelines encourage this attitude. Doctors, however, lack the resources to deliver ideal health care and currently take much of the blame. Inevitably we will all fail in our duty of care towards individual patients occasionally and in the UK there have been some recent notorious examples. The tide of dissatisfaction runs deep and is exemplified by the fact that in March 2000 the National Audit Office stated that 23 000 claims amounting to a total value of £2.6 billion were outstanding against the NHS.[10] Settlements of a further £1.3 billion were expected for claims not yet received. In 1998 it was estimated that £84 million was spent on clinical negligence claims by hospitals in England although the confidence intervals were wide. The increasing cost of medical negligence may not be as alarming as the above figures suggest; after allowing for hospital activity the annual rate of increase for closed claims during the 1990s was 7%. Most claims are legally aided and of those only 17% are successful. The Medical Defence Union (MDU) experience indicates that only 1% of cases end up in court, 70% do not proceed or run out of time, and in 29% of cases some sort of settlement is reached. It is difficult to escape the conclusion that the unregulated granting of legal aid is currently propelling the tide of litigation and that other approaches such as mediation and/or no-fault compensation merit re-examination.

Data from the Physician Insurers Association of America and the MDU indicate that missed heart attacks are the third most expensive type of claim, after brain damaged babies and breast cancer. Of 349 claims analysed over 10 years, 160 were against general practitioners, 70% involved patients with no previous evidence of coronary heart disease, 47% were under 50 years of age, and 77% died; the average cost per case in the UK was £27 000. Invasive and interventional cardiologists are potentially liable to larger claims against them and this is reflected in their medical insurance premiums.

What can the cardiologist do to avoid litigation? The first rule is to keep good records. "No notes = no defence" is a well tested aphorism. The second is to maintain competence. History shows that this is best achieved by practising in an environment where audit, peer review, and related activities are the norm. The single handed or isolated practitioner is the most susceptible to error. In undertaking procedures the cardiologist or institution with low volumes is vulnerable, especially if these fall below the numbers recommended by advisory bodies such as the British Cardiac Society.

Publications by the GMC explain what to do when things go wrong which, in essence, boil down to a frank explanation to the patient and/or relatives in the first place. All NHS hospitals nowadays have a department devoted to the handling of complaints who must be informed as soon as possible. If the matter cannot be resolved locally, the complainant then has two options. The first is to go to an "independent review" in which senior staff from an unrelated hospital examine the allegations, interview those concerned, produce a report, and make recommendations. In the author's experience these are a rather cumbersome and time consuming method of giving the complainants a chance to express their grievances. This is often all that is required. Sometimes it is difficult to escape the conclusion that the complainants are motivated by a desire, not just for an apology and a wish to see that the mis-

take will not be repeated, but rather by a desire to humiliate senior medical staff. Some doctors find this difficult to accept but they should remind themselves that humility is a virtue.

Sadly the implementation of any recommendations—for example, faster access to coronary artery bypass surgery—may be frustrated by lack of resources.

The complainant's second option is take legal advice, and then action. Nowadays the first clue that such action is being contemplated is a request for release of the patient's notes. In order to succeed the complainant must first show that harm has been done—"but for the cardiologist's action I would be alright now". Death is generally indisputable. Chronic leg pain and immobility following a femoral haematoma are, however, more difficult to evaluate unless there are convincing neurological signs, which might persuade a judge. Secondly, the complainant has to show that the doctor "failed in his duty of care" and that his action or negligence caused harm (liability). In order to succeed a complainant does not have to prove a causal relationship beyond all reasonable doubt as in criminal law, but merely to show that it was "more likely than not" (causation). Thirdly, when it comes to a settlement, the complainant must be able to show that he has been disadvantaged by the harm and to what extent (quantum).

These steps in the process of litigation explain why so few cases proceed. Most cardiologists should have little to fear. But even the threat of litigation is a very unsettling experience. A few doctors find it difficult to carry on but, with help, most do, and most find that patients still have enormous confidence in the profession. The tide of litigation may ebb somewhat because complainants are now subject to closer scrutiny before being granted legal aid, and the register of solicitors permitted to undertake medicolegal work is diminishing the availability of the opportunistic solicitor.

In defending an action a doctor will rely on the Bolam test. This was a case in which the defence successfully argued that the doctor's actions were in keeping with a reasonable body of medical opinion, as follows: "In the realm of diagnosis and treatment, there is ample scope for genuine difference of opinion and one man clearly is not negligent merely because his conclusion differs from that of other professional men, nor because he has less skill or knowledge than others would have shown. The true test for establishing negligence in diagnosis or treatment on the part of a doctor is whether he has been proved to be guilty of such failure as no doctor of ordinary skill would be guilty of acting with ordinary care".

This judgment has not been challenged for 45 years but there is a rider, as a result of a judgment handed down in the Bolitho case in 1997, since when it has also been necessary to demonstrate that the doctor's action would "stand up to analysis". It is thus not necessary to demonstrate that the cardiologist practised perfect medicine but simply that he acted rationally and logically according to a body of opinion among his peers.

The concept of the "non-negligent loser" should be familiar to all doctors. This is the case in which liability is not admitted but a financial settlement is negotiated with the complainant's representatives, because it is the cheapest option. No fault is admitted by the defendants and the doctor's professional status is unimpaired. Some doctors find this difficult to accept and want to fight on. The only gainers in that event are the lawyers.

Heart disease, guidelines, regulations, and the law: key points

- ▶ International (European) influences are playing an increasingly important role in the practice of cardiology
- ▶ Guidelines are intended to help practitioners and must be read with care; in specialist practice such as cardiology their application can be difficult
- ▶ Regulations and protocols are imposed by institutions; any violation must be supported by a very good reason
- ▶ Regulations that affect drivers are an interpretation of the law that states that you must not drive if you are liable to "sudden attacks of disabling giddiness or faintness"
- ▶ The GMC's booklets should be kept near to hand
- ▶ To establish that a cardiologist was medically negligent the plaintiff must prove causation and liability

Witnesses and experts

Solicitors approach doctors for assistance in two circumstances. The most common reason is for a factual statement relating to an involvement in a case. This should be prepared with professional help, should state who you are, be set out in short numbered paragraphs, should stick to the facts, and not offer an opinion.

Many cardiologists offer themselves as expert witnesses. The British Cardiac Society keeps a register. When this was set up in 1992 the legal and ethical committee was surprised that so many cardiologists wished to undertake this sort of work. The Society did not wish to impose restrictions on individuals who wished to provide expert opinions, but the committee did advise that cardiologists should not be over the age of 70 years and/or retired from active practice for more than five years.

Those who wish to provide a service as an expert will generally have been consultant cardiologists for 15 years or so because the courts and lawyers expect experts to have experience and standing. Expert witnesses must undergo further training, must acquaint themselves with the evolving literature on the subject, and should examine their motives. The profession is best served by those experts who are motivated by a desire to see justice done, rather than those whose interests are pecuniary. Serious experts will usually submit their names to the Law Society's register.

The duties of the expert lie beyond the scope of this article. The standard reference works[11][12] should be consulted. The initial and often sole task of the expert is to prepare a medical report. This must be impartial. The ultimate responsibility of the expert witness is to the court. Medical reports which are biased and which encourage the complainant or defendant to believe that an action may succeed do a disservice and are unhelpful in the long run. It should be unnecessary to point out that an expert should only give an opinion which is within his field of expertise, and can only comment with authority on his peers—for example, a cardiologist should not pass comment on a general practitioner.

The reform of the civil procedure rules recommended by the report of Lord Woolf came into force in 1998.[13] The aims are to improve access to justice, to speed up the process of litigation, and to reduce costs. Part 35 deals with experts and assessors; 35.1 describes the court's duty to restrict expert evidence; 35.4 describes its power to achieve this; and 35.7 describes its ability to instruct a single joint expert. This reform therefore reinforces need for impartiality in the preparation of expert reports.

Human Rights Act 1998

The impact that this legislation will have on the practice of cardiology is uncertain. The Act is likely to affect practice in several ways. A fundamental tenet is that humans have an absolute right to life. This may be at variance with sensible cardiological opinion—for example, a decision not to resuscitate. Consent to treatment protocols may have to be amplified. The allocation of scarce NHS resources may be become subject to judicial review—for example, a patient who dies while awaiting coronary artery bypass grafting might be said to have been denied his basic right to life which he would have been afforded had he lived in another country.

The difficulty in predicting the effect of this Act is that English law has been built on precedents and piecemeal legislation, not the grand and sometimes internally inconsistent principles of the Act. We can only wait and see what view our judiciary will take when interpreting the Act in the light of our considerable body of case law.

Social security law

This is a little known but important aspect of legal practice. The law is mainly concerned with issues related to social security, but this includes accidents at work which may entitle the victim to compensation. These are not obviously matters for the cardiologist, but there is one important exception, namely an event that might have triggered a heart attack. This stems from a case in 1967 when unaccustomed strenuous work was judged to be such a trigger. Since then this judgment has usually been upheld, and compensation been granted, although there are continuing areas of uncertainty.[14]

Social security law has established precedents which find application in insurance medicine. Victims of heart disease commonly discuss the option of retirement on grounds of ill health, and indeed may be encouraged to do so by their medical advisers, and personnel manager. Most permanent sickness policies, however, state that an employee should be "wholly incapable of continuing their former employment" in order to claim benefit. This is a difficult argument for the cardiologist to sustain if, for example, the individual has made a full recovery following a coronary bypass procedure. These policies were originally devised to compensate victims of accidents at work, not those whose illness results from natural causes. Hence there are insufficient funds to meet all claims and each is scrutinised both at the time of application, and subsequently. Patients may find themselves financially disadvantaged if they retire on medical grounds without first checking the terms of their policy.

CONCLUSION

Despite the foregoing, cardiologists still have immense freedom to interpret guidelines, regulations, and the law provided that they always act in the best interests of their patients and record the reasons for their actions.

REFERENCES

1 **Hampton JR**. The end of clinical freedom? *BMJ* 1983;**287**:1237–8.
▶ **An editorial which marked a turning point in clinical practice.**
2 **Petch MC**. Training cardiologists in Europe. *Heart* 1999;**81**:107–8.
3 **Woolf SH**, Grol R, Hutchinson A, *et al.* Potential benefits, limitations, and harms of clinical guidelines. *BMJ* 1999;**318**:527–30.
4 **Hurwitz B**. Legal and political considerations of clinical practice guidelines. *BMJ* 1999;**318**:661–4.
▶ **This and the previous reference are the first and third in a series of four helpful articles on issues in the development and use of clinical guidelines.**

5 **Raine R**, Streetly A, Maryon Davis A. Variation in local policies and guidelines for cholesterol management: national survey. *BMJ* 1996;**313**:1368–9.

6 **Grill R**, Magrini N, Penna A, *et al*. Practice guidelines developed by specialist societies: the need for a critical appraisal. *Lancet* 2000;**355**:103–5.

7 **Joy MD**. Second European workshop in aviation cardiology. *Eur Heart J* 1999;suppl D.
▶ **A supplement which deals with the assessment of pilots suspected of suffering from cardiovascular disease and details the logic behind the 1% rule (Chamberlain D19–24).**

8 **Taylor J**. In: *The medical aspects of fitness to drive*. London: Medical Commission on Accident Prevention, 1995.

9 **Kurbaan AS**, Smith S, Mills P. Consent in cardiac practice. *Heart* 2001;**86**:593–4.
▶ **One of three editorials in a recent issue of** *Heart* **which discuss the nature of, and offer practical advice on, obtaining informed consent.**

10 **Fenn P**, Diacon S, Gray A, *et al*. Current cost of medical negligence in NHS hospitals: analysis of claims database. *BMJ* 2000;**320**:1567–71.

11 **Powers MJ**, Harris NH. *Medical negligence*. London and Edinburgh: Butterworths, 1990.

12 **Kennedy I**, Grubb A. *Medical law: text and materials*. London: Butterworths, 1989.

13 **Anon**. *The civil procedure rules*. London: Sweet and Maxwell, 1999.

14 **Petch MC**. Triggering a heart attack. *BMJ* 1996;**312**:459–60.

30 APOPTOSIS IN THE CARDIOVASCULAR SYSTEM

Martin R Bennett

Apoptosis, or programmed cell death, is a process through which multicellular organisms dispose of cells efficiently. Much has been discovered about the molecular control of apoptosis since its initial description as a series of morphological events.[1] Apoptosis defines a type of cell death distinct from the more conventional necrotic death, seen classically in myocardial infarction, on the basis of characteristic morphological features (table 1, fig 1). Although these descriptions and distinctions are useful, there is a great deal of overlap between apoptosis and necrosis in morphological features and biochemical events. Indeed, apoptosis is frequently followed by secondary necrosis of cells, especially if there is failure of clearance or ingestion of apoptotic bodies.

▶ DETECTION OF APOPTOSIS

Apoptotic cells undergo a characteristic cascade of biochemical events (see Regulation of apoptosis), many of which are useful in detecting apoptotic cells. In particular, apoptotic cells expose specific membrane phospholipids that can be detected with labelled marker proteins (for example, phosphatidylserine detected with fluorescently labelled annexin V) and cleave their DNA into specific fragments that are the basis for the enzyme linked assays to detect fragmented DNA (for example, terminal UTP nick end labelling, or TUNEL). Biochemical signalling during apoptosis, such as activation or cleavage of specific caspase enzymes (see below) can also be used on both cells and tissue samples. While helpful, the gold standard for detecting apoptosis is still based on morphology at both the light and particularly the electron microscopic level, where the features outlined in table 30.1 are easily distinguished.

APOPTOSIS IN THE HEART

The adult cardiomyocyte has limited (if any) ability to proliferate. Correspondingly, apoptosis is observed infrequently in adult hearts. In contrast, cardiomyocyte apoptosis plays a critical role in heart formation, such as formation of septa between cardiac chambers and valves. This evidence suggests that defects in apoptosis can result in congenital heart disease. Major foci of apoptosis include zones of fusion of the atrioventricular or bulbar cushions, and both aortic and pulmonary valves in non-myocytes. Myocyte apoptosis also occurs in the interventricular septum and right ventricular wall after birth, during the transition from fetal to adult circulations. The conducting tissue also undergoes apoptosis, and aberrant apoptosis is implicated in congenital heart block and long QT syndrome or the persistence of accessory pathways.

Apoptosis in ischaemia/infarction

Ischaemia is a potent inducer of both myocyte necrosis and apoptosis in vitro. Thus, deprivation of oxygen alone, or in addition to serum withdrawal and deprivation of glucose, induces neonatal myocyte apoptosis. Ischaemia alone can induce apoptosis in the ischaemic territory in vivo, and this may be reduced by reperfusion. However, although reperfusion may limit ischaemia induced apoptosis, reperfusion itself may accelerate the appearance of apoptosis in the reperfused regions.[2]

Myocardial infarction has been considered to be a prime example of necrotic cell death, because of the breakdown of cellular energy metabolism. However, apoptosis of cardiomyocytes also occurs in a temporally and spatially specific manner. Thus, acute myocardial infarction manifests both forms of cell death,[3] with apoptosis particularly occurring at the hypoperfused "border" zones, between a central area of necrosis and viable myocardium. The central, unperfused region[4] also manifests apoptosis, particularly within the first six hours, although between 6–24 hours necrosis is more common. Apoptosis in the remote non-infarcted myocardium may be partly responsible for myocardial remodelling and dilatation after myocardial infarction, and may be amenable to treatment.

Apoptosis in heart failure

The finding that cardiomyocyte apoptosis occurs in the end stage human heart indicates that apoptosis may contribute to heart failure in a variety of situations.[5][6] Aging is associated with

Table 30.1 Characteristic features of apoptosis versus necrosis

Apoptosis	Necrosis
Condensation/clumping of nuclear chromatin	Nuclear chromatin non-specifically degraded
Loss of cell–cell contact, cell shrinkage, and fragmentation, with formation of membrane bound processes and vesicles containing fragments of nuclear material or organelles	Cell volume increases
Adjacent cells phagocytose the end product, the apoptotic body	
Minimal disruption of cell membranes or release of lysosomal enzymes, with consequently little inflammatory reaction	Cell membrane integrity lost early, release of lysosomal enzymes and subsequent inflammation
Organelle structure and function maintained until late into the process	Organelle structure and function lost early

myocardial cell loss, and cardiomyocyte apoptosis may be the mechanism of the gradual deterioration in cardiac function. In humans undergoing transplantation, apoptosis can be observed,[6] with some studies suggesting higher levels in ischaemic versus idiopathic dilated cardiomyopathy.[5] The transition from compensated to decompensated hypertrophy is also associated with myocyte apoptosis in animals,[7] and high levels of apoptosis are seen in arrhythmogenic right ventricular dysplasia, a condition characterised by myocardial replacement with fibrofatty material. Finally, there is increasing evidence that toxic cardiomyopathies, such as that induced by doxorubicin (Adriamycin), are associated with cardiomyocyte apoptosis.

Although the evidence that apoptosis promotes heart failure is persuasive, the present problem is defining by what extent. Vastly different rates of apoptosis have been reported in both human and animal heart failure, with rates of up to 35.5%.[5] While these death rates may be seen only in very localised areas, given that apoptosis takes less than 24 hours to complete, such rates would result in rapid involution of the heart. More recently, rates of < 0.5% have been consistently reported in end stage heart failure, which make far more physiological sense. In addition, in end stage heart failure necrosis is still (up to seven times) more frequent than apoptosis.

APOPTOSIS IN THE VESSEL WALL

Vascular smooth muscle cells (VSMCs) within the vessel wall can both divide and undergo apoptosis throughout life. However, the normal adult artery shows very low apoptotic and mitotic indices. In diseased tissue additional factors are present both locally, such as inflammatory cytokines, inflammatory cells, and the presence of modified cholesterol, and systemically, such as blood pressure and flow. These factors substantially alter the normal balance of proliferation and apoptosis, and apoptosis in particular may predominate in many disease states.

Remodelling

Remodelling defines a condition in which alterations in vessel size can occur through processes that do not necessarily require large changes in overall cell number or tissue mass. For example, physiological remodelling by cell proliferation/ apoptosis results in closure of the ductus arteriosus and reduction in lumen size of infra-umbilical arteries after birth, and remodelling occurs in primary atherosclerosis, after angioplasty and in restenosis. Although surgical reduction in flow results in compensatory VSMC apoptosis, the role of VSMC apoptosis per se in determining the outcome of remodelling is unclear.

Arterial injury and aneurysm formation

Acute arterial injury at angioplasty is followed by rapid induction of medial cell apoptosis. In animal models injury results in medial cell apoptosis 30 minutes to six hours after injury[8] with adventitial and neointimal apoptosis occurring later. In humans, restenosis after angioplasty has been reported to be associated with either an increase or decrease in VSMC apoptosis, and again the role of VSMC apoptosis in either the initial injury or the remodelling process in restenosis in humans requires further study.

The most common form of arterial aneurysm in humans is characterised by a loss of VSMCs from the vessel media, with fragmentation of elastin and matrix degradation, leading to progressive dilatation and eventually rupture. Apoptosis of VSMCs is increased in aortic aneurysms compared with normal aorta, associated with an increase in expression of a number of pro-apoptotic molecules. In particular, the presence of macrophages and T lymphocytes in aneurysms suggests that inflammatory mediators released by these cells may promote VSMC apoptosis. Moreover, the production of tissue metalloproteinases by macrophages may accelerate apoptosis by degrading the extracellular matrix from which VSMCs derive survival signals (see below).

Atherosclerosis

Rupture of atherosclerotic plaques is associated with a thinning of the VSMC-rich fibrous cap overlying the core. Rupture occurs particularly at the plaque shoulders, which exhibit lack of VSMCs and the presence of inflammatory cells. Apoptotic VSMCs are evident in advanced human plaques including the shoulder regions, prompting the suggestion that VSMC apoptosis may hasten plaque rupture. Indeed, increased VSMC apoptosis occurs in unstable versus stable angina lesions.

Although loss of VSMCs would be expected to promote plaque rupture, there is no direct evidence of the effect of apoptosis per se in advanced human atherosclerosis. Most apoptotic cells in advanced lesions are macrophages next to the lipid core.[9] Loss of macrophages from atherosclerotic lesions would be predicted to promote plaque stability rather than rupture, since macrophages can promote VSMC apoptosis by both direct interactions and by release of cytokines. However, macrophage apoptosis is found at sites of plaque rupture,[10] although it is not known if death directly promotes rupture, or simply that macrophages are the most common cell types found at rupture sites.

Effect of VSMC apoptosis

The effect of VSMC apoptosis is clearly context dependent. Thus, intimal VSMC apoptosis in advanced atherosclerotic plaques may promote plaque rupture, or medial apoptosis may promote aneurysm formation. In neointima formation post-injury, VSMC apoptosis of both intima and media can limit neointimal formation at a defined time point. However, apoptosis is also associated with a number of deleterious effects. Exposure of phosphatidylserine on the surface of apoptotic cells provides a potent substrate for the generation of

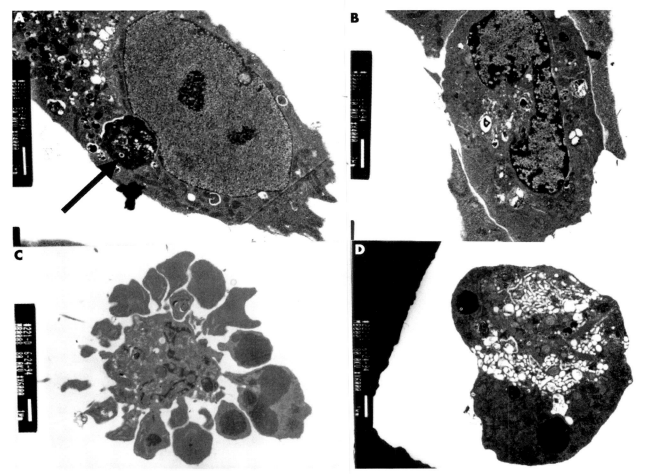

Figure 30.1 Electron microscopic appearances of a human vascular smooth muscle cell (VSMC) undergoing apoptosis in culture. (A) Normal appearance of a human VSMC. VSMC also contains an apoptotic body (arrow). (B) Peripheral condensation of nuclear chromatin. (C) Intense membrane blebbing and vesicle formation in apoptosis, with condensation of the nuclear chromatin into clumps. (D) An apoptotic body, the end product of apoptosis.

thrombin and activation of the coagulation cascade,[11] and apoptotic cells release membrane bound microparticles that are systemically procoagulant. Finally, VSMC apoptosis may be directly pro-inflammatory, with release of chemoattractants and cytokines from inflammatory cells.

REGULATION OF APOPTOSIS
Apoptosis via death receptors

Many stimuli can trigger apoptosis, but in vascular disease specific alterations within the cell elicit sensitivity to a particular stimulus that is disease associated. Thus, remodelling may trigger apoptosis following reduction in blood flow, the major stimulus being flow dependent stimuli such as nitric oxide or shear stress. In contrast, VSMC apoptosis in atherosclerosis or aneurysm formation may be caused by inflammatory cells that express surface death ligands or secrete pro-apoptotic cytokines. Whatever the stimulus, most downstream pathways that signal apoptosis are similar.

The regulation of apoptosis can be simplified into two major pathways (figs 30.2 and 30.3). First, membrane bound death receptors of the tumour necrosis receptor family (TNF-R), such as Fas (CD95), TNF-R1, or death receptors (DR) 3–6, bind their trimerised ligands causing receptor aggregation, and subsequent recruitment of adapter proteins (Fas-FADD, TNF-R1-TRADD, etc) through protein:protein interactions[12][13]

Diseases in which apoptosis has been implicated

► Cardiac (myocyte)
  – idiopathic dilated cardiomyopathy
  – ischaemic cardiomyopathy
  – acute myocardial infarction
  – arrhythmogenic right ventricular dysplasia
  – myocarditis
► Cardiac (conducting tissues)
  – pre-excitation syndromes
  – heart block, congenital complete atrioventricular heart block, long QT syndromes
► Vascular
  – atherosclerosis
  – restenosis after angioplasty/stenting
  – vascular graft rejection
  – arterial aneurysm formation

Abbreviations

AKT: cellular homologue of transforming oncogene of AKT8 retrovirus
ERK: extracellular signal related kinase
FLIP: Fas-like inhibitory protein
IAP: inhibitor of apoptosis protein
SAPK: stress activated protein kinase
TNF: tumour necrosis factor
TUNEL: terminal UTP nick end labelling
VSMC: vascular smooth muscle cell

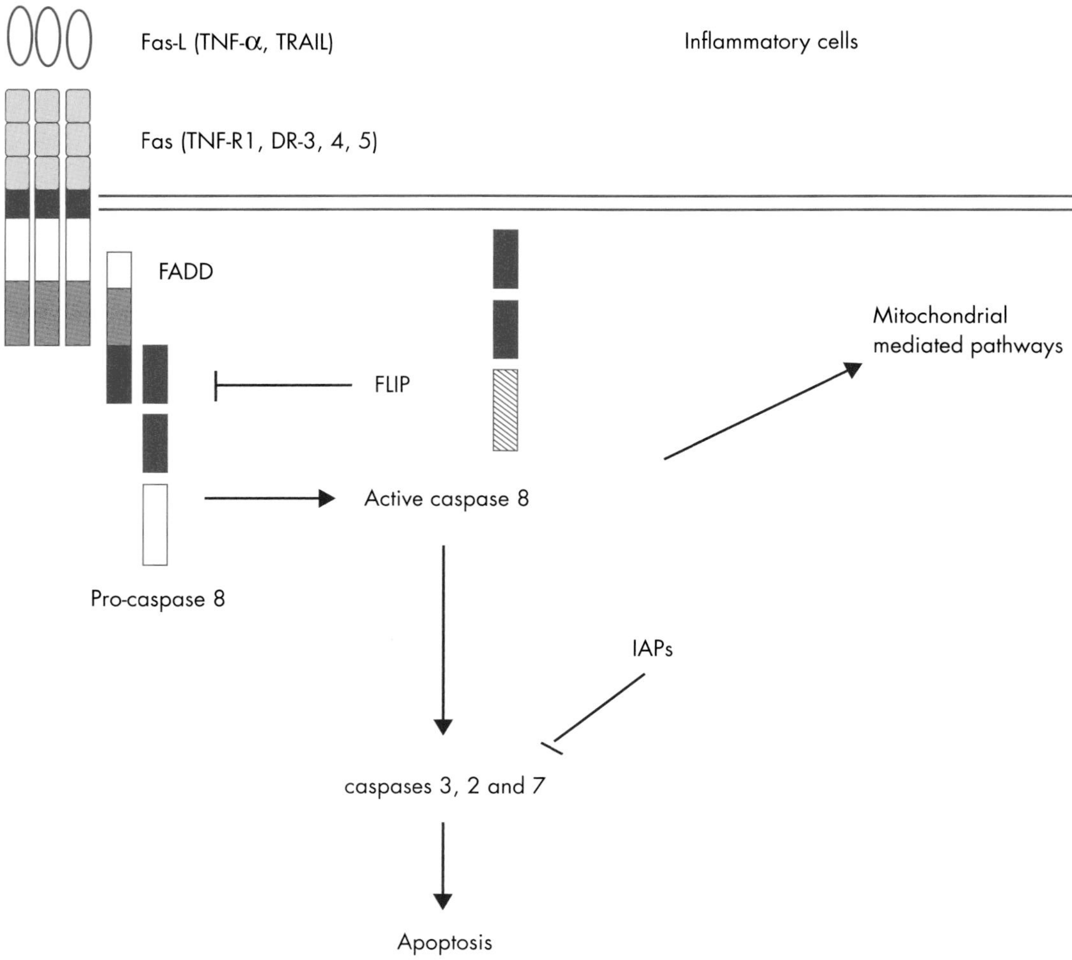

Figure 30.2 Schematic of Fas death signalling pathways. Fas, the prototypic member of the tumour necrosis factor (TNF) death receptor family, binds to its cognate ligand. Recruitment of the adapter molecule FADD and pro-caspase 8 results in activation of the latter. Caspase 8 activation directly activates downstream caspases, (3, 6, and 7) which results in DNA fragmentation and cleavage of cellular proteins. This pathway is thought to occur in type I cells and does not involve mitochondrial pathways. Caspase 8 activation also results in cleavage of Bid, which translocates and interacts with other Bcl-2 family members (see fig 30.3).

(fig 30.2). In turn, adapters recruit cysteine proteases (caspases) such as caspase 8 (FLICE) and caspase 2 to the complex.[14] Within the complex of Fas, FADD, and caspase 8 (known as the death inducing signalling complex (DISC)), caspase 8 becomes proteolytically activated by oligomerisation.[15] This in turn activates the terminal effector caspases (caspases 3, 6, and 7) responsible for cleavage of intracellular substrates required for cellular survival, architecture, and metabolic function.

Apoptosis via mitochondrial amplification
In addition to direct activation of caspases, caspase 8 activation causes cleavage of *bcl-2* family proteins such as *bid* (fig 30.3). Bcl-2 family members are either pro-apoptotic (Bax, Bid, Bik, Bak) or anti-apoptotic (Bcl-2, Bcl-X$_L$). Activation of pro-apoptotic Bcl-2 family members causes their translocation to mitochondria, where they interact with anti-apoptotic members that are mitochondrial membrane components. This interaction depolarises voltage dependent mitochondrial channels and releases mitochondrial mediators of apoptosis such as cytochrome c[16] and Smac/DIABLO. The association of cytochrome c with an adapter molecule apaf-1 and caspase 9 activates caspase 3, and the caspase cascade. In contrast, Smac/DIABLO promotes apoptosis by directly antagonising inhibitor of apoptosis proteins (IAPs) (see below).

Apoptosis can also be blocked by expression of several intracellular proteins, including FLIPs (FLICE inhibitory proteins) and IAPs (fig 30.2). FLIPs have the same pro-domain structure as caspase 8, but do not the active caspase site within the C-terminus. Binding of FLIP to caspase 8 therefore prevents its activation. In contrast, IAPs inhibit the enzymatic activity of downstream caspases, or they can mediate anti-apoptotic signalling pathways through the activation of nuclear transcription factor κβ.

REGULATION OF CARDIOMYOCYTE APOPTOSIS
The stimulus for cardiomyocyte apoptosis clearly depends upon the clinical or experimental setting. Ischaemia is associated with many changes in the intracellular and extracellular milieu of cardiomyocytes, many of which are potent apoptotic stimuli. Thus, hypoxia promotes cardiomyocyte apoptosis, both in vitro and in vivo, and ischaemia/reperfusion and hypoxia/reoxygenation are associated with increased expression of Fas. Decreased serum and glucose concentrations trigger cytochrome c release from mitochondria in cardiomyocytes, suggesting that ischaemia induced apoptosis may be mediated by mitochondrial amplification. Indeed oxygen species promote apoptosis by triggering pathways involving mitochondrial release of cytochrome c and caspase activation.

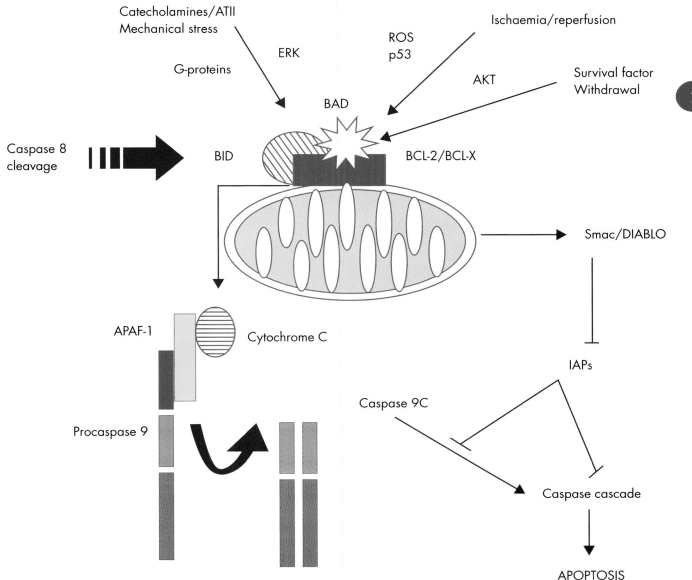

Figure 30.3 Schematic of mitochondrial death signalling pathways. Anti-apoptotic members of the Bcl-2 family, such as Bcl-2 and Bcl-X, are located on the mitochondrial outer membrane. Here they act to prevent the release of apoptogenic factors from the inner mitochondrial space. Binding of the pro-apoptotic proteins Bid (after cleavage by caspase 8) or Bad (after dephosphorylation) to Bcl-2 mitigates the protective effect of Bcl-2 and triggers release of cytochrome c and Smac/DIABLO. Cytochrome c, in concert with the adapter protein apaf-1 and caspase 9, activates caspase 3 and the downstream caspase cascade. Smac/DIABLO inhibits IAPs (inhibitor of apoptosis proteins), which in turn inhibit caspase activities, thus propagating apoptosis. Stimuli such as growth factor withdrawal or activation of p53 and Fas activation in type II cells act through this mitochondrial pathway.

In heart failure, a huge variety of initial stimuli have been propounded. In vitro, mechanical stretch can induce apoptosis, indicating a possible role for volume overload and raised ventricular end diastolic pressure; pressure overload following aortic banding also induces early myocyte apoptosis, before significant hypertrophy. Both four weeks of rapid ventricular pacing and catecholamines induce myocytes apoptosis in dogs associated with heart failure, suggesting that catecholamine responses may be directly toxic to myocytes.

REGULATION OF VASCULAR SMOOTH MUSCLE CELL APOPTOSIS

Human VSMCs express death receptors, and inflammatory cells within the atherosclerotic plaque express death ligands; interaction between membrane bound ligands and receptors may therefore induce VSMC death. In contrast, soluble ligand binding to death receptors is a very weak inducer of VSMC apoptosis, and does not induce apoptosis in the absence of "priming" of the cell. Some of this resistance can be explained by intracellular location of death receptors in VSMCs,[17] and priming may be associated with increased receptor expression. Physiologically, combinations of cytokines such as interleukin (IL) β (IL-1β), interferon γ (IFNγ) and tumour necrosis factor α (TNFα) increase surface death receptors, possibly via nitric oxide and p53 stabilisation.

Irrespective of the local environment, VSMCs derived from atherosclerotic plaques are intrinsically sensitive to apoptosis,[18] compared with cells from normal vessels. Heterogeneity of sensitivity between VSMCs in the vessel wall is also seen in animal vessels after injury, and in medial VSMCs from normal human arteries, This reflects differences in expression of pro- and anti-apoptotic molecules, specifically those regulating signalling from survival cytokines, cell:cell and cell:matrix interactions, and members of the *bcl-2* family. This may underlie observations that despite (apparently) the same stimulus for apoptosis, VSMC apoptosis in either normal or diseased vessels wall is highly localised. Indeed, insulin-like growth factor 1 receptor concentrations (IGF-1R), a potent survival signalling system for normal VSMCs, are downregulated in plaque VSMCs.

The *bcl-2* family members are critical in regulating VSMC apoptosis, both in vitro and in vivo. Human VSMCs express low levels of Bcl-2, but Bax is expressed in atherosclerotic plaques; reduced levels of VSMC apoptosis seen after cholesterol lowering in rabbit models of atherosclerosis is accompanied by a loss of Bax immunoreactivity. In vivo, rat VSMCs express minimal Bcl-2, but high levels of Bcl-X can be found after injury. Indeed, inhibition of Bcl-X dramatically induces apoptosis of VSMCs after balloon injury[19] and differences in expression of Bcl-X may account for differences in apoptosis sensitivity of intimal versus medial VSMCs. Regulation of sensitivity to apoptosis in VSMCs is also mediated by expression of IAP proteins and individual caspases.

THERAPEUTIC OPTIONS FOR APOPTOSIS TREATMENT

The prevention of cardiomyocyte apoptosis is now a very important therapeutic aim. However, critical to determining therapeutic benefit is not just inhibiting apoptosis markers at a single defined time point, but actually improving cardiac function. Many agents prevent the development of the morphological appearance of apoptosis or a biochemical marker (for example, DNA fragmentation) without inhibiting cell death. The ability to delay death may serve no useful purpose and may even be deleterious if that cell undergoes subsequent necrosis, with concomitant inflammation. In contrast, some studies have indicated that inhibition of apoptosis improves ventricular remodelling and contractility after infarction.[20] Although the long term effects of this inhibition are unknown, clinically meaningful improvements in cardiac function have been achieved.

Apoptosis can be interrupted at many points in the signalling pathway. Prevention of apoptotic myocyte death may be directed at (1) inhibiting/preventing the stimulus, (2) inhibiting the regulatory mechanisms determining the decision to die, or (3) inhibiting the pathways executing apoptosis. The cascade of events leading to cardiomyocyte apoptosis, and also the point at which a cell is irreversibly committed to die, crucially determine the approach to inhibiting apoptosis. Clearly, many signalling pathways are activated in ischaemia and heart failure. Interruption of a single pathway may therefore not inhibit apoptosis if there are multiple, redundant pathways inducing apoptosis.

In contrast, mediators that act beyond convergence of multiple signalling pathways may be better targets to inhibit apoptosis. However, many of the identified downstream mediators are enzymes required for effective cell disintegration and packaging, and may be beyond the point at which the cell is committed to die. Inhibition here would prevent the cellular appearances and markers of apoptosis, but the cell would still die. In addition, these molecules are critical to apoptosis in many tissues and such non-cardiac specificity may be unwelcome. From this argument, inhibiting the stimulus to apoptosis, particularly if specific to the heart at one point in time, would be more effective. The timing and delivery of treatment is also dependent upon the clinical situation. Clearly, it is easier to inhibit apoptosis transiently in an acute situation, such as myocardial infarction, than with chronic treatment in heart failure.

Inhibiting/preventing the pro-apoptotic stimulus

Ischaemia/reperfusion, hypertrophy caused by increased afterload, and myocardial remodelling following infarction all are associated with myocyte apoptosis. This suggests that current treatment of proven benefit in these diseases may already act by inhibition of apoptosis. The beneficial effects of β blockers in chronic heart failure and ischaemic heart disease may counteract the pro-apoptotic effect of excess catecholamines. Indeed, carvedilol can inhibit ischaemia/reperfusion induced myocyte apoptosis, and angiotensin converting enzyme inhibitors may protect against angiotensin II induced apoptosis. Clearly, approaches aimed at reducing myocardial stretch, or oxidative stress, or improving myocardial perfusion may have the same effect. Finally, many pathways leading to apoptosis are triggered by specific death ligands, with either apoptosis or the disease itself manifesting upregulation of death receptors. Inhibition of delivery of death ligands—for example, by scavenging ligands through soluble receptors or receptor antagonists—may reduce apoptosis mediated though these pathways. However, it should be noted that other signals emanate from death receptors. For example, Fas activation reduces the membrane potential and induces afterdepolarisations in cardiac myocytes; inhibiting Fas induced apoptosis may allow escape of other Fas signalling, promoting arrhythmias.

Protection against apoptosis

Many molecules protect cells from apoptosis, including anti-apoptotic Bcl-2 family members, IAPs, and decoys for death receptors. Although these agents inhibit apoptosis mediated by many stimuli, and may therefore be clinically useful, at present they cannot be selectively expressed without gene transfer into the heart, with all its inherent problems. More promising is the potential administration of soluble survival factors following the apoptotic stimulus. Many growth factors, including IGF-1, cardiotrophin-1, and the neuregulins, inhibit apoptosis following ischaemia, serum withdrawal,

Table 30.2 Potential inhibitors and signalling pathways of cardiomyocyte apoptosis

Stimulus	Signalling pathway	Potential inhibitor
Ischaemia/reperfusion	ERK/SAPK	Activation of ERK, inhibition of SAPK signalling
Pressure overload	ERK/SAPK	
Neurohormonal factors (e.g. catecholamines)	G protein coupling	β Blockers
Ischaemia	Lack of growth factor signalling	Activation of Akt/ERK pathways (for example, by IGF-1)
Death receptor ligands	Adapter molecules/caspases	Decoy receptors/receptor antagonists
		IAPs/caspase inhibitors

ERK, extracellular signal related kinase; IAP, inhibitor of apoptosis protein; SAPK, stress activated protein kinase.

Apoptosis in the cardiovascular system: key points

▶ Apoptosis of cardiomyocytes is seen in acute myocardial infarction where it may contribute to infarct size, and also in chronic heart failure, where it may be responsible for the gradual decline in cardiac function

▶ Apoptosis of vascular smooth muscle cells is both physiological, in vessel remodelling, and pathological, in disease states such as atherosclerosis and arterial aneurysm formation

▶ Apoptosis is regulated by both pro- and anti-apoptotic stimuli, and both activators and inhibitors of apoptosis signalling within the cell

▶ Treatment to inhibit apoptosis in the heart can be targeted to inhibit ischaemia or reperfusion injury, to enhance endogenous protective mechanisms within cardiomyocytes, or to disrupt apoptosis signalling

▶ The benefits of conventional heart failure treatment may be due in part to the inhibition of cardiomyocyte apoptosis

myocyte stretch, and cytotoxic drugs. Indeed, overexpression of IGF-1 reduces apoptosis in non-infarcted remote zones and promotes favourable remodelling postmyocardial infarction.[20] Activation of the cardiotrophin-1 receptor also inhibits cardiac dilatation following aortic banding, suggesting that reduced cardiomyocyte apoptosis can be translated into improved function. These agents signal through the AKT and ERK pathways, respectively, that are known to be anti-apoptotic in many cell types (table 30.2).

In contrast, some agents are potential therapeutics for long term administration. Heart failure is characterised by increased plasma concentrations of catecholamines and TNFα. The beneficial effects of β blockers in heart failure may therefore be achieved by prevention of myocyte apoptosis. Licensed inhibitors of TNFα are now available, although recent randomised controlled trials (RENAISSANCE and RECOVER) suggest that a soluble TNF receptor antagonist (etanercept) does not benefit patients with heart failure. In contrast, evidence identifying the type 2 angiotensin II receptor as inducing apoptosis in models of heart failure has suggested that its inhibition may be beneficial.

Preventing execution of apoptosis

Execution of apoptosis and cellular disintegration and packaging requires the activation of downstream signalling pathways, including mitochondrial amplification and activation of caspases. Augmentation of endogenous inhibitors of caspases, such as the IAPs, could therefore inhibit apoptosis induced by many stimuli. Pharmacological inhibition of caspases using cell permeable analogues of cleavage sites can inhibit myocyte apoptosis over the short term. However, their long term benefits are unknown, as cells that are destined to die may do so anyway, and delaying apoptosis may not provide long term benefit.

CONCLUSION

VSMC apoptosis occurs in the vasculature in both physiological and pathological contexts. Deaths are regulated by specific proteins that serve either to induce or protect against apoptosis. We are now beginning to understand the complex pro- and anti-apoptotic factors that lead to cell loss from the vasculature. Sensitivity to apoptosis is determined by expression of cell death receptors and ligands, and by multiple protein species below receptor level. In addition, sensitivity is determined by the presence and response to survival cytokines, mitogens, and local cell and matrix interactions, and by the growth status of the cell. Although much research has been performed in vitro, future studies in vivo should identify which pro- and anti-apoptotic factors are functional in vivo.

Apoptosis of cardiac myocytes is part of many disease states, including myocardial infarction and heart failure. At present, the precise role of cardiomyocyte apoptosis in the pathogenesis of these diseases is unknown, and therefore the benefit from anti-apoptotic treatment is unproven. Prevention of cardiomyocyte apoptosis may involve inhibiting both the pro-apoptotic stimulus and apoptosis signalling within the cell. Given the lack of cardiac specificity of apoptosis signalling, such strategies may benefit short lived insults, such as myocardial infarction or unstable angina, rather than heart failure. However, it is also highly likely that proven conventional treatment for heart failure works at least in part by inhibiting apoptosis.

REFERENCES

1 Kerr JF, Wyllie AH, Currie AR. Apoptosis: a basic biological phenomenon with wide-ranging implications in tissue kinetics. Br J Cancer 1972;**26**:239–57.
▶ The original (morphological) description of apoptosis. The features described are characteristic also of vascular cells, and morphological characterisation remains the "gold standard" for detecting apoptosis.

2 Gottlieb RA, Burleson KO, Kloner RA, et al. Reperfusion injury induces apoptosis in rabbit cardiomyocytes. J Clin Invest 1994;**94**:1621–8.

3 Saraste A, Pulkki K, Kallajoki M, et al. Apoptosis in human acute myocardial infarction. Circulation 1997;**95**:320–3.
▶ Detailed description of the timing and spatial characteristics of apoptosis and necrosis after human myocardial infarction.

4 Kajstura J, Cheng W, Reiss K, et al. Apoptotic and necrotic myocyte cell deaths are independent contributing variables of infarct size in rats. Lab Invest 1996;**74**:86–107.

5 Narula J, Haider N, Virmani R, et al. Apoptosis in myocytes in end-stage heart failure. N Engl J Med 1996;**335**:1182–9.
▶ This study (and reference 6 below) describe the evidence of cardiomyocyte apoptosis in end stage heart failure in humans, although the quantification of apoptotic index is both studies is now considered impossibly high.

6 Olivetti G, Abbi R, Quaini F, et al. Apoptosis in the failing human heart. N Engl J Med 1997;**336**:1131–41.

7 Li Z, Bing OH, Long X, et al. Increased cardiomyocyte apoptosis during the transition to heart failure in the spontaneously hypertensive rat. Am J Physiol 1997;**272**:H2313–9.

8 Perlman H, Maillard L, Krasinski K, et al. Evidence for the rapid onset of apoptosis in medial smooth muscle cells after balloon injury. Circulation 1997;**95**:981–7.
▶ The first description indicating that acute artery injury is associated with profound loss of VSMCs from the vessel media, by apoptosis. This observation has allowed subsequent studies to examine the mechanism of injury induced death.

9 Kockx MM. Apoptosis in the atherosclerotic plaque – quantitative and qualitative aspects. Arterioscler Thromb Vasc Biol 1998;**18**:1519–22.

10 Kolodgie FD, Narula J, Burke AP, et al. Localization of apoptotic macrophages at the site of plaque rupture in sudden coronary death. Am J Pathol 2000;**157**:1259–68.

11 Flynn P, Byrne C, Baglin T, et al. Thrombin generation by apoptotic vascular smooth muscle cells. Blood 1997;**89**:4373–84.

12 Ashkenazi A, Dixit V. Death receptors: signalling and modulation. Science 1998;**281**:1305–8.
▶ Detailed review of signalling from death receptors (and subsequent articles covering all aspects of apoptosis).

13 Chinnaiyan A, O'Rourke K, Tewari M, et al. FADD, a novel death domain-containing protein, interacts with the death domain of fas and initiates apoptosis. Cell 1995;**81**:505.

14 Cohen GM. Caspases: the executioners of apoptosis. Biochem J 1997;**326**:1–16.

15 Muzio M, Chinnaiyan A, Kischkel F, et al. FLICE, a novel FADD-homologous ice/ced-3-like protease, is recruited to the CD95 (Fas/Apo-1) death-inducing signaling complex. Cell 1996;**85**:817–27.

16 Shimizu S, Narita M, Tsujimoto Y. Bcl-2 family proteins regulate the release of apoptogenic cytochrome c by the mitochondrial channel VDAC. Nature 1999;**399**:483–7.
▶ Seminal study establishing the role of mitochondrial regulation of apoptosis, and the critical role of the Bcl-2 family proteins in regulating apoptosis signalled through mitochondria.

17 Bennett M, Macdonald K, Chan S-W, et al. Cell surface trafficking of Fas: a rapid mechanism of p53-mediated apoptosis. Science 1998;**282**:290–3.

18 **Bennett MR**, Evan GI, Schwartz SM. Apoptosis of human vascular smooth muscle cells derived from normal vessels and coronary atherosclerotic plaques. *J Clin Invest* 1995;**95**:2266–74.
▶ **The first demonstration that VSMCs in atherosclerotic plaques may be intrinsically sensitive to apoptosis, establishing that phenotypic modulation of VSMCs in atherosclerosis regulates apoptosis.**
19 **Pollman MJ**, Hall JL, Mann MJ, *et al.* Inhibition of neointimal cell bcl-x expression induces apoptosis and regression of vascular disease. *Nature Med* 1998;**4**:222–7.
▶ **This study showed that manipulation of apoptosis in the vessel wall may reduce neointimal formation, validating the use of pro-apoptotic strategies to inhibit the response to vessel injury in disease states such as restenosis after angioplasty or stenting.**
20 **Li Q**, Li B, Wang X, *et al.* Overexpression of insulin-like growth factor-1 in mice protects from myocyte death after infarction, attenuating ventricular dilation, wall stress, and cardiac hypertrophy. *J Clin Invest* 1997;**100**:1991–9.
▶ **This report was one of the first to show clinically meaningful effects of inhibiting apoptosis on cardiac function, thereby validating anti-apoptotic strategies as clinically useful.**

31 TO WHOM DO THE RESEARCH FINDINGS APPLY?

Curt D Furberg

When a new intervention (drug, procedure or device) becomes mainstream care, one hopes that all groups of patients for whom this intervention is intended have been properly studied and, thus, are well defined. This ideal situation rarely applies. The clinical trials conducted to determine efficacy and safety of new interventions are typically designed to be feasible and time and cost efficient. As a consequence, trial populations are typically highly selected and may represent only a subset of the patients for whom the intervention is targeted. Thus, the applicability of the trial findings to other subpopulations has to be based on extrapolations. Some of these extrapolations are reasonable, while others are debatable.

Five considerations often influence trial design[1]: the desire for a study population that (1) is aetiologically homogeneous, (2) is most likely to respond favourably to the intervention, (3) is least likely to suffer adverse events, (4) has no or limited co-morbidity, and (5) most likely will consist of good compliers. The inclusion and exclusion criteria in the trial protocol define those patients with a given condition who are eligible for trial participation or the so-called study population. In addition, all trial participants, by definition, must consent to participate in a research project. Those enrolled constitute the study sample.

This article highlights the conflict between the needs of an optimal research design and a desire from the clinical perspective to determine if all patient groups stand to benefit from a new intervention. The outcome chosen for a clinical trial often influences the interpretation of results. The problem of application of research findings will be illustrated by examples from the literature.

HOW ELIGIBILITY CRITERIA LIMIT THE ABILITY TO GENERALISE FINDINGS

From the point of view of generalisability, the ideal trial would have no exclusion criteria, other than exclusions that reflect known contraindications to the study intervention. All other patients with a given condition would be eligible for enrolment. In addition, the sample size chosen would allow enrolment of sufficient numbers of participants in defined subgroups of interest, so that adequately powered subgroup analyses could be conducted. Unfortunately, such trials are not feasible. Rarely do we have enough statistical power to determine the efficacy and safety of an intervention in even major subgroups that are defined by co-variates such as age, sex, ethnicity, disease severity and stage, co-morbidity, use of other major interventions (interactions), and presence of specific genetic polymorphism that may influence treatment response. Readers of scientific articles should be aware of the "leaps of faith" that are inherent in interpreting research findings.

Homogeneity
Patients who could potentially benefit the most from a new intervention represent the preferred candidates for enrolment into a trial. Decisions regarding eligibility are often based on knowing the mechanism(s) of action of an intervention, thus enabling investigators to identify those most likely to respond favourably. Knowledge of the microorganism causing a specific infection is an important consideration when designing a trial of a new antibiotic agent. Those with the same clinical diagnosis caused by other types and strains of bacteria may be excluded. Exclusion of otherwise eligible patients based on age, impaired renal or liver function, and other co-morbidity creates a more homogeneous group that is more likely to benefit maximally. The desire to create a well defined, homogeneous study population that optimises the likelihood of a favourable trial outcome, however, may limit the ability to generalise the findings.

Likelihood of benefit
Behind the careful selection of study participants is also the desire to obtain results within a reasonable time and with a finite amount of funding. For a new anti-anginal drug, one would probably exclude those with mild angina as well as those with the most severe pain, thus focusing on patients who fall between these extremes. It could be difficult to demonstrate benefit in a patient who only has chest pain once a month. Patients at the other end of the disease spectrum—those with very severe or intractable chest pain—may be too incapacitated to respond to a typical new

224

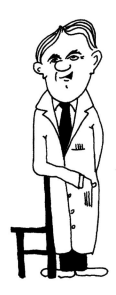

— RESEARCH SOMETIMES
ADVANCES THE SCIENTIST
MORE THAN SCIENCE.

anti-anginal agent. The aetiology behind their pain may be different from that of ambulatory patients with modest angina pectoris. This selection of a study population most likely to respond favourably may come at the expense of not knowing whether and to what extent the drug works in the mildest and most severe cases. Once again, the desire to optimise the outcome of a research study could limit the ability to generalise study findings.

Avoiding adverse effects

Since most (all?) interventions have adverse effects, investigators who design trials prefer excluding patients who are likely to experience these. This consideration is in accordance with the ethical guidelines defined in the Declaration of Helsinki. Many exclusion criteria in a randomised clinical trial indeed reflect potential safety problems. Because such exclusions include various types and severities of potential adverse effects of the intervention, these constitute relative and absolute contraindications. Teratogenicity is a common concern, and pregnant women are typically excluded from trial participation. Excluding patients who are at increased risk for developing adverse events makes sense. Patients with a history of gastric bleeding are typically excluded from trials testing agents that may cause gastric bleeding, such as anti-inflammatory drugs. Thus, trials are designed to enroll uncomplicated cases, in which the risk of adverse effects is small. Low rates also help in the regulatory approval process and in the subsequent marketing of the new product. Co-morbidity is avoided, which often means an under representation of older patients in the study population. In real life, the most likely candidates for prescription of a newly marketed drug are those with some form of co-morbidity or more advanced disease. They may have failed to respond to existing drugs or developed adverse effects. Thus, the desire for a well defined study population with no or limited co-morbidity comes with a cost, in terms of general applicability and an underestimation of adverse effects.

Avoidance of competing risk

A related issue is that of so-called competing risk. A general principle in trial design is to exclude certain patients who are at increased risk of developing the clinical outcome that investigators are trying to prevent. For example, in a lipid lowering trial with all cause mortality as the primary outcome, patients with an increased risk of dying from reasons unrelated to lipids/lipoproteins are excluded. This would, for example, apply to those with cancer or serious kidney or liver damage who can be expected to have shortened life expectancy. Inclusion of patients who are dying from other conditions during a trial will add background "noise" to the trial findings by diluting any mortality effect of the new lipid lowering agent. Thus, the ability to ascertain the true effect of an intervention is lessened in the presence of competing risk.

Avoiding potential non-compliers

Every investigator's nightmare is the patient who stops taking the study medication, especially shortly after he or she has been enrolled. The impact of non-compliers as well as poor compliers on sample size can be substantial. These patients also require major staff commitment during the trial. For analytic purposes, they have to be contacted and monitored for the occurrence of trial outcomes. For proper reporting of trial findings, events in all randomised patients are expected to be collected and reported. Therefore, investigators endeavour to exclude from trial participation anticipated non-compliers or poor compliers. This would include those with a history of adherence problems, alcohol and drug abusers, and those with mental problems. It makes sense from a design efficiency perspective to enrich the study population with potentially good compliers. However, it should be noted that poor and good compliers might differ in other respects. Canner and colleagues[2] reported that the risk of major coronary events differed among compliers and non-compliers in the placebo group of the coronary drug project. The non-compliers were at a significantly higher risk. It is not known why non-compliers on placebo have more coronary events. Thus, the focus in clinical trials on good compliers can overestimate the favourable findings of a trial.

Volunteers

Finally, clinical trial participants all volunteer to enroll by signing an informed consent. It has been argued that volunteers and non-volunteers (those who qualify but decline an invitation to participate) differ. There is scientific evidence to support either side of that argument. Efforts were made to address this question in the coronary artery surgery study.[3] The event rate in the non-surgical (medically treated) control group of the trial was comparable to that of patients who met the inclusion criteria, but declined randomisation. In contrast, Smith and Arnesen[4] found that non-consenters had a higher mortality than consenters in a postinfarction trial.

In summary, clinical trials are typically designed to test an intervention in patients: (1) who are carefully chosen to respond optimally based on the presumed mechanism(s) of action of the intervention and disease severity, (2) who are at low risk of adverse effects and free of co-morbid conditions, and (3) who are likely to be compliant. Compared to an unselected population with the same condition, one could expect trials to provide results in terms of both efficacy and safety that are more favourable to the new intervention. Extrapolation of the research findings to patients with characteristics that disqualified them from trial participation may present a challenge. Readers of scientific reports need to consider carefully the eligibility criteria and accept that the benefit versus risk balance may differ for patients not meeting these criteria. Clinical trials with few exclusion criteria (other than major contraindications) are more applicable to clinical practice.

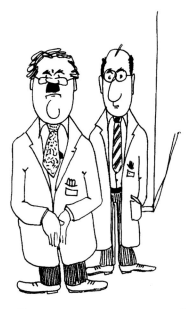

— THE TRIAL WAS SO EXCLUSIVE THAT
NO ONE WAS EVER RANDOMIZED.

HOW THE TYPE OF INTERVENTION OUTCOME INFLUENCES APPLICABILITY

Most medical interventions are aimed at alleviating an existing symptom or sign, such as pain. Others directed at acute conditions such as an infection may accelerate cure or recovery. A third type of intervention is directed at altering the future course of a disease by preventing its complications, including premature death. Antihypertensive treatment is prescribed to prevent or reduce the risks of developing the devastating cardiovascular complications of hypertension.

Intervention trials assume varying designs, depending, in part, on whether they address existing conditions or endeavour to prevent complications that may occur. Of paramount importance are sample size requirements, which can differ enormously. It takes fewer patients to document a symptomatic benefit of a new agent. Whether such a treatment is beneficial in individual patients is easy to determine clinically. The patient can serve as his or her own control and an improvement may be "credited" to the intervention. This concept is behind the "trial of n = 1" approach.[5]

Preventing a future stroke in a hypertensive subject is a different story. If the risk of stroke is 2% per annum and the risk is reduced by half, of 100 hypertensive subjects treated, on average, one stroke will be prevented, one subject will suffer a stroke in spite of effective treatment, and the other 98 subjects will experience no strokes during the year of treatment. The problem with prevention is that no one can project who will suffer a complication that is preventable, who will suffer a complication in spite of treatment, and who will be treated unnecessarily and only be at risk of possible adverse events. Until we learn how to predict the course of a disease in individual patients better, prevention will always involve playing the odds.

Applying research findings to individual patients is more straightforward for interventions that alleviate symptoms or accelerate recovery from an acute condition. The individual patient's response after exposure to the intervention will tell whether it "works". There is no such direct feedback in prevention. Typically a large number of patients have to be treated for extended periods in order to help a few.

HOW CHANGES IN SURROGATE MARKERS PREDICT CLINICAL OUTCOMES

To avoid large and lengthy clinical trials, investigators and trial sponsors often resort to surrogate markers in the testing of an intervention. The blood pressure lowering effect of a new antihypertensive agent can be documented in a placebo controlled trial of 50–100 hypertensive subjects treated for 8–12 weeks. A stroke prevention trial of the same agent would require 4–5000 subjects treated for 4–5 years. Thus, small, short term trials with surrogate markers offer obvious advantages. Other examples of common surrogates in the cardiovascular field include low density and high density lipoprotein (LDL and HDL) cholesterol, Hb_{A1C}, premature ventricular depolarisations, ejection fraction, other haemodynamic measures, and angiographic changes.

A valid surrogate marker is one whose response to an intervention *closely* mimics that of the real (clinical) outcome it is supposed to represent. Unfortunately, this requirement is seldom met. The Veterans Affairs high density lipoprotein intervention trial[6] reported that gemfibrozil reduced the risk of major coronary events in coronary patients with normal LDL cholesterol, but low HDL cholesterol. The assumption was that benefit was mediated through gemfibrozil induced increases in HDL cholesterol. When the investigators analysed the trial data to determine how much of the health benefit could be explained by individual changes in the surrogate marker (HDL cholesterol), they came up with the surprising finding that only 22% of the benefit could be attributed to gemfibrozil induced increases in HDL cholesterol. Similar observations have been reported for raised blood pressure (CD Furberg, unpublished data).

By contrast, sometimes drugs have favourable effects on surrogates, but actually cause harm. The cardiac arrhythmia suppression trial[7] reported that even though encainide and flecainide notably reduced the number of premature ventricular depolarisations (a surrogate for sudden death), these drugs increased the risk of sudden death. A handful of inotropic agents have been shown to improve haemodynamic parameters in patients with congestive heart failure, but they were later shown to increase mortality.

The magnitude of the "improvement" of a surrogate marker cannot be assumed to predict, with high precision, the magnitude of a health benefit in individual patients. The expectation

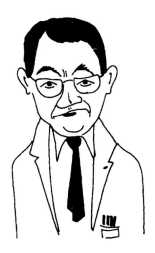

— DARN, THIS TRIAL WOULD BE SIGNIFICANT
IF I COULD JUST EXCLUDE ONE MORE
EVENT FROM THE TREATMENT GROUP.

that common surrogates are clinically useful and predictive rests on the assumptions that drugs have only one mechanism of action (that of the surrogate) and that the development of clinical complications evolves through a single mechanism (mediated through the surrogate). All antihypertensive drugs lower raised blood pressure, but they differ greatly in their blood pressure independent actions. Hypertension is not just high blood pressure. Thus, there are good scientific reasons to expect that different classes of antihypertensive agents differ in how they reduce risk.[8]

It is important to remember that clinical trials investigate and report results for groups of subjects, not individual subjects. When we interpret trials, we assume that the group data apply equally to all individuals. Two recent articles[9 10] highlight the issues of interpreting and applying research findings to individuals. Caution is advised in inferring that a large change in a surrogate marker in an individual automatically translates to a greater clinical benefit than a small marker change. Subjects with small changes may also stand to benefit clinically.

ILLUSTRATIONS FROM CLINICAL TRIALS

To illustrate how highly selected the cohort of eligible trial patients are, Kääriäinen and colleagues[11] analysed 397 consecutively hospitalised cases of gastric ulcer to determine what proportion would be eligible for participation in drug trials and how the eligibility criteria affected generalisability. When the commonly used exclusion criteria were applied, 282 patients (71%) met at least one of them. Several patients had two or more reasons for exclusion. The most troubling findings came from an extended follow up of all 397 patients. Major complications of gastric ulcer—bleeding, perforation, gastric retention, and deaths—occurred in 71 patients, and only two of those were observed in the 115 patients who met the typical eligibility criteria for trials of gastric ulcer. Patients with the worst prognosis would have been excluded. The authors concluded: "when many patients are excluded, the applicability of the results to the whole material is questionable."

Under representation of certain subgroups of patients in randomised clinical trials is another problem. Women and minorities are often under represented.[12 13] So are patients aged 65 years or older,[14] who are the most likely to develop adverse effects. This failure to enroll certain groups of patients has led to a change in federal policies in the USA. It is important that patients enrolled in a trial represent the entire spectrum of patients with a given condition, to enhance the clinical applicability of the results.

ILLUSTRATIONS FROM OTHER TYPES OF RESEARCH STUDIES

Many of the methodological issues of randomised clinical trials also apply to other types of research studies. The latter studies are susceptible to additional problems/biases caused by lack of randomisation, comparable control groups, and blinding. This is illustrated by the following example.

In early July 1997, the US Food and Drug Administration (FDA) reported that it had received 33 reports of unusual valvar morphology and regurgitation among users of combined fenfluramine and phentermine, "fen-phen".[15 16] Half of the cases, all women, who had used the drug combination from one month to more than 16 months (mean 10 months) also had pulmonary hypertension.

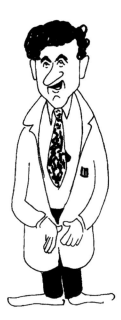

– SOMETIMES I HAVE TO GO THROUGH MANY DIFFERENT STATISTICIANS TO GET THE RIGHT RESULTS.

To determine the magnitude of the problem nationwide, the FDA strongly encouraged all healthcare professionals to report suspected cased of cardiac valvar disease associated with fen-phen use. It was know that between 1.2–4.7 million persons had been "exposed" (14 million prescriptions). Obesity clinics from five states reported echocardiographic findings from 284 subjects. The prevalence of valvulopathy was a staggering 32.8%; 22% in those with exposures < 6 months and 35% in those with longer exposures. Multiplying the number of persons exposed with the risk of valvulopathy gives a number of persons affected ranging from 130 000–500 000. These estimates, of epidemic proportions, raised several questions regarding their reliability.

A closer look at the data revealed a sampling bias. The cases in the Mayo Clinic report[15] and the FDA sample had a much longer exposure than the 1.2–4.7 million users. Expectation bias created by all the publicity was another factor. The sonographers and the readers were not blinded and the readings were subjective (non-standardised). No consideration was given to the fact that valvulopathy is not uncommon in obese, middle aged persons.

Interestingly, the *Wall Street Journal*[17] subsequently conducted its own survey, which among 746 persons found 57 leaky valves (8%). Subsequent scientific studies confirmed an even lower prevalence and also concluded that most cases were mild, with a large majority of confirmed cases having an exposure duration > 3 months.

Several methodologic lessons were learned: (1) defined cohorts, including unexposed persons, are more reliable sources of data than case series, (2) random sampling is preferable to self selection, (3) standardisation (explicit diagnostic criteria) trumps non-standardisation, and (4) blinded readings are superior to unblinded readings. Adjustment for "background noise" is another important consideration. Routine clinical echocardiograms are rarely of the highest scientific quality and should not be relied on for estimation of prevalence rates.

To whom do the research findings apply? Key points

- Design considerations tend to limit the broad applicability of findings from randomised clinical trials
- Trials of new interventions are typically designed to optimise the benefit-versus-harm balance
- The application of research findings to individual patients in clinical practice often requires leaps of faith, some being reasonable, others less so
- Reliance on surrogate markers in lieu of health outcomes can be misleading
- Poorly standardised clinical data from selected case series may be highly biased

ACKNOWLEDGEMENTS

The cartoons appearing in this article are reproduced from *All that glitters is not gold: what clinicians need to know about clinical trials*, by B Furberg and C Furberg, with permission.

REFERENCES

1 **Friedman LM**, Furberg CD, DeMets DL. *Fundamentals of clinical trials*, 3rd ed. St. Louis: Mosby, 1996; New York: Springer-Verlag, 1998.
- **One of the leading texts on clinical trials methodology.**
2 **The Coronary Drug Project Research Group**. Influence of adherence to treatment and response of cholesterol on mortality in the Coronary Drug Project. *N Engl J Med* 1980;**303**:1038–41.
- **Classic paper showing that poor compliers to placebo had a worse survival experience than good compliers.**
3 **CASS Principal Investigators**. Coronary artery surgery study (CASS): a randomized trial of coronary artery bypass surgery. Comparability of entry characteristics and survival in randomized patients and non-randomized patients meeting randomization criteria. *J Am Coll Cardiol* 1984;**3**:114–28.
4 **Smith P**, Arnesen H. Mortality in non-consenters in a post-myocardial infarction trial. *J Intern Med* 1990;**228**:253–6.
5 **Guyatt GH**, Keller JL, Jaeschke R, *et al*. The n-of-1 randomized controlled trial: clinical usefulness. Our three-year experience. *Ann Intern Med* 1990;**112**:293–9.
6 **Robins SJ**, Collins D, Wittes J, *et al*. Relation of gemfibrozil treatment and lipid levels with major coronary events. VA-HIT: a randomized controlled trial. *JAMA* 2001;**285**:1585–91.
- **Examined how much of the mortality/morbidity benefit of gemfibrozil could be explained by individual changes in HDL cholesterol. Only one quarter of the benefit was explained, thus concluding that gemfibrozil has important HDL cholesterol independent mechanism(s) of action.**
7 **Echt DS**, Liebson PR, Mitchell LB, *et al*. Mortality and morbidity in patients receiving encainide, flecainide, or placebo. The cardiac arrhythmia suppression trial. *N Engl J Med* 1991;**324**:781–8.
- **CAST surprised the cardiology community by showing that drug induced suppression of premature ventricular depolarisations increased rather than decreased the risk of sudden death. The findings were a setback for believers in surrogate markers.**
8 **Furberg CD**, Psaty BM, Pahor M, *et al*. Clinical implications of recent findings from the antihypertensive and lipid-lowering treatment to prevent hearth attack trial (ALLHAT) and other studies of hypertension. *Ann Intern Med* 2001;**135**:1074–8.
- **A recent review of comparative trials strongly suggesting that it matters how raised blood pressure is lowered.**
9 **Davey Smith G**, Egger M. Incommunicable knowledge? Interpreting and applying the results of clinical trials and meta-analyses. *J Clin Epidemiol* 1998;**51**:289–95.
- **A thoughtful review of the central role clinicians have in applying trial results to individual patients.**
10 **Chalmers I**. A patient's attitude to the use of research evidence for guiding individual choices and decisions in health care. *Clinical Risk* 2000;**6**:227–30.
- **An interesting commentary from the perspective of the patient.**
11 **Kääriäinen I**, Sipponen P, Siurala M. What fraction of hospital ulcer patients is eligible for prospective drug trials? *Scand J Gastroenterol* 1991;**26**:73–6.
- **One of the few studies that documented how trial eligibility criteria can undermine generalisability.**
12 **Schmucker DL**, Vesell ES. Underrepresentation of women in clinical drug trials. *Clin Pharmacol Ther* 1993;**54**:11–15.
13 **El-Sadr W**, Capps L. The challenge of minority recruitment in clinical trials for AIDS. *JAMA* 1992;**267**:954–7.
14 **Hutchins LF**, Unger JM, Crowley JJ, *et al*. Underrepresentation of patients 65 years of age or older in cancer-treatment trials. *N Engl J Med* 1999;**341**:2061–7.
15 **Connolly HM**, Crary JL, McGoon MD, *et al*. Valvular heart disease associated with fenfluramine-phentermine. *N Engl J Med* 1997;**337**:581–8.
16 **US Food and Drug Administration**. FDA Public Health Advisory. Reports of valvular heart disease in patients receiving concomitant fenfluramine and phentermine. *FDA Medical Bulletin* 8 July 1997.
- **A premature alarm overstating the magnitude of the fen-phen epidemic.**
17 **Anon**. WSJ Survey, *The Wall Street Journal*. 31 October 1997.
- **An example of balanced investigative reporting.**

32 MANAGEMENT OF MARFAN SYNDROME

John C S Dean

Marfan syndrome is a variable, autosomal dominant connective tissue disorder, affecting mainly the cardiovascular system, eyes, and skeleton. The incidence is approximately 1 in 9800, and around 26% of cases have no family history, the condition resulting from a new mutation.[1] Characteristic features include progressive aortic dilatation associated with aortic valve incompetence, mitral valve prolapse and incompetence, lens dislocation and myopia, and a tall and thin body (fig 32.1) with long limbs, arachnodactyly, pectus deformities, and sometimes scoliosis. Further less specific features are often detectable in the clinic, such as a high palate with dental crowding, and skin striae distensae, and other characteristic findings may be sought by radiological imaging, such as protrusio acetabulae and dural ectasia. A history of recurrent pneumothorax may be found in some cases. The clinical features have been codified into the so-called Ghent diagnostic nosology,[2] as the clinical variability of the condition can otherwise make diagnosis difficult.

Life expectancy is primarily determined by the severity of cardiovascular involvement, and has improved substantially in the past 30 years as a result of improved medical and surgical management. In particular, β blockade reduces the rate of aortic dilatation in some patients, and, perhaps not surprisingly, the outcome of prophylactic aortic root surgery has been shown in several recent series to be superior to that of emergency surgery for dissecting aneurysm. The timing of prophylactic surgical intervention depends on a number of factors including the aortic diameter and its rate of dilatation, implying a need for regular aortic root surveillance. The optimal management of Marfan patients may therefore require lifelong medical treatment, and lifelong aortic surveillance with a view to potential aortic root surgery, representing a major commitment for patient and doctor alike. At the same time, a diagnosis of Marfan syndrome may have serious social consequences for the patient, in terms of lifestyle, employment, and insurance.

Marfan syndrome almost always results from mutation in the fibrillin 1 gene on chromosome 15,[3] although in one family the disease was linked to an unknown gene on chromosome 3. Molecular testing for Marfan syndrome has proved less useful than was hoped for two main reasons. Firstly, very few fibrillin 1 mutations have been observed more than once, so the detection of a mutation yields little prognostic information beyond that available from the patient's own family history. Secondly, fibrillin 1 mutations have also been detected in Marfan related disorders whose cardiovascular involvement is milder or non-existent. These include MASS syndrome, a disorder with some Marfan-like features (*m*yopia, *m*itral valve prolapse, *a*ortic dilatation, *s*kin involvement, *s*keletal involvement) but mild and apparently stable aortic dilatation, and isolated ectopia lentis.[4] The importance of a careful clinical assessment and accurate clinical diagnosis cannot therefore be overstated, if appropriate targeting of medical and surgical resources in Marfan patients is to be achieved. In this article, I will review current approaches to diagnosis of Marfan syndrome and cardiovascular management.

► MAKING THE DIAGNOSIS OF MARFAN SYNDROME

Much effort has been expended over the years in devising agreed diagnostic criteria for Marfan syndrome. The currently accepted criteria, known as the Ghent nosology,[2] were defined in 1996 as a revision of the earlier Berlin criteria of 1988. In the Ghent nosology, clinical features in the skeletal, ocular, cardiovascular, pulmonary, and integumentary systems are used to define either a major criterion or only involvement of a particular organ system (table 32.1). The dura and the genetic findings count as two further systems, with lumbosacral dural ectasia on imaging studies, and aspects of the family history or genetic testing being classified as a major criterion in each respectively. A diagnosis of Marfan syndrome requires, as a minimum, a major criterion in two systems and involvement of a third.

In the skeletal system, arachnodactyly may be assessed (fig 32.2) using the Steinberg thumb sign (the entire thumbnail projects beyond the ulnar border of the hand) and the Walker-Murdoch wrist sign (the thumb and fifth finger overlap around the wrist). An upper to lower segment ratio in an adult of less than 0.86, or a span to height ratio of greater than 1.05, are objective measures of a marfanoid body habitus. The lower segment is measured as the distance from the symphysis

Table 32.1 Ghent diagnostic nosology

System	Major criterion	Involvement
Skeletal	At least 4 of the following features: ▶ pectus carinatum ▶ pectus excavatum requiring surgery ▶ ULSR < 0.86 or span:height >1.05 ▶ wrist and thumb signs ▶ scoliosis > 20° or spondylolisthesis ▶ reduced elbow extension (<170°) ▶ pes plenus ▶ protrusio acetabulae	2 of the major features, or 1 major feature and 2 of the following: ▶ pectus excavatum ▶ joint hypermobility ▶ high palate with dental crowding ▶ characteristic face
Ocular	Lens dislocation (ectopia lentis)	Flat cornea Increased axial length of globe (causing myopia) Hypoplastic iris or ciliary muscle (causing decreased miosis)
Cardiovascular	Dilatation of the aortic root Dissection of the ascending aorta	Mitral valve prolapse Dilatation of the pulmonary artery, below age 40 Calcified mitral annulus, below age 40 Other dilatation or dissection of the aorta
Pulmonary	None	Spontaneous pneumothorax Apical blebs
Skin/integument	None	Striae atrophicae Recurrent or incisional hernia
Dura	Lumbosacral dural ectasia	None
Genetic findings	Parent, child or sibling meets these criteria independently Fibrillin 1 mutation known to cause Marfan syndrome Inheritance of DNA marker haplotype linked to Marfan syndrome in the family	None

Having one of the features listed constitutes a major criterion or system involvement for all systems except the skeletal system, where more than one feature is needed.
ULSR, upper to lower segment ratio

pubis to the floor, and the upper segment calculated by subtracting this distance from the height. One of the eight major skeletal features in the Ghent nosology (four must be present for the skeletal system to contribute a major criterion) is protrusio acetabulae, detected by pelvic x ray. To avoid unnecessary x ray exposure, this investigation should only be undertaken when a positive finding would make the diagnosis of Marfan syndrome under the Ghent nosology. Lumbosacral magnetic resonance imaging (MRI) scanning for dural ectasia should be considered in similar circumstances.

In the ocular system, only lens dislocation is regarded as a major criterion, other less specific findings such as myopia being regarded as eye involvement.

Aortic dilatation or dissection are the major criteria in the cardiovascular system. Aortic diameter should be measured by transthoracic echocardiogram at the sinuses of Valsalva (fig 32.3) and related to normal values based on age and body surface area (BSA).[2][5] The risk of aortic dissection rises as the aortic root diameter increases.[6] Other imaging techniques such as transoesophageal echocardiography, MRI or computed tomographic scanning (fig 32.4) may be helpful in some cases.

Many Marfan features such as echocardiographic findings,[7] ectopia lentis, scoliosis, upper to lower segment ratio, and protrusio acetabulae are age dependent in their occurrence.[8] For younger patients with a family history of Marfan syndrome who do not fulfil the diagnostic criteria, and for younger Marfan-like patients with no family history who only fail to meet the diagnostic criteria by one system, repeat evaluations should be considered until age 18 (see box). This is to avoid missing the evolving diagnosis, while not stigmatising children and adolescents who may be unaffected. From the foregoing discussion, it can be seen that initial

evaluation of patients with possible Marfan syndrome requires a multidisciplinary approach involving clinical genetics, cardiology, ophthalmology, and radiology.

DIFFERENTIAL DIAGNOSIS

There are a number of disorders with similar features to Marfan syndrome, but some can be easily distinguished by their

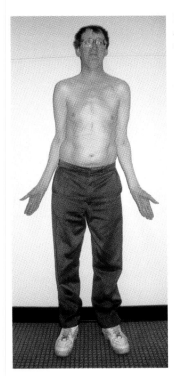

Figure 32.1 Patient with Marfan syndrome. Note aesthenic or marfanoid body habitus, pronounced myopia (thick glasses), previous thoracic surgery (composite aortic root/aortic valve replacement). Residual evidence of pectus carinatum can be seen. Photograph reproduced with patient's permission.

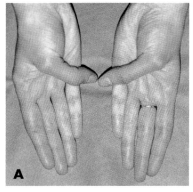
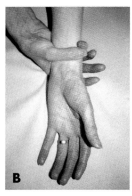

Figure 32.2 Arachnodactyly. (A) Steinberg thumb sign. Entire thumb nail protrudes beyond ulnar border of hand. (B) Walker-Murdoch wrist sign. Thumb and fifth finger can overlap around wrist. Both signs must be present to diagnose arachnodactyly according to the Ghent Marfan diagnostic criteria.

Assessment of a patient with possible Marfan syndrome

► The diagnosis should be based on the Ghent diagnostic nosology

► The initial assessment should include a personal history, detailed family history, and clinical examination including ophthalmology examination and transthoracic echocardiogram

► The aortic diameter at the sinus of Valsalva (fig 32.3) should be related to normal values based on age and body surface area

► The development of scoliosis and protrusio acetabulae is age dependent, commonly occurring following periods of rapid growth. Radiographic examination for these features is indicated, depending on age, if a positive finding would make the diagnosis of Marfan syndrome

► A pelvic MRI scan to detect dural ectasia is indicated if a positive finding would make the diagnosis of Marfan syndrome

► Younger patients with suspected Marfan syndrome, who do not fulfil the Ghent diagnostic criteria, should be offered repeat clinical evaluations pre-school, before puberty, and at age 18, if they fall into one of the groups below. Additional evaluations may be clinically indicated around puberty:

(1) Children or adolescents with a positive family history in whom DNA testing is not possible

(2) Children or adolescents with no family history, who fall short of fulfilling the diagnostic criteria by one system only.

---

other clinical features or by biochemical testing. Lujan-Fryns syndrome is an unusual X-linked mental handicap disorder with marfanoid features, while in the autosomal dominant Shprintzen-Goldberg syndrome, craniosynostosis is also evident. Some Shprintzen-Goldberg cases have fibrillin 1 mutations, so this might be regarded as an unusual variant of Marfan syndrome. Homocystinuria (autosomal recessive) is characterised by raised urinary homocysteine excretion, while in congenital contractural arachnodactyly or Beals syndrome (autosomal dominant, associated with mutation in fibrillin 2) joint contractures and ear anomalies are evident in addition to a marfanoid appearance. In other disorders, the distinction from Marfan syndrome is more difficult. The best known of these is the MASS syndrome, which may be considered a

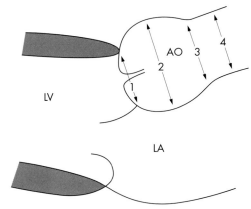

Figure 32.3 Diagram of the aortic root as seen at echocardiography. The aortic diameter may be measured at the aortic annulus (1), the sinuses of Valsalva (2), the supra-aortic ridge (3), and the proximal ascending aorta (4). In Marfan syndrome, dilatation usually starts at the sinuses of Valsalva, so this measurement is critical in monitoring the early evolution of the condition. Diameters must be related to normal values for age and body surface area. After Roman et al, *Ann Intern Med* 1987;**106**:800–7, with permission.

forme fruste of Marfan syndrome. The name is an acronym for the clinical features (*m*yopia, *m*itral valve prolapse, *a*ortic dilatation, *s*kin involvement, *s*keletal involvement), the skin and skeletal features being similar to those seen in Marfan syndrome, but less pronounced. The disorder may be associated with fibrillin-1 mutation,[3 4] but the aortic dilatation is mild, and the risk of aortic aneurysm rupture seems low.

A condition of mitral valve prolapse with thoracic skeletal anomalies (often pectus excavatum) but without other Marfan features has also been described, and in one case a fibrillin 1 mutation was found.[4] Molecular investigation of this disorder has not been widely undertaken, and it is not clear whether it is truly distinct from MASS syndrome. Autosomal dominant ectopia lentis may occur with Marfan-like skeletal findings, fibrillin 1 mutation, but no cardiac involvement. There are also forms of hereditary aortic aneurysm without other Marfan features, which have been associated with as yet unidentified genes on chromosomes 5 and 11. Other hereditary connective tissue disorders, such as Ehlers-Danlos syndrome and Stickler syndrome, may also cause confusion because of their overlapping features. Skin laxity and easy bruising are prominent in the Ehlers-Danlos syndrome while myopia with retinal detachment but not ectopia lentis is a feature of Stickler syndrome. Stickler syndrome patients also have a distinctive facial appearance (midface hypoplasia), and the condition is sometimes associated with cleft palate and hearing loss.

CARDIOVASCULAR COMPLICATIONS IN MARFAN SYNDROME

Cardiovascular complications of Marfan syndrome include mitral valve prolapse and regurgitation, left ventricular dilatation and cardiac failure, and pulmonary artery dilatation, but aortic root dilatation is the most common cause of morbidity and mortality. Aortic valve incompetence usually arises in the context of a dilated aortic root, and the risk of aortic rupture increases substantially when the diameter at the sinus of Valsalva exceeds 5.5 cm.[5 9] Myocardial infarction may occur if an aortic root dissection occludes the coronary ostia. Marfan syndrome mortality from complications of aortic root dilatation has decreased (70% in 1972, 48% in 1995) and life

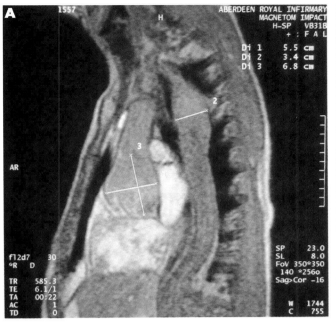

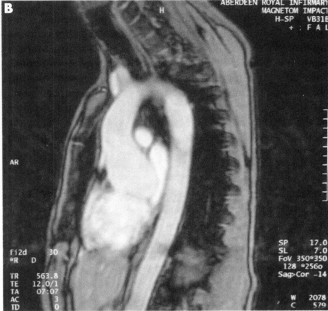

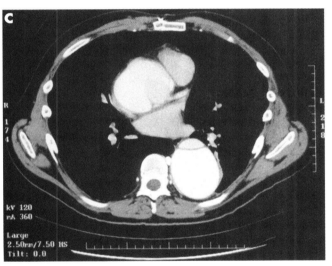

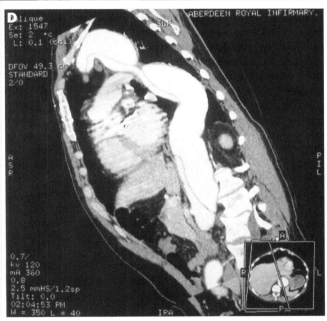

Figure 32.4 (A) Parasagittal breath hold T1 magnetic resonance (MR) image showing pronounced dilatation of the aortic root with slight dilatation of the descending aorta in a young adult with Marfan syndrome. Line 1 represents the diameter at the sinuses of Valsalva. (B) Parasagittal cine MR angiogram showing dilated aortic root but with normal upper ascending arch and descending aorta in a young adult. (C) Axial computed tomographic (CT) scan at T7 of a Marfan patient showing dilated ascending and descending aorta with dissection flap anteriorly in the descending aorta and previous surgery to the ascending aorta. (D) Parasagittal reformatted CT of chest and abdomen in the same patient with contrast showing dilatation of the whole of the aorta with a spiral dissection from the arch through to the lower abdominal aorta. MR and CT images courtesy of Professor J Weir, Department of Radiology, Grampian University Hospitals NHS Trust.

expectancy has increased (mean (SD) age at death 32 (16) years in 1972 versus 45 (17) years in 1998),[1] associated with increased medical and surgical intervention. Risk factors for aortic dissection include increased aortic diameter, extent of aortic dilatation, rate of aortic dilatation, and family history of aortic dissection.[7 9]

LABORATORY FINDINGS
Histologically, the Marfan aorta is characterised by elastic fibre fragmentation and disarray, paucity of smooth muscle cells, and deposition of collagen and mucopolysaccharide between the cells of the media. These appearances are

sometimes described as "cystic medial degeneration" although there are no true cysts present. Mucopolysaccharide deposition in the valves may cause valve leaflet thickening. The molecular basis for these changes is abnormality of fibrillin, an important component of the elastic microfibril. Fibrillin is a 350 kD glycoprotein, synthesised as a 375 kD precursor which is processed and secreted into the matrix. It is encoded by the fibrillin 1 gene which maps to chromosome 15q21.1. Mutation in another fibrillin gene (fibrillin 2, mapping to chromosome 5q23–31) causes Beals syndrome. With current techniques, fibrillin 1 mutations can be detected in about 66% of Marfan patients, diagnosed by the Ghent nosology.[4] Most mutations are missense, suggesting that the phenotype is usually cause by a dominant negative effect of the mutant gene product on microfibrillar assembly. Some nonsense and frameshift mutations are also seen, suggesting that reduced amount of fibrillin (haploinsufficiency) can also cause Marfan syndrome. Wide variability in severity has been documented with different mutations, even in the same codon, causing either severe neonatal Marfan syndrome or classical adult Marfan syndrome. Similarly, mutations in the central region of the gene (exons 24–32), sometimes called the "neonatal region", may be associated with phenotypes ranging from severe neonatal Marfan syndrome to isolated ectopia lentis.

PATHOPHYSIOLOGY AND MEDICAL MANAGEMENT

The pathophysiological consequence of the elastic fibre degeneration seen in the Marfan aorta is reduced distensibility in response to the pulse pressure wave or increased stiffness, and this can be detected at any age by echocardiography[10] or gated MRI scanning, although it is less pronounced in children. This abnormal aortic compliance is associated with an increased pulse wave velocity. The normal aorta dilates gradually with age, and becomes stiffer, but these changes are more notable at any age in Marfan syndrome. In the early 1970s, it was suggested that reduction of the systolic ejection impulse (dP/dt, the rate of change of central arterial pressure with time) using β blocker treatment might reduce the risk of aortic dissection in Marfan syndrome.[7] Studies in turkeys prone to aortic dissection had shown improved survival following treatment with propranolol. A randomised trial of propranolol treatment in 70 adolescent and young adult Marfan patients demonstrated a reduced rate of aortic dilatation and fewer aortic complications in the treatment group, although some patients seemed to respond better than others.[7] A retrospective historically controlled trial of propranolol or atenolol treatment in 113 patients found similar effects.[11] Recent studies have shown that β blockade with propranolol, atenolol or metoprolol increases aortic distensibility, and reduces aortic stiffness and pulse wave velocity[9 12 13] in a subgroup of Marfan patients, although in the "non-responders" a minor deterioration in aortic distensibility was seen, the clinical significance of which is unclear. Those who responded to β blockade tended to have smaller aortic diameters[12] (< 4 cm in one study[10]), in keeping with other studies suggesting that the reduction in rate of aortic dilatation with β blockade is greatest in younger patients with smaller aortas.[7 11] These studies provide strong evidence that β blockade should be considered in all Marfan patients, but particularly in the younger age group (see box).

Although remarkably few withdrawals because of side effects were recorded in these studies, β blockers are not suitable for everyone—for example, patients with asthma, cardiac failure or bradyarrhythmias. Other treatments aimed at reducing the ejection impulse, such as calcium antagonists or angiotensin converting enzyme (ACE) inhibitors, have been suggested for such cases. Unfortunately, there are no reported clinical trials to confirm the benefit or otherwise of these drugs in Marfan syndrome. There may be theoretical reasons to consider ACE inhibitors or angiotensin II receptor blockers for future clinical study. Vascular smooth muscle cell apoptosis has been implicated in the cystic medial degeneration seen in the Marfan aorta, and both types of drug have been shown to inhibit vascular smooth muscle cell apoptosis in cultured Marfan aortic media cells.[14] In addition, one small study demonstrated abnormal flow mediated vasodilation of the brachial

Cardiovascular management of Marfan syndrome

▶ β Blocker treatment should be considered in any Marfan patient with aortic dilatation at any age, but prophylactic treatment may be more effective in those with an aortic diameter of < 4 cm

▶ Risk factors for aortic dissection in Marfan syndrome include aortic diameter > 5 cm, aortic dilatation extending beyond the sinus of Valsalva, rapid rate of aortic dilatation (> 5% per year, or 2 mm/year in adults), and family history of aortic dissection

▶ Marfan patients of all ages should be offered at least annual evaluation with clinical history, examination, and transthoracic echocardiography. In children, serial transthoracic echocardiography at 6–12 month intervals is recommended, the frequency depending on the aortic diameter (in relation to body surface area) and the rate of increase

▶ Marfan patients should be referred for prophylactic aortic root surgery when the diameter at the sinus of Valsalva exceeds 5.5 cm in an adult or 5.0 cm in a child

▶ Pregnant patients with Marfan syndrome are at increased risk of aortic dissection if the aortic diameter exceeds 4 cm. Such cases warrant frequent cardiovascular monitoring throughout pregnancy and into the puerperium

artery in Marfan patients, although agonist mediated vasodilation was normal. This was attributed to abnormal endothelial cell mechanotransduction associated with abnormal fibrillin. This could lead to alternative molecular targets for future pharmacological interventions. There is much scope for further laboratory and clinical trial work in this area.

SURGICAL MANAGEMENT

Aortic root dilatation leading to aortic dissection and/or aortic valve dysfunction usually occurs first at the sinus of Valsalva.[5] There is general agreement, based on a number of comparative studies, that there is a better outcome with early aortic root surgery than with later or emergency surgery,[9 15] and prophylactic surgery is recommended when the diameter at the sinus of Valsalva exceeds 5.5 cm in an adult[2 9] and 5.0 cm in a child. Other factors such as the rate of growth of the aortic diameter and family history of aortic dissection may be taken into account, and it may be that assessment of aortic distensibility will become a useful prognostic indicator. Survival data also show improved longevity of Marfan patients who undergo prophylactic surgery, compared with their untreated relatives.[16] Not surprisingly, part of this is attributable to death before reaching hospital in untreated patients with acute dissection. Until recently, the procedure of choice for most cardiothoracic surgeons would have been the Bentall composite graft repair, in which both the aortic root and the aortic valve are replaced. This procedure has a low operative mortality in experienced hands, with long term survival of around 80% at five years and 60% at 10 years.[17] In 1979, Yacoub and colleagues described a valve conserving (remodelling) technique which therefore avoids the need for long term anticoagulants, and in 1992 David and Feindell described an alternative valve conserving procedure in which the native aortic valve is re-implanted in a Dacron tube (re-implantation technique).

Application of these methods in Marfan syndrome has been controversial, as it has been suggested that further deterioration of the aortic valve leaflets will inevitably require reoperation for valve replacement at a later date. Case series currently being reported suggest that when use of these procedures is restricted to cases where the aortic valve appears structurally normal and valve incompetence is largely caused by annular ectasia, the long term outcome is as good as the Bentall procedure, without the hazards of anticoagulation.[18] There is certainly a case for considering this option for children (where future growth is also a consideration), women, and in those in whom anticoagulation may be hazardous. As Marfan patients survive longer, reoperation for new aneurysms developing elsewhere in the arterial tree are becoming common (for example, see fig 32.4C,D)—in one series, 70% developed second aneurysms requiring surgery.[16] Partly for this reason, continuation of long term β blockade after surgery is strongly recommended in most Marfan centres.[17] Marfan syndrome may also affect the function of other heart valves and give rise to symptoms for which valve surgery may be indicated in children and adults.[2] For example, mitral valve replacement may be required in up to 10% of those requiring aortic root surgery.[16]

CARDIOVASCULAR FOLLOW UP

It is clear that with the need for life long β blocker treatment, the possible development of other medical therapies for those who cannot tolerate β blockers, and the advantages of prophylactic aortic root surgery based on the size and rate of change of the aortic diameter, lifelong follow up is advisable for Marfan patients. At least annual evaluation with clinical history and examination and transthoracic echocardiography[5] is recommended, with additional assessments as clinically indicated (see box). The rate of change of the aortic diameter should clearly influence follow up intervals.

MARFAN SYNDROME AND PREGNANCY

The two major issues in pregnancy are the risk of cardiovascular complications in an affected mother and the 50% risk of transmission of Marfan syndrome to the fetus. The risk of aortic dissection in pregnancy is increased, and may be caused by inhibition of collagen and elastin deposition in the aorta by oestrogen, and the hyperdynamic hypervolaemic circulatory state of pregnancy. Gestational hypertension and pre-eclampsia may increase the risk of aortic rupture. Most complications occur in women with pre-existing cardiac disease. In three recent studies, two retrospective and one prospective, nine women in 83 (11%) had severe complications, mostly aortic rupture, although endocarditis was also reported. Cardiovascular complications appear more likely if the aortic root is greater than 4 cm at the start of pregnancy, or dilates rapidly.[19] β Blockers should be continued throughout pregnancy. With regard to the risk of transmission of Marfan syndrome to the fetus, genetic counselling should be offered to women of childbearing age with Marfan syndrome. Mutation detection or linkage can be used for prenatal diagnosis in some families if the parents wish, but fetal ultrasound scanning is unreliable.

MARFAN SYNDROME AND SPORTS

The risks of sports in patients with Marfan syndrome depend on which organ systems are involved and to what degree, in a particular patient. Low to moderate activity levels have been regarded as acceptable for Marfan patients. Contact sports involving a likelihood of bodily collision (for example rugby, high diving, equestrian events) may not be advisable, both because of cardiovascular risks and because of the risk of exacerbating lens dislocation. Patients who have undergone aortic root or valve replacement, or both, will have more severe restrictions, particularly if taking anticoagulants. Scuba diving carries a risk of precipitating pneumothorax in Marfan patients and should be avoided.

CONCLUSION

The investigation, management, and long term follow up of patients with Marfan syndrome is complex and requires a multidisciplinary approach. Although many studies have been carried out into the delineation and management of Marfan syndrome, the trials and case series generally involve relatively few patients, the largest being in the hundreds. For those used to evidence based clinical management based on trials of thousands, this may present a difficulty, which has been recognised in a recent discussion of evidence based management of genetic conditions.[20] Despite this, the outlook for Marfan patients has improved dramatically since the 1970s, and this should inspire further endeavours for Marfan patients as there are many aetiological and management issues still to be resolved.

ACKNOWLEDGEMENTS

This article is based on work undertaken in conjunction with colleagues from many disciplines who formed the Marfan syndrome Guideline Development Group (see below) as part of a project funded by the Clinical Resources and Audit Group of the Scottish Executive Department of Health.

Membership of the Marfan Syndrome Guideline Development Group
Clinical genetics: JCS Dean, NE Haites, E Hobson, Z Miedzybrodzka, S Moore, S Simpson. *Anaesthetics*: P Martin. *Cardiology*: P Booth (paediatrics), S Walton (adults). *Cardiothoracic surgery*: JS Cockburn, R Jeffrey. *Obstetrics*: M Hall. *Ophthalmology*: W Church. *Orthopaedics*: T Scotland. *Respiratory medicine*: JAR Friend (adults), G Russell (paediatrics), *Rheumatology*: D Reid. *Scottish Guideline Steering Group*: N Bradshaw, H Campbell, M Porteous.

REFERENCES

1 **Gray JR**, Bridges AB, West RR, *et al*. Life expectancy in British Marfan syndrome populations. *Clin Genet* 1998;**54**:124–8.
▶ This article describes life expectancy and risk factors in a British Marfan population, and reviews previous work on the natural history of Marfan syndrome.
2 **De Paepe A**, Devereux RB, Dietz HC, *et al*. Revised diagnostic criteria for the Marfan syndrome. *Am J Med Genet* 1996;**62**:417–26.
▶ This article describes the Ghent clinical diagnostic criteria for Marfan syndrome and considers the differential diagnosis.
3 **Dietz HC**, Pyeritz RE. Mutations in the human gene for fibrillin-1 (FBN1) in the Marfan syndrome and related disorders. *Hum Mol Genet* 1995;**4**:1799–809.
▶ This is a good review of molecular information about fibrillin 1 and the diseases caused by mutations therein.
4 **Loeys B**, Nuytinck L, Delvaux I, *et al*. Genotype and phenotype analysis of 171 patients referred for molecular study of the fibrillin-1 gene FBN1 because of suspected Marfan syndrome. *Arch Intern Med* 2001;**161**:2447–54.
▶ This article describes a series of patients in whom fibrillin mutation studies were requested, and the outcome of the investigations. It discusses current molecular information, hypotheses about how fibrillin mutation causes disease, and information about genotype–phenotype correlations.
5 **Roman MJ**, Rosen SE, Kramer-Fox R, *et al*. Prognostic significance of the pattern of aortic root dilation in the Marfan syndrome. *J Am Coll Cardiol* 1993;**22**:1470–6.
▶ This article includes discussion of how to assess the aortic root by echocardiography in Marfan syndrome, the significance of the appearance of the root, and of the longitudinal extent of any dilatation.
6 **Legget ME**, Unger TA, O'Sullivan CK, *et al*. Aortic root complications in Marfan's syndrome: identification of a lower risk group. *Heart* 1996;**75**:389–95.
7 **Shores J**, Berger KR, Murphy EA, *et al*. Progression of aortic dilatation and the benefit of long-term beta-adrenergic blockade in Marfan's syndrome. *N Engl J Med* 1994;**330**:1335–41.
▶ This is the only prospective randomised trial of β blocker treatment in Marfan syndrome and discusses possible mechanisms of action.

8 **Lipscomb KJ**, Clayton-Smith J, Harris R. Evolving phenotype of Marfan's syndrome. *Arch Dis Child* 1997;**76**:41–6.

9 **Groenink M**, Lohuis TAJ, Tijssen, *et al.* Survival and complication free survival in Marfan's syndrome: implications of current guidelines. *Heart* 1999;**82**:499–50.

▶ **An excellent discussion of current guidelines for surgical intervention in Marfan syndrome and their implications for management and survival in a patient cohort.**

10 **Rios AS**, Silber EN, Bavishi N, *et al.* Effect of long-term beta-blockade on aortic root compliance in patients with Marfan syndrome. *Am Heart J* 1999;**137**:1057–61.

▶ **Describes a study of the effects of long term treatment on aortic distensibility and compliance and notes that while some patients respond well, others do not.**

11 **Salim MA**, Alpert BS, Ward JC, *et al.* Effect of beta-adrenergic blockade on aortic root rate of dilation in the Marfan syndrome. *Am J Cardiol* 1994;**74**:629–33.

12 **Haouzi A**, Berglund H, Pelikan PCD, *et al.* Heterogeneous aortic response to acute beta-adrenergic blockade in Marfan syndrome. *Am Heart J* 1997;**133**:60–3.

13 **Groenink M**, de Roos A, Mulder BJM, *et al.* Changes in aortic distensibility and pulse wave velocity assessed with magnetic resonance imaging following beta-blocker therapy in the Marfan syndrome. *Am J Cardiol* 1998;**82**:203–8.

14 **Nagashima H**, Sakomura Y, Aoka Y, *et al.* Angiotensin II type 2 receptor mediates muscle cell apoptosis in cystic medical degeneration associated with Marfan's syndrome. *Circulation* 2001;**104**(suppl I):I-282–7.

▶ **This paper describes an in vitro study showing a theoretical reason why ACE inhibitors or angiotensin 2 receptor blockers might be an alternative treatment for Marfan patients who cannot tolerate β blockers.**

15 **Gott VL**, Greene PS, Alejo DE, *et al.* Replacement of the aortic root in patients with Marfan's syndrome. *N Engl J Med* 1999;**340**:1307–13.

16 **Finkbohner R**, Johnston D, Crawford S, *et al.* Marfan syndrome. Long-term survival and complications after aortic aneurysm repair. *Circulation* 1995;**91**:728–33.

17 **Treasure T**. Elective replacement of the aortic root in Marfan's syndrome. *Br Heart J* 1993;**69**:101–3.

18 **Bassano C**, De Matteis GM, Nardi P, *et al.* Mid-term follow-up of aortic root remodelling compared to Bentall operation. *Eur J Cardiothorac Surg* 2001;**19**:601–5.

▶ **A helpful discussion comparing aortic root remodelling surgery with the conventional Bentall procedure in Marfan syndrome.**

19 **Lind J**, Wallenburg HCS. The Marfan syndrome and pregnancy: a retrospective study in a Dutch population. *Eur J Obstet Gynaecol Reprod Biol* 2001;**98**:28–35.

20 **Campbell H**, Bradshaw N, Davidson R, *et al.* Evidence based medicine in practice: lessons from a Scottish clinical genetics project. *J Med Genet* 2000;**37**:684–91.

Additional references appear on the *Heart* website–www.heartjnl.com

33 DEVELOPMENT AND STRUCTURE OF THE ATRIAL SEPTUM

Robert H Anderson, Nigel A Brown, Sandra Webb

Most cardiologists would probably consider that, during their training, they had received appropriate instruction concerning the mode of development and structure of the atrial septum. This is likely to be founded on the diagrams that exist in most standard textbooks of cardiac embryology. These illustrate the formation of primary and secondary atrial septums as overlapping muscular sheets that grow into the common atrium. This type of illustration implies that similar morphological mechanisms of development lead to the formation of these two "septums". This is not so. To the best of our knowledge, there is no evidence existing which supports this concept of growth of a second muscular shelf into the developing atriums so as to overlap the primary atrial septum, and to provide the rims of the definitive oval fossa. On the contrary, it has long been established[1][2] that the superior border of the "septum secundum", in other words the superior rim of the oval fossa, is an infolding of the atrial roof. In this respect, case reports are to be found that describe the formation of lipomas within the supposed "septum secundum".[3] Careful study of such lipomas,[4] along with scrutiny of the published images,[3] reveals that the fat accumulates within the deeply infolded superior interatrial groove.

All the "classical" accounts of atrial septal development have also ignored totally the contribution to atrial septation made by the "spina vestibuli", a structure first described by His in the 19th century.[5] Similarly, they take no account of the contributions made by the mesenchymal cap which clothes the leading edge of the muscular primary atrial septum.[6] In reality, therefore, more structures contribute to division of the atriums than the so-called primary and secondary septums.[7] It is appreciation of the roles of all these various components that provides the basis for understanding the proper structure of the muscular walls interposed between the right and left atriums.[8] This information, in this burgeoning era of interventional catheterisation, is now of major practical importance to the cardiologist.[9] In this review, we will describe all the building blocks that contribute to the walls that separate the definitive right and left atrial chambers, showing how knowledge of their position provides the basis for understanding the definitive anatomy.

▶ DEVELOPMENT OF THE ATRIAL SEPTUM

During early development, the initially tubular heart is suspended along its length by a dorsal mesocardium. It is at this stage that the so-called "straight tube" can be recognised, albeit that it has been shown that, with time, this part of the tube gives rise only to the ventricular component of the definitive heart.[10][11] At the stage when the developing heart tube is straight, the outflow tract, the atrioventricular canal, and the primary atrium have all still to form.

With continued growth, the ventricular component of the tube liberates itself from the body wall in the process called looping, thus losing most of its dorsal mesocardial connection. Concomitant with looping, there is expansion of the caudal inlet, part of the tube to form the primary atrium. At the same time, there is recruitment of extracardiac cells to expand the outlet portion of the tube at the arterial pole.[11] The newly formed atrial component is directly continuous with the systemic venous tributaries. These wide venous channels, which carry the blood back to the heart from both the right and left sides of the body, are from the outset connected directly to the primary atrial component. In man, however, from the earliest stages we have been able to study, there is a pronounced asymmetry in the connections of the right and left sided venous channels to the heart. From the outset, the left sinus horn is incorporated within the developing left atrioventricular junction as it extends to terminate in the atrium. Despite the asymmetry, at this stage the primary atrial component initially receives large systemic venous tributaries from both sides of the embryo (fig 33.1). It communicates with the ventricular loop through the atrioventricular canal. Towards the developing spinal column, the atrial cavity, now receiving the systemic venous tributaries, abuts directly on the body wall. In this area, the myocardial and mesenchymal tissues retain their continuity, persisting as a dorsal mesocardium (fig 33.1A). This connection between heart and body will, eventually, provide the portal of entry for the pulmonary vein.[6] At this stage, however, the lungs are only just starting to bud from the trachea. Also, at this stage, the endothelium lining the heart tube separates the lumen of the atrium from the mesenchyme of the body wall (fig 33.1B). In the

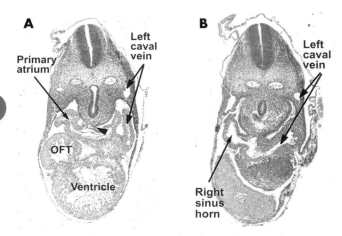

Figure 33.1 These sections are taken from a human embryo at Carnegie stage 12, sectioned in the short axis of the body. Section A shows how the walls of the primary atrium are continuous with the body of the embryo through the so-called "dorsal mesocardium" (arrowhead). Section B shows the continuity between the primary atrial component and the sinus horns, which are asymmetrical as they join the heart, the left horn being continuous with the left cardinal vein, which becomes the left superior caval vein.

human, this stage of development is reached when the entire embryo is less than 5 mm long. This is in the sixth week of development, and is representative of the 12th horizon within the temporal sequence established from the Carnegie collection of embryos.[12]

The primary atrium at this early stage is a common cavity. As a prelude to division of the cardiac cavities by formation of muscular septums, endocardial cushions have already formed within the atrioventricular canal, and also within the outflow tract which leads from the ventricular loop to supply the arteries of the developing branchial arches. As already shown (fig 33.1), initially the systemic venous tributaries join with the primary atrium from both sides of the embryo. These channels are the horns of the systemic venous sinus, the "sinus venosus", or the ducts of Cuvier. At this early stage, there are no discrete anatomical landmarks that mark boundaries between the venous horns and the primary atrium. Furthermore, at this stage, as also explained, the lung buds are only just starting to develop, and the pulmonary vein has yet to appear. The left sinus horn diminishes in size through and beyond this period, becoming more fully

incorporated into the left atrioventricular junction as the coronary sinus. Throughout its development, the coronary sinus, and its precursor, the left sinus horn, possesses its own discrete walls (figs 33.1 and 33.2). These walls form a discrete bifurcation with the right sinus horn at their junction with the developing right atrium, which persist as the part of the right atrium called the "sinus septum".

Subsequent to rearrangements in the structure of the systemic venous tributaries, the entire systemic venous compartment comes to drain exclusively to the right side of the primary atrium. As it does so, valve-like structures are produced at the right and left borders of its junction with the primary atrial component of the heart tube (fig 33.2). The appearance of these valves permits, for the first time, the boundaries of the systemic venous sinus to be located with certainty relative to the other parts of the developing atriums. While the systemic venous component has been establishing its own identity in this fashion, further important changes have occurred in the primary atrial segment. Expansions to right and left have formed the atrial appendages (fig 33.2A); concomitant with development of the lungs in the body wall behind the heart, a venous channel, the primary pulmonary vein canalises within the dorsal mesocardium (fig 33.2C). Canalisation of this channel brings the pulmonary venous plexuses into continuity with the cavity of the developing left atrium. Initially, a solitary pulmonary venous channel enters the left atrial part of the primary atrial component inferiorly and posteriorly, the entrance being bounded by two ridges which demarcate the site of the persisting dorsal mesocardium. The right of these two ridges becomes particularly prominent (fig 33.3). It is this structure that His[5] nominated as the "spina vestibuli".

All of these changes and remodellings relative to the primary atrium set the scene for atrial septation. The first indication of this septation is the formation of the primary atrial septum, first seen as a muscular crescent in the atrial roof. As it grows into the atrial cavity, it carries a mesenchymal cap on its leading edge (fig 33.2B). With continued growth, septum and cap move towards the atrioventricular endocardial cushions which, at the same time, are dividing the atrioventricular canal. The space between the mesenchymal cap on the leading edge of the primary atrial septum and the fusing atrioventricular cushions is the primary atrial foramen.

The primary septum, from the outset, is continuous inferiorly with the right pulmonary ridge, now prominent as the vestibular spine (fig 33.3). As it grows into the primary atrial

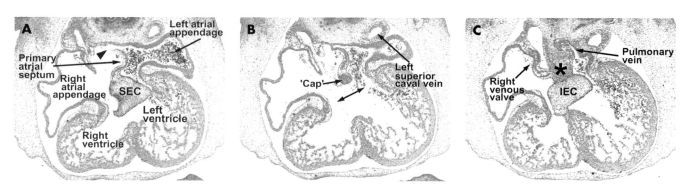

Figure 33.2 These three sections are from a human embryo at Carnegie stage 16, and are cut in the frontal plane of the heart. Section A is through the superior atrioventricular endocardial cushion (SEC). Note that the upper end of the primary septum has broken down to form the secondary foramen (arrowhead). The endocardial cushions have yet to fuse at this stage, and section B is taken between the cushions. Note the mesenchymal cap on the leading edge of the primary septum. Section C is through the inferior cushion (IEC) and shows how tissue from the body of the embryo enters the heart through the vestibular spine (asterisk). Note the solitary pulmonary vein joining the left side of the primary atrium.

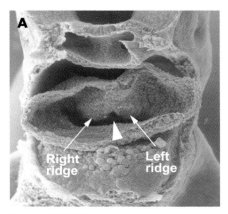
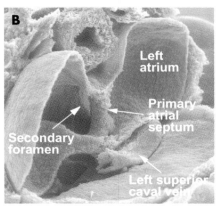
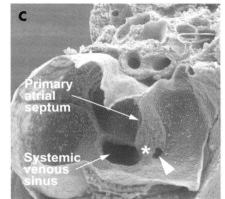

Figure 33.3 These pictures are scanning electron micrographs of the developing mouse heart. Picture A, from a mouse at embryonic day 9.5, with 28 somites, shows the stage before canalisation of the pulmonary vein. When formed, the vein will enter heart through the so-called "pulmonary pit", arrowed, which at this stage is flanked by prominent right and left pulmonary ridges. Picture B, at embryonic day 10.5, when the embryo has 42 somites, shows the primary septum growing down towards the atrioventricular cushions. Its upper edge has broken down to form the secondary foramen. Note that the left superior caval vein, now formed from the left cardinal vein, is a discrete structure within the left atrioventricular groove. Picture C, again from an embryo of 10.5 days, but now with 45 somites, shows the pulmonary vein opening as a solitary channel inferiorly to the left atrium, the systemic venous sinus, enclosed by the venous valves, now having become incorporated into the right atrium. The right pulmonary ridge has now expanded to become the vestibular spine (asterisk).

chamber, and fuses with the atrioventricular endocardial cushions, the primary atrial septum interposes between the right sided systemic venous component and the orifice of the pulmonary vein (fig 33.2). At this stage, the 16th horizon within the Carnegie system,[12] the pulmonary vein is a solitary channel at its junction with the primary atrium, with its mouth positioned posteriorly, inferiorly, and to the left of the vestibular spine (fig 33.4). Accompanying the growth of the primary septum into the atrium, there has been expansion of the vestibular spine, by now covered by its own mesenchymal cap, with additional tissues entering the heart from the body wall through the spine (fig 33.2C). It is the expansion of the spine which unifies the mesenchymal cap on the primary atrial septum with the fused atrioventricular cushions, obliterating the primary atrial foramen in the process, and forming the basis of the fibrous septal structures of the heart (fig 33.5).

Before closure of the primary foramen, the upper edge of the primary septum, close to its site of origin from the atrial roof, breaks down to form the secondary interatrial communication (figs 33.3 and 33.5). Such establishment of a secondary foramen is essential if the systemic venous return is to

continue to reach the left side of the heart during the remainder of fetal development. Within this period, the atrioventricular canal has also expanded rightward, establishing the connection between the newly formed morphologically right atrium and the distal part of the ventricular loop, which has now become the right ventricle.[13] The musculature of the atrioventricular canal itself becomes incorporated into the atrial chambers as the vestibules of the atrioventricular valves. Forward growth of the vestibular spine, binding the base of the primary septum to the upper surface of the fused

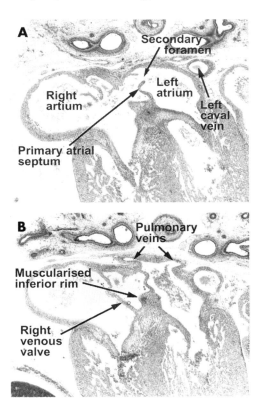

Figure 33.5 These sections are from a human embryo at Carnegie stage 20/21, showing the beginnings of the infolding of the atrial wall which will produce the rims of the oval fossa. Section A is taken cranial to section B. Note the ongoing muscularisation of the antero-inferior rim of the oval fossa (see also fig 33.10).

Figure 33.4 This section, taken in the sagittal plane from a human embryo at the 20th Carnegie stage, shows the solitary pulmonary vein entering inferiorly to the left atrium. Only with subsequent growth do four pulmonary veins enter that atrial roof, but this process is necessary to produce the so-called "septum secundum", in reality the infolded atrial roof (see fig 33.6).

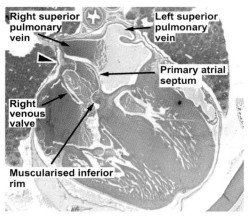

Figure 33.6 This section, from a human embryo at 11 weeks of development, shows the continuing infolding of the atrial roof as the pulmonary veins become incorporated into the left atrium.

atrioventricular cushions, has also carried forward the inferior ends of the valves of the systemic venous sinus (fig 33.5). The expanded vestibular spine itself then becomes muscularised to form a bulbous structure that reinforces the base of the primary atrial septum. The thinner upper margin of the primary septum itself persists as the flap valve of the oval foramen. At this stage, representing the 21st stage of the Carnegie horizons, the pulmonary vein continues to drain inferiorly to the left atrium, but has divided into its right and left branches.[12] As yet, there is no formation of a "secondary" septum within the roof of the dividing atrial chambers adjacent to the mouth of the superior caval vein, although evidence of infolding has begun to appear more inferiorly (fig 33.5).

Only subsequent to the eighth week of development does the initially solitary pulmonary vein begin fully to become incorporated into the body of the primary atrium, itself now largely part of the developing left atrium. By the 12th week of development,

the superior right sided pulmonary vein has become a separate tributary of the left atrium. Concomitant with this change, the atrial roof has infolded adjacent to the mouth of the superior caval vein to form the antero-superior margin of the oval foramen.[14] This process of infolding, when complete (fig 33.6), provides the buttress against which the flap valve can close in postnatal life. Concomitant with incorporation of the pulmonary veins to form the extensive posterior left atrial wall, the two atrioventricular junctions, now discrete and separate structures incorporating the insulating tissues of the atrioventricular grooves, have expanded posteriorly and inferiorly. The expansion of the right atrial wall relative to the base of the ventricular mass sandwiches the inferior atrioventricular groove as a layer of fibroadipose tissue between the atrial and ventricular musculatures in the floor of the triangle of Koch.[15]

Thus, subsequent to the completion of septation, the definitive atriums each possess a part of the body of the primary atrium, an appendage, a vestibule, and a venous component. They remain in continuity with each other through the oval foramen. The newly muscularised antero-inferior margin of the oval foramen, derived from the vestibular spine, is anchored to the fibrous skeleton, itself formed from the atrioventricular cushions. The primary atrial septum persists as the flap valve of the oval foramen. The antero-superior rim, against which the flap valve abuts, and which is usually described as the "septum secundum", is the infolding now existing between the junction of the superior caval vein to the right atrium and the right pulmonary veins to the left atrium.

DEFINITIVE STRUCTURE OF THE ATRIAL SEPTUM

Concepts of development, if correct, must provide the basis for understanding definitive atrial structure. When the right atrium is opened parietally, there is, at first sight, an extensive area of potential communication with the cavity of the left atrium (fig 33.7). Sectioning across this area (fig 33.8), however, shows that only a small part is a septal structure, when a septum is defined as that part which can be removed without exiting from the cavities of the heart.[16] The parts that can be removed to provide an interatrial communication are the floor of the oval fossa, the flap valve, and the part of the antero-inferior rim of the fossa which abuts on the vestibule of the tricuspid valve (fig 33.9). The floor of the oval fossa represents the embryonic primary atrial septum, while the antero-inferior margin of the fossa has been produced by muscularisation of the vestibular spine (fig 33.10). The extensive area extending between the superior margin of the oval fossa and

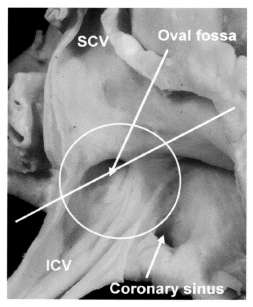

Figure 33.7 This picture of the human right atrium, taken from posteriorly and the right, shows how, at first sight, an extensive septal area, within the circle, separates the right from the left atrium. The true situation is shown in fig 8, which is a cross section along the line shown in the figure. SCV, superior caval vein; ICV, inferior caval vein.

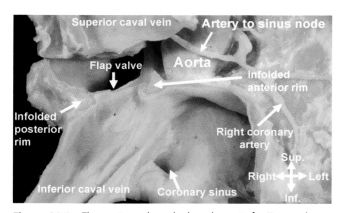

Figure 33.8 This section, along the line shown in fig 7, reveals how the rims of the oval fossa anteriorly and posteriorly are folds of the atrial wall. Note the relation of the anterior atrial wall to the aortic root.

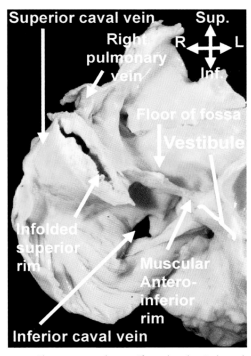

Figure 33.9 This section, taken in "four chamber" plane through an adult human heart, shows how the so-called "septum secundum" is a deep infolding between the connections of the pulmonary veins to the left atrium, and the superior caval vein to the right atrium. The "compass" shows the orientation. Sup, superior; Inf, inferior; R, right; L, left.

the mouth of the superior caval vein, although usually described as the "septum secundum", is a deep infolding of the atrial wall. This infolding, which is positioned between the connections of the systemic venous tributaries to the right atrium and the right pulmonary veins to the left atrium, is filled with extracardiac adipose tissue (figs 33.9 and 33.10). The flap valve of the septum, a fibromuscular structure in adult life, abuts against the fold to close the oval foramen. As long as the flap valve is of greater dimensions than the floor of the oval fossa, and the left atrial pressure exceeds that in the

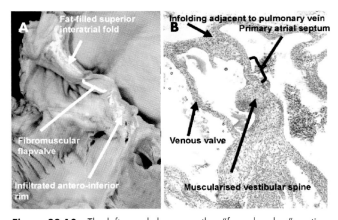

Figure 33.10 The left panel shows another "four chamber" section through an adult human heart. It shows not only the accumulation of fat within the superior interatrial fold, but also the fat which is infiltrating through the inferior atrioventricular groove into the inferior rim of the oval fossa. The right panel shows a section from a human embryo of 7–8 weeks' development, when two pulmonary veins have been incorporated into the left atrium. It shows the muscularisation of the vestibular spine, which forms the inferior rim of the oval fossa.

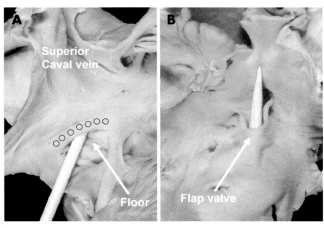

Figure 33.11 The pictures show a probe-patent oval foramen in a human heart, viewed from the right (left panel) and left (right panel) atrial aspects. The probe is placed through the foramen, separating the flap valve in the left atrium from the rims of the oval fossa (yellow dots).

right atrium, there will be no potential for interatrial shunting even if the two structures are not mechanically fused. This is of major clinical significance, since such anatomic fusion has occurred only in between two thirds and three quarters of individuals, even in the eighth or ninth decades of life.[17] Thus, in that minority in which fusion has not occurred, or in other words, those with a probe-patent oval foramen (fig 33.11), there is the potential for interatrial shunting should right atrial pressure exceed left, and hence the potential for paradoxical embolism. The true atrial septum, therefore, is made up of the flap valve of the oval foramen and its bulbous antero-inferior base.

Antero-superiorly, the right atrial wall itself directly overlies the aortic root (fig 33.9). The bulbous antero-inferior margin is perforated by the tendon of Todaro, this being the extension of the inferior junction of the valves of the systemic venous sinus. The valves themselves regress to greater or lesser extent in the postnatal heart. The atrial wall itself continues anteriorly beyond the bulbous inferior rim of the oval foramen as the smooth vestibule of the tricuspid valve, which superiorly forms the border of the atrioventricular membranous septum, an integral part of the central fibrous body. In the definitive heart, this fibrous area has become incorporated into the aortic root. It is perforated by the atrioventricular conduction axis as it passes from the atrioventricular node to become the bundle of His (fig 33.12). This transition from node to bundle marks the initial position of that part of the embryonic atrioventricular canal musculature which persisted as the atrioventricular bundle, the conduction tissue itself being a specialised part of the canal musculature.[18]

The extensive vestibule of the tricuspid valve seen inferiorly is derived from expansion of the right atrioventricular junction subsequent to the completion of embryonic septation. This is confirmed by the extent of the fibroadipose tissue to be found in the inferior atrioventricular groove between the atrial and ventricular musculatures. As already discussed, this incorporation of fibroadipose tissue between layers of myocardium produces the muscular atrioventricular sandwich,[15] an area which we previously considered, incorrectly, to represent a true muscular septal structure.[19] Also opening into this inferior corner of the right atrium is the mouth of the coronary sinus, a remnant of the embryonic left sinus horn. The mouths of the inferior and superior caval veins represent the remaining tributaries of the right sinus horn, with the prominent

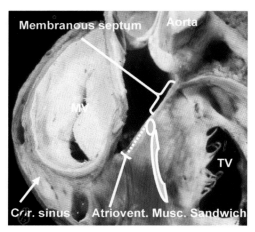

Figure 33.12 This dissection of a human heart shows the relations between the right and left atrioventricular junctions and the subaortic outflow tract. It has been made by removing the atrial walls, along with the non-coronary sinus of the aortic root. It shows the location of the membranous septum, which is penetrated by the atrioventricular conduction axis as it passes from the atrioventricular node (blue oval) to reach the crest of the muscular ventricular septum. The dots show the tissues of the inferior atrioventricular groove which interpose between the atrial and ventricular layers of the muscular atrioventricular sandwich. The red cross hatched area is the vestibule of the tricuspid valve (TV). MV, mitral valve; Cor sinus, coronary sinus.

terminal crest and the remnants of the right venous valve marking their boundary with that part of the right atrium derived from the primary atrial component of the heart tube. Most of this primary atrium is made up of the pectinated atrial appendage. The so-called "sinus septum" is no more than the fold of the atrial walls between the mouths of the inferior caval vein and the coronary sinus.

The location of the flap valve of the septum is much better appreciated when viewed from the left side, with two horns anchoring the flap to the left side of the infolded superior rim, albeit often without anatomic fusion (fig 33.11). The left atrium has its own appendage, with its pectinated walls, positioned anteriorly and superiorly. The posterior wall is exclusively smooth walled, being derived by incorporation of the extensive pulmonary venous component between the vestibule and the body of the atrium, the latter forming the extensive atrial dome.

COMMENT

It was HL Mencken who pointed out that, for every complex question, there was a simple and straightforward answer, which was usually wrong! This is certainly the case with the development of the atrial septum. There is no evidence of which we are aware to substantiate the notion that primary and secondary septums grow into the developing atrium, becoming perforate and overlapping so as to produce the definitive oval foramen. It is certainly the case that the primary septum grows into the primary atrial component of the heart tube, and that it persists as the flap valve of the definitive oval foramen. The bulbous muscular antero-inferior rim of the septum, in contrast, has a much more complex mode of development. It represents muscularisation of an area of mesenchyme which grows into the heart. The mesenchyme is derived from the cap that is carried on the leading edge of the primary septum, along with the mass known as the vestibular spine. Intriguingly, the mechanism of muscularisation of this population of cells, which grow into the heart at

the venous pole, has much in common with similar muscularisation recently shown to be involved with transformation of the ingrowth of cells through the aortopulmonary septum at the arterial pole of the heart.[20] Be that as it may, this part of the septum can reasonably be equated with the inferior part of the "septum secundum" depicted in standard textbooks. The position of this septal component, located as it is between the vestibules of the mitral and tricuspid valves, may well explain why His named its primordium as the "spina vestibuli".[5] If this bulbous base of the septum can justifiably be considered to be a secondary septal structure, the deeply infolded antero-superior rim certainly cannot. And this is the area most usually depicted as the "septum secundum" in classical texts! Lipomas in this area are usually held to involve this "secondary" septum.[3]

Much of any disagreement regarding this issue, of course, depends on the definition used for a "septum". As we have explained, we define a septum as a structure that can be removed without exiting from the cavities of the heart.[16] The distinction between structures fulfilling this definition, and those folds or sandwiches which can similarly interpose between cardiac cavities, is important to the clinician working in the heart, be his or her discipline surgery or interventional catheterisation. The surgeon needs to be aware that, if cuts are made through a fold or sandwich, they pass outside the heart. The congenital cardiac surgeon is certainly aware that incisions through the deep superior interatrial groove offer a good access to the left atrium. In the days of surgical procedures producing atrial redirection, it was equally well established that dissections of the walls of the groove provided increased lengths of atrial wall for use in the subsequent reconstruction. Nowadays, the interventional cardiologist is well aware of the difference in structure between the firm antero-inferior base of the atrial septum, which provides a firm foundation for anchorage of devices used for interventional closure, as opposed to the superior rim, which can often be effaced.[9] It is our hope that, in this review, we have shown how these important clinical differences between septums, flaps, folds, and sandwiches are well explained once it is established properly how the atrial chambers develop.

REFERENCES

1 **Röse C**. Zur Entwicklungsgeschichte des Saugerthierherzens. *Morphol Jahr* 1899;**15**:436–56.

2 **Christie GA**. The development of the limbus fossae ovalis in the human heart: a new septum. *J Anat* 1963;**97**:45–54.
► These works show that it has long been recognised that the so-called "septum secundum" is, in reality, no more than an infolding between the connections of the pulmonary veins to the left atrium, and the caval veins to the right atrium.

3 **Basso C**, Barbazza R, Thiene G. Images in cardiovascular medicine. Lipomatous hypertrophy of the atrial septum. *Circulation* 1998;**97**:1423.
► Although the authors claim that their image demonstrates the collection of fat within the atrial septum, in fact it is clear that the fat has accumulated within the superior interatrial groove.

4 **Li J**, Ho SY, Becker AE, *et al.* Multiple cardiac lipomas and sudden death – a case report and literature review. *Cardiovasc Pathol* 1998;**7**:349–52.
► The authors review an amazing heart which shows multiple lipomas, and show how the fat accumulates within the grooves of the heart, albeit that there is also infiltration of the myocardium.

5 **His W**. Die Area interposita, die Eustachi'sche Klappe und die Spina vestibuli. In: *Anatomie Menschlicher Embryonen*. Leipzig: von FCW Vogel, 1880:49–152.
► The initial description of the "spina vestibuli". His's reconstructions are remarkably accurate, although he does not specify the nature of the vestibule in which the spine is formed.

6 **Webb S**, Brown NA, Wessels A, *et al.* Development of the murine pulmonary vein and its relationship to the embryonic venous sinus. *Anat Rec* 1998;**250**:325–34.
► An experimental study of the mouse heart, using scanning electron microscopy, showing that the pulmonary vein canalises in the so-called "dorsal mesocardium", and not originating, as has been claimed, from the systemic venous sinus.

7 **Webb S**, Brown NA, Anderson RH. Formation of the atrioventricular septal structures in the normal mouse. *Circ Res* 1998;**82**:645–56.

▶ **An extension of the work published in reference 6, emphasising that several primordiums are needed to achieve appropriate separation of the right and left atriums along with their atrioventricular junctions.**

8 **Anderson RH**, Webb S, Brown NA. Clinical anatomy of the atrial septum with reference to its developmental components. *Clin Anat* 1999;**12**:362–74.

▶ **A review of the structure of the atrial septum, emphasising that the so-called "septum secundum" is no more than an infolding of the atrial roof.**

9 **Ferreira Martins JD**, Anderson RH. Anatomy of the interatrial communication – what does the interventionist need to know? *Cardiol Young* 2000;**10**:464–73.

▶ **A review of atrial septal structure in the light of the increasing use of devices inserted on catheters to close holes within the oval fossa.**

10 **de la Cruz MV**, Sanchez-Gomez C, Palomino MA. The primitive cardiac regions in the straight tube heart (stage 9) and their anatomical expression in the mature heart: an experimental study in the chick embryo. *J Anat* 1989;**165**:121–31.

11 **Kelly RG**, Brown NA, Buckingham ME. The arterial pole of the mouse heart forms from *Fgf-10* expressing cells in pharyngeal mesoderm. *Developmental Cell* 2001;**1**:1–20.

▶ **Two studies which question the classical concept that the heart develops as a series of segments within an initially straight primary heart tube. In fact, at no stage in normal development is there such a straight tube with venous, atrial, ventricular, and arterial components.**

12 **O'Rahilly R**, Müller F. *Developmental stages in human embryos.* Washington: Carnegie Institution of Washington Publication 637, 1987.

▶ **The classical study which provided the landmarks for categorising the stages of development of the human embryo.**

13 **Lamers WH**, Wessels A, Verbeek FJ, *et al.* New findings concerning ventricular septation in the human heart. *Circulation* 1992;**86**:1194–205.

▶ **A study which used an antibody to the nodose ganglion of the chick to chart the development of the atrioventricular junctions of the human heart, showing that the right ventricle was formed exclusively from the distal component of the ventricular loop.**

14 **Webb S**, Kanani M, Anderson RH, *et al.* Development of the human pulmonary vein and its incorporation in the morphologically left atrium. *Cardiol Young* 2001;**11**:632–42.

▶ **An examination of serial sectioned human embryos which showed that, as in the mouse, the pulmonary vein canalised within the dorsal mesocardium. No evidence was found to support the concept that the vein originated from the systemic venous sinus. The study showed that the subsequent incorporation of four pulmonary veins to the atrial roof was a relatively late event during development.**

15 **Anderson RH**, Ho SY, Becker AE. Anatomy of the human atrioventricular junctions revisited. *Anat Rec* 2000;**260**: 81–91.

16 **Anderson RH**, Brown NA. The anatomy of the heart revisited. *Anat Rec* 1996;**246**:1–7.

▶ **These two studies questioned the definitions used for septal structures, emphasising that true septums are the walls of the heart which can be removed without exiting from the cardiac cavities. The first study also reviewed the relationships of the conduction axis to the atrioventricular junctions.**

17 **Hagen PT**, Scholz DG, Edwards WD. Incidence and size of patent foramen ovale during the first 10 decades of life: an autopsy study of 965 normal hearts. *Proc Staff Meet Mayo Clin* 1984;**59**:1489–94.

▶ **An important study which showed that, irrespective of age, about one third of the population retains probe patency of the oval foramen.**

18 **Kim J-S**, Viragh Sz, Moorman AFM, *et al.* Development of the myocardium of the atrioventricular canal and the vestibular spine in the human heart. *Circ Res* 2001;**88**:395–402.

▶ **A study of the development of the human heart, showing how the vestibular spine becomes muscularised to form the antero-inferior margin of the oval foramen.**

19 **Becker AE**, Anderson RH. What's in a name? *J Thorac Cardiovasc Surg* 1982;**83**:461–9.

▶ **The initial study which emphasised that a common atrioventricular junction was the pathognomonic feature of hearts with so-called "atrioventricular canal malformations". The study also showed that the hole between the four cardiac chambers was, in reality, an atrioventricular septal defect.**

20 **van den Hoff MJ**, Moorman AFM, Ruijter JM, *et al.* Myocardialization of the cardiac outflow tract. *Dev Biol* 1999;**212**: 477–490.

▶ **The embryological study which had first demonstrated the importance of myocardialisation of the endocardial cushions, this investigation concentrating of the formation of the outflow segments.**

34 ARTERIOSCLEROTIC RENAL ARTERY STENOSIS: CONSERVATIVE VERSUS INTERVENTIONAL MANAGEMENT

Christlieb Haller

Renal artery stenosis is the most common cause of secondary hypertension. Over 90% of renal artery stenoses are caused by arteriosclerosis, the remainder resulting from fibromuscular dysplasia which usually does not lead to progressive azotemia and end stage renal disease. Renal angioplasty is the treatment of choice for fibromuscular dysplastic disease and has the potential of curing hypertension if performed early.

The situation is quite different for arteriosclerotic renal artery disease which generally occurs in older patients with longstanding hypertension. The stenotic lesions are typically localised at the ostium of the renal artery, respectively in the aortic wall. Reconstructive surgery has been the classical treatment for these lesions,[1] particularly since the initial experience with renal artery angioplasty for arteriosclerotic ostial lesions was disappointing. However, a prospective randomised study has demonstrated that reconstructive surgery offers no definite advantage over interventional treatment of renal artery stenosis.[2] Since most patients with arteriosclerotic renal artery disease have coronary and cerebral atherosclerosis and other significant comorbid conditions which increase the risk of surgery, the interventional treatment of renal artery stenosis has become the preferred method of renal revascularisation in many centres. This development has been reinforced by the more recent introduction of renal arterial stent implantation, which may improve the outcome of renal artery interventions, although there have been no randomised prospective comparisons between renal artery stenting and other forms of treatment. Most reports on renal angioplasty with stent implantation have been based on relatively few patients with only a short follow up period. However, a recently published paper from a multicentre registry of 1058 patients reports a benefit from renal artery stenting on both blood pressure control and renal function after four years of follow up.[3]

The treatment of renal artery disease has recently been reviewed.[4] The present paper summarises the arguments and evidence for interventional versus conservative treatment of arteriosclerotic renal artery disease, focusing on the indications for interventional treatment to provide interventional cardiologists with criteria for patient selection.

▶ ## RENAL ARTERY STENOSIS: WHY IS IT IMPORTANT FOR THE CARDIOLOGIST?

Renal artery stenosis is a particularly relevant comorbid condition in cardiological practice, since the risk factors for coronary artery disease and renal artery disease are identical. Consequently both vascular beds are commonly affected by atherosclerosis in the same patient.[5] Renal artery stenosis causes or aggravates hypertension and/or interferes with its treatment. Renal artery stenosis therefore has a negative impact on both primary and secondary prevention of coronary heart disease. In patients undergoing cardiac catheterisation renal artery stenosis is an independent risk factor for mortality which correlates with the severity of the renal artery disease.[6] Moreover, ischaemic renal disease is the most rapidly increasing cause of end stage renal disease in the USA.[7] Renal failure impairs the outcome of coronary artery bypass grafting and percutaneous coronary interventions.

Because of the interrelation between arteriosclerotic renal and coronary artery disease cardiologists are frequently confronted with "cardiorenal" problems. They are not only experts in the conservative treatment of atherosclerosis, but they also have the expertise necessary for interventional treatment of the complications of atherosclerosis. The angioplasty/stent implantation of ostial renal artery lesions can be performed effectively with equipment adapted from coronary artery interventions (fig 34.1). Indeed, the largest single centre series on primary renal artery stenting comes from a group of cardiologists.[8] This team treated 363 renal artery stenoses in 300 patients between 1993 and 1998 with stent implantation. The procedural success rate was 100% without procedural deaths or emergency surgical procedures. The overall restenosis rate during a median follow up of 16 months was 21%, 12% in renal arteries with a diameter > 4.5 mm These results show that primary renal artery stenting can be performed safely and effectively.

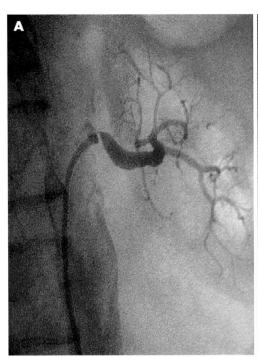
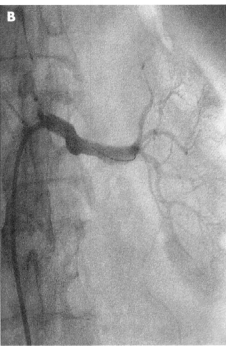

Figure 34.1 Arteriosclerotic renal artery stenosis in a 69 year old male patient. (A) Subtotal occlusion of the ostium of the left renal artery. (B) After percutaneous angioplasty with stent implantation. A guiding catheter (FR 3.5, 7 French) and a steerable 0.014 inch guidewire were used to advance a 12 mm balloon expandable stent over the lesion. The stent was deployed by inflating the balloon (6 mm diameter) for 30 seconds.

However, what is the evidence that percutaneous renal revascularisation benefits patients? This central question is particularly pertinent as recent studies suggest that blood pressure can be controlled conservatively in most patients with arteriosclerotic renal artery stenosis. What is the evidence that renal revascularisation improves/preserves renal function? Who should undergo renal revascularisation? What are the most effective methods for diagnosis and follow up?

RENAL ARTERY INTERVENTION FOR THE TREATMENT OF HYPERTENSION

Most patients with arteriosclerotic renal artery disease do not have renovascular hypertension. Rather they have essential hypertension that has been complicated by atherosclerosis and the development of a stenotic renal artery lesion. Therefore the correction of renal artery stenosis is unlikely to cure the hypertension, since the exposure of the non-stenotic kidney to the increased blood pressure results in (subclinical) renal injury. Such subtle renal damage is increasingly recognised as an important cause of persistent hypertension.[9] Nevertheless the data from a multicentre registry on renal artery stenting in 1058 patients over a four year period show a beneficial effect of renal revascularisation on blood pressure control.[3]

The indication of renal artery intervention for blood pressure control has been challenged. A randomised study comparing medical treatment with angioplasty in 55 patients with atheromatous renal artery stenosis showed a mild reduction of blood pressure after angioplasty only in patients with bilateral disease without improvement in renal function, but with a significant complication rate.[10] Another study involving 49 patients with unilateral renal artery stenosis showed a similar reduction in blood pressure in patients treated with renal angioplasty compared with conservative management.[11] A larger multicentre randomised trial in 106 patients with arteriosclerotic renal artery stenosis compared pharmacological treatment with renal angioplasty (only two patients received a stent). Twenty two patients initially assigned to drug treatment underwent renal angioplasty after three

months. After 12 months the blood pressure was not significantly different between the two treatment groups, but the interventionally treated patients required fewer drugs. The authors concluded that angioplasty offers little advantage over antihypertensive drug treatment alone.[12]

In an individual patient the blood pressure response to renal revascularisation is uncertain. However, most published studies and the data from the large registry[3] are in agreement that blood pressure is better controlled with fewer medications after successful angioplasty.

Lowering blood pressure with any medication reduces renal perfusion pressure and can cause a deterioration of renal function. This is particularly true for drugs that interfere with the renin angiotensin system because of their specific effects on the regulation of glomerular haemodynamics. The reduced renal perfusion pressure distal of a stenotic renal artery is counterbalanced by a decreased tone of the afferent glomerular arteriole and an increased tone of the efferent vessel. This results in an increased filtration pressure which maintains the glomerular filtration rate at a higher filtration fraction (fig 34.2). The increased resistance of the efferent arteriole is mediated by angiotensin II. Thus, angiotensin converting enzyme (ACE) inhibitors can cause a deterioration of renal function, particularly in patients with severe bilateral disease or a high grade stenosis of an artery supplying a single functioning kidney. On the other hand, ACE inhibitors are highly effective in the treatment of renovascular hypertension, particularly when combined with a diuretic. Therefore they are the treatment of choice for renovascular hypertension provided patients do not develop rapidly worsening azotemia. By extrapolation, the same should apply for angiotensin II receptor blockers, but there are fewer published data. Close monitoring of the serum creatinine concentration is essential upon initiation of ACE inhibitor treatment in patients with renal artery stenosis. During maintenance treatment periodic measurement of renal size and ("split" renal) function is prudent for the early detection of atrophy of the post-stenotic kidney under ACE inhibition. This should be regarded as an indication to proceed with revascularisation of the stenotic kidney.

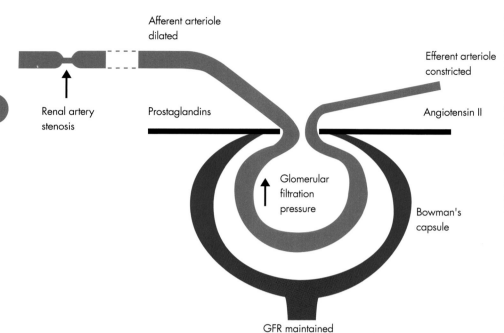

Figure 34.2 Regulation of glomerular haemodynamics. Reduction of the glomerular perfusion pressure behind a stenosis of the renal artery induces dilatation of the afferent arteriole and constriction of the efferent arteriole. The decreased resistance of the afferent arteriole is mediated by vasodilatory prostaglandins, the constriction of the efferent vessel by angiotensin II. These changes result in the increase of the filtration pressure. The higher filtration fraction maintains the glomerular filtration rate despite the lower perfusion pressure.

RENAL ARTERY INTERVENTION FOR PRESERVATION OF RENAL FUNCTION

There is increasing consensus that blood pressure can be managed medically in most patients with renal artery stenosis. Therefore the preservation/improvement of renal function has become the most important indication for renal revascularisation. Patients with generalised atherosclerosis may have a variety of conditions causing renal failure including (essential) hypertension, renal hypoperfusion due to congestive heart failure, atheroembolic disease, diabetes mellitus, radiocontrast nephrotoxicity from (repeat) percutaneous coronary interventions, and ischaemic nephropathy from arteriosclerotic renal artery disease. Recently it has been argued that many patients with renal artery stenosis do not have critical ischaemia/hypoxia of the renal parenchyma, but rather a relative hypoperfusion which limits the glomerular filtration rate without causing true tissue ischaemia. Therefore, the more appropriate term "chronic azotemic renovascular disease" has been proposed.[13]

Compared with the excellent procedural results of renal artery stenting[8] the clinical outcome of this procedure is less certain. In particular, the impact on renal function is complex; in addition to the general risks of invasive arterial procedures, renal artery interventions themselves carry a significant renal risk, mainly related to radiocontrast nephropathy and cholesterol embolisation from atheromatous plaques. Hence it is not surprising that renal function often fails to improve, despite technically successful revascularisation; in a substantial portion of patients it may even deteriorate. The registry report on renal artery stenting in 1058 patients showed overall a significant reduction of the mean (SD) serum creatinine concentration from 1.7 (1.1) mg/dl (150 (97) µmol/l) to 1.3 (0.8) mg/dl (115 (71) µmol/l) over a four year follow up period, suggesting that renal artery revascularisation is beneficial in the long term in the majority of patients.[3]

However, there are no published randomised controlled studies in which the effect of renal artery stenting is compared to optimal conservative treatment with modern antihypertensive agents. Such studies are very difficult to conduct, as patients with advanced renal dysfunction are more likely to die of other (cardiovascular) causes before a potential benefit of the renal revascularisation can be detected. On the other hand, patients with normal or only mild renal dysfunction may require very long follow up periods to show a significant benefit.

The functional results of 10 descriptive studies have been reviewed by Isles and colleagues: renal function improved in 26%, remained stable in 48%, and deteriorated in 26% of stented patients.[14] In the large single centre series on primary renal artery stenting by Lederman and colleagues, renal function improved in 19% of patients with renal insufficiency before the intervention, remained stable in 54%, and decreased in 27%.[8] Thus, despite the 100% procedural success rate reported by this group, from the renal function point of view the procedure was detrimental in more patients than it was beneficial; in most patients it was inconsequential.

Watson and associates published the results of a prospective study on renal artery stenting in 33 patients with deteriorating renal function before the intervention.[15] Stenting was technically successful in all patients. During 20 (11) months of follow up, renal function improved in 18 patients and the deterioration of renal function was stopped or slowed in the remainder of the patients. The preservation/improvement of renal function was accompanied by a preservation of renal size. Another recent prospective study on the effect of renal artery stenting on renal function in 63 patients with renal insufficiency is consistent with these results, demonstrating that patients with declining renal function, but not with stable renal dysfunction, benefit from stenting.[16] However, in this study five patients reached end stage renal failure within six months of stent implantation, in two cases because of stent implantation. Patients with stable renal insufficiency derived no benefit from stenting during a median follow up period of 23 months.

Taken together these studies suggest that renal revascularisation is most beneficial in patients with progressive renal failure. Its overall usefulness in patients with stable renal (dys)function is less certain, since the procedure itself is not innocuous and can cause a rapid deterioration of renal function. Hence, careful patient selection and meticulously documented informed consent are important.

Table 1 Factors influencing the treatment decision of renal artery stenosis

> ▶ Favouring renal revascularisation:
> Refractory hypertension despite >3 drugs
> Progressive azotemia
> Acute renal failure on ACE inhibitors (angiotensin II receptor blockers)
> Recurrent "flash" pulmonary oedema
> "Salvage" therapy in recent onset end stage renal disease
> ▶ Favouring conservative treatment/watchful waiting:
> Hypertension controlled on <3 drugs
> Normal renal function
> Stable mild/moderate renal insufficiency
> Advanced renal atrophy (<7.5 cm)
> Doppler ultrasonographic renal resistance index >80
> History or clinical evidence of cholesterol embolisation

ACE, angiotensin converting enzyme.

Arteriosclerotic renal artery stenosis: key points

> ▶ Arteriosclerosis is the most common cause of renal artery stenosis
> ▶ Hypertension can be treated safely and effectively with anti-hypertensive drugs in most patients with renal artery stenosis
> ▶ The treatment of arteriosclerotic renal artery stenosis with angioplasty and stenting is safe and effective with a low risk of restenosis
> ▶ Correction of arteriosclerotic renal artery stenosis generally fails to cure hypertension, but control of blood pressure requires fewer drugs
> ▶ The preservation of renal function through the interventional treatment of arteriosclerotic renal artery stenosis is less certain; patients with deteriorating renal function seem to derive greater benefit than patients with stable renal insufficiency

WHO SHOULD BE EVALUATED FOR RENAL ARTERY STENOSIS?

General screening of hypertensive patients for the presence of renal artery stenosis is not indicated for two reasons: (1) the prevalence of renal artery stenosis in the general hypertensive population is too low; and (2) even if renal artery stenosis is present, this finding does not need to influence patient management provided blood pressure is controlled by medication and renal size and function remain stable. Therefore only patients who potentially benefit from renal revascularisation should be worked up for renal artery revascularisation. There are several clinical clues to identify these patients (table 1). Unusually severe hypertension or hypertension refractory to more than three medications should prompt an evaluation for renal artery stenosis, especially if a renal ultrasound shows asymmetric and/or small kidneys. Patients with hypertension, other arteriosclerotic manifestations, and renal failure should have a work up for renal artery stenosis, particularly if the renal insufficiency is progressive and/or aggravated by ACE inhibitors or angiotensin II antagonists.

Patients with severe hypertension, good systolic left ventricular function, and recurrent "flash" pulmonary oedema are a distinct subgroup in whom it is important to exclude renal artery stenosis.[17] This clinical syndrome of recurrent episodes of sudden onset non-ischaemic pulmonary oedema can be caused by severe bilateral renal artery stenosis or a critically stenosed artery to a single functioning kidney. Because of the compromised renal perfusion a rise in blood pressure is not accompanied by a pressure natriuresis. The ensuing hypertensive crisis induces pronounced diastolic dysfunction and pulmonary oedema. Correction of the stenosis permits the excretion of sodium and prevents the hypertensive crisis and the recurrence of the pulmonary oedema.

The renal risk of angioplasty is increased in proportion to the severity of the renal insufficiency because of the greater susceptibility to radiocontrast nephropathy and possibly the greater arteriosclerotic burden, adding to the risk of cholesterol embolisation. This increased risk has to be taken into account when obtaining informed consent, and patients should be warned that the interventional procedure can hasten the course towards dialysis. On the other hand, there are several anecdotal reports that even patients with severe renal failure on dialysis may recover sufficient renal function from renal "salvage" revascularisation to discontinue renal replacement therapy. Therefore, treatment of renal artery disease should not be denied simply because a patient is on dialysis, particularly if kidney size is relatively preserved and renal replacement therapy has just begun.

Since renal atrophy is irreversible, no significant functional improvement can be expected in atrophic kidneys, and patients with renal artery stenosis in kidneys < 7.5 cm should be treated conservatively (or by nephrectomy, if blood pressure cannot be controlled pharmacologically).[13] Recently Doppler ultrasound has been proposed as a valuable tool to discriminate between patients who benefit from renal revascularisation and those who can be spared this potentially dangerous and expensive procedure.[18] However, the discriminating value of the Doppler sonographic renal resistance index in routine clinical practice is still uncertain. Other indicators of parenchymal renal disease, including a urinary protein excretion > 1 g/day, hyperuricaemia, and a creatinine clearance < 40 ml/min, may identify a subgroup of patients who are less likely to benefit from renal revascularisation.

HOW IS RENAL ARTERY STENOSIS DIAGNOSED?

The diagnosis of renal artery stenosis is established by functional and/or morphological studies. The current diagnostic gold standard is arterial digital subtraction angiography (DSA). Arterial DSA requires cannulation of the aorta and exposes the patient to potentially nephrotoxic iodinated radiocontrast agents. This is pertinent, since renal function is often compromised in these patients putting them at an increased risk of radiocontrast induced nephropathy.

Spiral computed tomographic angiography allows the three dimensional reconstruction of the abdominal aorta and its branches, including the renal arteries. However, it requires about the same volume of intravenous iodinated radiocontrast material as arterial DSA; therefore it also carries the risk of nephrotoxicity.

Nuclear magnetic resonance angiography is becoming increasingly popular for imaging renal arteries, since it is relatively non-invasive and does not require iodinated radiocontrast agents. In addition to imaging the renal arteries, enabling direct detection of a stenosis, this technique allows the evaluation of renal function and perfusion. Hence it can provide information on the haemodynamic relevance of the stenosis. The assessment of perfusion is potentially useful for follow up after stent implantation, since imaging by magnetic resonance is usually not possible after stent implantation because of the metal artefact.

A totally non-invasive tool for the diagnosis of renal artery stenosis is renal duplex ultrasonography. However, even under optimal circumstances this technique is time consuming and in a substantial group of patients not satisfactory because of obesity, bowel gas, and other patient factors. Because duplex ultrasonography does not expose the patient to nephrotoxic contrast agents or ionising radiation it can be readily repeated and is the method of choice for follow up after renal artery interventions, including stent implantation in suitable patients.

Renal scintigraphy, especially in combination with the administration of captopril, is a standard technique to evaluate renal perfusion for the diagnosis of renovascular hypertension. The captopril challenge is based on the substantial reduction of the glomerular filtration rate in the post-stenotic kidney after reducing angiotensin II by blocking the angiotensin converting enzyme (fig 2). Renal scintigraphy can be useful not only for the estimation of the functional significance of the stenosis, but also for follow up after interventions to exclude a haemodynamically relevant restenosis. A disadvantage of the method is that it does not provide anatomical information and has only a limited diagnostic accuracy, even when used in combination with captopril.

Many patients with renal artery stenosis undergo coronary angiography. In selected patients it may be appropriate to proceed directly to renal arteriography after the coronary procedure with little additional risk, provided the radiocontrast volume stays within reasonable limits. However, most patients with morphological evidence of renal artery stenosis do not have renovascular hypertension and are not likely to benefit from angioplasty. Therefore the routine imaging of renal arteries during coronary angiography in all hypertensive patients as a screening tool for renal artery disease and especially immediate angioplasty/stenting is not indicated.

CONCLUSIONS AND OUTLOOK

Renal artery angioplasty with stent implantation has become a standard procedure in the management of patients with arteriosclerotic renal artery disease. The procedure is safe and effective and results in the reduction of blood pressure and/or medication requirement. With regards to renal function its benefit is less clear. Patients with progressive renal dysfunction appear to be more likely to benefit from the procedure than patients with stable renal failure. The procedure has a definite risk of worsening renal function through radiocontrast nephrotoxicity and/or atheroembolism. Therefore patient selection is critical (table 1). In appropriately selected patients the diagnosis and treatment of renal artery stenosis is not only clinically beneficial, but also cost effective.[19]

All patients with arteriosclerotic renal artery stenosis should be evaluated for coronary artery disease and most patients should receive an ACE inhibitor and a statin. The latter not only reduces cardiac risk but may induce a regression of renal artery stenosis.[20] The role of pharmacological treatment in the management of renal artery disease is likely to increase in the future.

REFERENCES

1 **Allenberg J-R**, Hupp T. Endovasculäre und offene rekonstruktive Chirurgie der Nierenarterienläsion. Chirurg 1995;**66**:101–11.
2 **Weibull H**, Bergqvist, Bergentz SE, et al. Percutaneous transluminal angioplasty versus surgical reconstruction of atherosclerotic renal artery stenosis: a prospective randomized study. J Vasc Surg 1993;**18**:841–52.
▶ **Important study showing that interventional treatment is as effective as surgery for the treatment of arteriosclerotic renal artery stenosis.**
3 **Dorros G**, Jaff M, Mathiak L, et al. Multicenter Palmaz stent renal artery stenosis revascularization registry report: four-year follow-up of 1,058 successful patients. Catheter Cardiovasc Interv 2002;**2**:182–8.
▶ **Largest series on renal artery stenting. In patients with normal or only mildly impaired renal function renal artery stenting was beneficial for blood pressure control and preservation of renal function. Though not from a randomised study, this is pertinent information.**
4 **Plouin P-F**, Rossignol P, Bobrie G. Atherosclerotic renal artery stenosis: to treat conservatively, to dilate, to stent, or to operate? J Am Soc Nephrol 2001;**12**:2190–6.
▶ **Excellent recent review of the subject focusing on the comparison between conservative and interventional treatment, including stents.**
5 **Gross CM**, Kramer J, Waigand J, et al. Renovascular illness: prevalence and therapy in patients with coronary heart disease. Z Kardiol 2000;**89**:747–53.
6 **Conlon PJ**, Little MA, Pieper K, et al. Severity of renal vascular disease predicts mortality in patients undergoing coronary angiography. Kidney Int 2001;**60**:1490–7.
7 **Fatica RA**, Port FK, Young EW. Incidence trends and mortality in end-stage renal disease attributed to renvascular disease in the United States. Am J Kidney Dis 2001;**37**:1184–90.
8 **Lederman RJ**, Mendelsohn FO, Santos R, et al. Primary renal artery stenting: characteristics and outcomes after 363 procedures. Am Heart J 2001;**142**:314–23.
▶ **Largest single centre study on arteriosclerotic renal artery stenting: 363 renal artery stenoses were treated in 300 patients between 1993 and 1998 with a 100% procedural success rate. The overall restenosis rate during a median follow up of 16 months was 21%. There were no procedural deaths or surgical emergencies.**
9 **Johnson RJ**, Herrera-Acosta J, Schreiner GF, et al. Mechanisms of disease: subtle acquired renal injury as a mechanism of salt-sensitive hypertension. N Engl J Med 2002;**346**:913–23.
▶ **Review article developing the pathophysiological concept that a variety of factors, including renal artery stenosis, induce subtle renal injury which can cause salt sensitive (essential) hypertension.**
10 **Webster J**, Marshall F, Abdalla M, et al. Randomised comparison of percutaneous angioplasty vs continued medical therapy for hypertensive patients with atheromatous renal artery stenosis. Scottish and Newcastle renal artery stenosis collaborative group. J Hum Hypertens 1998;**12**:329–35.
11 **Plouin PF**, Chatellier G, Darne B, et al. Blood pressure outcome of angioplasty in atherosclerotic renal artery stenosis: a randomized trial. Essai Multicentrique medicaments vs angioplastie (EMMA) study group. Hypertension 1998;**31**:823–9.
12 **van Jaarsveld BC**, Krijnen P, Pieterman H, et al. The effect of balloon angioplasty on hypertension in atherosclerotic renal artery stenosis. N Engl J Med 2000;**342**:1007–14.
▶ **Important randomised study involving 106 patients treated either conservatively or by angioplasty. Interventional treatment had little advantage over drug therapy, but angioplasty resulted in a reduction of antihypertensive medication. There was a relatively high crossover rate of patients initially treated conservatively who later received angioplasty.**
13 **Textor SC**, Wilcox CS. Renal artery stenosis: a common, treatable cause of renal failure? Annu Rev Med 2001;**52**:421–42.
▶ **Excellent review of renal artery stenosis and its effect on renal (dys)function. The term chronic azotemic renovascular disease describes the pathophysiology more accurately than ischaemic nephropathy, since there is usually no true tissue ischaemia.**
14 **Isles CG**, Robertson S, Hill D. Management of renovascular disease: a review of renal artery stenting in ten studies. Q J M 1999;**92**:159–67.
▶ **A useful meta-analysis of the outcome of renal artery stenting, particularly with respect to renal function.**
15 **Watson PS**, Hadjipetrou P, Cox SV, et al. Effect of renal artery stenting on renal function and size in patients with atherosclerotic renovascular disease. Circulation 2000;**102**:1671–7.
16 **Beutler JJ**, van Ampting JMA, van de Ven PJG, et al. Long-term effects of arterial stenting on kidney function for patients with ostial atherosclerotic renal artery stenosis and renal insufficiency. J Am Soc Nephrol 2001;**12**:1475–81.
17 **Missouris CG**, Belli A-M, MacGregor GA. "Apparent" heart failure: a syndrome caused by renal artery stenosis. Heart 2000;**83**:152–5.
18 **Radermacher J**, Chavan A, Bleck J, et al. Use of doppler ultrasonography to predict the outcome of therapy for renal-artery stenosis. N Engl J Med 2001;**344**:410–17.
▶ **This study examines the value of renal Doppler ultrasound to distinguish patients who might benefit from renal revascularisation from those who do not. A renal resistance index > 80 identifies a subgroup of patients who do not benefit from renal revascularisation. Although still subject to validation in routine application, this finding may be included in clinical decision processes.**
19 **Nelemans PJ**, Kessels AG, de Leeuw P, et al. The cost-effectiveness of the diagnosis of renal artery stenosis. Eur J Radiol 1998;**27**:95-107.
▶ **This study stresses the importance of a careful clinical evaluation, since the cost effectiveness of the diagnosis of renal artery stenosis is critically dependent on a pre-test likelihood > 20%.**
20 **Khong TK**, Missouris CG, Belli AM, et al. Regression of atherosclerotic renal artery stenosis with aggressive lipid lowering therapy. J Hum Hypertens 2001;**15**:431–3.

Additional references appear on the Heart website–www.heartjnl.com

35 EFFECT OF PARTIAL COMPLIANCE ON CARDIOVASCULAR MEDICATION EFFECTIVENESS

Joyce A Cramer

The typical assessment of mediation compliance by physicians is similar to the assessment of an iceberg from the ship captain's window. The difference is that when a captain sees ice in the water, he assumes that what he sees might be only the "tip of the iceberg" requiring attention. In contrast, patients who inadvertently omit many doses and doctors who attribute poor control to lack of drug efficacy may have no concept that the underlying problem is poor compliance with the prescribed regimen. If the captain fails to recognise an iceberg in advance, he knows that he must turn his immense vessel rapidly to avoid disaster. Failing to recognise inadequate compliance as the source of the patient's problem, the physician is unaware of the appropriate action to be taken. Instead, the physician typically prescribes even more medication as a higher dose, or an alternative or second drug. Unfortunately, the patient often remains on a potentially fatal collision course. Why is this scenario so common in medical practice?

Inherent in the answers to these questions is a message for every clinician who prescribes medications: Look under the surface. Don't assume that you know which patients take their medication regularly. Don't assume that failure to control hypertension, hyperlipidaemia or other measures of cardiovascular disease is caused by lack of efficacy of the prescribed medications.

In daily practice, after the physician determines the diagnosis and selects an appropriate treatment, the burden of achieving a good outcome is shifted to the patient. Depending on the setting, patients might be left to accomplish this important task of self management with little guidance. Both physicians and patients need to understand that key factors affecting outcome are "compliance" (that is, attempting to take the medication each day as prescribed) and "persistence" (that is, continuing to take the medication long term).[1] We know that the current treatment style does not work well because national surveys continue to demonstrate that only 23% of people with diagnosed hypertension have blood pressure measurements within the target range. Why is effectiveness so low? The diagnoses and prescribed treatments probably are appropriate. The patients heard the diagnosis and received the prescriptions. Why were the prescriptions not filled, or refilled? Why were doses not taken daily or long term? Where is the weak link in the system? Compliance with medication regimens is the link between disease management and attainment of the desired treatment outcomes.

Drugs don't work for patients who don't take them

▶ DEFINITIONS

Compliance in the medical setting can be defined as when a patient follows mutually agreeable instructions prescribed by a healthcare provider. Another aspect of compliance is treatment persistence, with a focus on long term continuation of treatment. Both definitions include the concept of partial compliance ranging from the occasional missed dose to the occasional extra dose. The pattern for partial compliance may be erratic, or it may be consistent but different from what the physician prescribed. Patients who are partial compliers are making an effort to participate in their treatment, but neither achieve their intention nor receive the full effect of their treatment. Common reasons are forgetfulness and feeling that treatment is not necessary. Persistence is an issue when patients feel that they no longer need medication. Some people test themselves by purposefully omitting doses, while others simply become lax about daily dosing. Medication compliance for symptomatic and asymptomatic disorders is highly variable among the adult population. Approximately three quarters of medication is taken as prescribed,[2] across a wide range of medical disorders. Simple dose regimens are easier to follow. However, compliance rates are most highly correlated with the number of doses rather than the number of medications or tablets that must be taken daily. The core issue for patients is: "How many times a day must I remember to take a dose?"

MEASURING COMPLIANCE

Physicians have been concerned about whether patients were following their medical instructions since the time of Hippocrates. Unfortunately, the simple method of asking patients whether they took their medication is not a very accurate measure of compliance. Patients who know they have missed doses tend to tell physicians what they think the physician wants to hear to avoid embarrassment.[2] If forgetfulness about dosing has been the main problem, the patient might not realise the frequency of missed doses. Reporting good compliance is not deceit, but lack of awareness of the problem. Large medical centres have the capacity to assess compliance based on the frequency of prescription refills. Analyses of large databases can provide an estimate of overall compliance long term without the details of whether doses were omitted occasionally or whether the pattern included long periods with no doses.

The newest technology to assess compliance is continuous electronic monitoring[3] (MEMS, Medication Event Monitoring Systems, AARDEX, Zug, Switzerland). These units use a standard prescription bottle that has a microprocessor in the cap to record the date and time whenever the bottle is opened.[3 4] Data from the units can be downloaded to a computer for a visual representation of how often the patient took the medication, the number of hours between doses, and periods of missed dosing. Electronic monitoring has given us a window on patient behaviour and the opportunity to study the link between compliance and treatment outcome. Most patients take approximately 50–90% of doses, although the overall range is 0–100%. On average, patients treated for a variety of medical disorders take approximately 75% of medication as prescribed, irrespective of the potential for negative consequences.[2 5] Neuropsychological correlates showed that compliance does not correlate with intelligence, memory, personality disorder, age, or education. The number of drugs a patient takes also does not correlate with compliance. Patients who are prescribed several medications tend to take all types of drugs together (for example, three medications, six pills with breakfast) or forget all of them when they miss that dose.[2] The conclusion is that the number of medications is not as important as the number of times a day doses must be remembered.

Electronic monitoring has proven the widely help belief that compliance diminishes when the number of doses per day increases. An overview of 76 reports using electronic monitoring showed mean (SD) compliance rates of 79 (14)% for once daily, 69 (15)% for twice daily, 65 (16)% for three times daily, and 51 (20)% for four times daily dosing (p < 0.001) for treatment of a variety of medical disorders.[1] Precision of dosing was even lower with only 59% of doses taken at appropriate time intervals. A review of 13 studies showed that compliance rates for once daily antihypertensive medications ranged from 55–86%, averaging 76%.[5]

People take approximately 75% of doses as prescribed, across a variety of medical disorders

PATTERNS OF COMPLIANCE

Cardiovascular disease is a chronic disorder, requiring long term treatment. Medication taking behaviour starts with the first prescription and continues for a lifetime. Prescriptions for antihypertensive and lipid lowering medications are often given to patients based on the assumption that people are reluctant to participate in lifestyle modification. Physicians seem to think that patients who will not diet and exercise to improve their health will be willing to take medication. The result is that even simple once daily medications are not taken regularly.[5] When blood pressure and lipids have been maintained at target levels for a long time, patients might feel that the medication is no longer necessary. A study of elderly patients newly treated for hypertension revealed that they filled prescriptions covering only 49% of days during the first year.[6] Studies of treatment persistence have shown that half of patients discontinue lipid lowering treatment within five years.[7] However, patients with comorbid diagnoses of hypertension, diabetes or coronary artery disease had significantly better compliance rates than those with only hyperlipidaemia.

Patients who take medication can be categorised as near optimal compliers, partial compliers, or non-compliers.[8] The proportion of patients who have been prescribed an antihypertensive or lipid lowering medication but do not fill or refill the prescription is unknown, but assumed to be large. Among compliers, dosing can vary from day to day, or month to month, resulting in periods without treatment. I found that compliance was significantly higher during five day periods before and after medical appointments, compared to 30 days after a visit,[9] a phenomenon I call "white-coat compliance". These data suggest that attention to dosing was enhanced in anticipation of the visit when health behaviour was a prominent issue. This behaviour was maintained for at least a brief period after the visit. Fading of health behaviour was associated with erratic compliance within a few weeks and the potential for medical problems because of under dosing. Thus, blood pressure readings in the medical office are likely to be the result of recent dosing but might not reflect a steady state measurement. Similarly, lipid concentrations might reflect careful dieting for a few days before the blood test.

Did the drug fail, or did the patient fail to take the drug?

COMPLIANCE AND OUTCOMES

The relation between compliance with lipid lowering drugs and cardiovascular risk was demonstrated in the Lipid Research Clinic's coronary primary prevention trial.[10] The more doses taken, the lower the cardiovascular risk, with the greatest benefit achieved for patients who took full doses of cholestyramine daily. These data are included in the medication label to explain the value of full compliance. The Helsinki heart study demonstrated that lipid reductions were linearly related to gemfibrozil compliance.[11] Effectiveness was greatly reduced among patients who took less than 70% of prescribed doses. Other studies have shown that patients readmitted to the hospital because of uncontrolled blood pressure had used significantly less medication than patients who were not readmitted (26% v 9% of days without medications).[12] A small study with electronic monitoring showed a significant correlation between ambulatory diastolic blood pressure and mean compliance.[13]

CONSEQUENCES OF ERRATIC COMPLIANCE

Stopping and restarting an antihypertensive medication can be dangerous. Studies have demonstrated that omission of dose of a short acting calcium channel blocker or β blocker resulted in significantly increased systolic and diastolic pressure and heart rate during the following two days, with three patients developing rebound hypertension.[14] Abrupt discontinuation of non-intrinsic sympathomimetic activity blockers can also result in rebound hypertension.[15] Doxazosin, a peripheral vasodilator, can cause severe problems if doses are omitted for several days. The risk of a cardiovascular event was fourfold higher among patients who took less than 80% of

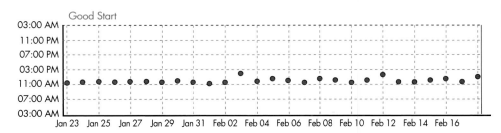

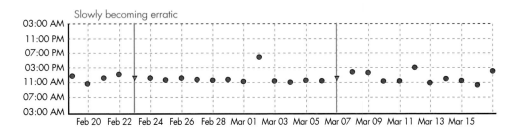

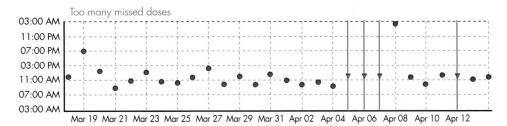

Figure 35.1 Example of initially good compliance, followed by erratic dose timing and many dose omissions (PowerView software, AARDEX Ltd, Zug, Switzerland).

their β blocker medication, and twofold higher among those taking 80–90% of doses than patients who took more than 90% of doses.[16] Note also that some cardiac antiarrhythmic drugs have a proarrhythmic effect when not taken as directed. This is an important lesson when prescribing medication that might do more transient harm than the overall beneficial effect of treatment for patients who are erratic compliers.

> What can doctors do? Teach your patients simple skills on how to follow a dosing plan, and reinforce the message at every visit

STRATEGIES FOR IMPROVING MEDICATION COMPLIANCE

Some of the essential aspects of prescribing that will enhance patient compliance are:

▶ selecting the fewest number of doses to be taken daily
▶ taking into consideration other medications the patient must take
▶ scheduling when doses are to be taken
▶ helping the patient select a reminder cue.[17]

A cue can be any activity that patients perform regularly that can be mentally associated with a scheduled dose. Basic cues are clock times, meal times, or daily rituals. For example, recommend that patients select specific clock times as dose times (for example, 7 am and 7 pm), or plan to take doses with meals (if they eat meals regularly). Other good cues are shaving, fixing one's hair, walking the dog, or listening to the news broadcast. Making the suggestion at the time the prescription is written will emphasise the importance of regular dosing, and takes minimal extra time. Everyone in the clinic or practice should reinforce the need for daily dosing with every patient, at every visit. Ask patients about their cue and how well it reminds them to take their medication. If the cue is not helping, suggest they choose another type of reminder. The message should stress the need for long term treatment to maintain persistence.

A combination of reminder cues and visual feedback of compliance data from electronic monitors is an effective method for improving compliance. I developed a Medication Usage Skills for Effectiveness Program as a rapid, simple teaching programme that can be initiated by non-medical personnel spending a few minutes with the patient.[18] The

Table 35.1 Electronic dosing record for a patient prescribed a medication to be taken three times a day. The calendar plot reveals erratic compliance on weekdays, and neglect on weekends

Sunday	Monday	Tuesday	Wednesday	Thursday	Friday	Saturday
	3	3	2	3	2	1
1	3	3	3	2	2	0
0	0	3	2	2	2	1
0	2	2	2	2	1	0
0	0	1	2	0		

250

patients sees a record of all doses taken on a computer screen in a calendar format listing the number of doses taken each day, the dose times, or a figure showing dosing over several months. The report (fig 35.1 and table 35.1) is reviewed with the patient, asking about special problems on days when doses were missed, and how reminders can be used to improve compliance. This technique takes only minutes by any staff person to teach skills that might be useful for a lifetime.

> Patients should develop a personalised plan to take their medication every day, 365 day a year, including holidays

SUMMARY

Physicians can picture themselves in the role of the ship's captain who sees ice in the water. Having learned about the high incidence of inadequate compliance and persistence, it is clear that every ice floe must be investigated to avoid potential disaster. We do not have the sonar system that helps the ship's captain scan under the water, but we can use other methods to avoid problems. We know that:

- taking three quarters of doses as prescribed leaves a wide window for potential cardiac disaster that is further increased when treatment is discontinued
- interruptions in the pharmacodynamic action of antihypertensive medications may compromise health in the short term or long term
- efficacy of some lipid lowering drugs is dose related.

The collision course includes target organ damage over time.

The American Heart Association has recommended use of strategies to enhance compliance to decrease morbidity and mortality from cardiovascular disease and stroke.[19] The first task should be to help partial compliers develop better dosing habits to help to achieve this goal. Physicians who routinely discuss compliance and dose schedules, and who help patients select personalised cue reminders, can engage patients in their own care.[20] Attention to compliance is a simple way to demonstrate special attention to patient care as well as improve medical success.

REFERENCES

1 **Claxton AJ**, Cramer JA, Pierce C. Medication compliance: the importance of the dosing regimen. *Clin Therapeutics* 2001;**23**:1296–310.
- ▶ **Overview of 76 studies with electronic compliance monitoring describes dose taking and dose timing deficits across a wide variety of medical disorders.**
2 **Cramer JA**, Mattson RH, Prevey ML, *et al.* How often is medication taken as prescribed? A novel assessment technique. *JAMA* 1989;**261**:3273–7.
- ▶ **The first report of variable compliance using electronic monitoring demonstrated that compliance was imperfect despite potentially disastrous consequences.**
3 **Cramer JA**. Microelectronic systems for monitoring and enhancing patient compliance with medication regimens. *Drugs* 1995;**49**:321–7.

- ▶ **Spending a few minutes to show patients how to tailor their medication regimens to fit into their schedules enhances compliance. Electronic monitoring systems allow clinicians to better understand patient dose taking behaviours, and to utilise those data to help patients develop schedules that meet individual lifestyles.**
4 **Cramer JA**. Medication use by the elderly: enhancing patient compliance in the elderly: role of packaging aids and monitoring. *Drugs & Aging* 1998;**12**:7–15.
5 **Cramer JA**. Consequences of intermittent treatment for hypertension: the case for medication compliance and persistence. *Am J Managed Care* 1999;**4**:1563–8.
6 **Monane M**, Bohn R, Gurwitz J, *et al.* Compliance with antihypertensive therapy among elderly medicaid enrollees: the roles of age, gender, and race. *Am J Public Health* 1996;**86**:1805–8.
- ▶ **Despite the efficacy of antihypertensive treatment, non-compliance may contribute to suboptimal cardiovascular outcomes.**
7 **Avorn J**, Monette J, Lacour A, *et al.* Persistence of use of lipid-lowering medications: a cross-national study. *JAMA* 1998;**279**:1458–62.
- ▶ **A comparison of US and Canadian populations for persistence with lipid lowering medications.**
8 **Rudd P**. Compliance with antihypertensive therapy: a shifting paradigm. *Cardiol Rev* 1994;**25**:230–40.
9 **Cramer JA**, Scheyer RD, Mattson RH. Compliance declines between clinic visits. *Arch Intern Med* 1990;**150**:1509–10.
10 **Coronary Drug Project Research Group**. Influence of adherence to treatment and response of cholesterol on mortality in the coronary drug project. *N Engl J Med* 1980;**303**:1038–41.
- ▶ **Demonstration of the link between compliance and cardiovascular benefit from lipid lowering treatment.**
11 **Manninen V**, Elo MO, Frick H, *et al.* Lipid alterations and decline in the incidence of coronary heart disease in the Helsinki heart study. *JAMA* 1988;**260**:641–51.
12 **Maronde RF**, Chan LS, Larsen FJ, *et al.* Underutilization of antihypertensive drugs and associated hospitalization. *Med Care* 1989;**27**:1159–66.
13 **Burnier M**, Schneider MP, Chiolero A, *et al.* Electronic compliance monitoring in resistant hypertension: the basis for rational therapeutic decisions. *J Hypertension* 2001;**19**:335–41.
- ▶ **A demonstration of the usefulness of compliance intervention to bring previously uncontrolled hypertension under control.**
14 **Johnson BF**, Whelton A. A study design for comparing the effects of missing daily doses of antihypertensive drugs. *Am J Therapeutics* 1994;**1**:260–7.
- ▶ **A controlled simulation of the effect of missing a few doses of antihypertensive medication.**
15 **Rangno RE**, Langlois S. Comparison of withdrawal phenomena after propranolol, metroprolol, and pindolol. *Br J Clin Pharmacol* 1982;**13**(suppl 2):345S–51S.
16 **Psaty BM**, Koepsell TD, Wagner EH, *et al.* The relative risk of incident coronary heart disease associated with recently stopping use of beta blockers. *JAMA* 1990;**263**:1653–7.
17 **Cramer JA**. Overview of methods to measure and enhance patient compliance. In: Cramer JA, Spilker B, eds. *Patient compliance in medical practice and clinical trials.* New York: Raven Press, 1991.
18 **Cramer JA**, Rosenheck R. Enhancing medication compliance for people with serious mental illness. *J Nervous Mental Dis* 1999;**187**:52–4.
- ▶ **Patients randomised to a brief compliance feedback programme had significantly higher compliance rates than those assigned to usual care.**
19 **Miller NH**, Hill M, Kottke T, *et al.* The multilevel compliance challenge. Recommendations for a call to action: a statement for healthcare professionals. *Circulation* 1997;**95**:1085–90.
20 **Waeber B**, Burnier M, Brunner HR. How to improve adherence with prescribed treatment in hypertensive patients? *J Cardiovasc Pharmacol* 2000;**35**(suppl 3):S23–6.
- ▶ **Various strategies to improve compliance concludes that the "motivation of the patient to follow the treatment requires the doctor to be equally motivated".**

36 MYOTONIC DYSTROPHY AND THE HEART

G Pelargonio, A Dello Russo, T Sanna, G De Martino, F Bellocci

Myotonic dystrophy (dystrophia myotonica, DM) is the most frequently inherited neuromuscular disease of adult life. DM is a multisystem disease with major cardiac involvement. Core features of myotonic dystrophy are myotonia, muscle weakness, cataract, and cardiac conduction abnormalities. Classical DM (first described by Steinert and called Steinert's disease or DM1) has been identified as an autosomal dominant disorder associated with the presence of an abnormal expansion of a CTG trinucleotide repeat on chromosome 19q13.3 (the DM 1 locus). A similar but less common disorder was later described as proximal myotonic myopathy, caused by alterations on a different gene on chromosome 3q21 (the DM2 locus). This article will mainly focus on DM1. It will provide an insight into the epidemiology and genetic alterations of the disease and provide up-to-date information on postmortem and clinical findings and on diagnostic and therapeutic options in patients presenting cardiac involvement.

▶ EPIDEMIOLOGY AND CLASSIFICATION OF DM1

The incidence of DM1 is estimated to be 1 in 8000 births and its worldwide prevalence ranges from 2.1 to 14.3/100 000 inhabitants.[1] Based on the age of onset and on its clinical features, DM1 can be divided into three forms: congenital, classical, and minimal, which may occur in the same kindred.

Congenital DM1 presents at birth or during the first year of life in a severe form. It is characterised by neonatal hypotonia, facial diplegia, joint contractures, frequent and often fatal respiratory failure, feeding difficulties, and developmental delay. The risk of dying from congenital DM1 in the neonatal period is high.[1] Patients who survive exhibit non-progressive psychomotor retardation and may subsequently exhibit the features of the adult-type, classical form of DM1.

In the classical form, which is the most common, symptoms become evident between the second and the fourth decade of life, showing a slow progression over time (table 36.1). The key feature of the disease is myotonia, which is characterised by delayed relaxation after muscular contraction (fig 36.1A,B); progressive muscular weakness (dystrophy) and wasting are also typical findings; facial, axial, semi-distal, and distal compartments are predominantly involved. DM1 is, however, a multisystem disorder; indeed, affected patients can manifest abnormalities of other organs and systems including the eye (cataract), the endocrine system (diabetes, thyroid dysfunction, hypogonadism), the central nervous system (cognitive impairment, mental retardation, attention disorders), the gastrointestinal system (dysphagia, constipation, gallbladder stones, pseudo-obstruction), and the heart (table 36.2).

Minimal DM1 begins later in life, usually after 50 years of age, with a very mild degree of muscle weakness and myotonia or only cataracts, associated with a normal lifespan.

GENETIC ALTERATIONS OF DM1

DM1 is an autosomal dominant disorder with incomplete penetrance and variable phenotypic expression. The genetic basis of DM1 is known to include mutational expansion of a repetitive trinucleotide sequence (CTG) in the 3′-untranslated region of the DMPK gene (myotonic dystrophy protein kinase gene) on chromosome 19q13.3. While 5-34 CTG repeats are observed in normal alleles, their number may reach 50–2000 in DM1.[2] The process which leads from abnormal expansion of CTG repeats in a non-coding region of DMPK gene to cellular dysfunction is still incompletely understood. However, the localisation of DMPK in the heart muscle at the level of intercalated discs, combined with the observation that DMPK reduction in animal models compromise conduction both at the level of the atrioventricular node and of the His-Purkinje system,[3] suggest impairment of intercellular impulse propagation as a possible mechanism of disease.

Pathologic expansion of the CTG repeats is unstable both during mitotic and meiotic divisions. Mitotic instability explains the presence of somatic mosaicism, a common feature of DM1. Meiotic instability represents the mechanism underlying the phenomena of "anticipation" and "reverse mutation" observed during parent-to-child transmission in DM1 pedigrees. "Anticipation" occurs in earlier onset and a greater severity of symptoms in succeeding generations is caused by a meiotic increase in the size of CTG repeats, while the less common "reverse mutation", possibly

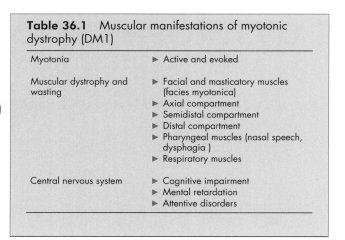

Table 36.1 Muscular manifestations of myotonic dystrophy (DM1)

Myotonia	▸ Active and evoked
Muscular dystrophy and wasting	▸ Facial and masticatory muscles (facies myotonica) ▸ Axial compartment ▸ Semidistal compartment ▸ Distal compartment ▸ Pharyngeal muscles (nasal speech, dysphagia) ▸ Respiratory muscles
Central nervous system	▸ Cognitive impairment ▸ Mental retardation ▸ Attentive disorders

Table 36.2 Systemic involvement in DM1

Eye	▸ Cataract
Endocrine system	▸ Diabetes ▸ Thyroid dysfunction ▸ Hypogonadism
Gastrointestinal tract	▸ Dysphagia ▸ Constipation ▸ Gallbladder stones ▸ Pseudo-obstruction
Central nervous system	▸ Cognitive impairment ▸ Mental retardation ▸ Attentive disorders
Heart	

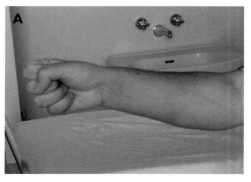

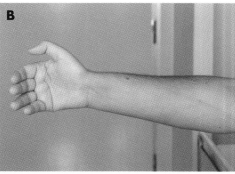

Figure 36.1 The grip test is a quick and easy way to determine the presence of active myotonia. After contraction of the fist (A) the patient is unable to relax the muscles of the hand (B). Photographs courtesy of Dr Gabriella Silvestri, Unione Italiana Lotta alla Distrofia Muscolare, Sezione Lazio, Italy.

accounting for incomplete penetrance of DM1, is caused by a meiotic regression in the size of the expansion bringing the number of the CTG repeats towards normal range.[2]

Many attempts have been made to find a possible correlation between the number of CTG repeats and severity of clinical manifestations of DM1. Despite earlier controversial results, evidence is accumulating in favour of a correlation between cardiac involvement and CTG expansion.[2 4 5] Indeed, the number of CTG repeats seems on average to influence the timing of cardiac complications,[6] to predict the presence and the progression of ECG abnormalities,[5] and the risk of major cardiac events,[7] but it does not predict abnormal findings at electrophysiological study (EPS).[8] Analysis of CTG repeats is, however, of limited predictive value in individual patients because of the overlap between expansion sizes seen in different phenotypic groups, somatic mosaicism, and current analysis of CTG repeats from peripheral blood leucocyte DNA instead of skeletal and cardiac muscle DNA.[2]

CARDIAC INVOLVEMENT IN DM1
Pathology and mechanisms of cardiac death
Endomyocardial biopsies and postmortem studies performed on patients with DM1 have documented various degrees of non-specific changes, such as interstitial fibrosis, fatty infiltration, hypertrophy of myocardiocytes, and focal myocarditis. A selective and extensive impairment of the conduction system is the most common finding.[9]

During a 10 year follow up study of 367 DM1 patients,[1] mortality was 7.3 times higher than that in an age matched reference population, with a mean age at death of 53 years and a positive correlation between age at onset of DM1 and age of death. In this series, respiratory failure and cardiovascular disease were the most prevalent causes of death, accounting for about 40% and 30% of fatalities, respectively. Cardiac mortality occurred because of progressive left ventricular dysfunction, ischaemic heart disease, pulmonary embolism, or as a result of unexpected sudden death.[1] Relative contribution of sudden death ranges from about 2–30% in different published series, according to selection criteria. The hypothesis that cardiac arrhythmias may represent the most prevalent cause of sudden death in DM1 patients is supported by the absence of other causes of sudden death at necropsy studies. Sudden cardiac death may be caused by ventricular asystole, degeneration of ventricular tachycardia (VT), ventricular fibrillation (VF) or electromechanical dissociation. The consistent evidence of the degeneration of the conduction system in DM generated the hypothesis that bradyarrhythmias might represent the most prevalent mechanism of SD. However, ventricular tachyarrhythmias are increasingly recognised as a common finding in these patients (fig 36.2A,B), possibly explaining some cases of sudden death after pacemaker implant.

Clinical presentation
Heart disease is common in DM1 but its prevalence is difficult to estimate precisely, as different definitions have been used in the literature. Neuromuscular alterations are usually the initial clinical manifestation of DM1 (with or without subclinical cardiac involvement), but cardiac symptoms may be occasionally the first to appear. Cardiac involvement is characterised by conduction system abnormalities, supraventricular and ventricular arrhythmias and, less frequently, myocardial dysfunction and ischaemic heart disease (table 36.3). At variance with other neuromuscular diseases, patients with DM1 rarely present overt clinical manifestations of cardiomyopathy ("myotonic" heart disease).[10]

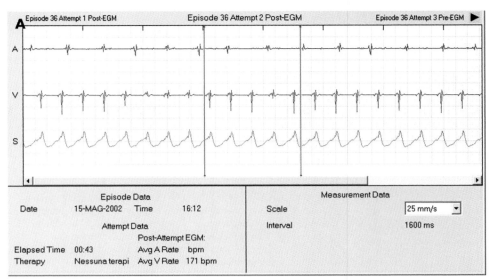

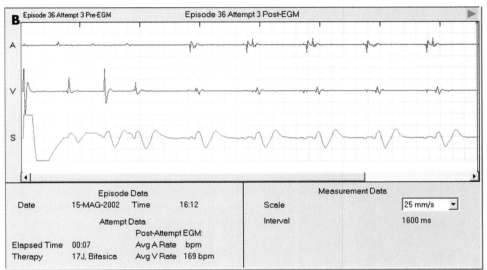

Figure 36.2 (A) Intracardiac electrograms (EGM) of a spontaneous episode of sustained ventricular tachycardia as recorded from the cardioverter-defibrillator (ICD) implanted in a 32 year old male patient affected by DM1. From top to bottom the tracings show the atrial EGM, the ventricular EGM, and a pseudo-surface lead II derived from signals recorded between the shock coils and the ICD. Atrioventricular dissociation, enabling a diagnosis of ventricular tachycardia, is evident. (B) Resumption of sinus rhythm after a 17 J biphasic DC shock.

Conduction system defects

Conduction system abnormalities are commonly observed in DM1. Any part of the conduction system may be affected, but the His-Purkinje system is most frequently involved. Minor conduction defects are often present in 12 lead ECG in asymptomatic DM1 patients in the early stages of disease; their progression towards more severe conduction defects may cause shortness of breath, dizziness, fainting, syncope, and sudden death. Rate of progression of conduction abnormalities is usually slow,[11] but fast progression has been occasionally observed thus making the clinical course of individual patients rather unpredictable. Delayed impulse propagation along the conduction system can be associated with a long PR interval (prevalence ranging from 20–40% in different studies, depending on patient selection criteria) and/or with a wide QRS complex (prevalence ranging from 5–25% in different studies, depending on patient selection criteria). Unfortunately, the presence of a long PR interval does not give any clue as to the site of the conduction delay, as it may occur at any level from the atrium to the His bundle, through the atrioventricular node. However, when a wide QRS is also present (for example, right or left bundle brunch block), the probability of an infrahissian (below the His bundle) conduction impairment is higher. Of note, prolongation of the HV interval has been observed in about half of unselected patients with DM1.[9 12]

In patients with DM1, analysis of late potentials has unique implications. Late potentials are expression of delayed myocardial activation usually caused by abnormal tissue (for example, myocardial fibrosis or necrosis, as typically observed in ischaemic heart disease after myocardial infarction), and are considered predictors of ventricular arrhythmias. Delayed myocardial activation in DM1 is not a consequence of inhomogeneous conduction through scattered areas of fibrosis but rather of delayed activation along the His-Purkinje system.[13] In DM1, abnormal late potentials are thus an expression of a conduction defect, and represent an important non-invasive clue to the presence of a long HV interval. QRS duration ≥ 100 ms and low amplitude signals in the last 40 ms of QRS complex ≥ 36 ms can predict a prolonged HV interval at EPS with good sensitivity and specificity (80% and 83.3%, respectively).

Tachyarrhythmias

In DM1 patients, supraventricular tachyarrhythmias are a common finding on 12 lead ECG or during 24 hour Holter monitoring, and may be asymptomatic. Most common arrhythmias are atrial flutter or fibrillation, observed in up to 25% of patients both as unsustained and sustained forms. Atrial flutter, atrial fibrillation, and atrial tachycardia are also easily inducible at EPS even in the absence of previously documented spontaneous episodes, but the clinical implications of these findings are still uncertain.

Table 36.3 Cardiac involvement in DM1

Conduction system	▶ Atrioventricular block, any degree

Arrhythmias	▶ Supraventricular
	   –atrial premature complexes
	   –atrial tachycardia
	   –atrial flutter
	   –atrial fibrillation
	▶ Ventricular
	   –ventricular premature complexes
	   –ventricular tachycardia
	   –ventricular fibrillation

Ventricular function	▶ Systolic function impairment ▶ Diastolic function impairment
Ischaemic heart disease Mitral valve prolapse	

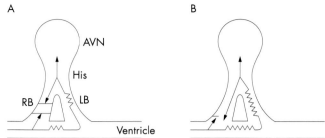

Figure 36.3 Bundle branch re-entry. (A) A ventricular premature impulse is blocked retrogradely in the right bundle branch (RB); conduction proceeds retrogradely through the left bundle branch (LB) up to the His bundle (His); from the His bundle, the impulse travels anterogradely over the right bundle branch which is still refractory, thus blocking propagation. (B) Conversely, if the right bundle branch has enough time to recover, the impulse can be conducted anterogradely to the ventricles, then retrogradely through the left bundle branch up to the His bundle, thus maintaining a macro-reentry. AVN, atrioventricular node.

Ventricular arrhythmias are frequent. Spontaneous episodes of both monomorphic and polymorphic VT and even VF have been consistently reported.[14] Therefore, in patients with clinical symptoms suggestive of ventricular tachycardia (for example, lipothymia, syncope) and/or with a family history of sudden death, an EPS is strongly advised.[7 8] The prognostic value of inducible VT in patients without a history of spontaneous VT and without symptoms suggestive of VT is still uncertain. In a seminal study on DM1 and cardiac disease, VT could be induced at EPS in 18% of patients referred for conduction abnormalities in the absence of ventricular arrhythmias during Holter monitoring.[8] Inducible VT is most commonly represented by unsustained polymorphic VT, but sustained polymorphic VT, VF, and both sustained and unsustained monomorphic VT have also been reported. Given the risk of sudden death in these patients, the prognostic significance of inducible VTs, even when polymorphic and unsustained, should be carefully considered, as risk stratification criteria used in other subsets of patients may not apply to DM.[15]

Mechanisms of monomorphic VT in DM are:
▶ re-entry around areas of fibro-fatty degeneration of the myocardium (possible)
▶ bundle brunch re-entry (typical)
▶ triggered activity.

In bundle branch re-entry ventricular tachycardia (BBRVT) the loop of the re-entrant circuit runs around the two ramifications of His bundle, which represent the anterograde and the retrograde limb (fig 36.3). Cardiac involvement in DM1 represents an ideal substrate for this type of re-entry, due to the common presence of a delayed conduction along the His bundle branch (prolonged HV interval) which is essential for BBRVT to occur.[16] Identification of bundle branch re-entry VT is important because it can be cured by radiofrequency ablation of one of the two limbs of the circuit. BBRVT is not easily inducible by standard programmed ventricular stimulation, while it is induced by short-long-short sequences which should be performed during the assessment of DM1 patients.[16] VT originating from the left posterior fascicle of His bundle (with characteristic RBBB and superior axis appearance on 12 lead ECG), which can be cured by radiofrequency ablation, has also been reported in these patients.

Myocardial dysfunction, ischaemia, and other features of cardiac involvement

Overt myocardial dysfunction (myotonic heart disease) is not frequent. However, subclinical, mild myocardial dysfunction

may be detected. Symptoms of heart failure are infrequent because of the limited level of activity of these patients and of their difficulties in reporting symptoms caused by mental retardation. The existence of a myocardial equivalent of skeletal muscle myotonia (myocardial myotonia) has been confirmed by assessment of diastolic function by echo Doppler parameters.[17] Ischaemic heart disease is sometimes observed as chronic stable angina, unstable angina, and acute myocardial infarction. Microvascular dysfunction has also been described in DM1 patients suffering from chest pain, exhibiting a positive thallium scan and normal coronary arteries.[18] Mitral valve prolapse has been reported in 25–40% of most DM1 series.[9] Hypertrophic cardiomyopathy and left ventricular hypertrabeculation have been described in case reports.

Management of cardiac involvement in DM

A careful cardiac evaluation including basal ECG, 24 hour Holter monitoring, echocardiogram, and signal averaged ECG should be routinely performed in all patients presenting with DM1. A history of fainting, palpitation, shortness of breath, lipothymia, and syncope should be carefully searched by interviewing not only the patient but also his or her relatives. Indications for EPS in DM1 patients are still debated but, given the risk of sudden death, we suggest an early invasive approach in selected subsets of patients as summarised in table 36.4. When classical indications[19] are met, pacemaker implant is needed and should not be delayed. Asymptomatic AV conduction delay, in particular in the presence of a prolonged HV interval, represents one of the major therapeutic challenges in DM1, as data on the rate of progression to complete atrioventricular block are conflicting. Which degree of HV interval prolongation should be considered an indication for prophylactic pacing in the absence of clinically relevant bradyarrhythmias is still an open issue. Recent findings, however, suggest that a prolongation of HV interval beyond 70 ms may warrant a prophylactic pacemaker implant even in the absence of symptoms.[20]

Treatment of ventricular arrhythmias is also an area of considerable debate. When classical criteria are met,[19] an implantable cardioverter-defibrillator should be implanted without delay. A major effort is needed for identification of BBRVT which can be cured by radiofrequency ablation alone. When a VT is induced in an asymptomatic patient, the appropriate treatment strategy is as yet undetermined.

Table 36.4 Suggested indications for electrophysiological study in DM1 patients

Disturbances and/or symptoms suggestive of arrhythmias	Syncope, lipothymia, dizziness, palpitations
Family history	Sudden death Ventricular fibrillation Sustained VT Pacemaker implant

Non-invasive findings suggestive of intra- or infrahissian AV conduction disturbances (with or without symptoms)	LBBB
	RBBB + LAFH
	RBBB + LPFH
	
	First degree AV block with:
	   PR interval >240 ms
	   LAFH
	   LPFH
	
	Second or third degree AV block
	
	Signal averaged ECG positive for late potentials

Sinus node dysfunction (with or without symptoms)	Sinus pause >3 seconds Sinus bradycardia <40/min
Ventricular arrhythmias (with or without symptoms)	Frequent ventricular premature beats Non-sustained VT Sustained VT

AV, atrioventricular; LAFH, left anterior fascicular hemiblock; LBBB, left bundle branch block; LFPH, left posterior fascicular hemiblock; RBBB, right bundle branch block; VT, ventricular tachycardia.

255

Myotonic dystrophy and cardiac involvement: key points

▶ Cardiac involvement is mainly represented by conduction abnormalities at ECG
▶ Conduction abnormalities are progressive, but the rate of progression is not clear
▶ Ventricular arrhythmias are common
▶ The unusual bundle branch re-entry ventricular tachycardia should be actively sought as radiofrequency ablation may be curative
▶ Sudden death represents 2–30% of fatalities in patients with DM1. Possible mechanisms are ventricular asystole, degeneration of ventricular tachycardia, ventricular fibrillation or electromechanical dissociation. The respective prevalence of these mechanisms is unknown
▶ Overt myocardial dysfunction is rare; however, impairment of ventricular systolic and diastolic functions may be part of the cardiac scenario

CONCLUSION

Conduction system abnormalities, arrhythmias and, less commonly, myocardial dysfunction and angina are observed in patients with DM1 and may occasionally represent the initial manifestations of disease, even in the absence of overt neuromuscular involvement. Thus, cardiologists should be aware of this diagnosis. Conversely, in all patients presenting with DM1 a careful clinical and diagnostic evaluation needs to be performed for the identification of patients at risk of major cardiac events. An attitude of a low threshold for invasive procedures is suggested, considering the unclear rate of cardiac disease progression and the risk of sudden death in some subsets of patients (table 36.4). Several questions are still unanswered. Future studies are needed in order to improve the identification of patients at risk of sudden death. A prospective, long term multicentre study (RAMYD, risk of arrhythmia in myotonic dystrophy) is now ongoing which will

hopefully contribute to the formulation of evidence based guidelines for the management of cardiac conditions associated with DM1.

REFERENCES

1 **Mathieu J**, Allard P, Potvin L, et al. A 10 year study of mortality in a cohort of patients with myotonic dystrophy. *Neurology* 1999;**52**:1658–62.
▶ This is a recent longitudinal study involving a large population of DM patients, followed for 10 years, which extensively investigates the natural history and the causes of death associated with the disease.

2 **Melacini P**, Villanova C, Menegazzo E, et al. Correlation between cardiac involvement and CTG trinucleotide repeat length in myotonic dystrophy. *J Am Coll Cardiol* 1995;**25**:239–45.
▶ This excellent work points out the possible predictive value of CTG repeats size on cardiac conduction abnormalities and their severity, adding also important information on the role of late potentials in predicting VT.

3 **Saba S**, Vanderbrink BA, Luciano B, et al. Localization of the sites of conduction abnormalities in a mouse model of myotonic dystrophy. *J Cardiovasc Electrophysiol* 1999;**10**:1214–20.
▶ This is one of the few experimental control studies in a mouse model of DM where affected mice underwent complete EPS, showing the higher predilection to the infrahissian tissue for conduction abnormalities related to DMPK loss.

4 **Jaspert A**, Fahsold R, Grehl, et al. Myotonic dystrophy correlation of clinical symptoms with the size of CTG repeats. *J Neurol* 1995;**25**:239–45.

5 **Groh W**, Lowe M, Zipes D. Severity of cardiac conduction involvement and arrhythmias in myotonic dystrophy type 1 correlates with age and CTG repeat length. *J Cardiovasc Electrophysiol* 2002;**13**:444–8.

6 **Antonini G**, Giubilei F, Mammarella A, et al. Natural history of cardiac involvement in myotonic dystrophy: correlation with CTG repeats. *Neurology* 2000;**55**:1207–9.

7 **Clarke NRA**, Kelion AD, Nixon J, et al. Does cytosine-thymine-guanine (CTG) expansion size predict cardiac events and electrocardiographic progression in myotonic dystrophy? *Heart* 2001;**86**:411–16.

8 **Lazarus A**, Varin J, Ounnoughene Z, et al. Relationships among electrophysiological findings and clinical status, heart function, and extent of DNA mutation in myotonic dystrophy. *Circulation* 1999;**99**:1041–6.
▶ This study is the largest EP observation reported in DM, which confirms the predominance of infrahissian conduction impairment, and underlines easy inducible arrhythmias, without finding any relation between ECG or EP abnormalities and DNA mutation size.

9 **Phillips MF**, Harper PS. Cardiac disease in myotonic dystrophy. *Cardiovasc Res* 1997;**33**:13–22.
▶ This comprehensive review of the literature concerns all the aspects of cardiac involvement in DM and the clinical cardiac hints to be remembered when dealing with such patients.

10 **Church S**. The heart in myotonia atrophica. *Arch Intern Med* 1967;**119**:176–81.

11 **Prystowsky EN**, Pritchett EIC, Roses A, *et al*. The natural history of conduction system disease in myotonic muscular dystrophy as determined by serial electrophysiologic studies. *Circulation* 1979;**60**:1360–4.
► **This is the first and only study which describes nine patients with DM who underwent EPS twice to look for any progression of the electrophysiological abnormalities over a three year period of follow up, and to test if EPS might predict them.**

12 **Oloffson B**, Forsberg H, Andersson S, *et al*. Electrocardiographic findings in myotonic dystrophy. *Br Heart J* 1988;**59**:47–52.

13 **Babuty D**, Fauchier L, Tena-Carbi D, *et al*. Significance of late potentials in myotonic dystrophy. *Am J Cardiol* 1999;**84**:1099–101.

14 **Hadian D**, Lowe MR, Scott LR, *et al*. Use of an insertable loop recorder in a myotonic dystrophy patient. *J Cardiovasc Electrophysiol* 2002;**13**:72–3.

15 **Grigg LE**, Chan W, Mond HG, *et al*. Ventricular tachycardia and sudden death in myotonic dystrophy: clinical, electrophysiologic and pathologic features. *J Am Coll Cardiol* 1985;**6**:254–6.

16 **Merino JL**, Carmona JR, Fernandez-Lozano I, *et al*. Mechanisms of sustained ventricular tachycardia in myotonic dystrophy. *Circulation* 1998;**98**:541–6.
► **This article provides evidence for the possible role of BBRVT in the mechanism of VT in DM and the appropriate therapeutic strategy.**

17 **Fragola PV**, Calo L, Luzi M, *et al*. Doppler echocardiographic assessment of left ventricular diastolic function in myotonic dystrophy. *Cardiology* 1997;**88**:498–502.
► **The authors find, in a large population of asymptomatic DM patients with normal left ventricular systolic function, several impaired diastolic indices, suggesting a possible intrinsic myocardial abnormality in this disease, beside conduction system defect.**

18 **Itoh H**, Shimizu M, Horita Y, *et al*. Microvascular ischemia in patients with myotonic dystrophy. *Jpn Circ J* 2000;**64**:720–2.

19 **Gregoratos G**, Cheitlin MD, Conill A, *et al*. ACC/AHA guidelines for implantation of cardiac pacemakers and antiarrhythmia devices: a report of the American College of Cardiology/American Heart Association task force on practice guidelines (committee on pacemaker implantation). *J Am Coll Cardiol* 1998;**31**:1175–209.

20 **Lazarus A**, Varin J, Duboc D. Final results of the French diagnostic pacemaker study in myotonic dystrophy [abstract]. *PACE* 2002;**25**:599.
► **This study involved 49 DM1 patients with HV interval > 70 ms who underwent a prophylactic pacemaker implant. During 51 months of follow up the diagnostic pacemaker algorithm was able to identify spontaneous severe brady/tachyarrhythmias (complete atrioventricular block in 51%, and ventricular arrhythmias in 26.5%); 20% DM1 patients (10) died during follow up, four of them suddenly.**

INDEX

Page numbers in **bold** refer to figures, and page numbers in *italic* refer to tables and boxed material.

CITATION INDEX

SECTION I: CORONARY DISEASE

1. Lane I, Byrne J. Carotid artery surgery for people with existing coronary artery disease. *Heart* 2002;**87**:86-90.

2. Reffelmann T, Kloner RA. The "no-reflow" phenomenon: basic science and clinical correlates. *Heart* 2002;**87**:162-8.

3. Thompson GR. Screening relatives of patients with premature coronary heart disease. *Heart* 2002;**87**:390-4.

4. Ribichini F, Wijns W. Acute myocardial infarction: reperfusion treatment. *Heart* 2002;**88**:298-305.

5. De Jaegere PP Th, Suyker WJL. Off-pump coronary artery bypass surgery. *Heart* 2002;**88**:313-8.

6. Menon V, Hochman JS. Management of cardiogenic shock complicating acute myocardial infarction. *Heart* 2002;**88**:531-7.

SECTION II: HEART FAILURE

7. Deng MC. Cardiac transplantation. *Heart* 2002;**87**:177-84.

8. Ward C. The need for palliative care in the management of heart failure. *Heart* 2002;**87**:294-98.

9. Lainchbury JG, Richards AM. Exercise testing in the assessment of chronic congestive heart failure. *Heart* 2002;**88**:538-43.

SECTION III: CARDIOMYOPATHY

10. McKenna WJ, Behr ER. Hypertrophic cardiomyopathy: management, risk stratification and prevention of sudden death. *Heart* 2002;**87**:169-76

SECTION IV: VALVE DISEASE

11. Enriquez-Sarano M. Timing of mitral valve surgery. *Heart* 2002;**87**:79-85.

12. Boon NA, Bloomfield P. The medical management of valvar heart disease. *Heart* 2002;**87**:395-400.

13. Bloomfield P. Choice of heart valve prosthesis. *Heart* 2002;**87**:583-9.

SECTION V: ELECTROPHYSIOLOGY

14. Schilling RJ. Which patient should be referred to an electrophysiologist: supraventricular tachycardia. *Heart* 2002;**87**:299-304.

15. Triedman JK. Arrhythmias in adults with congenital heart disease. *Heart* 2002;**87**:383-9.

16. Sears Jr SF, Conti JB. Quality of life and psychological functioning of ICD patients. *Heart* 2002;**87**:488-92.

17. Friedman PA. Novel mapping techniques for cardiac electrophysiology. *Heart* 2002;**87**:575-82.

18. Blaauw Y, Van Gelder IC, Crijns HJGM. Treatment of atrial fibrillation. *Heart* 2002;**88**:432-7.

19. Morgan JM. Patients with ventricular arrhythmias: who should be referred to an electrophysiologist? *Heart* 2002;**88**:544-50.

SECTION VI: CONGENITAL HEART DISEASE

20. Burch M. *Heart* failure in the young. *Heart* 2002;**88**:198-202.

21. Wren C. Sudden death in children and adolescents. *Heart* 2002;**88**:426-31.

22. Haworth SG. Pulmonary hypertension in the young. *Heart* 2002;**88**:658-64.

SECTION VII: IMAGING TECHNIQUES

23. Schoenhagen P, Nissen S. Understanding coronary artery disease: tomographic imaging with intravascular ultrasound. *Heart* 2002;**88**:91-6.

24. Greaves SC. Role of echocardiography in acute coronary syndromes. *Heart* 2002;**88**:419-25.

25. Thomas JD. Doppler echocardiographic assessment of valvar regurgitation. *Heart* 2002;**88**:651-7.

SECTION VIII: HYPERTENSION

26. Wallis EJ, Ramsay LE, Jackson PR. Cardiovascular and coronary risk estimation in hypertension management. *Heart* 2002;**88**:306-12.

SECTION IX: GENERAL CARDIOLOGY

27. Froehlich JB, Eagle KA. Anaesthesia and the cardiac patient: the patient versus the procedure *Heart* 2002;**87**:91-96.

28. Brand NJ, Barton JR. Myocardial molecular biology: an introduction. *Heart* 2002;**87**:284-93.

29. Petch MC. *Heart* disease, guidelines, regulations, and the law. *Heart* 2002;**87**:472-9.

30. Bennett MR. Apoptosis in the cardiovascular system. *Heart* 2002;**87**:480-7.

31. 31. Furberg CD. To whom do the research findings apply? *Heart* 2002;**87**:570-4.

32. Dean JCS. Management of Marfan syndrome. *Heart* 2002;**88**:97-100.

33. Anderson RH, Brown NA, Webb S. Development and structure of the atrial septum. *Heart* 2002;**88**:104-10.

34. Haller C. Arteriosclerotic renal artery stenosis: conservative versus interventional management. *Heart* 2002;**88**:193-7.

35. Cramer JA. Effect of partial compliance on cardiovascular medication effectiveness. *Heart* 2002;**88**:203-6.

36. Pelargonio G, Russo AD, Sanna T, De Martino G, Belloci F. *Heart* 2002;**88**:665-70.

Thank you for purchasing *Education in Heart* Volume III

This purchase entitles you to online access to ALL *Education in Heart* material on the *Heart* website—www.heartjnl.com—for one year (US$50 value).

Education in Heart was launched in January 2000 and publishes three articles per issue (36 articles per year), which have associated multiple choice questions—these are also available online through BMP Publishing Group Online Learning (cpd.bmjjournals.com).

The *Heart* website has full text (HTML) and pdf full text versions. There is additional material available only through the website.

To access these articles online you need to complete and return the order form below—THERE IS NO ADDITIONAL CHARGE FOR THIS SERVICE.

Once you receive your customer number you should activate your subscription online and choose a user name and password (www.bmjjournals.com/sub/activate/basic).

Please provide my customer number for FREE ACCESS to *Education in Heart* Online

Name:

Address:

County: Zip/Postcode:

Email address::   Telephone:

Place of work (optional)   Level, eg, Consultant (optional):

Return this form by mail to:
Subscriptions Department
BMJ Publishing Group
PO Box 299
London WC1H 9TD, UK

For enquiries please telephone: +44 (0) 20 7383 6270 or email: subscriptions@bmjgroup.com

The *Education in Heart* articles published during 2000 and 2001 are also available as a compilation
Further details available from www.bmjbookshop.com